AF449121

HEMOPHILIA

Strange it is that our bloods
Of colour, weight and heat, pour'd all together
Would quite confound distinction, yet stand off
In differences so mighty

William Shakespeare
All's Well That Ends Well
Act 2, Scene 3

HEMOPHILIA

EDITED BY

C.D. *Forbes*
University Department of Medicine, Ninewells Hospital and Medical School, Dundee, UK

L.M. *Aledort*
Mount Sinai School of Medicine, New York, USA

and

R. *Madhok*
Centre for Rheumatic Diseases, The Royal Infirmary, Glasgow, UK

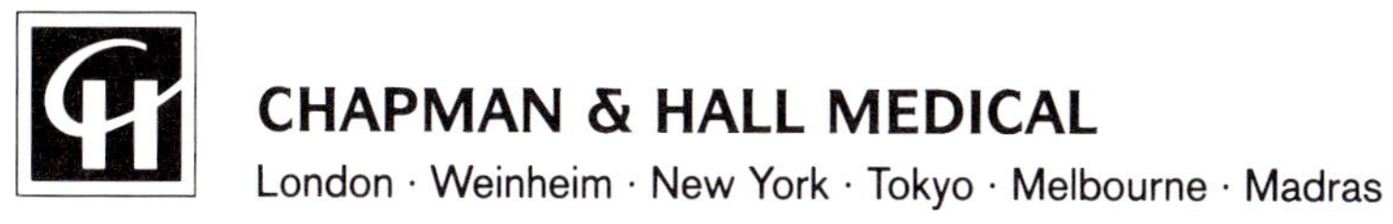

CHAPMAN & HALL MEDICAL
London · Weinheim · New York · Tokyo · Melbourne · Madras

Published by Chapman & Hall, 2–6 Boundary Row, London SE1 8HN, UK

Chapman & Hall, 2–6 Boundary Row, London SE1 8HN, UK

Chapman & Hall GmbH, Pappelallee 3, 69469 Weinheim, Germany

Chapman & Hall USA, 115 Fifth Avenue, New York, NY 10003, USA

Chapman & Hall Japan, ITP-Japan, Kyowa Building, 3F, 2-2-1 Hirakawacho, Chiyoda-ku, Tokyo 102, Japan

Chapman & Hall Australia, 102 Dodds Street, South Melbourne, Victoria 3205, Australia

Chapman & Hall India, R. Seshadri, 32 Second Main Road, CIT East, Madras 600 035, India

First edition 1997

© 1997 Chapman & Hall

Typeset in 10/12 pt Sabon by Gray Publishing

Printed in Great Britain by Alden Press Ltd, Osney Mead, Oxford

ISBN 0 412 63820 7

A catalogue record for this book is available from the British Library

Library of Congress Catalog Card Number: 96-86288

∞ Printed on acid-free text paper, manufactured in accordance with ANSI/NISO Z39.48-1992 (Permanence of Paper).

CONTENTS

Part Four: Psychosocial Aspects

Index   371

CONTRIBUTORS

L.M. Aledort
Mount Sinai School of Medicine, One Gustave L. Levy Place, New York, NY 10029-6574, USA

E. Berntorp
Dept for Coagulation Disorders, University of Lund, University Hospital, Malmö, S-205 02 Malmö, Sweden

P.H.B. Bolton-Maggs
University Dept of Haematology, Manchester Royal Infirmary, Oxford Rd, Manchester, UK.

B.M. Buzzard
Newcastle Haemophilia Comprehensive Care Centre, Royal Victoria Infirmary, Queen Victoria Rd, Newcastle upon Tyne, NE1 4LP, UK.

D. Cardi
New York Hospital–Cornell Medical Center, 525 East 68th Street, New York, NY 10021, USA

J.M. Connor
Dept of Medical Genetics, University of Glasgow, Yorkhill Hospitals, Glasgow G3 8SJ, UK.

B. Cuthbertson
Protein Fractionation Centre, Scottish National Blood Transfusion Service, 21 Ellen's Glen Rd, Edinburgh EH17 7QT, UK

B.L. Evatt
Hematologic Diseases Branch, Division of HIV/AIDS, National Center for Infectious Diseases, Centers for Disease Control and Prevention, Atlanta, GA 30333, USA

M.E. Eyster
Division of Hematology, Dept of Medicine, Pennsylvania State University College of Medicine, The Milton S Hershey Medical Center, PO Box 850, Hershey, PA 17033, USA

C.D. Forbes
University Dept of Medicine, Ninewells Hospital and Medical School, Dundee DD1 9SY, UK

P.R. Foster
Protein Fractionation Centre, Scottish National Blood Transfusion Service, 21 Ellen's Glen Rd, Edinburgh EH17 7QT, UK

M.S. Gilbert
1100 Park Ave, New York, NY 10128, USA

J.J. Goedert
National Cancer Institute, 6130 Executive Boulevard Suite 434, Rockville, MD 20892, USA

I. Goldberg
New York Hospital–Cornell Medical Center, 525 East 68th Street, New York, NY 10021, USA

A.C. Goodeve
Section of Moleclar Genetics, Dept of Medicine and Pharmacology, Royal Hallamshire Hospital, Sheffield S10 2JF, UK

I.A. Greer
Dept of Obstetrics and Gynaecology, Glasgow Royal Infirmary University NHS Trust, Glasgow G12 8QQ, UK

L.J. Haas
Dept of Family and Preventive Medicine, University of Utah School of Medicine, 50 N Medical Drive, Salt Lake City, UT 84132 USA

J.P. Hanley
Dept of Rheumatology, Royal Infirmary, Lauriston Place, Edinburgh EH3 9YW, UK

C.R.M. Hay
University Dept of Haematology, Manchester Royal Infirmary, Oxford Rd, Manchester, UK

M.W. Hilgartner
New York Hospital–Cornell Medical Center, 525 East 68th Street, New York, NY 10021, USA

W.C. Hooper
Hematologic Diseases Branch, Division of HIV/AIDS, National Center for Infectious Diseases, Centers for Disease Control and Prevention, Atlanta, GA 30333, USA

L.W. Hoyer
Holland Laboratory, American Red Cross, 15601 Crabbs Branchway, Bethesda, MD 20855, USA

M.J. Inwood
South Western Ontario Regional Hemophilia Program, St Joseph's Health Centre, London, Ontario, Canada

P.M. Jones
Newcastle Haemophilia Comprehensive Care Centre, Royal Victoria Infirmary, Queen Victoria Rd, Newcastle upon Tyne, NE1 4LP, UK

G. Kemball-Cook
Haemostasis Research Group, MRC Clinical Sciences Centre, Royal Postgraduate Medical School, Hammersmith Hospital, Du Cane Rd, London W12 0NN, UK

N.L. Kobrinsky
Roger Maris Cancer Center, 820 4th Street North, Fargo, ND 58122, USA

B.L. Kroner
Research Triangle Institute, 6101 Executive Boulevard Suite 365, Rockville, MD 20852, USA

S. Lethagen
Dept for Coagulation Disorders, University of Lund, University Hospital, Malmö, Sweden.

D.K. Liles
Dept of Medicine, Division of Hematology/Oncology; The Center for Thrombosis and Hemostasis, University of North Carolina, Chapel Hill, NC 27599, USA

R.A. Lipton
11 Devon Rd, Rockville Center, New York, NY 11570, USA

C.A. Ludlam
Dept of Rheumatology, Royal Infirmary, Lauriston Place, Edinburgh EH3 9YW, UK

J.M. Lusher
Division of Hematology–Oncology, Children's Hospital of Michigan, 3901 Beaubien, Detroit, MI 48201, USA

R.V. McIntosh
Protein Fractionation Centre, Scottish National Blood Transfusion Service, 21 Ellen's Glen Rd, Edinburgh EH17 7QT, UK

A.J. MacLeod
Protein Fractionation Centre, Scottish National Blood Transfusion Service, 21 Ellen's Glen Rd, Edinburgh EH17 7QT, UK

R. Madhok
Centre for Rheumatic Diseases, The Royal Infirmary, 84 Castle St, Glasgow G4 0SF, UK

I. Marková
Dept of Psychology, University of Stirling, Stirling FK9 4LA, UK

I.R. Peake
Section of Molecular Genetics, Dept of Medicine and Pharmacology, Royal Hallamshire Hospital, Sheffield S10 2JF, UK

O.D. Ratnoff
University Hospitals of Cleveland, 204 Abington Rd, Cleveland, OH 44106, USA

K.A. Rickard
Haemophilia Centre and Haematology Dept, Royal Prince Alfred Hospital, Sydney 2050, Australia

M.A. Rigdon
Dept of Family and Preventive Medicine, University of Utah School of Medicine, 50 N Medical Drive, Salt Lake City, UT 84132, USA

H.R. Roberts
Dept of Medicine, Division of Hematology/Oncology; The Center for Thrombosis and Hemostasis, University of North Carolina, Chapel Hill, NC 27599, USA

J.R. Schultz
Dept of Family and Preventive Medicine, University of Utah School of Medicine, 50 N Medical Drive, Salt Lake City, UT 84132, USA

S.V. Seremetis
Division of Hematology and Regional Comprehensive Hemophilia Program, Mount Sinai Hospital and Medical Center, New York, NY 10029, USA

S. Sindet-Pedersen
Dept of Oral and Maxillofacial Surgery, Aarhus University and University Hospital, Aarhus, Denmark

D.A. Stegman
Roger Maris Cancer Center, 820 4th Street North,
Fargo, ND 58122, USA

E.G.D. Tuddenham
Haemostasis Research Group, MRC Clinical Sciences
Centre, Royal Postgraduate Medical School,
Hammersmith Hospital, Du Cane Rd, London
W12 0NN, UK

I.D. Walker
Dept of Haematology, Glasgow Royal Infirmary
University NHS Trust, Glasgow G12 UQQ, UK

D.E. Wilcox
Dept of Medical Genetics, University of Glasgow,
Yorkhill Hospitals, Glasgow G3 8SJ, UK

P. Wilkie
Division of General Practice, St George's Hospital
Medical School, Blackshaw Rd, London SW17 0QT,
UK

PREFACE

Hemophilia is unique among diseases in that it is generally well known to members of the general public because of its royal connections. Few people do not know the story of the descendants of Queen Victoria, especially those of the Russian and Spanish royal families and the subsequent catastrophic social, personal and political results.

Early case reports documented the bleeding sagas of individuals or their families and later reports collected series of clinical cases, special bleeding events and their heroic treatment. It is probably true to say that all of clinical medicine is encapsulated in the study of hemophilia and related disorders and its investigation and treatment.

This book sets out to produce a comprehensive review of the current status of the important clinical and laboratory aspects of these diseases. The authors were invited to make their contributions because of their established pre-eminence in their specialist fields and have been chosen equally from Europe and the USA.

The subject coverage is comprehensive with 31 chapters, divided into four sections. The first section covers the historical introduction and the philosophy of why hemophiliacs bleed, followed by the molecular and genetic defects which have now been described. The second section covers the laboratory diagnosis and bleeding into or from special sites. The third section concentrates on comprehensive care and specific management issues with appropriate plasma concentrates and other therapeutic agents. Complications of treatment regimes, particularly human immunodeficiency virus (HIV) and hepatitis, are given special prominence.

The final section deals with family, social and psychological aspects of the diseases in all their aspects.

The book has been written to appeal to all who care for patients with hemophilia and their families and it is our hope that this volume will enhance the spread of knowledge and so improve hemophilia management.

C. Forbes
L. Aledort
R. Madhok

PART ONE

Understanding Hemophilia

[Hebrew quotation, Babylonian Talmud]

Babylonian Talmud, 4th century
Yevamoth 64b

1 THE EARLY HISTORY OF HEMOPHILIA

C.D. Forbes

The word hemophilia is derived from two Greek words *haima*, blood, and *philein*, to love – and, despite being senseless in the description of excess bleeding, it remains in general use. In the older literature various names have been used, e.g. hemorrhaphilia, hematophilia, hemorrhea, hemorrhagophilia, idiosyncrasia haemorrhagica and morbus haematicus. The first use of the word 'hemophilia' is attributed to Schönlein (Virchow, 1854) but the first written use was by Hopf, a student of Schönlein, who gave a dissertation entitled *Die Hamophiliet* at Wurzburg in 1828 (Brinkhous, 1975).

The disease is now called hemophilia A or classic hemophilia and is due to deficient activity of antihemophilic factor (AHF, antihemophilic globulin (AHG) or factor VIII). A variety has been described which is called Christmas disease in the UK but in Europe and the USA is often called hemophilia B or plasma thromboplastin component (PTC) deficiency. This is due to deficient activity of Christmas factor (CF, PTC or factor IX).

The clinical manifestations of these two diseases are essentially similar and no differentiation is made between them with regard to bleeding tendency. It is probable that genetically determined bleeding disorders are as old as time but they seem to have been neglected by the Egyptian, Roman and Greek physicians. The earliest documented case of a familial bleeding disorder occurs in the fourth-century Talmud and in Rabbinic writings thereafter. The Babylonian Talmud in the tractate Yevamoth 64b states:

> For it was taught: if she circumcised her first child and he died (as a result of bleeding from the operation), and a second one also died, she must not circumcise her third child.

This decree of Rabbi Judah (redactor of the Mishneh) recognized the familial and sex-linked nature of the bleeding defect and variations of his edict have been incorporated into Rabbinic law through the centuries and commented on by others (e.g. Alfasi, 1013–1103; Maimonides, 12th century).

Apart from this legal debate, no cases suggestive of a bleeding disorder were described in medieval times, except for a reference by Abul El Kassam (Albucasis), an Arabian physician who lived in Cordoba in 1107. He described that in a certain village there were men who, when wounded or phlebotomized, suffered an uncontrollable hemorrhage which ended only in the death of the patient.

Thereafter sporadic case reports of patients with excess bleeding may be found in the scientific literature. Philip Höchstetter, a physician practicing in Augsburgh at the beginning of the 17th century, speaks of a boy who hemorrhaged from the navel at birth; later in life he had repeated epistaxis, bloody stools and spontaneous ecchymosis. Banyer (1743) described the case of a 24-year-old gardener from Wisbech, in the Isle of Ely, who bled profusely from a puncture wound of his foot and then nearly exsanguinated from the site of a phlebotomy performed by his physician. This boy had epistaxis, recurrent melena and hematuria and eventually died in 1738, aged 33 years, following a trivial wound of the leg. In neither of these cases was there a documented family history.

The first probable case of hemophilia in the USA was recorded in an obituary in the Salem (Massachusetts) Gazette of 22 March 1791 and described the case of Isaac Zoll who died in Frederick County, Virginia, at the age of 19 from:

> a slight cut in one of his feet, with an axe. From the time of his receiving the wound, till he expired, no method could be devised to stop the bleeding.

This obituary goes on to describe the deceased's five brothers who had all died of exsanguination following minor trauma:

Hemophilia. Edited by C.D. Forbes, L. Aledort and R. Madhok. Published in 1997 by Chapman & Hall, London. ISBN 0 412 63820 7

one received a prick with a thorn – another, a scratch with a comb – a third, a prick with a needle – a fourth, bruised his cheek against a stove – and a fifth, received a cut in one of his thumbs.

It is of great interest that this boy's father, Henry Zoll, was twice married and only the children of the first wife were affected by this bleeding tendency.

In 1803, John C. Otto of Philadelphia described a family of bleeders by the name of Smith who had settled in the vicinity of Plymouth, New Hampshire, about 1720. Otto recorded that only the males were subject to this strange affliction and the females were exempt, although they were still capable of transmitting it to their male children. Unfortunately, Otto never saw or examined the patients but learned of them from Samuel Livermore, a lawyer who represented New Hampshire in the Continental Congress. The first pedigree of hemophilia was published by Hay (1813), who followed the disease in the Appleton-Swain family through six generations spanning 172 years and containing 20 hemophilic males. This family has been reinvestigated since then (McKusick, 1962) and has now been traced over 400 years and 13 generations. The disease in this family was originally identified in a male born in Bristol, UK, in 1630; this man went to Newbury, Massachusetts in 1639.

The first European notices of the disease are case reports by the editor of *Sammlung Auserlesener Abhandlungen* (1805) and by Consbruck (1810; quoted by Bulloch and Fildes, 1911), followed by careful clinical and postmortem observations by Blagden (1817) and Wilson (1819). It is of interest that the first report of a coagulation defect in hemophilic blood was by Ward (1819), but his suggestion was ignored for 80 years.

The next publication marks the transition from isolated case reports to an attempt at scientific description of the disease. In 1820, Nasse published a collection of the cases available at that time and gave a general review of the disease. He was of the opinion that the blood was of 'unusual fluidity' and this was due to 'hyperoxidation'. From study of the family histories came 'Nasse's law' which stated that hemophilia occurs only in males and is transmitted by unaffected females.

After 1820, the history of hemophilia is almost totally contained in the German literature and between 1830 and 1860 complete descriptions of the disease are met within the textbooks of Schönlein, Constatt, Neumann and Fuchs. At this time there was no real clue to the etiology of the disease but it was thought by Schönlein to be due to 'cyanosis and malformation of the heart' and by others to be due to 'anomalous gout' or 'scrofula' – despite the adequate postmortem examinations reported by Virchow (1854).

Grandidier (1855) collected all cases published up to that time of abnormal bleeding and found that there were 452 males and 32 females. These numbers are difficult to evaluate, as they contain cases of umbilical hemorrhage, menorrhagia and hemorrhage after circumcision, as well as cases of hemorrhagic disease suggestive of hemophilia.

In 1872 Legg wrote an excellent *Treatise on Hemophilia* describing the genetic transmission of the disease:

> The daughters ... possess in a very high degree the faculty of transmitting haemophilia to their sons. The women may appear perfectly healthy; they may marry perfectly healthy husbands; and yet bear a family, all the boys of which shall be bleeders.

He also described in detail the bleeding problems associated with the disease, the causes of mortality, the psychiatric aspects, the episodic bleeding and the current treatment. All this seems to have been neglected until it was rediscovered by later authors.

In 1893 Wright discovered that the clotting time of the patient's blood was prolonged and in 1911 Addis, then Minot and Lee (1916), observed that the addition of normal blood could correct the clotting defect in the hemophiliac blood.

In their classical monograph, Bulloch and Fildes (1911) surveyed the disease in 235 patients and their relatives. They re-emphasized the limitation of the disease to males but gave no credence to earlier descriptions of hemophilia in the female, despite case reports strongly suggestive of a bleeding tendency. Indeed, the female patient described by Treves in 1886 has subsequently been shown to belong to a family afflicted with classic hemophilia (Merskey, 1951).

In the first few years of this century the diagnosis of hemophilia depended on the clinical and family history, plus the finding of prolongation of the whole blood clotting time (Liston, 1839; Wright, 1893) in patients with normal levels of prothrombin (Howell and Cekada, 1926).

Treatment of the bleeding episodes up to this point varied from the bizarre to the lethal, despite the demonstration by Lane (1840) of the beneficial value of blood transfusion. This was rediscovered by Weil (1906) and Minot and Lee in the USA (1916). The use of plasma was then shown to be superior to whole blood by Feissly (1923) and Payne and Steen (1929) and this treatment became standard practice for 30 years.

The first major biochemical advance occurred in 1935 when Bendien and van Creveld, then Patek and Taylor (1937) found that platelet-free plasma, precipitated with water at a pH of 5.3–5.8, yielded a substance which was capable of correcting the clotting abnormality. This was confirmed by Lewis *et al.* (1946) and Brinkhous (1947) and the protein further characterized.

Until 1947, hemophilia was considered to be a single disease entity, then Pavlovsky observed that blood from one hemophiliac could correct the clotting defect in another. This phenomenon was demonstrable both *in vivo* and *in vitro* (Koller, Krusi and Luchsinger, 1950; Schulman and Smith, 1952). Coincident with these clinical findings, the development of tests of thromboplastin generation (Biggs *et al.*, 1952) confirmed that there were two separate groups of patients. This observation was confirmed clinically by the finding of a group of 'hemophilic' patients whose defect could be corrected by the infusion of haemophilic blood plasma (Aggeler *et al.*, 1952; Biggs *et al.*, 1952). This new disease was called Christmas disease and is associated with lack of a factor found in serum called Christmas factor (CF, factor IX or PTC).

As knowledge increased and new clotting tests were devised, it became apparent that there were other bleeding disorders besides the hemophilias. In 1947, a clotting deficiency was described by Owren in a patient with normal prothrombin and fibrinogen levels. This plasma would not clot readily with tissue extract and calcium ions and the defect was called factor V deficiency. In the course of time it became apparent that this factor was identical with the 'labile' factor described by Quick (1943).

Further investigations have shown the need for two additional factors participating in clotting with tissue thromboplastin, factor VII (de Vries, Alexander and Goldstein, 1949; Alexander, Goldstein and Landwehr, 1951) and factor X (Telfer, Denson and Wright, 1956; Hougie, Barrow and Graham, 1957). All these defects present with bleeding which is clinically indistinguishable from that of hemophilia and it is probable that early case records included patients with these defects.

As the pathways of blood coagulation have become better understood, it is apparent that other defects can be found in the laboratory which are not manifested clinically; for example, Hageman factor deficiency (Ratnoff and Colopy, 1955) is not usually associated with bleeding and deficiency of plasma thromboplastin antecedent (Rosenthal, Dreskin and Rosenthal, 1953) is associated with bleeding in only about two-thirds of cases. Deficiency of fibrinogen may be associated with only a mild bleeding defect.

Classical hemophilia probably exists in about 3–4 per 100 000 of the population in the UK (Biggs and Macfarlane, 1966). A similar figure is found in Europe (Hardisty and Ingram, 1965) and in the USA (Ratnoff, 1960; Lewis *et al.*, 1963). It is important to remember the dictum of Legg (1872):

> the number of cases in a given country depends upon the previous education of the medical men, and the interest which they take in the disease.

He points out that in 1872 Germany had 50% of cases, England fewer than 20% and France, USA and Switzerland 10% each.

The disease has now been described in every racial group (Prentice and Ratnoff, 1967) but is said to be uncommon in the American Negro (Lewis *et al.*, 1963), the Japanese (Yoshida, 1961) and the Bantu (Merskey, 1958). This last statement is probably correct and may apply to other negroid stock. In a recent study of East African negroes from various Kenyan tribes we found only three families with Christmas disease and five families with hemophilia (Forbes, MacKay and Khan, 1966). This observation has been confirmed by other investigators working in Uganda (Lothe, 1968). As laboratory facilities are extremely deficient in both these countries it is difficult to draw definite conclusions, but if the incidence of these diseases was similar to that in Europe and the USA, one would expect about 270 patients in Kenya alone. It is possible that the number of adult hemophiliacs is in fact low due to the high mortality expected following ritual circumcision carried out at puberty.

There are also wide variations in the incidence of bleeders within certain countries, e.g. in the Tenna valley in Switzerland (Moor-Jankowski *et al.*, 1957); in the Amish communities in Ohio and Pennsylvania (Wall, McConnell and Moore, 1967) the incidence of Christmas disease is high due to inbreeding.

Only about two-thirds of patients with these disorders have a family history of excess bleeding (Aggeler *et al.*, 1961; Macfarlane, 1962; Schulman, 1962). The interpretation of this figure is difficult, as few people know the medical history of their forebears beyond two generations and many of the cases could have been transmitted through successive generations of female carriers. When extremely active attempts are made to trace family histories, a higher incidence (80%) of positive histories is found (Ramgren, 1962; Quick, 1966). Occasionally the patient's disorder must be due to a fresh gene mutation.

Perhaps the most famous hemophilic family internationally is that of Queen Victoria, who in 1853 gave birth to her eighth child, Leopold, Duke of Albany, and he was a hemophiliac. In addition to this, two of her daughters proved to be carriers. It can truly be said that the result of the transmission of hemophilia into the royal families of Europe had a profound effect on the course of European history. Nowhere is this more poignant than in the case of Alexandra, who became the consort of Tsar Nicholas the Second of Russia, who produced Alexis, a severely affected hemophiliac, in 1904. In Victoria's family there was no evidence of any ancestor with hemophilia and it must be presumed that the disease was due to a mutant gene.

It is from these humble beginnings that the pace of research in hemophilia has increased exponentially and the following chapters will update the reader in the clinical, therapeutic and molecular areas. In addition, during the production of better concentrates, there have been devastating infections with hepatitis B, hepatitis C and human immunodeficiency virus (HIV). Production of recombinant factor VIII and factor IX is now available and for the new generation of hemophiliacs and those not infected with hepatitis or HIV there is the potential for a life which should be normal in span and free of the long-term complications of bleeding.

References

Abul El Kassam in 'Al-Tasrif' written about 1100 AD. Translated by Grimm S. (1519) in *Liber Theoriacae ne non Practicae Alsaharavii*.

Addis, T. (1911) The pathogenesis of hereditary haemophilia. *Journal of Pathology and Bacteriology*, **15**, 427–452.

Aggeler, P.M., White, S.G., Glendining, M.B. *et al.* Plasma thromboplastin component deficiency (PTC): a new disease resembling haemophilia. *Proceedings of the Society for Experimental Biology and Medicine*, **79**, 692–694.

Aggeler, P.M., Hoag, M.S., Wallerstein, R.O. and Whissell, D. (1961) The mild haemophilias. Occult deficiencies of AHF, PTC and PTA frequently responsible for unexpected surgical bleeding. *American Journal of Medicine*, **30**, 84–94.

Alexander, B., Goldstein, R. and Landwehr, G. (1951) The labile factor of prothrombin conversion: its consumption under normal and pathological conditions affecting blood coagulation. *Journal of Clinical Investigation*, **30**, 252–262.

Alfasi, L. (1957) On tractate Yevamoth 64b in the Babylonian Talmud; see edition of Otzar Hasefarim, New York (1957).

Anon (1805) *Sammlung Auserlesener Abhandlungen*, **22**, 275–279.

Banyer, H. (1743) Two remarkable medical cases; one of an extraordinary haemorrhage, the other an ascites caused by tapping. *Philosophical Transactions of the Royal Society, London*, **42**, 628–633.

Bendien, W.M. and van Creveld, S. (1935) Investigations of haemophilia. *Acta brevia Neerlandica de physiologia, pharmacologia, microbioligia e.a*, **5**, 135–138.

Biggs, R. and Macfarlane, R.G. (1966) *Treatment of Haemophilia and Other Coagulation Disorders*, Blackwell Scientific Publications, Oxford.

Biggs, R., Douglas, A.S., Macfarlane, R.G. *et al.* (1952) Christmas disease: a condition previously mistaken for haemophilia. *British Medical Journal*, **2**, 1378–1382.

Blagden, R. (1817) Case of a fatal haemorrhage from the extraction of a tooth. *Medico-Chirurgical Transactions*, **8**, 224–227.

Brinkhous, K.M. (1947) Clotting defect in haemophilia: deficiency in a plasma factor required for platelet utilisation. *Proceedings of the Society for Experimental Biology and Medicine*, **66**, 117–120.

Brinkhous, K.M. (1975) A short history of hemophilia with some comments on the word 'hemophilia', in *Handbook of Hemophilia*, (eds K.M. Brinkhace and H.C. Hemker), American Elsevier, New York, pp. 3–19.

Bulloch, W. and Fildes, P. (1911) In *Treasury of Human Inheritance*. Parts V and VI, Section XIV(a) on haemophilia. Cambridge University Press, London, pp. 169–347.

Consbruch, G.W. (1810) *Hufeland's Journal*, **30**, 116; quoted in Bulloch and Fildes (1911).

de Vries A., Alexander, B. and Goldstein, R. (1949) Factor in serum which accelerates conversion of prothrombin to thrombin: its determination and some physiologic and biochemical properties. *Blood, The Journal of Hematology*, **4**, 247–258.

Feissly, R. (1923) Études sur l'hémophilia. *Bulletin et mémoires de la Société de Médicine de Paris*, **47**, 1778–1783.

Forbes, C.D., MacKay, N. and Khan, A.A. (1966) Christmas disease and haemophilia in Kenya. *Transactions of the Royal Society of Tropical Medicine and Hygiene*, **60**, 777–781.

Grandidier, L. (1855) *Die Hämophilie oder die Bluterkrankheit nach eigenen und fremden Biobachtungen monographisch bearbeitet*, O. Wigand, Leipzig, p. 158.

Hardisty, R.M. and Ingram, G.I.C. (1965) *Bleeding Disorders. Investigation and Management*, Davis, Philadelphia.

Hay, J. (1813) Account of a remarkable haemorrhagic disposition, existing in many individuals of the same family. *New England Journal of Medicine and Surgery (Boston)*, **2**, 221–225.

Höchstetter, P. (1674) *Rarum Observationum Medicinalium Decades Sex*, Francofurti et Lipsiae, Tom 1, Decas ii, Casus nonus, 170.

Hopf, F. (1828) *Uber die Hämophilie oder die erbliche Anlage zu tödtlichen Blutungen*, C.W. Becker, Wurzerg.

Hougie, C., Barrow, E.M. and Graham, J.B. (1957) Stuart clotting – defect I. Segregation of an hereditary haemorrhagic state from the heterogeneous group heretofore called stable factor (SPCA, proconvertin, factor VII) deficiency. *Journal of Clinical Investigation*, **36**, 485–496.

Howell, W.H. and Cekada, E.B. (1926) The cause of the delayed clotting of hemophilic blood. *American Journal of Physiology*, **78**, 500–511.

Koller, F., Krusi, G. and Luchsinger, G. (1950) Uber eine besondre Form hämorrhagischer Diathese. *Schweizerische medizinische Wochenschrift*, **80**, 1101–1103.

Lane, S. (1840) Successful transfusion of blood. *Lancet*, **1**, 185–188.

Legg, W. (1872) *A Treatise on Haemophilia*. H.K. Lewis, London.

Lewis, J.H., Tagnon, H.J., Davidson, C.S. *et al.* (1946) The relation of certain fractions of the plasma globulins and the coagulation defect in haemophilia. *Blood, The Journal of Hematology*, **1**, 166–172.

Lewis, J.H. Didisheim, P. Ferguson, J.H. and Li, C.C. (1963) Genetic considerations in familial hemorrhagic disease I. The sex-linked recessive disorders hemophilia and PTC deficiency. *American Journal of Human Genetics*, **15**, 53–61.

Liston, J.R. (1839) Haemorrhagic idiosyncrasy. *Lancet*, **2**, 137–138.

Lothe, F. (1968) Haemophilia in Uganda. *Transactions of the Royal Society of Tropical Medicine and Hygiene*, **62**, 3561.

Macfarlane, R.G. (1962) Purification of factor X, its activation by Russel's viper venom and also by physiological factors. *Thrombosis et Diathesis Haemorrhagica*, **7**, 222–228.

McKusick, V.A. (1962) Hemophilia in early New England. *Journal of the History of Medicine*, **17**, 342–365.

Maimonides, M. (1957) Laws of circumcision, Book of Adoration (Sefer Ahavah), in *Code of Maimonides* (Mishneh Torah). Pardes Publishers, Jerusalem, Chapter 1, paragraph 18.

Merskey, C. (1958) The occurrence of haemophilia in the human female. *Quarterly Journal of Medicine* (NS), **79**, 299–312.

Minot, G.R. and Lee, R.I. (1916) The blood platelets in hemophilia. *Archives of Internal Medicine*, **18**, 474–495.

Moor-Jankowski, J.K., Truog, G., Rosin, S. and Huser, H.J. (1957) Der Bluterstamm von Tenna und seine Nachkommen. *Acta Genetica et Statistica Medica*, **1**, 597–601.

Nasse, C.F. (1820) Vor einer erblichen Neigung zu tödtlichen Blutungen. *Archiv für Medizin Erfahr (Berlin)*, **1**, 385–434.

Otto, J.C. (1803) An account of an hemorrhagic disposition existing in certain families. *The Medical Repository*, **6**, 1–4.

Owren, P.A. (1947) Coagulation of blood; investigations on a new clotting factor. *Acta edica Scandinavica*, **128** (suppl. 194), 1–327.

Patek, A.J. and Taylor, F.H.L. (1937) Haemophilia: some properties of a substance obtained from normal human plasma effective in accelerating the coagulation of hemophilic blood. *Journal of Clinical Investigation*, **16**, 113–124.

Pavlovsky, A. (1947) Contribution to the pathogenesis of haemophilia. *Blood, The Journal of Hematology*, **2**, 185–181.

Payne, W.W. and Steen, R.E. (1929) Haemostatic therapy in haemophilia. *British Medical Journal*, **1**, 1150–1152.

Prentice, C.R.M. and Ratnoff, O.D. (1967) Genetic disorders of blood coagulation. *Seminars in Hematology*, **4**, 93–132.

Quick, A.J. (1943) On constitution of prothrombin. *American Journal of Physiology*, **140**, 212–220.

Quick, A.J. (1966) *Haemorrhagic Disease and Thrombosis*, 2nd edn, Lea and Febiger.

Ramgren, O. (1962) Haemophilia in Sweden. Hereditory investigations. *Acta Medica Scandinavia*, **379** (suppl), 759–769.

Ratnoff, O.D. (1960) *Bleeding Syndromes*, C.C. Thomas, Springfield, Illinois.

Ratnoff, O.D. and Colopy, J.E. (1955) Familial haemorrhagic trait associated with deficiency of clot-promoting fraction of plasma. *Journal of Clinical Investigation*, **34**, 602–613.

Rosenthal, R.L., Dreski, O.H. and Rosenthal, M. (1953) New hemophilia-like disease caused by deficiency of third plasma thromboplastin factor. *Proceedings of the Society for Experimental Biology and Medicine*, **82**, 171–174.

Schulman I. and Smith, C.H. (1952). Haemorrhagic disease in an infant due to deficiency of a previously undescribed clotting factor. *Blood, The Journal of Hematology*, **7**, 794–807.

Schulman, I. (1962) Pediatric aspects of the mild hemophilias. *Medical Clinics of North America*, **46**, 93–105.

Telfer, T.P., Denson, K.W.E. and Wright, D.R. (1956) A new coagulation defect. *British Journal of Haematology*, **2**, 308.

Treves, F. (1886) A case of haemophilia pedigree through five generations. *Lancet*, **2**, 533.

Wall, R.L., McConnell, J.L. and Moore, D. (1967) Christmas disease, colour blindness and the Xg[a] blood group. *American Journal of Medicine*, **43**, 214–226.

Virchow, R. (1854). Die Bluterkrankheit. *Handbuch der speciellen Pathologie und Therapie*, Berlin, pp. 263–270.

Ward, Mr (1819) quoted by Wardrop J. On the curative effects of the abstraction of blood. A. Waldie, Philadelphia, 1837, pp. 9–10.

Weil, P.E. (1906) Étude du sang chez les hémophilies. *Bulletin et Mémoires de la Societé de Médicine de Paris*, **23**, 1001–1005.

Wilson, J. (1819) *Lectures on the Blood and on the Anatomy, Physiology and Surgical Pathology of the Vascular System of the Human Body*, Burgess and Hill, London, p. 410.

Wright, A.E. (1893) On the method of determining the condition of blood coagulability for clinical and experimental purposes and on the effects of administration of calcium salts in haemophilia and actual or threatened haemorrhage. *British Medical Journal*, **2**, 223–225.

Yoshida, K. (1961) Hemophilia and related diseases. *Acta Haematologica Japonica*, **24**, 109–139.

2 HEMOSTATIC MECHANISMS: WHY HEMOPHILIACS BLEED

O.D. Ratnoff

The ability to stem blood loss after vascular injury is vital for all vertebrate species. In human beings, an early response to vascular damage is transient vasoconstriction in the area of the wound, but this is probably of little benefit. Vasoconstriction may be brought about by local release of thromboxane A2 and 5-hydroxytryptamine (serotonin) from platelets, and polypeptide endothelins derived from vascular endothelial cells; whether the endothelins contribute to hemostasis is not certain (Simonson and Dunn, 1991; Levin, 1995; Saito, 1996). Essentially simultaneously, escape of blood through the gap created by minimal vascular damage is normally staunched by platelets, anuclear cells that arise from the break-up of the cytoplasm of megakaryocytes, a process stimulated by a trace plasma polypeptide, thrombopoei-tin, that promotes both the proliferation and differentiation of megakaryocyte progenitor cells (Kelemen, Cserháti and Tanos, 1958; Levin *et al.*, 1982; Kaushansky, 1995). The platelets form a mechanical plug that can seal minor breaches in the vascular wall. Platelets do this by sticking to the edges of severed vessels, to exposed subendothelial structures such as collagen, and to each other (Marcus, 1996). Adhesion of platelets to these structures is enhanced by plasma von Willebrand factor, a protein deficient in von Willebrand's disease that reacts with a specific receptor on platelet membranes, glyco-protein Ib. Contact of platelets with collagen induces activation of these cells which release biologically active agents from their cytoplasmic granules that enhance the formation of platelet aggregates.

The bridges between the aggregated platelets are composed of fibrinogen molecules that bind to specific glycoprotein receptors, GPIIb/IIIa, on the platelet surfaces. The adherent and aggregated platelets clump rapidly, forming a hemostatic plug that can close small gaps in the walls of blood vessels. Platelet aggregation is brought about by a cyclic endoperoxide, thromboxane A2, a derivative of arachidonic acid that is released from platelet membrane phospholipids when these cells have been stimulated by collagen, adenosine diphosphate (ADP) or other agonists. Essentially simultaneously, gaps in the vascular wall are closed by generation of a blood clot, that is, by transformation of liquid blood to a gel-like coagulum that consolidates the platelet aggregates. Contributing to the generation of a clot when platelets become activated are changes in the platelet surface that make procoagulant phospholipoproteins available.

Coagulation of blood at the site of injury can diminish or halt blood loss from vascular defects larger than those that can be controlled by platelets alone. When bleeding occurs into a closed space such as the tip of a finger or toe, blood loss is minimized by the back-pressure of extravasated blood; the importance of this device can be appreciated by the extensive loss of blood that may occur in otherwise normal individuals after injury to periorbital tissues or to an intraperitoneal vessel. In these situations, the accumulated shed blood usually does not provide sufficient back-pressure to stop blood flow. Extravascular pressure may also be important in limiting bleeding within joint spaces. In the special case of the uterus, bleeding after delivery is further controlled by contraction of the myometrium, applying external pressure on blood vessels at the site of the avulsed placenta. A similar mechanism may participate in the control of menstrual bleeding (Christianes, Sixma and Haspels, 1982).

The importance of blood coagulation for the control of bleeding is readily understood from the hemorrhagic tendency of individuals with hereditary clotting defects. Clotting is the end-result of a series of chemical events that are initiated upon contact of blood with either injured tissue or with negatively charged surfaces such as glass. Perturbation of blood in these ways starts

Hemophilia. Edited by C.D. Forbes, L. Aledort and R. Madhok. Published in 1997 by Chapman & Hall, London. ISBN 0 412 63820 7

sequential reactions that result, in the end, in the release of a plasma protease, thrombin, that brings about coagulation. At each step, a plasma protein clotting factor undergoes limited proteolysis that results in its conversion to a form with enzymatic activity until, in the end, prothrombin is cleaved proteolytically, releasing enzymatically active thrombin (Davie and Ratnoff, 1964; Macfarlane, 1964). A characteristic of these clotting factors is that they may have multiple functions, suggesting that their role has been determined by the forces of evolution.

The formation of fibrin

Normally, clotting comes about because the thrombin released from prothrombin transforms a soluble plasma protein, fibrinogen (factor I), into a network of insoluble protein strands, fibrin (Mosesson, 1992; Fig. 2.1). Blood cells and serum (that is, the liquid part of blood after clotting takes place) are trapped within the fibrin meshwork, bringing about a typical clot.

Fibrinogen, the plasma protein from which fibrin is derived, has a molecular weight of about 340 000 and is synthesized largely, or more probably, solely in the parenchymal cells of the liver.

Fibrinogen is a dimer, each half of which is made up of three disulfide-linked dissimilar polypeptides chains, designated Aα, Bβ and γ. When blood is shed, the transformation of fibrinogen to fibrin is brought about enzymatically by thrombin, a serine protease that is generated from its precursor in plasma, prothrombin (factor II). Thrombin, a protein with a molecular weight of 28 000,

cleaves a pair of small polypeptides, described as fibrinopeptides A and B, from each Aα and Bβ polypeptide chain of fibrinogen respectively, reducing its molecular weight by about 2%. The monomeric units of fibrin that remain polymerize into the insoluble protein strands that comprise the clot. Studies with coagulant snake venoms that cleave the Aα or Bβ chains selectively indicate that it is the separation of fibrinopeptide A that is critical for fibrin formation.

Fibrin strands that are prepared from purified fibrinogen and thrombin are held together by weak electrostatic forces that, in the test tube, can be disrupted by dispersing agents such as 1% monochloroacetic acid or 5 mol/l urea, bringing about dissolution of the clot. When fibrin forms in normal plasma, however, the monomeric molecules are quickly linked covalently one to another, end-to-end and side-to-side, by a plasma transamidase, activated fibrin-stabilizing factor (factor XIIIa), that forms γ-glutamyl-ϵ-lysine links between adjacent fibrin monomers. Fibrin-stabilizing factor is a tetrameric protein with a molecular weight of about 320 000 and is composed of two a (or α) and two b (or β) chains. It is synthesized in hepatic parenchymal cells and in megakaryocytes; about half the fibrin-stabilizing factor in blood is found in platelets where it is composed only of α chains. Inert in circulating blood, fibrin-stabilizing factor is converted by thrombin to its enzymatically functional state (factor XIIIa) by cleavage of a small peptide from each of its subunits. Calcium ions are not needed for the formation of fibrin by thrombin, but, at the concentration found in plasma, they greatly accelerate polymerization of fibrin monomers. Calcium ions are also needed for the activation of fibrin-stabilizing factor.

The formation of thrombin: overview

Thrombin does not circulate in any significant amount in normal plasma, but when blood is shed it is generated locally from its plasma precursor, prothrombin (Schmidt, 1892). Prothrombin, a single-chain protein with a molecular weight of 70 000 that is synthesized in the liver, is the prototype for several plasma proteins that require vitamin K for their synthesis. Synthesis of these vitamin K dependent proteins occurs in two stages. In the first, amino acids are assembled into a polypeptide that seems to have no function in clotting. In the second stage, vitamin K directs the insertion of a second carboxyl group into the γ carbon of certain glutamic acid residues at the amino-terminal end of the polypeptide. These unique tricarboxylic glutamic acid residues are needed to create a functionally competent molecule (p. 13).

Schmidt (1892) believed that the *vis a tergo* that brings about release of thrombin is contact of shed blood with injured tissue. The agent (or agents) furnished by injured cells, now called tissue factor or tissue thromboplastin,

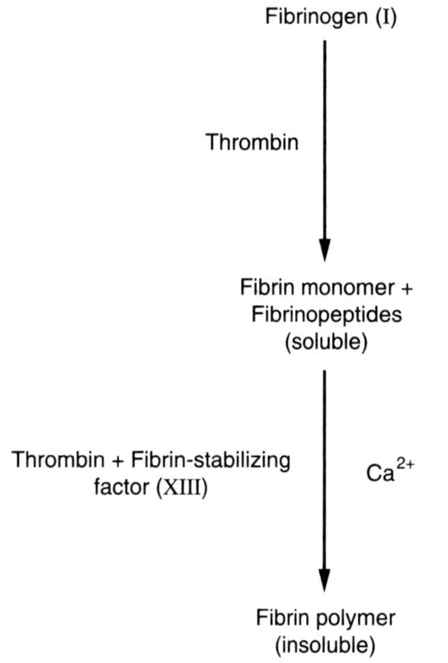

Fig. 2.1 The formation of fibrin in human plasma. Redrawn from Beeson, P.B., McDermott, W. and Wyngaarden, J.B. (eds) (1979) *Cecil Textbook of Medicine*, 15th edn. W.B. Saunders, Philadelphia, with permission.

is a non-enzymatic phospholipoglycoprotein found by immunostaining to be in highest concentration in brain, lung and placental tissue (Fleck *et al.*, 1990). Among other cell types that may furnish thromboplastic activity are fibroblasts, smooth-muscle cells and endothelial cells, all components of vascular walls. Tissue factor requires calcium ions to function and, as Bordet (1921) showed, additional plasma substances. These additional agents, later identified as factors V (proaccelerin), VII and X (Stuart–Prower factor), are necessary cofactors for optimal generation of thrombin from prothrombin.

Physiologic thrombin generation is more complex than Schmidt envisioned. Elaboration of thrombin, the enzyme immediately responsible for fibrin formation, is the end-result of either of two sequential and interlocking chains of chemical reactions, designated the extrinsic and intrinsic pathways of thrombin formation. These reactions involve the participation of a number of plasma protein clotting factors, most of them proenzymes that

are synthesized in hepatic parenchymal cells. The sequence of reactions described as the **extrinsic pathway** begins when blood comes into contact with injured tissues, as it might after a wound is inflicted (Fig. 2.2). The injured tissues furnish one or more agents, called generically **tissue factor** or **tissue thromboplastin**, that bring about clotting upon contact with blood (Nemerson, 1992). Tissue factor is a lipoprotein whose protein component is synthesized under the direction of a gene that has been localized to chromosome 1 and its DNA sequence determined (Carson, Henry and Shons, 1985; Mackman *et al.*, 1989). Synthesis has been induced experimentally in aortic smooth muscle and umbilical vein endothelial cells subjected to physical or chemical stimulation (Galdal, 1984; Marmur *et al.*, 1993).

Blood also clots via reactions described as **the intrinsic pathway of thrombin formation** when it comes into contact with certain negatively charged agents, of which glass, a non-biologic substance, is a prototype.

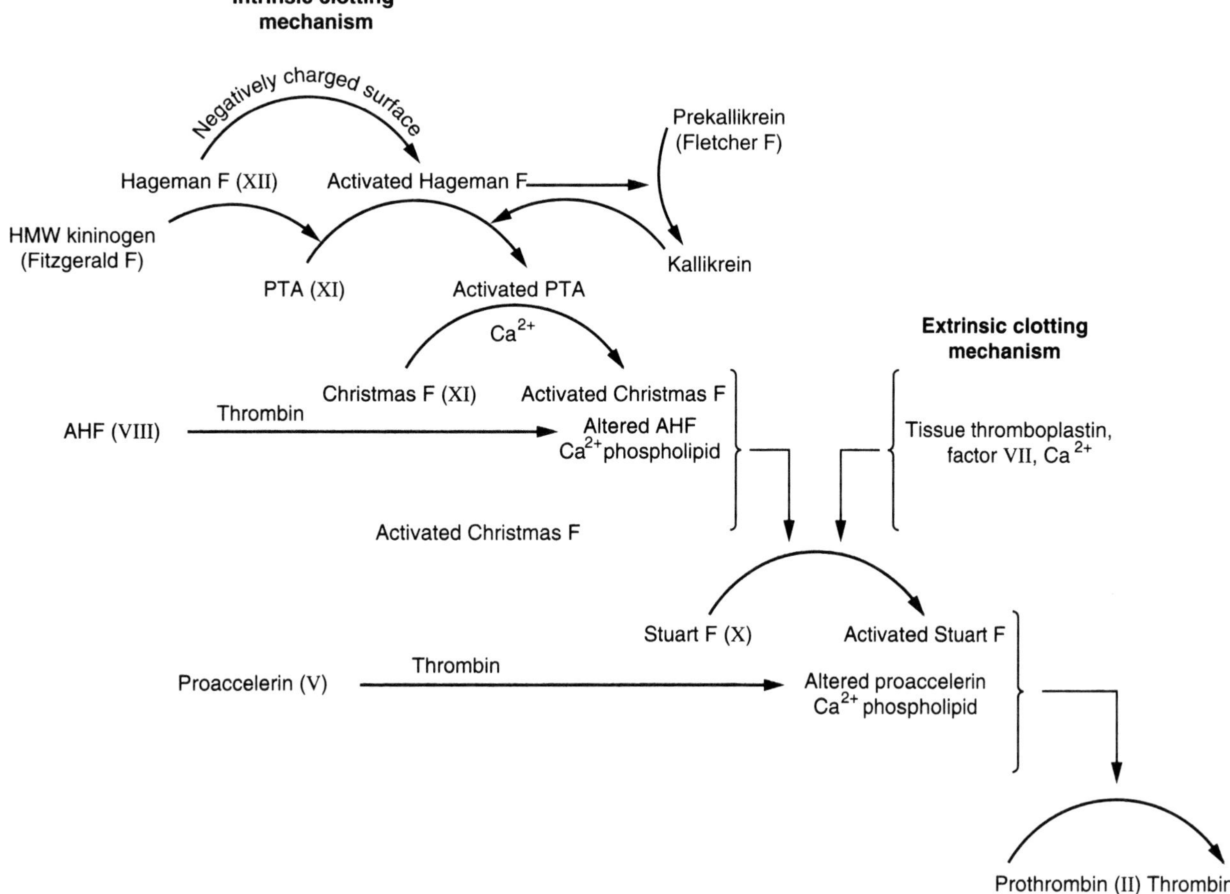

Fig. 2.2 The intrinsic and extrinsic pathways for the formation of thrombin. Omitted from the diagram are inhibitors of the various steps. The phospholipid portion of tissue thromboplastin may function in the activation and action of factor X (Stuart factor). The phospholipid for the intrinsic pathway is furnished by platelets and by the plasma itself. Augmentation of the action of factor VII by thrombin, activated Hageman factor and activated Stuart factor, and activation of Christmas factor by the tissue factor–factor VII complex are not depicted. HMW = High-molecular-weight; PTA = plasma thromboplastin antecedent; AHF = antihemophilic factor. Redrawn from Beeson P.B., McDermott, W. and Wyngaarden, J.B. (eds) (1979) *Cecil Textbook of Medicine*, 15th edn, W.B. Saunders, Philadelphia, with permission.

The extrinsic pathway of thrombin formation

A current view of the extrinsic pathway of thrombin formation is that in the presence of calcium ions tissue thromboplastin combines with and activates a plasma proenzyme, factor VII (Broze, 1982; Broze *et al.*, 1985; Kang and Niemetz, 1988; Nemerson, 1988). Tissue factor is localized to the membranes of most cells, including vascular endothelium (Zeldis, Nemerson and Lentz, 1972; Maynard *et al.*, 1977; Galdal, 1984; Østerud *et al.*, 1986) and subendothelial structures (Weiss *et al.*, 1989). Tissue factor is a complex of a glycoprotein with a molecular weight of about 45 000 and phospholipid, principally phosphatidyl choline and phosphatidyl ethanolamine. Platelets, striated muscle cells and synovial membranes have relatively little thromboplastic activity (Astrup and Sjølin, 1958; Astrup, 1965).

Factor VII, like prothrombin, a vitamin K-dependent clotting factor, is synthesized in hepatic parenchymal cells; its molecular weight is 48 000. In the presence of calcium ions, tissue factor binds to factor VII through the latter's tricarboxylic acid glutamic acid (Gla) residues (Nemerson, 1966a). As a consequence, factor VII, which is a one-chain polypeptide with weak enzymatic properties, is cleaved to form hemostatically active factor VIIa. In turn, factor VIIa, bound to tissue factor, cleaves factor X (Stuart factor), another plasma vitamin K-dependent proenzyme with a molecular weight of 59 000, changing it to its proteolytically active state, activated factor X (factor Xa; Nemerson, 1988). Reciprocally, factor Xa converts factor VII to its two-chain form, enhancing its clotting activity. Abetted by a non-enzymatic protein cofactor, **factor V (proaccelerin)**, factor Xa also cleaves thrombin from its parent molecule, prothrombin (Rao *et al.*, 1985; Peterson *et al.*, 1995).

Factor V, synthesized principally in the liver but also in endothelial cells and probably megakaryocytes, is a single-chain protein with a molecular weight of about 330 000 (Cerveny, Fass and Mann, 1984; Nichols *et al.*, 1985). Its activity is enhanced by limited proteolysis by either factor Xa or thrombin (Ware and Seegers, 1948; Rapaport *et al.*, 1963; Foster, Nesheim and Mann, 1983). Activation of factors VII and X and the release of thrombin from prothrombin require the presence of calcium ions and of phospholipid, the latter furnished by tissue factor itself. Factor Xa may have the additional property of stimulating cellular growth (Altion, 1995).

The importance of the extrinsic pathway of thrombin formation, an elaboration of Schmidt's original construction of the steps leading to clotting, was not challenged in a major way for many years, despite many reported confounding observations that could not be fitted into his paradigm. Two major obstacles prevented generalization of Schmidt's hypothesis. It did not explain either the pathogenesis of hemophilia nor the long-known clot-promoting properties of agents such as glass. A minimal expansion of Schmidt's ideas required envisioning a second pathway leading to the formation of thrombin. Knowledge about this second pathway gradually evolved from study of patients in whom clotting, as measured *in vitro*, was impaired.

The intrinsic pathway of thrombin formation

Although loose usage abounds, the term hemophilia should be restricted to hereditary, X chromosome-linked deficiencies of factor VIII (antihemophilic factor) or factor IX (Christmas factor) and still more carefully, to classic hemophilia (factor VIII deficiency, hemophilia A). Classic hemophilia and Christmas disease, both inherited as sex-linked disorders and therefore almost entirely restricted to males, are essentially indistinguishable clinically; rupture of the spleen, virtually limited to patients with Christmas disease, may be the consequence of injuries common among Amish patients with this malady. In severe cases of classic hemophilia or Christmas disease, bleeding may occur almost anywhere and bleeding into joints is a prominent feature; normal synovial fluid and tissues appear to be devoid of clot-promoting properties (Astrup and Sjølin, 1958; Astrup, 1965; Ratnoff, unpublished studies). Indeed, in the early 19th century, patients who would now be said to have hemophilia or Christmas disease were believed to have a form of rheumatism because of the prominence of joint deformities brought about by recurrent hemarthrosis, that is, bleeding into joint spaces. In 1837 Ward recognized that in such patients blood clotting was delayed, and in 1840 Lane added that blood transfusion seemed to control epistaxis in a patient who may have had hemophilia.

The first substantive contribution to the mechanism underlying the bleeding tendency in hemophilia was provided by Wright in 1893, when he pointed out that, in comparison to normal individuals, the clotting of whole blood was delayed in some patients who had a bleeding tendency; in modern terms, the clotting time was abnormally long. The defect in certain patients with a hereditary bleeding tendency was localized more sharply by Addis (1910) to a defect in plasma that impeded generation of thrombin in shed blood. Addis attributed the clotting abnormality to lack of a normal plasma constituent. In retrospect, it is unclear whether Addis was studying Christmas disease (factor IX deficiency) or classic hemophilia. Measurement of the slow generation of thrombin in hemophilic blood *in vitro* emerged as a diagnostic tool, the prothrombin consumption test. But Addis interpreted his data to mean that the basic defect in hemophilia was an abnormality of prothrombin itself when he correctly observed that the conversion of prothrombin to thrombin was retarded.

The nature of the abnormality in classic hemophilia was clarified further by Frank and Hartmann (1927) and Govaerts and Gratia (1936) who found that normal plasma contained a thermolabile agent distinct from prothrombin that shortened the abnormally long clotting time of hemophilic plasma. Their observations were confirmed and extended by Patek and his associates (Patek and Stetson, 1936; Patek and Taylor, 1937). A fraction of normal plasma shortened the abnormally long clotting time of hemophilic blood, whereas a comparable fraction of hemophilic plasma lacked this property. Moreover, intravenous infusion of the fraction prepared from normal plasma shortened the clotting time of patients with hemophilia. Similar results were reported by Bendien and van Creveld (1937).

By the end of the 1930s, it was evident that in classic hemophilia, the plasma was deficient in an agent needed for the generation of thrombin in shed blood, but the function of this agent, variously called antihemophilic factor, antihemophilic globulin or factor VIII, was not yet apparent (Brinkhous, 1939). Years earlier, von Manteuffel (1893) had reported that hemophilic blood clotted normally upon addition of tissue factor or tissue thromboplastin. Thus, the function of factor VIII appeared to be localized to a pathway other than that initiated by tissue factor.

Two other observations both confused and extended this interpretation. The first resulted from studies of a peculiar familial bleeding disorder among inhabitants of the Åland Islands in the Baltic sea. Hemorrhagic manifestations occurred in affected individuals of both sexes who seemed to inherit their malady as an autosomal dominant trait. Von Willebrand (1931) distinguished this disorder, which he named eponymously von Willebrand's disease, from classic hemophilia not only because it affected both men and women but because the bleeding time (that is, the time elapsing until bleeding stops from a deliberately incised cutaneous wound) was prolonged. Years later, several investigators (Alexander and Goldstein, 1953; Larrieu and Soulier, 1953; Quick and Hussey, 1953) added the critical observation that patients with von Willebrand's disease, like those with classic hemophilia, were functionally deficient in antihemophilic factor (factor VIII). Since the bleeding time is normal in classic hemophilia, the deficiency of factor VIII alone could not explain the abnormally long bleeding time in von Willebrand's disease. Subsequently, patients with von Willebrand's disease were found to be deficient in an additional plasma protein, now called von Willebrand factor, that participates in controlling bleeding from small vascular wounds by fostering adhesion of platelets to the wounded endothelial surface. Deficiency of this protein seems responsible for the long bleeding time in von Willebrand's disease. Von Willebrand factor, a heterogeneous protein with molecular weights ranging from about 500 000 to about 20 000 000, is synthesized in vascular endothelial cells and megakaryocytes (Jaffe, Hoyer and Nechman, 1977; Nachman, Levine and Jaffe, 1977) and has a substructure made up largely of identical disulfide-linked polypeptide subunits, each with a molecular weight of 265 000, that are essential to its hemostatic function (Chopek et al., 1986). The concentration of von Willebrand factor is normal or even elevated in patients with classic hemophilia. Additionally, von Willebrand factor agglutinates normal or formalin-fixed platelets in the presence of ristocetin, an antibiotic withdrawn from use because it induced thrombocytopenia (Howard and Firkin, 1971). This property has been exploited to measure von Willebrand factor quantitatively (Weiss et al., 1973).

Factor VIII, functionally deficient in the plasma in both classic hemophilia and von Willebrand's disease, has now been purified and its structure determined. It is a polymeric protein composed of a variable number of single-chain glycoproteins, each with a molecular weight of about 265 000, made up of an amino-terminal heavy chain and a carboxy-terminal light chain that are held together with calcium ions (Foster and Zimmerman, 1989). It circulates in plasma in a non-covalent complex with von Willebrand factor (Poon and Ratnoff, 1976), the plasma protein that is deficient in von Willebrand's disease. Von Willebrand's factor appears to prolong the half-disappearance time of factor VIII from plasma. The coagulant activity of factor VIII is enhanced by its partial proteolysis by thrombin (Ware and Seegers, 1948; Hoyer and Trabald, 1981; Puttman and Kaufman, 1988). In the test tube, further incubation with thrombin leads to loss of the coagulant function of factor VIII (Fulcher, Roberts and Zimmerman, 1983).

The second observation confounding Schmidt's construction of the clotting process was recorded by Pavlovsky (1947), who reported that a mixture of the plasmas of two patients, both of whom appeared to have typical hemophilia, behaved like normal plasma; further, infusion of the plasma of one hemophilic patient into another corrected the clotting defect of the recipient. These studies could be explained by assuming that the **clinical** syndrome of hemophilia might be the consequence of either of two distinct plasma defects. This supposition was soon confirmed by Schulman and Smith (1952), Aggeler et al. (1952) and Biggs and colleagues (1952), all of whom studied apparently typical hemophiliacs whose defect was corrected by the plasma of patients with classic hemophilia. These patients, then, appeared to be functionally deficient in another plasma agent, a protein that was originally called plasma factor X (not to be confused with Stuart factor, now designated factor X) or plasma thromboplastin component, and was later renamed factor IX. Using the trivial name, Christmas factor (Biggs et al., 1952), after Biggs' index patient, may help to avert therapeutic accidents arising from the sometimes confusing nature of the numerical nomenclature.

These newly discovered clotting factors could find no place in the classic hypothesis that had been promulgated in the late 19th century to explain blood clotting that is now described as the extrinsic pathway of thrombin formation. As early as the mid-19th century, other observations made clear that Schmidt's paradigm for the steps leading to blood clotting was incomplete. Clotting could be delayed or prevented by collecting normal blood in such a way that it did not come into contact with glass or porcelain, using syringes and needles coated with petrolem jelly or silicone. Plasma separated from such blood then coagulated upon touching the walls of a glass-like container. The effect of glass was localized to an action upon a plasma protein, now called Hageman factor, named after the first patient in whom a functional deficiency of this protein was recognized, or factor XII (Ratnoff and Rosenblum, 1958). Hageman factor, a single-chain glycoprotein with a molecular weight of about 80 000 that is apparently made in the liver, can be split by trypsin into a carboxy-terminal fragment with a molecular weight of about 28 000 and an amino-terminal fragment with a molecular weight of about 52 000. The amino-terminal fragment contains the amino acid sequences that react with negatively charged agents, bringing about activation of the clotting factor, whereas the carboxy-terminal fragment contains the sequences responsible for the catalytic functions of Hageman factor.

Through a series of chemical steps involving at least two other proteins, Hageman factor, activated by contact with glass or other negatively charged agents, acquires proteolytic properties and can then transform three other clotting factors, plasma thromboplastin antecedent or factor XI (PTA), factor VII and plasma prekallikrein (Fletcher factor) to their enzymatically active states, factor XIa, factor VIIa and plasma kallikrein respectively. Activation of Hageman factor can also bring about conversion of prorenin to renin and of plasminogen to the fibrinolytic enzyme, plasmin. The latter reaction, under appropriate conditions, results in transformation of the first component of complement (C1) to its enzymatically active form, C1 esterase or C$\overline{1}$ (Sumi, Muramutu and Fijii, 1973).

Activation of PTA by activated Hageman factor (factor XIIa) is enhanced by the presence of a non-enzymatic plasma protein with which its circulates as a non-covalent complex, high-molecular-weight kininogen (Fitzgerald, Flaujeac or Williams factor). High-molecular-weight kininogen has an additional role, serving as a source of biologically active small polypeptide kinins such as bradykinin that under experimental conditions can bring about reactions associated with inflammation (Wuepper, 1972). The release of kinins results from partial digestion of high-molecular-weight kininogen by proteolytically active plasma kallikrein, generated by activated Hageman factor from its precursor, plasma prekallikrein. Like factor XI, plasma prekallikrein circulates in normal plasma in non-covalent linkage with high-molecular-weight kininogen. Plasma kallikrein reciprocally activates Hageman factor. Thus, activated Hageman factor (factor XIIa) can activate factor XI both by a direct action and indirectly by its conversion of prekallikrein to kallikrein, a reaction that enhances activation of Hageman factor. Factor XIa, thrombin and trypsin can all directly change factor XI to its active form in the absence of Hageman factor (Saito *et al.*, 1973; Mannhalter, Schiffman and Jacobs, 1980; Gailani and Broze, 1991; Naito and Fujikawa, 1991; Rapaport, 1993; von dem Borne *et al.*, 1994). And, at least *in vitro*, factor XIa, like plasma kallikrein, can release kinins from high-molecular-weight kininogen (Scott *et al.*, 1985).

In the test tube, factor XIa's principal role is conversion of factor IX, the agent deficient in Christmas disease, to its proteolytically active form (factor IXa), a reaction enhanced by phospholipids (Ratnoff and Davie, 1962; Mannhalter, Schiffman and Deutsch, 1984). Activation of factor IX is brought about by scission of its molecule. Activation of factor IX can also be brought about by the tissue factor–factor VII complex, an example of the interlocking nature of the pathways to thrombin generation (Østerud and Rapaport, 1977). Once generated, factor IXa binds via its carboxy-terminal heavy chain to anti-hemophilic factor (factor VIII), a non-enzymatic cofactor (Hamaguchi *et al.*, 1994). In this configuration, factor IXa catalyzes transformation of factor X to enzymatically active factor Xa. Activation requires the presence of calcium ions and negatively charged phospholipids and comes about because factor IXa cleaves an amino-terminal peptide from factor X, allowing it to express its proteolytic properties. In turn, factor Xa, again abetted by calcium ions and phospholipids, cleaves thrombin from the prothrombin molecule and thereby brings about the formation of fibrin.

Plasma kallikrein has multiple functions, among them, activation of factor XII, enhancement of the activity of factor VII and separation of biologically active polypeptide kinins from their plasma precursors, the kininogens. The steps leading to clotting upon contact of plasma with glass or other negatively charged agents are described as the intrinsic pathway of thrombin formation.

Needless to say, this review of the steps leading to the formation of a clot represents an oversimplificaton. Many studies demonstrate the intertwining nature of the reactions of the extrinsic and intrinsic pathways of thrombin formation. For example, activated Hageman factor (factor XIIa) not only initiates thrombin formation via the intrinsic pathway, but it also converts factor VII, a participant in formation of thrombin by the extrinsic pathway, to an enzymatically active form (factor VIIa). Activation of factor VII in this way provides a route to the formation of fibrin under conditions in which some of the early steps of the intrinsic pathway may be impaired. Similarly, both factors IXa and Xa can bring about activation of factor VII while factor VIIa (or the factor VIIa–tissue factor complex), like activated PTA (factor XIa), can activate Christmas factor (factor IX) (von Manteuffel, 1893; Sumi, Muramutu and Fijii, 1973; Zur and Nemerson, 1980; Rao, Bajaj and Rapaport, 1985; Gailani and Broze, 1991; Naito and Fujikawa, 1991; Rapaport, 1993). Plasma kallikrein, the product of the activation of plasma prekallikrein by factor XIIa, can reciprocally enhance activation of factor XII. And in certain experimental situations, thrombin, like factor XIIa, can convert factor XI to factor XIa (Gailani and Broze, 1991). Thus, reactions of the intrinsic and extrinsic pathways are intertwined, presumably improving the opportunity to provide hemostasis.

Activated Hageman factor (factor XIIa) has other identified functions, including conversion of prorenin to renin, transformation of plasminogen to plasmin (*vide infra*) and release of interleukin-1 from human peripheral blood monocytes, but whether these properties are biologically significant remains to be determined.

These various interactions are not surprising, as factor XIIa, XIa, VIIa, Xa and thrombin are all similarly constructed serine proteases, and non-enzymatic factors V and VIII have structural homologies with each other (Church *et al.*, 1984; Fass *et al.*, 1985; Kane and Davie, 1988).

Synthesis of factors VII, IX and X and prothrombin requires the availability of vitamin K, as if these proteins had evolved from a common ancestral polypeptide. Each of these clotting factors is synthesized in the liver as a non-functional polypeptide. Vitamin K is a necessary cofactor for a carboxylase that directs the insertion of carbon dioxide into the γ carbon of certain glutamic residues. The resultant tricarboxylic glutamic acid residues are needed for the physiologic roles of the vitamin K-dependent clotting factors. Vitamin K is also needed for the synthesis of two related plasma proteins, proteins C and S (p. 14).

Repeated reference has been made to the importance of phospholipids in the reactions leading to the formation of a clot. In the extrinsic pathway of thrombin formation, phospholipids are an integral part of the tissue thromboplastin complex. In whole blood, additional phospholipid is furnished by the membranes of platelets and other cells and by the plasma itself.

The dissolution of clots

Teleologically, one might anticipate that mechanisms might exist to remove intravascular clots in order to minimize tissue damage from the resultant ischemia. Indeed, the phenomenon of fibrinolysis, the dissolution of clots, was recognized more than a century ago. Fibrinolysis is, for the most part, the result of the digestion of fibrin by a plasma enzyme, plasmin, which normally circulates as an inert precursor, plasminogen. Plasminogen is a protein with a molecular weight of 92 000 that is synthesized in the liver. Conversion of plasminogen to plasmin can be brought about by activators derived from vascular endothelial cells that are readily liberated into the circulation by a variety of stimuli. Activation can also be brought about by other tissues and by activated Hageman factor (factor XIIa) and activated PTA (factor XIa) (Goldsmith, Saito and Ratnoff, 1978; Mandle and Kaplan, 1979; Saito, 1980). Two activators of therapeutic importance are urokinase, an enzyme synthesized by renal cells, and streptokinase, a non-enzymatic protein elaborated by β-hemolytic streptococci. Plasma also contains several agents that inhibit the conversion of plasminogen to plasmin. **Plasminogen activator inhibitor-1**, made at least in part within vascular endothelial cells, impedes the induction of fibrinolytic activity and can itself be inhibited by activated protein C (van Hinsbergh *et al.*, 1985; Sakata *et al.*, 1986; Lee and Mann, 1989).

Once activated, plasmin can digest fibrin, the basis for fibrinolytic therapy of thromboembolic disorders. Like thrombin, plasmin can enhance the activity of factor V (Lee and Mann, 1989). Among other substrates of plasmin that are of interest are fibrinogen, complement components C1 and C3, and antihemophilic factor (factor VIII). Plasmin can also cleave biologically active polypeptide kinins from plasma kininogens and can fragment Hageman factor (factor XII).

Inhibitors of clotting and fibrinolysis

The congeries of enzymes participating in the formation and dissolution of clots suggest that plasma must be rich in agents retarding their activation or activity. Several such inhibitors have been described, most of them multifunctional. The principal inhibitor of thrombin is a plasma glyco-protein with a molecular weight of 63 000 designated as **antithrombin III**. This protein is synthesized in the liver and additionally participates in inhibition of other plasma proteases of the clotting system, notably factor Xa (Olds, Lane and Mille, 1994; Pizzo, 1994). The inhibitory properties of antithrombin III are enhanced by heparin, a complex sulfated polysaccharide that is synthesized by many tissues, but particularly by the liver. Heterozygosity for hereditary deficiency of antithrombin III is associated with familial recurrent thrombosis in both arteries and veins (Perry, 1994). Heparin is required for inhibition of thrombin by a second plasma protein, **heparin cofactor 2** (van Deerlin and Tollefsen, 1992).

The function of thrombin may also be impeded by its adsorption to fibrin, an example of one way that a protease can be influenced by the product of its own proteolytic activity (Seegers, 1955).

Another important plasma inhibitor of proteases, designated **C$\bar{1}$ inhibitor** or C$\bar{1}$ inactivator because it inactivates the enzymatically active form of the first component of complement (C$\bar{1}$), neutralizes a broad spectrum of plasma proteases, among them activated Hageman factor (factor XIIa), activated PTA (factor XIa), plasma kallikrein, plasmin and tissue plasminogen activator (Ratnoff and Lepow, 1957; Ratnoff and Saito, 1979). Hereditary angioneurotic edema, in which affected individuals have episodic, sometimes life-threatening urticarial lesions, is associated with a functional deficiency of C$\bar{1}$ inhibitor (Donaldson and Evans, 1963).

Protein C, a vitamin K-dependent plasma protein originally described by Seegers and Ulutin (1961) and Stenflo (1976), participates in inhibition of the activated forms of factors V and VIII (Kisiel *et al.*, 1977). It is synthesized in the liver as a proenzyme with a molecular weight of 62 000. Its activation is complex (Fig. 2.3 Esmon, 1994; Dahlbäck, 1995). Thrombin generated in the vicinity of vascular endothelium binds to a protein bound to the cell membrane, **thrombomodulin** (Esmon, 1981). In this configuration, thrombin binds protein C and cleaves this protein, changing it to an enzymatically active form. Thus activated, protein C can then inhibit thrombin-altered factors V and VIII so that they no longer serve as enzymatic cofactors (Kisiel *et al.*, 1977; Vahar and Davie, 1980; Marlar, Kleiss and Griffin, 1982; Fulcher *et al.*, 1984; Kalafatis and Mann, 1993). Alternatively, protein C can be activated by the plasma protease **plasmin** (Varadi *et al.*, 1994) and by the proteolytically active form of factor X (factor Xa; Haley *et al.*, 1989). Activated protein C serves to enhance fibrinolysis both *in vitro* and *in vivo*. This process is brought about both by release of an activator of plasminogen, presumably from vascular endothelial cells, and by neutralization of plasminogen activator inhibitor-1 by activated protein C (Seegers *et al.*, 1972; Comp and Esmon, 1981; Sakata *et al.*, 1985).

The functional activity of protein C depends upon the presence of yet another vitamin K-dependent plasma protein, designated **protein S**, which binds to and enhances the effect of surface-bound activated protein C upon factors Va and VIIIa (Walker, 1980; Griffin *et al.*, 1981; Church *et al.*, 1984; Comp *et al.*, 1984; Fass *et al.*, 1985). Protein S is a non-enzymatic protein that circulates in plasma partially bound to an inhibitor of complement, C4b-binding protein; it is unbound protein S that serves as a cofactor to protein C (Dahlbäck and Stenflo, 1981; Shen and Dahlbäck, 1994). Further increasing this complexity, factor V appears to serve as a cofactor for the degradation of factor VIIIa by protein C (Scott *et al.*, 1982; Comp *et al.*, 1984). Inactivation of activated protein C is brought about by α_1-antitrypsin

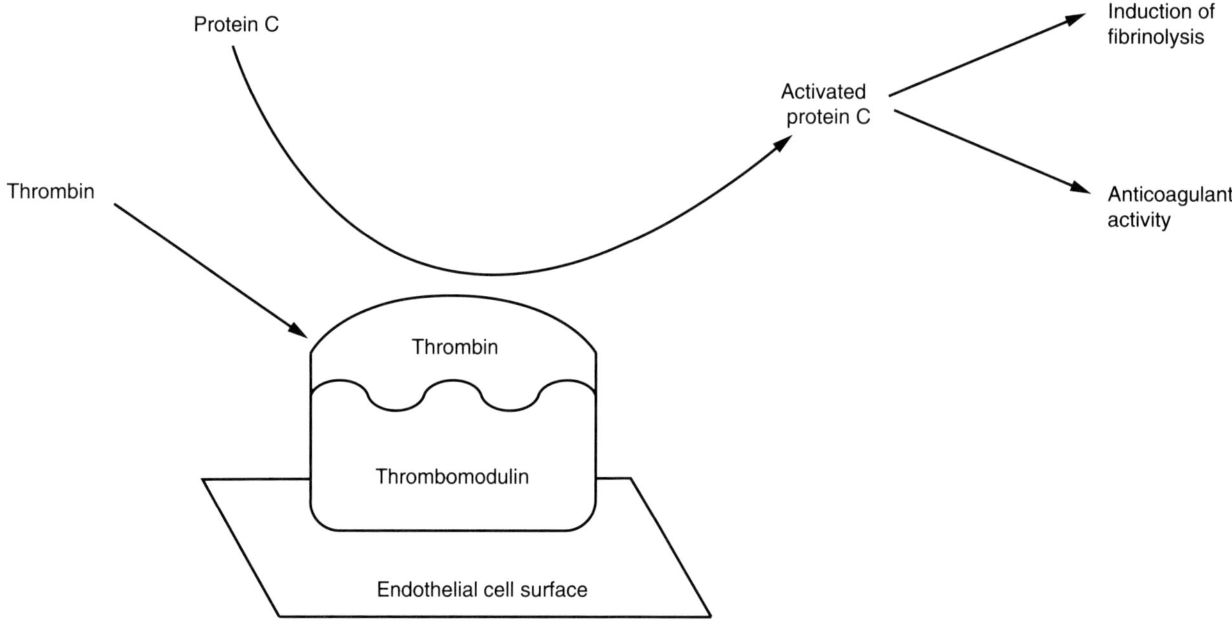

Fig. 2.3 Proposed model of *in vitro* protein C activation. Redrawn from Comp, P.C. *et al.* (1982) Activation of protein C *in vivo*. *J Clin Invest*, **70**, 127–134, by permission of the American Society for Clinical Investigation.

and by a plasma protein C inhibitory protein (Suzuki, Nishioka and Hashimoto, 1983; España and Griffin, 1989). An unusual disorder in which recurrent thrombosis is associated with combined functional deficiencies of factors V and VIII has been attributed to impaired inhibition of protein C (Marlar and Griffin, 1980).

Even partial deficiencies of proteins C and S may be manifested by thrombotic episodes, often apparently spontaneous in origin but sometimes clearly following surgery or injury (Esmon, 1994; Dahlbäck, 1995). Experimentally, a decrease in free activated protein S, brought about by elevation of C4b-binding protein, has been related to induction of intravascular coagulation (Taylor *et al.*, 1991).

α_1-**Antitrypsin** (α_1-antiproteinase) blocks the function of activated PTA (factor XIa), activated factor X (factor Xa), plasmin, activated protein C and possibly thrombin and plasma kallikrein, actions **not** enhanced by heparin (van der Meer, van Tijburg and van Wijngaargen, 1989). Hereditary deficiency of this inhibitor has been correlated with the development of chronic pulmonary obstruction and hepatic cirrhosis (Talamo *et al.*, 1968; Morse, 1978).

α_2-**Macroglobulin** inhibits thrombin, activated factor X, plasmin, plasma kallikrein and activated protein C (Harpel, 1970; Cummings and Castellino, 1984; Meijers, Tijburg and Bouma, 1987; Hoogendorne *et al.*, 1991).

Additional plasma inhibitors are directed against activated protein C (Heeb, España and Griffin, 1989; España *et al.*, 1991) and against tissue factor (tissue thromboplastin) or the thromboplastin-factor VIIa complex (Schneider, 1947).

Inhibition of the clot-promoting properties of tissue factor by one or more plasma agents was described some years ago by Thomas (1947), Schneider (1947) and others. Hjort (1957) demonstrated that the responsible agent, earlier called lipoprotein-associated coagulation inhibitor (Broze *et al.*, 1988) or extrinsic pathway inhibitor (Rapaport, 1991), and now referred to as **tissue factor pathway inhibitor**, is directed against the clot-promoting complex of factor VII and tissue factor; as Thomas (1947) and Lanchantin and Ware (1953) had proposed, inhibition required the presence of calcium ions. Further, Sanders (1986) observed that inhibition requires the additional presence of activated Stuart factor (factor Xa), whose activity is blocked by the plasma inhibitor of tissue factor(Schneider, 1947; Broze and Miletich, 1985; Hubbard and Jennings, 1986; Rao and Rapaport, 1987; Sandset, Abildgaard and Pettersen, 1987; Warn-Cramer *et al.*, 1988; Broze, 1992; Wesselschmidt *et al.*, 1992; Rapaport, 1993). This inhibitor is also said to block the action of plasmin (Cerveny, Fass and Mann, 1984). Tissue factor pathway inhibitor can be identified immunologically in megakaryocytes, macrophages, the villi of the placenta at term, and in the endothelium of small but not multilayered blood vessels (Werling *et al.*, 1993; Green, 1994; Østerud, Bajaj and Bajaj, 1995). This agent's inhibitory properties have been related to the presence of amino acid sequences resembling those of Kunitz-type protease inhibitors (Wun *et al.*, 1988). From an evolutionary point of view, the multiplicity of inhibitors seems to serve as a protection against inadvertent activation of the clotting system within our vessels.

Disordered hemostasis

When patients with defective blood coagulation sustain overt injury such as a deep cut, they may bleed excessively because the process of adhesion and aggregation of platelets at the site of vascular damage is inadequate to provide hemostasis and that of blood coagulation proceeds too slowly to allow timely closure of the defect. Excessive bleeding after surgery is the rule in patients with coagulative defects who have not been protected by timely transfusion of normal blood or blood products. Particularly instructive are those patients with **parahemophilia**, the hereditary deficiency of factor V; such patients may bleed severely after tonsillectomy or dental extraction even though the initial steps of the intrinsic pathway of thrombin formation are apparently normal (Owren, 1947; Friedman *et al.*, 1961). Surprisingly, lethal exsanguination is unusual except, perhaps, in such rare disorders as deficiency of fibrin-stabilizing factor (XIII) or afibrinogenemia, the virtual absence of plasma fibrinogen. A much more likely and more frequent event in patients with hereditary disorders of blood coagulation is bleeding into the skin, muscles or other soft tissues, often after trauma that may seem relatively trivial and would not cause significant bleeding in normal individuals. Indeed, the patient is usually unaware of any preceding injury that might bring on an episode of bleeding. The presumption must be made that hemostatic devices independent of the clotting factors that may be missing from the patient's blood cannot stem bleeding from even those trivial vascular injuries that occur in the normal course of life. For example, in patients with classic hemophilia, in whom the clotting defect is localized to the middle steps of the intrinsic pathway, when blood that flows from an injured vessel comes into contact with injured tissue, and therefore with tissue thromboplastin or tissue factor, the thrombin that evolves via the extrinsic pathway of coagulation may be insufficient to prevent hemorrhage. Thus, in patients with classic hemophilia or von Willebrand's disease (both functional deficiencies of factor VIII) or Christmas disease (the functional deficiency of factor IX), trauma can result in cutaneous or intramuscular bleeding despite test tube evidence that the extrinsic pathway is intact.

That this is at best a superficial explanation for the occurrence of bleeding in patients with classic hemophilia or Christmas disease is seen in the usual absence of any evidence of a hemorrhagic tendency in patients with isolated deficiencies of Hageman factor, plasma prekallikrein or high-molecular-weight kininogen, and the relatively minor bleeding tendency of most patients deficient in PTA (factor XI). In these individuals, more subtle devices must provide hemostatic control. Indeed, some investigators, noting that in the test tube PTA can be activated by thrombin itself, believe that the early steps of the intrinsic pathway are unimportant for normal clotting; perhaps their role relates to other reactions of the intrinsic pathway.

Consideration must be given to the pathogenesis of bleeding in certain sites or situations. For example, bleeding into joint spaces is common in patients with severe classic hemophilia or Christmas disease, as if injury to the synovial surface may not be sufficient to initiate clotting after trauma. In agreement with this, normal synovial membranes or fluid itself have little or no clot-promoting activity (Astrup and Sjølin, 1958; Manuel *et al.*, 1993; Chang *et al.*, 1995; Ratnoff, unpublished studies). Similarly, the joint fluid of patients with osteoarthritis had less than 1% of the factor V, factor VIII and von Willebrand factor titers of normal plasma. In contrast, however, individuals with severe defects of the extrinsic or common pathways are less likely to bleed into their joints, as if their intact intrinsic pathway were adequate for the task of hemostasis, and joint bleeding is a problem only in the severest forms of von Willebrand's disease. Often, the patient with hemophilia or Christmas disease is unaware of any injury or unusual activity that might have brought about joint hemorrhage. Similarly, episodes of both cutaneous and soft tissue bleeding often seem to occur without significant injury. Hemarthrosis is most likely to occur in the elbow, shoulder, hip and knee, whereas bleeding into the joints of the hands and toes is more unusual and into the vertebral joints, distinctly rare (Rizza, 1994). A distressing feature of hemarthrosis is its tendency to recur in joints that have previously been the site of bleeding, leading inexorably to permanent damage to the joint and surrounding structures.

Other sites of bleeding present special problems. Particularly to be feared is intracranial bleeding, for the accumulation of even small amounts of blood within the rigid cranium may bring about irreversible brain damage. In patients with hereditary hemostatic defects, a history of recent trauma is elicited in only about half of cases of central nervous system bleeding (Eyster *et al.*, 1978). In a few instances, hypertension or the presence of congenital vascular malformations may be contributing factors. In those who recover, recurrent bleeding is not unusual.

Bleeding into the urinary tract also seems to be spontaneous in most patients, but careful urologic examination may uncover the presence of infection, renal calculi, neoplasm or chronic nephritis (Broze, 1992; Greer *et al.*, 1985). Often, bleeding continues for several days, even though apparently adequate replacement therapy has been instituted. Perhaps the persistence of bleeding into the urinary tract has its origin in the presence of urokinase in urine. Presumably this enzymatic activator of plasminogen may foster dissolution of clots in the urinary tract, exacerbating the bleeding tendency.

No such simple explanation accounts for the pathogenesis of bleeding from the gastrointestinal tract, a common complication of both classic hemophilia and Christmas disease and occasionally a problem in von Willebrand's disease. Peptic ulceration, particularly duodenal, and gastritis are said to be common among patients with hemophilia, particularly those with severe disease (Forbes *et al.*, 1973). Perhaps this reflects the chronic stress experienced by most patients; as Mittal *et al.* speculate (1985), painful hemarthropathy may be met by excessive consumption of alcohol and aspirin. In other patients, bleeding from esophageal varices is attributable to portal hypertension complicating the hepatic cirrhosis that is a sequel of the infectious hepatitis common in hemophiliacs treated with blood products. Bleeding from the colon may reflect underlying angiodysplasia or telangiectasis (Ewenstein and Handlin, 1995).

Epistaxis is commonplace in patients with severe classic hemophilia, von Willebrand's diseases or Christmas disease. Sometimes this symptom occurs in the setting of an upper respiratory infection. Recurrent epistaxis is particularly liable to occur at sites earlier treated by cauterization. Recurrent nosebleeds, particularly during the first decades of life, should alert the physician examine the nasal septum for the characteristic telangiectatic lesions of the Osler–Rendu–Weber syndrome of hereditary hemorrhagic telangiectasia (Perry, 1987; Guttmacher *et al.*, 1995). Patients with this autosomal dominant disorder may have pulmonary arteriovenous fistulas, leading to hemoptysis and hemothorax among other symptoms, and cerebral vascular abnormalities that may result in intracranial hemorrhage and other neurologic problems. This disorder is not associated with alterations in peripheral blood-clotting mechanisms.

Other manifestations of a bleeding tendency occur in limited sets of patients who have hemostatic abnormalities that are demonstrable in the test tube. For example, in women with factor V deficiency, menorrhagia may be severe or even lethal, and postpartum and cerebral bleeding have been described (Brink and Kingsley, 1952; Mammen, 1983). In congenital afibrinogenemia, apparently spontaneous cerebral hemorrhage is sometimes the *coup de grâce*. In those with congenital dysfibrinogenemia, in whom plasma fibrinogen is qualitatively abnormal, episodes of thrombosis or hemorrhage and dehiscence of wounds may occur. And prominent manifestations of hereditary functional deficiencies of fibrin-stabilizing factor (factor XIII) include bleeding from the umbilicus in the neonatal period, spontaneous abortion during pregnancy and bleeding into the central nervous system.

References

Addis, T. (1910) The pathogenesis of hereditary haemophilia. *J Path Bact*, **15**, 427–452.

Aggeler, P.M., White, S.G., Glendenning, M.B. *et al.* (1952) Plasma thromboplastin component (PTC) deficiency: a new disease resembling hemophilia. *Proc Soc Exp Biol Med*, **79**, 692–694.

Alexander, B. and Goldstein, R. (1953) Dual hemostatic defect in pseudohemophilia. *J Clin Invest*, **32**, 55 (abstract).

Altiori, D.C. (1995) Xa receptor EPR-1. *FASEB J*, **9**, 860–865.

Astrup, T. (1965) Assay and content of tissue thromboplastin in different organs. *Thromb Diath Haemorrh*, **14**, 401–416.

Astrup, T. and Sjøli, K.E. (1958) Thromboplastic and fibronolytic activity of human synovial membrane and fibrous capsular tissue. *Proc Soc Exp Biol Med*, **97**, 852–853.

Benedien, W.M. and van Creveld, S. (1937) Investigations on hemophilia. *Am J Dis Child*, **54**, 713–725.

Biggs, R., Douglas, A.S., Macfarlane, R.G. *et al.* (1952) Christmas disease: a condition previously mistaken for haemophilia. *Br Med J*, **2**, 1378–1382.

Bordet, J. (1921) The theories of blood coagulation. *Bull Johns Hopkins Hosp*, **32**, 213–218.

Brink, A.J. and Kingsley, C.S. (1952) A familial disorder of blood coagulation due to deficiency of the labile factor. *Q J Med (ns)*, **21**, 19–31.

Brinkhous, K.M. (1939) A study of the clotting defect in hemophilia. The delayed formation of thrombin. *Am J Med Sci*, **198**, 509–516.

Broze, G.J. Jr. (1982) Binding of human factor VII and VIIa to monocytes. *J Clin Invest*, **70**, 526–535.

Broze, G.J. Jr. (1992) The role of tissue factor pathway inhibitor in a revised coagulation cascade. *Semin Hematol*, **29**, 159–169.

Broze, G.J. Jr. and Miletich, J.P. (1985) Characterization of the inhibitor of tissue factor in serum. *Blood*, **69**, 150–155.

Broze, G.J. Jr., Leykham, J.E., Schwartz, B.D. and Miletich, J.P. (1985) Purification of human brain tissue factor. *J Biol Chem*, **260**, 10917–10920.

Broze, G.J. Jr., Warren, L.A., Novotny, W.F. *et al.* (1988) The lipoprotein-associated coagulation inhibitor that inhibits the factor VII-tissue factor complex also inhibits factor Xa: insight into its possible mechanism of action. *Blood*, **71**, 335–343.

Carson, S.D., Henry, W.M. and Shons, T.B. (1985) Tissue factor gene localized to human chromosome 1 (1pter → 1p21). *Science*, **229**, 991–993.

Cerveny, T.J., Fass, D.N. and Mann, K.G. (1984) Synthesis of coagulation factor V by cultured aortic endothelium. *Blood*, **63**, 1467–1474.

Chang, P., Aronson, D.L., Borenstein, D.G. and Kessler, C.M. (1995) Coagulant proteins and thrombin generation in synovial fluid. A model for extravascular coagulation. *Am J Hemat*, **50**, 79–83.

Chopek, M.W., Girma, J.-P., Fujikawa, K. *et al.* (1986) Human von Willebrand factor: a multivalent protein composed of identical subunits. *Biochemistry*, **25**, 3146–3155.

Christianes, G.C.M.L., Sixma, J.J. and Haspels, A.A. (1982) Hemostasis in menstrual endometrium: a review. *Obst Gyn Surv*, **37**, 281–303.

Church, W.R., Jernigan, R.L., Toole, J.L. *et al.* (1984) Coagulation factors V and VIII and ceruloplasmin constitute a family of structurally related proteins. *Proc Natl Acad Sci USA*, **81**, 6934–6937.

Comp, P.C. and Esmon, C.T. (1981) Generation of fibrinolytic activity by infusion of activated protein C in dogs. *J Clin Invest*, **68**, 1221–1228.

Comp, P.C., Nixon, R.R., Cooper, M.R. *et al.* (1984) Familial protein S deficiency is associated with recurrent thrombosis. *J Clin Invest*, **74**, 2082–2088.

Cummings, H.S. and Castellino, F.J. (1984) Interaction of human plasmin with human α_2-macroglobulin. *Biochem*, **23**, 105–111.

Dahlbäck, B. and Stenflo, J. (1981) High molecular weight complex in human plasma between vitamin K-dependent protein S and complement C4b-binding protein. *Proc Natl Acad Sci USA*, **78**, 2512–2516.

Davie, E.W. and Ratnoff, O.D. (1964) Waterfall sequence for intrinsic blood clotting. *Science*, **145**, 1310–1312.

Donaldson, V.H. and Evans, R.R. (1963) A biochemical abnormality in hereditary angioneurotic edema. Absence of serum inhibitor of C′1-esterase. *Am J Med*, **35**, 37–44.

Esmon, C.T. (1994) Clinical and physiological manifestations of the protein C anticoagulant pathway, in *Anticoagulants: Physiologic, Pathologic and Pharmacologic* (ed. D. Green), CRC Press, Boca Raton, pp. 3–25.

Esmon, C.T. and Owen, W.G. (1981) Identification of an endothelial cell cofactor for thrombin catalyzed activation of protein C. *Proc Natl Acad Sci USA*, **78**, 2249–2252.

Espana, F. and Griffin, J.H. (1989) Determination of functional and antigenic protein C inhibitor and its complexes with activated protein C in plasma by ELISAs. *Thromb Res*, **55**, 671–682.

Espana, F. Gruber, A., Heeb, M.J. *et al.* (1991) *In vivo* and *in vitro* complexes of activated protein C with two inhibitors in baboons. *Blood*, **77**, 1754–1760.

Ewenstein, B.M. and Handin, R.I. (1995) von Willebrand's disease, in *Blood: Principles and Practice of Hematology* (eds R. Handin, E. Lux and T.P. Stossel), J.B. Lippincott, Philadelphia, pp. 1069–1094.

Eyster, M.E., Gill, F.M., Blatt, P.M. *et al.* (1978) Central nervous system bleeding in hemophiliacs. *Blood*, **51**, 1179–1188.

Fass, D.N., Hewick, R.M., Kutson, G.J. *et al.* (1985) Internal duplication and sequence homology in factors V and VIII. *Proc Natl Acad Sci USA*, **82**, 1658–1691.

Fleck, R.A., Rao, L.V.M., Rapaport, S.I. *et al.* (1990) Localization of tissue factor antigen by immuno-staining with monospecific, polyclonal, anti-human tissue factor antibody. *Thromb Res*, **57**, 765–781.

Forbes, C.D., Barr, R.D., Prentice, C.R.M. and Douglas, A.S. (1973) Gastro-intestinal bleeding in haemophilia. *Q J Med (ns)*, **42**, 503–511.

Foster, W.B., Nesheim, M.E. and Mann, K.G. (1983) The factor Xa-catalyzed activation of factor V. *J Biol Chem*, **258**, 13970–13977.

Foster, P.A. and Zimmerman, T.S. (1989) Factor VIII structure and function. *Blood Rev*, **3**, 180–191.

Frank, E. and Hartmann, E. (1927) Über das Wesen und die therapeutische Korrektur der hámophilen Gerinnungstörung. *Klin Wochenschr*, **6**, 435–439.

Friedman, I.A., Quick, A.J., Higgins, F. *et al.* (1961) Hereditary labile factor (factor V) deficiency. *JAMA*, **175**, 370–374.

Fulcher, C.A., Gardner, J.E., Griffin, J.H. and Zimmerman, T.S. (1984) Proteolytic inactivation of human factor VIII procoagulant protein by activated human protein C and its analogy with factor V. *Blood*, **63**, 486–489.

Fulcher, C.A., Roberts, J.R. and Zimmerman, T.S. (1983) Thrombin proteolysis of purified factor VIII procoagulant protein: correlation of activation with generation of a specific polypeptide. *Blood*, **61**, 807–811.

Gailani, D. and Bronze, G.J. (1991) Factor XI activation in a revised model of blood coagulation. *Science*, **253**, 909–912.

Galdal, K.S. (1984) Thromboplastin synthesis in endothelial cells. *Haemostasis*, **14**, 378–385.

Goldsmith, G.H. Jr, Saito, H. and Ratnoff, O.D. (1978) The activation of plasminogen by Hageman factor (factor XII) and Hageman factor fragments. *J Clin Invest*, **62**, 54–60.

Govaerts, P. and Gratia, A. (1936) Contribution á l'étude de l'hémophilie. *Rev Belge Sci Méd*, **3**, 689–696.

Green, D. (1994) *Anticoagulants. Physiologic, Pathologic, Pharmacologic*, CRC Press, Boca Raton.

Greer, I.A., Lowe, G.D.O., Yogarajah, S. *et al.* (1985) Haematuria in patients with haemostatic defects. *Brit MJ*, **290**, 1648–1649.

Griffin, J.H., Evatt, B., Zimmerman, T.S. *et al.* (1981) Deficiency of protein C in congenital thrombotic disease. *J Clin Invest*, **68**, 1370–1373.

Guttmacher, A.E., Marchuk, D.A. and White, R.I. Jr. (1995) Hereditary hemorrhagic telangiectasia. *N Engl J Med*, **333**, 918–924.

Haley, P.E., Doyle, M.F. and Mann, K.G. (1989) The activation of bovine protein C by factor Xa. *J Biol Chem*, **264**, 16303–16310.

Hamaguchi, N., Bajaj, S.P., Smith, K.J. *et al.* (1994) The role of amino-terminal residues of the heavy chain of factor IXa in the binding of its cofactor, factor VIIIA. *Blood*, **84**, 1837–1842.

Harpel, P.C. (1970) Human plasma alpha 2-macroglobulin – an inhibitor of plasma kallikrein. *J Exp Med*, **132**, 329–352.

Heeb, M.J. Espana, F. and Griffin, J.H. (1989) Inhibition and complexation of activated protein C by two major inhibitors in plasma. *Blood*, **73**, 446–454.

Hjort, P.F. (1957) Intermediate reactions in the coagulation of blood with tissue thromboplastin. *Scand J Clin Lab Invest*, **9**, (suppl 27), 76–97.

Hoogendoorne, H., Toh, C.H., Nesheim, M.E. and Giles, A.R. (1991) α_2Macroglobulin binds and inhibits activated protein C. *Blood*, **77**, 2283–2290.

Howard, M.A. and Firkin, B.G. (1971) Ristocetin – a new tool in the investigation of platelet aggregation. *Thromb Diath Haemorrh*, **26**, 362–369.

Hoyer, L.W. and Trabald, N.C. (1981) The effect of thrombin on human factor VIII. Cleavage of the factor VIII procoagulant protein during activation *J Lab Clin Med*, **97**, 50–64.

Hubbard, A.R. and Jennings, C.A. (1986) Inhibition of tissue thromboplastin-mediated blood coagulation. *Thromb Res*, **42**, 489–498.

Jaffe, E.A.L., Hoyer, L.W. and Nachman, R. (1977) Synthesis of antihemophilic factor by cultured human endothelial cells. *J Clin Invest*, **60**, 914–921.

Jesty, J., Wun, T.-C. and Lorenz, A. (1994) Kinetics of the inhibition of factor Xa and the issue factor–factor VIIa complex by the tissue factor pathway inhibitor in the presence and absence of heparin. *Biochemistry*, **33**, 12686–12694.

Kalafatis, M. and Mann, K.G. (1993) Role of the membrane in the inactivation of factor Va by activated protein C. *J Biol Chem*, **268**, 27246–27257.

Kane, W.H. and Davie, E.W. (1988) Blood coagulation factors V and VIII: structure and function similarities and their relationship to hemorrhagic and thrombotic disorders. *Blood*, **71**, 539–555.

Kang, S. and Niemetz, J. (1988) Purification of human brain tissue factor. *Thromb Haemostas*, **59**, 400–403.

Kaushansky, K. (1995) Thrombopoietin: the primary regulator of platelet production. *Blood*, **86**, 419–431.

Kelemen, E., Cserháti, I. and Tanos, B. (1958) Demonstration and some properties of human thrombopoietin in thrombocythaemic sera. *Acta Haemat (Basel)*, **20**, 350–355.

Kisiel, W., Canfield, A.M., Ericsson, L.H. and Davie, E.W. (1977) Anticoagulant properties of bovine plasma protein C following activation by thrombin. *J Biol Chem*, **16**, 5824–5831.

Lanchantin, G.P. and Ware, A.G. (1953) Identification of a thromboplastin inhibitor in serum and in plasma. *J Clin Invest*, **32**, 381–389.

Lane, S. (1840) Haemorrhagic diathesis. Successful transfusion of blood. *Lancet*, **1**, 185–188.

Larrieu, M.-J. and Soulier, J.P. (1953) Deficit en facteur anti-hemophilique a chez une fille associé un trouble de saignement. *Revue Hematol*, **8**, 361–370.

Lee, C.D. and Mann, K.D. (1989) Activation/inactivation of human factor V by plasmin. *Blood*, **73**, 185–190.

Levin, E.R. (1995) Endothelins. *N Engl J Med*, **333**, 356–363.

Levin, J., Levin, F.C., Hull, D.F. III and Penington, D.G. (1982) The effects of thrombopoietin on megakaryocyte-CFC, megakaryocytes, and thrombopoiesis: with studies of ploidy and platelet size. *Blood*, **60**, 989–998.

Macfarlane, R.G. (1964) An enzyme cascade in the blood clotting mechanism, and its function as a biochemical amplifier. *Nature*, **202**, 498–499.

Mackman, N., Morrissey, J.H., Fowler, B. and Edgington, T.S. (1989) Complete sequence of the human tissue factor gene, a highly regulated cellular receptor that initiates the coagulation protease cascade. *Biochemistry*, **28**, 1755–1762.

Mammen, E.F. (1983) Congenital coagulation disorders: factor V deficiency. *Semin Thromb Hemostas*, **9**, 17–21.

Mandle, R.J. Jr. and Kaplan, A.P. (1979) Hageman factor-dependent fibrinolysis: generation of fibrinolytic activity by the interaction of human activated factor XI and plasminogen. *Blood*, **54**, 850–862.

Mannhalter, C., Schiffman, S. and Jacobs, A. (1980) Trypsin activation of human factor XI. *J Biol Chem*, **255**, 2667–2669.

Mannhalter, L.C., Shiffman, S. and Deutsch, E. (1984) Phospholipids accelerate factor IX activation by surface bound factor XIa. *Br J Haemat*, **56**, 261–277.

Manuel, R.P., Hoogendorn, H., Giles, A.R. *et al.* (1993) Antigens of coagulation and fibrinolysis in synovial fluids in rheumatoid (RA) and osteo (OA) arthritis. *Thromb Haemostas*, **69**, 1048.

Marcus, A.J. (1996) Platelets and their disorders, in *Disorders of Hemostasis*, 3rd edn (eds O.D. Ratnoff and C.D. Forbes), W.B. Saunders, Philadelphia.

Marlar, R.A. and Griffin, J.H. (1980) Deficiency of protein C in combined factor V/VIII deficiency disease. *J Clin Invest*, **66**, 1186–1189.

Marlar, R.A., Kleiss, A.J. and Griffin, J.H. (1982) Mechanism of action of human activated protein C, a thrombin-dependent anticoagulant enzyme. *Blood*, **59**, 1067–1072.

Marmur, J.D., Rossikhina, M., Guha, A. *et al.* (1993) Tissue factor is rapidly induced in arterial smooth muscle after balloon injury. *J Clin Invest*, **91**, 2253–2259.

Maynard, J.R., Dreyer, B.E., Stemerman, M.B. and Pitlick, F.A. (1977) Tissue-factor coagulant activity of cultured human endothelial and smooth muscle cells and fibroblasts. *Blood*, **50**, 387–396.

Meijers, J.C.M., Tijburg, P.N.M. and Bourna, B.N. (1987) Inhibition of human blood coagulation factor Xa by α_2-macroglobulin. *Biochemistry*, **26**, 5932–5937.

Mittal, R., Spero, J.A., Lewis, J.H. *et al.* (1985) Patterns of gastrointestinal hemorrhage in hemophilia. *Gastroenterology*, **88**, 512–522.

Morse, J.O. (1978) Alpha$_1$-antitrypsin deficiency. *N Engl J Med*, **299**, 1045–1048; 1099–1105.

Mosesson, M.W. (1992) The role of fibrinogen and fibrin in hemostasis and thrombosis. *Semin Hemat*, **29**, 177–178.

Nachman, R., Levine, R. and Jaffe, E.A. (1977) Synthesis of factor VIII antigen by cultured guinea pig mega-karyocytes. *J Clin Invest*, **60**, 914–921.

Naito, K. and Fujikawa, K. (1991) Activation of human blood coagulation factor XI independent of factor XII. Factor XI is activated by thrombin and factor XIa in the presence of negatively charged surfaces. *J Biol Chem*, **266**, 7353–7358.

Nemerson, Y. (1966) The reaction between bovine brain tissue factor and factors VII and X. *Biochemistry*, **5**, 601–608.

Nemerson, Y. (1988) Tissue factor and hemostasis. *Blood*, **71**, 1–8.

Nemerson, Y. (1992) The tissue factor pathway in blood coagulation. *Semin Hemat*, **29**, 170–176.

Nichols, W.L., Gastineau, D.A., Solberg, L.A. Jr. and Mann, K.G. (1985) Identification of human megakaryocytic coagulation factor V. *Blood*, **65**, 1396–1406.

Novotny, W.F. (1994) Tissue factor pathway inhibitor. *Semin Thrombos Hemostas*, **20**, 101–108.

Olds, R.L., Lane, D.A. and Mille, B. (1994) Antithrombin: the principal inhibitor (TFPI) and tissue factor expression under physiologic and pathologic conditions. *Thromb Haemost*, **73**, 873–875.

Østerud, B., Bajaj, M.S. and Bajaj, S.P. (1995) Sites of tissue factor pathway inhibitor (TFPI) and tissue factor expression under physiologic and pathologic conditions. *Thromb Haemost*, **73**, 872–875.

Østerud, B. and Rapap ort, S.I. (1977) Activation of factor IX by the reaction product of tissue factor and factor VII: additional pathway for initiating of blood clotting. *Proc Natl Acad Sci USA*, **74**, 5260–5264.

Østerud, B., Tindall, A., Brox, J.H. and Olsen, I.O. (1986) Thromboplastin content in the vessel walls of different arteries and organs of rabbits. *Thrombos Res*, **42**, 323–329.

Owren, P.A. (1947) The coagulation of blood. Investigations on a new clotting factor. *Acta Med Scand*, **194** (suppl), 1–327.

Patek, A.J. Jr. and Stetson, R.H. (1936) Hemophilia. I. The abnormal coagulation of the blood and its relation to the blood platelets. *J Clin Invest*, **15**, 531–542.

Patek, A.J. Jr. and Taylor, F.H.L. (1937) Hemophilia. II. Some properties of a substance obtained from normal plasma effective in accelerating the clotting of hemophilic blood. *J Clin Invest*, **16**, 113–124.

Pavlovsky, A. (1947) Contribution to the pathogenesis of hemophilia. *Blood*, **2**, 185–181.

Peery, W.H. (1987) Clinical spectrum of hereditary hemorrhagic telangiectasia (Osler–Weber–Rendu disease). *Am J Med*, **82**, 989.

Perry, D.J. (1994) Antithrombin and its inherited deficiencies. *Blood Rev*, **8**, 37–55.

Petersen, L.C., Valentin, S. and Hedner, U. (1995) Regulation of the extrinsic pathway system in health and disease: the role of factor VIIa and tissue factor pathway inhibitor. *Thromb Res*, **79**, 1–47.

Pittman, D.D. and Kaufman, R.J. (1988) Proteolytic requirements for thrombin activation of anti-hemophilic factor (factor VIII). *Proc Natl Acad Sci USA*, **85**, 2429–2433.

Pizzo, S.V. (1994) The physiologic role of antithrombin III as an anticoagulant. *Semin Hematol*, **31** (suppl), 4–7.

Poon, M.-C. and Ratnoff, O.D. (1976) Evidence that functional subunits of antihemophilic factor (factor VIII) are linked by noncovalent bonds. *Blood*, **48**, 87–94.

Quick, A.J. and Hussey, C.V. (1953) Hemophilic condition in the female. *J Lab Clin Med*, **42**, 929–930.

Rao, L.V.M., Bajaj, S.P. and Rapaport, S.I. (1985) Activation of human factor VII during clotting *in vitro*. *Blood*, **65**, 218–226.

Rao, L.V.M. and Rapaport, S.I. (1987) Studies of a mechanism inhibiting the initiation of the extrinsic pathway of coagulation. *Blood*, **69**, 645–651.

Rapaport, S.I. (1991) The extrinsic pathway inhibitor: a regulator of tissue factor-dependent blood coagulation. *Thromb Haemostas*, **68**, 6–15.

Rapaport, S.I. (1993) Blood coagulation and its alterations in hemorrhagic and thrombotic disorders. *West J Med*, **158**, 153–161.

Rapaport, S.I., Schiffman, S., Patch, M.J. and Ames, S.P. (1963) The importance of activation of antihemophilic globulin and proaccelerin by traces of thrombin in the generation of intrinsic prothrombinase activity. *Blood*, **21**, 221–236.

Ratnoff, O.D. and Davie, E.W. (1962) The activation of Christmas factor (factor IX) by activated plasma thromboplastin antecedent (activated factor XI). *Biochemistry*, **1**, 677–685.

Ratnoff, O.D. and Lepow, I.H. (1957) Some properties of an esterase derived from preparations of the first component of complement. *J Exp Med*, **106**, 327–343.

Ratnoff, O.D. and Rosenblum, J.M. (1958) Role of Hageman factor in the initiation of clotting by glass. Evidence that glass frees Hageman factor from inhibition. *Am J Med*, **25**, 160–168.

Ratnoff, O.D. and Saito, H. (1979) Surface-mediated reactions. *Current Topics Hematol*, **2**, 1–57.

Rizza, C.R. (1994) Haemophilia and related inherited coagulation defects, in *Haemostasis and Thrombosis*, vol. 2, 3rd edn (eds A.L. Bloom, C.D. Forbes, D.P. Thomas and E.G.D. Tudenham), Churchill Livingstone, Edinburgh, 819–841.

Saito, H. (1980) The participation of plasma thromboplastin antecedent (factor XI) in contact-activated fibrinolysis. *Proc Soc Exp Biol Med*, **164**, 153–157.

Saito, H. (1996) Normal hemostatic mechanisms, in *Disorders of Hemostasis* (eds O.D. Ratnoff and C.D. Forbes), 3rd edn, W.B. Saunders, Philadelphia.

Saito, H., Ratnoff, O.D., Marshall, J.S. and Pensky, J. (1973). Partial purification of plasma thromboplasin antecedent (factor XI) and its activation by trypsin. *J Clin Invest*, **52**, 850–861.

Sakata, Y., Curriden, S., Lawrence, D. *et al.* (1985) Activated protein C stimulates the fibrinolytic activity of cultured endothelial cells and decreases antiactivator activity. *Proc Natl Acad Sci USA*, **80**, 1121–1125.

Sakata, Y., Loskutoff, J., Gladson, C.L. *et al.* (1986) Mechanism of protein C-dependent clot lysis. Role of plasminogen activator inhibitor. *Blood*, **68**, 1218–1223.

Sanders, N.L., Bajaj, S.P., Zwelin, A. and Rapaport, S.I. (1986) Inhibition of tissue factor/factor VII activity in plasma requires factor X and an additional plasma component. *Blood*, **66**, 204–212.

Sandset, P.M., Abildgaard, U. and Pettersen, M. (1987) A sensitive chromogenic substrate assay of extrinsic coagulation pathway inhibitor (EPI) in plasma and plasma fractions. *Thromb Res*, **47**, 389–400.

Schmidt, A. (1892) *Zur Blutlehre*, Vogel, Leipzig.

Schneider, C.L. (1947) The active principle of placental toxin: tissue thromboplastin; its inactivation by blood: antithromboplastin. *Am J Physiol*, **149**, 123–129.

Schulman, J. and Smith, C.H. (1952) Hemorrhagic disease in an infant due to deficiency of a previously undescribed clotting factor. *Blood*, **7**, 794–807.

Scott, C.F., Schapira, M. and James, H.L. (1982) Inactivation of factor XIa by plasma protease inhibitor and protective effect of high molecular weight kininogen. *J Clin Invest*, **69**, 844–852.

Scott, C.F., Silver, D., Purdon, A.D. and Colman, R.W. (1985) Cleavage of human high molecular weight kininogen by factor XIa *in vitro*. Effect on structure and function. *J Biol Chem*, **260**, 10856–10863.

Seegers, W.H. (1955) Coagulation of the blood. *Adv Enzymol*, **16**, 23–103.

Seegers, W.H., McCoy, L.E., Groben, H.D. (1972) Purification and some properties of autoprothrombin II-A: an anticoagulant perhaps also related to fibrinolysis. *Thromb Res*, **1**, 443–460.

Seegers, W.H. and Ulutin, O.N. (1961) Autoprothrombin II-anticoagulant (autoprothrombin II-A). *Thromb Diath Haemorrh*, **6**, 270–281.

Shen, I. and Dahlbäck, B. (1994) Factor V and protein S as synergistic cofactors to activated protein C in degradation of factor VIIIa. *J Biol Chem*, **269**, 18375–18378.

Simonson, M.S. and Dunn, M.J. (1991) Endothelins: a family of regulatory proteins. *Hypertension*, **17**, 856–863.

Stenflo, J. (1976) A new vitamin K-dependent protein: purification from bovine plasma and preliminary characterization. *J Biol Chem*, **251**, 355–366.

Sumi, H., Muramutu, M. and Fijii, S. (1973) The relation of C1s, a subunit of the activated first component of complement, to the other plasma enzymes. *Biochim Biophys Acta*, **327**, 207–212.

Suzuki, K., Nishioka, J. and Hashimoto, S. (1983) Protein C inhibitor. Purification from human plasma and characterization. *J Biol Chem*, **258**, 163–168.

Talamo, R.C., Allen, J.D., Kahan, M.G. and Austin, K.F. (1968) Hereditary alpha$_1$ antitrypsin deficiency. *N Engl J Med*, **278**, 345–351.

Taylor, F., Chang, A., Ferrell, G. *et al.* (1991) C4b-binding protein exacerbates the host response to *Escherichia coli*. *Blood*, **78**, 357–363.

Thomas, L. (1947) Studies on the intravascular thromboplastic effect of tissue suspensions in mice. II. A factor in normal rabbit serum which inhibits the thromboplastic effect of the sedimentable tissue component. *Bull Johns Hopkins Hosp*, **81**, 25–42.

van Deerlin, V.M.D. and Tollefsen, D.M. (1992) Molecular interactions between heparin cofactor II and thrombin. *Semin Thromb Hemostas*, **18**, 341–346.

van der Meer, F.J.M., van Tilburg, N.H. and van Wijngaarden, A. (1989) A second plasma inhibitor of activated protein C: α$_1$-antritrypsin. *Thromb Haemostas*, **6**, 756–762.

van Hinsbergh, V.W.Z.M., Bertina, R.M., van Wijngaarden, A. *et al.* (1985) Activated protein C decreases plasminogen activator-inhibitor in endothelial cell-conditioned medium. *Blood*, **65**, 444–451.

Váradi, K., Philapitsch, A., Santa, T. and Schwarz, H.P. (1994) Activation and inactivation of human protein C by plasmin. *Thrombos Haemostas*, **71**, 615–621.

Vehar, G.A. and Davie, E.W. (1980) Preparation and properties of bovine factor VIII (antihemophilic factor). *Biochemistry*, **19**, 401–410.

von dem Borne, P.A.Kr., Koppelman, S.J., Bourna, B.N. and Meijers, J.C.M. (1994) Surface independent factor XI activation by thrombin in the presence of high molecular weight kininogen. *Thrombos Haemostas*, **72**, 397–402.

von Manteuffel, Z. (1893) Bermerkungen zur blutstillung bei Hämophilie. *Dtsch Med Wochenschr*, **19**, 665–667.

von Willebrand, E.A. (1931) Über hereditare Pseudohämophilie. *Acta Med Scand*, **76**, 521–549.

Walker, F.J. (1980) Regulation of activated protein C by a new protein. A possible function for bovine protein S. *J Biol Chem*, **255**, 5521–5524.

Ward, M., quoted by Wardrup, J. (1837) *On the Curative Effects of the Abstraction of Blood*, A. Waldie, Philadelphia, pp. 9–10.

Ware, A.G. and Seegers, W.H. (1948) Serum Ac-globulin: formation from plasma Ac-globulin; role in blood coagulation; partial purification; properties, and quantitative determination. *Am J Physiol*, **152**, 567–576.

Warn-Cramer, B.J., Rao, L.V.M., Maki, S.L. and Rapaport, S.I. (1988) Modifications of the extrinsic pathway inhibitor (EPI) and factor Xa that affect their inability to interact and to inhibit factor VIIa/tissue factor: evidence for a two-step model of inhibition. *Thrombos Haemostas*, **60**, 453–456.

Weiss, H.J., Hoyer, L.W., Rickles, F.R. *et al.* (1973) Quantitative assay of a plasma factor deficient in von Willebrand's disease that is necessary for platelet aggregation. Relationship to factor VIII pro-coagulant activity and antigen content. *J Clin Invest*, **52**, 2708–2716.

Weiss, H.J., Turitto, V.T., Baumgartner, H.R. *et al.* (1989) Evidence for the presence of tissue factor activity on subendothelium. *Blood*, **73**, 968–975.

Werling, R.W., Zacharski, L.R., Kisiel, W. *et al.* (1993) Distribution of tissue factor pathway inhibitor in normal and malignant human tissue. *Thromb Haemost*, **69**, 366–369.

Wesselschmidt, R., Likert, K., Girard, T. *et al.* (1992) Tissue factor pathway inhibitor: the carboxy-terminus is required for optimal inhibition of factor Xa. *Blood*, **79**, 2004–2010.

Wright, A.E. (1893) On the method of determining the condition of blood coagulability for clinical and experimental purposes, and on the effect of the administration of calcium salts in haemophilia and actual or threatened haemorrhage. *Br Med J*, **2**, 223–225.

Wuepper, K.D. (1972) Biochemistry and biology of components of the plasma kinin-forming system, in *Inflammation: Mechanisms and Control* (eds I.H. Lepow and P.A. Ward), Academic Press, New York, pp. 93–117.

Wun, T.-C., Kretzmer, L.L., Girard, T.J. *et al.* (1988) Cloning and characterization of a cDNA coding for the lipoprotein-associated coagulation inhibitor. *J Biol Chem*, **263**, 6001–6004.

Zeldis, S.M., Nemerson, Y. and Lentz, T.L. (1972) Tissue factor (thromboplastin): localisation to plasma membranes by peroxidase-conjugated antibodies. *Science*, **175**, 766–768.

Zur, M. and Nemerson, Y. (1980) Kinetics of factor IX activation via the extrinsic pathway. *J Biol Chem*, **255**, 5703–5707.

3 THE MOLECULAR DEFECT IN HEMOPHILIA A

G. Kemball-Cook and E.G.D. Tuddenham

Introduction

Over the last decade there has been a dramatic increase in our understanding of the pathology of hemophilia A in molecular terms, at the levels both of nucleic acid sequence and, to a much lesser extent, protein structure. By 1983 factor VIII (FVIII), the protein absent or defective in hemophilia A, had been purified to homogeneity (Rotblat *et al.*, 1983) and shortly afterwards the gene was successfully cloned (Gitschier *et al.*, 1984). Previously, it was possible to carry out laboratory assays both for FVIII activity and for antigenic protein in the plasma of hemophilia A patients, allowing the distinction to be made between those lacking any FVIII protein and those with normal or reduced levels of a dysfunctional protein: however, in the absence of molecular genetic studies, there was little further analysis to be made of the molecular nature of the defects.

The cloning of the FVIII gene and the more recent adoption of the polymerase chain reaction (PCR; Saiki *et al.*, 1988) and other technical innovations to probe for missense mutations, insertion/deletions and other gene defects has now allowed the definition of the molecular defect in a large majority of patients with clinically significant bleeding due to hemophilia A. An overview of the molecular pathology of hemophilia A, together with some speculations on the structure–function aspects of FVIII revealed by these data, is presented below.

Structure and function of the factor VIII gene and protein

FACTOR VIII GENE

The human FVIII gene was cloned between 1982 and 1984 by Gitschier and colleagues at Genentech Inc.

(Gitschier *et al.*, 1984): at the time the gene was the largest described (186 kb). Mapping positions the FVIII gene in the most distal band (Xq28) of the long arm of the X chromosome (Poustka *et al.*, 1991; Freije and Schlessinger, 1992). As shown in Fig. 3.1, analysis of the gene reveals 26 exons, 24 of which vary in length from 69 to 262 bp: the remaining much larger exons, 14 and 26, contain 3106 and 1958 bp respectively (the large majority of exon 26 is 3′ untranslated sequence). The spliced FVIII messenger RNA (mRNA) is approximately 9 kb in length and predicts a precursor protein of 2351 amino acids. Of the introns, 6 are larger than 14 kb. Unusually, the intron separating exons 22 and 23 (IVS22) contains a CpG island associated with two additional transcripts, termed F8A (Levinson *et al.*, 1990) and F8B (Levinson *et al.*, 1992). F8B is a transcript of 2.5 kb and is transcribed in the same direction as the FVIII gene, using a private exon plus FVIII exons 23–26. F8A, however, contains no introns and is transcribed in the opposite direction to the FVIII gene: furthermore, two additional copies of F8A have been found approximately 400 kb telomeric to the FVIII gene (Levinson *et al.*, 1990): these F8A copies are implicated in almost half of severe hemophilia A via a partial inversion mechanism (p. 24) The functions, if any, of the F8A and F8B transcripts and their potential translated products are unknown, although F8A transcripts have been found in a wide variety of tissues.

STRUCTURE AND FUNCTION OF FACTOR VIII

FVIII circulates in plasma as a large glycoprotein complexed non-covalently to the giant multimeric adhesive protein von Willebrand factor (vWf) which acts as a carrier for FVIII both during its secretion and in the general circulation. Sequencing of FVIII complementary

Hemophilia. Edited by C.D. Forbes, L. Aledort and R. Madhok. Published in 1997 by Chapman & Hall, London. ISBN 0 412 63820 7

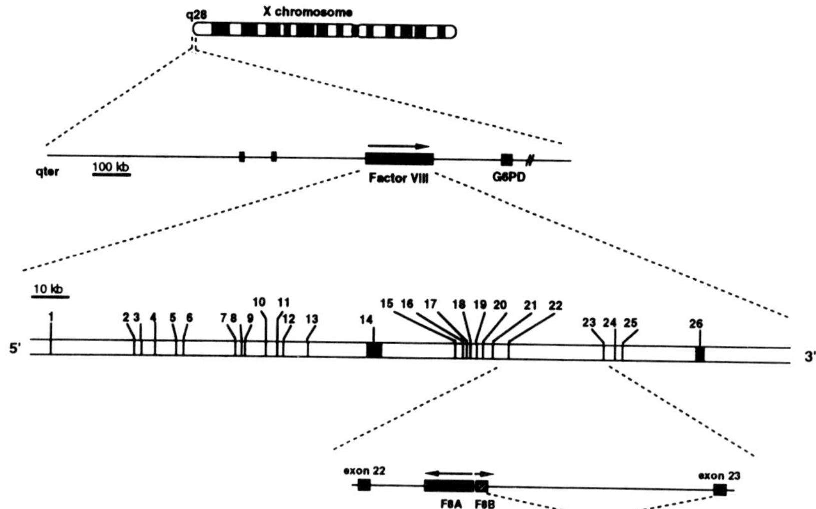

Fig. 3.1 Schematic representation of the chromosomal localization and structure of the factor VIII gene, located about 1000 kb from the Xq telomere (Xqter). The gene is 186 kb long and contains 26 exons. The large intron IVS22 contains two nested genes *F8A* and *F8B*, the latter using exon 23 of factor VIII as its second exon. There are two further copies of sequences homologous to *F8A* shown by the grey boxes on the second line. (Figure reproduced with permission from Kazazian *et al.*, 1995.)

DNA (cDNA) predicted a mature secreted protein consisting of 2332 amino acids with a calculated molecular weight of 265 kDa (without carbohydrate). Analysis of the sequence showed very clearly a repeating domain structure A1-A2-B-A3-C1-C2 (Vehar *et al.*, 1984). In addition, close homology was seen (Fig. 3.2) to coagulation factor V (also A1-A2-B-A3-C1-C2, although the B domains are apparently unrelated) and to the plasma protein ceruloplasmin (A1-A2-A3; Vehar *et al.*, 1984; Koschinsky *et al.*, 1986; Kane and Davie, 1986). Less obvious homology of the C domains has also been noted with milk fat globule membrane protein (Stubbs *et al.*, 1990), discoidin I (Vehar *et al.*, 1984) and a receptor

tyrosine kinase found in breast carcinoma cells (Johnson, Edman and Rutter, 1993). No significant homology has yet been identified between the B domain of FVIII and any other protein sequence in protein sequence databases.

FVIII is highly sensitive to proteolytic processing before and after secretion and only a small fraction of circulating FVIII is in the single-chain form: the majority consists of heavy chains of variable length (consisting of the A1 and A2 domains together with variable lengths of B domain) linked non-covalently to light chains consisting of the A3, C1 and C2 domains (Vehar *et al.*, 1984). Expression of active recombinant FVIII lacking the entire

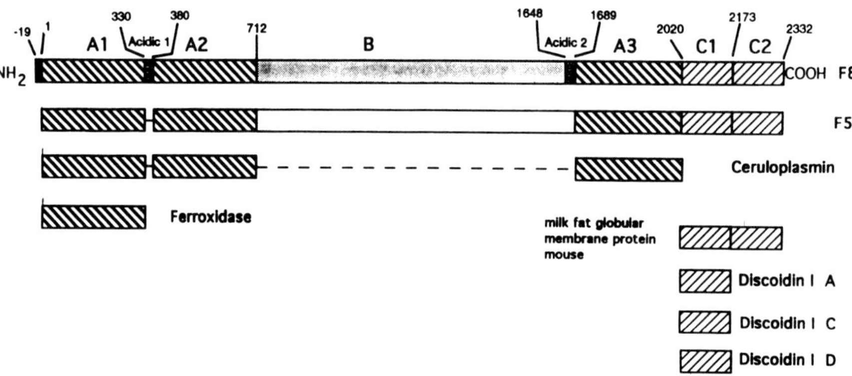

Fig. 3.2 Amino acid homologies of factor VIII domains. The A and C domains have significant homology with coagulation factor V. All three A domains have homology with ceruloplasmin and ferroxidase, while the C domains also have homology with discoidin lectins from *Dictyostelium discoides* and mouse milk fat globule membrane protein. (Figure reproduced with permission from Kazazian *et al.*, 1995.)

length of the B domain has confirmed that this domain is unnecessary for coagulation activity (Eaton, Rodriguez and Vehar, 1986): a cleavage after R740 (probably by thrombin) during coagulation serves to remove it.

The function of FVIII is to act as an essential cofactor for the activation of factor X (FX) by activated factor IX (FIXa) on a suitable phospholipid surface, thus amplifying the clotting stimulus manyfold (van Dieijen *et al.*, 1981; Mann *et al.*, 1990). Proteolytic processing mediates both the generation and destruction of this activity. Thus, in order to participate in this reaction plasma FVIII must first be proteolytically cleaved at two distinct sites which lie at the interfaces between domains – after R372 (A1/A2 junction) and after R1689 (B/A3 junction; Pittman and Kaufman 1988; Hill-Eubanks, Parker and Lollar, 1989). The first cleavage may serve to allow the short (~30 residue) acidic linker a1 between the A1 and A2 domains to function as a binding-site for A2 in the proposed heterotrimeric active FVIIIa species (Fay, Haidaris and Huggins, 1993), while the second allows the dissociation of FVIII from vWf by removing the 40-residue acidic peptide a3 bearing a vWf binding-site (Leyte *et al.*, 1991): it is thought that FVIIIa is then able to interact with a phospholipid surface via its C2 domain and form a macromolecular complex with membrane-bound factors IXa and X. Further proteolytic cleavage by activated protein C (APC), thrombin, FIXa or FXa may specifically inactivate FVIIIa by cleavage after R336 (all four enzymes) after 1719 (FIXa only), or after R562 (APC only; Vehar *et al.*, 1984; Walker, Chavin and Fay, 1987; O'Brien *et al.*, 1992): this latter may be the most important in the down-regulation of FVIII activity following coagulation. Additionally, the A2 subunit of highly purified heterotrimeric FVIIIa has been shown to dissociate spontaneously from the complex *in vitro* with

complete loss of activity, although the active complex may be stabilized against this dissociation when complexed with FIXa and phospholipid (Curtis *et al.*, 1994). Figure 3.3 shows in diagrammatic form a scheme for the activation and inactivation of FVIII.

EXPRESSION OF FACTOR VIII

The results of immunohistology with a monoclonal antibody against FVIII antigen (Zelechowska, van Mourik and Brodniewicz-Proba, 1985), the presence of FVIII mRNA in hepatocytes (Wion *et al.*, 1985) and liver transplantation studies in hemophiliacs (Bontempo *et al.*, 1987) suggest that in humans the primary site of production of FVIII is the liver, although other tissues do contain detectable FVIII mRNA (Wion *et al.*, 1985). Analysis of *in vitro* expression using cloned FVIII cDNA transfected into mammalian cells in tissue culture has shown that mRNA accumulation is grossly reduced by a dominant inhibitor of transcriptional elongation found in a 1.2 kb portion of the cDNA (Koeberl *et al.*, 1995). Following synthesis, the 19-amino-acid leader peptide is removed on translocation into the endoplasmic reticulum (ER; Kaufman, Wasley and Dorner, 1988). The precise fate of FVIII from this stage is unclear in that, in addition to glycosylations being added to asparagine residues, a proportion of the molecules associate tightly with an ER protein called BiP or GRP78 (Dorner, Bole and Kaufman, 1987; Munro and Pelham, 1986) and may not be successfully expressed. This binding to BiP appears to be mediated via the C-terminal portion of the A1 domain (Marquette, Pittman and Kaufman, 1995). In the Golgi apparatus, successfully exported molecules have further O-linked glycosylations carried out, six tyrosine residues are sulfated and a range of proteolytic cleavages made in

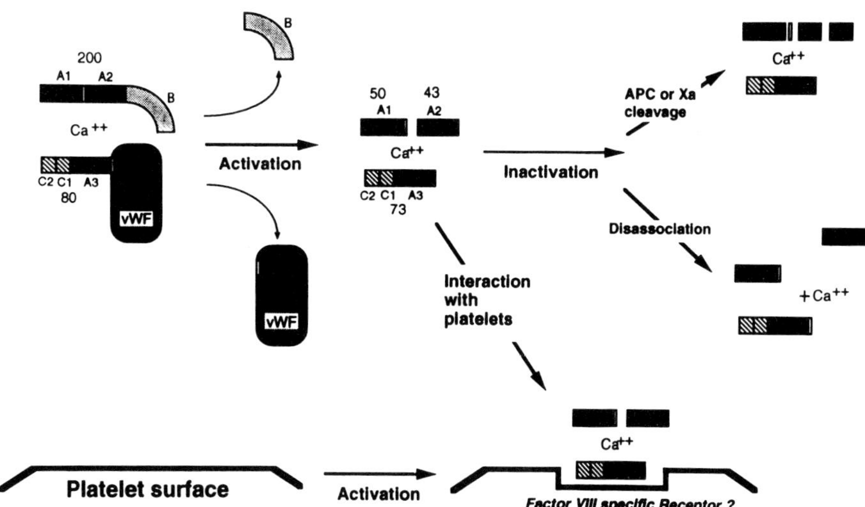

Fig. 3.3 A model for activation and inactivation of factor VIII. Activation involves protease cleavages and interaction with divalent cations and platelet surfaces. Inactivation requires either further proteolysis or dissociation of the subunits. (Figure reproduced with permission from Kazazian *et al.*, 1995.)

the B domain (Kaufman, Wasley and Dorner, 1988; Pittman, Wang and Kaufman, 1992). The resulting two-chain molecule consists of a C-terminal 80 kDa light chain and heavy chains ranging in size from 90 to 200 kDa, associated via metal ion interaction (Vehar *et al.*, 1984).

Molecular pathology of hemophilia A

Over 1000 DNA samples from hemophilia A patients have been examined for genetic defects and the results summarized in a mutation database updated in 1994 (Tuddenham *et al.*, 1994) and now accessible online on the World Wide Web (URL: http://europium.mrc.rpms.ac.uk). The results presented below constitute a selective summary: for full details readers should consult the online database. Defined FVIII gene defects may be broadly split into several categories:

1. Gross rearrangements of DNA sequence involving the FVIII gene.
2. Single DNA base substitutions leading to amino-acid replacement (missense), premature peptide chain termination (nonsense or stop mutations) or mRNA splicing defects.
3. Deletions of genetic sequence of a size varying from one bp up to the entire gene.
4. Insertions of DNA of varying size.

GENE REARRANGEMENTS

Gross gene rearrangements reported consist almost entirely of a unique inversion elaborated quite recently, yet now known to be responsible for more than 40% of all cases of severe hemophilia A. During intensive attempts to define the causative mutations in a population of severe patients by PCR amplification of all 26 exons, mutations were found in only about 50% of cases (Higuchi *et al.*, 1991): in the rest, all the exonic sequences appeared normal. However, on RT-PCR of FVIII mRNA from these cases it was found that no amplification was possible between exons 22 and 23 (Naylor *et al.*, 1992, 1993). It is now known that in all these patients there is a large inversion and translocation of exons 1–22 (together with introns) away from exons 23–26, the mechanism of which is homologous recombination between the *F8A* gene in intron 22 (Fig. 3.1) and one of the extragenic *F8A* copies 400 kb 5′ to the FVIII gene (Lakich *et al.*, 1993; Naylor *et al.*, 1993). Figure 3.4 shows how a simple cross-over event during the meiotic division of spermatogenesis can lead to fragmentation of the gene, with subsequent severe disease. Indeed, family studies show that the origin of such inversions is almost exclusively a gamete supplied by a normal male (Rossiter *et al.*, 1994).

SINGLE-BASE SUBSTITUTIONS

There have been 191 different single-base substitutions described, of which 155 (81%) predict a single amino-acid change from the wild-type sequence (missense). A further 27 lead to creation of preliminary peptide chain termination or STOP codons, while 14 may give rise to altered or absent splicing of the FVIII mRNA: of these latter, 5 also predict an amino acid substitution. Table 3.1 lists the different substitutions together with their predicted effect, the number of independent reports of the change in the database, any data available on FVIII activity or antigen levels, plus an indication of clinical severity and anti-FVIII inhibitor status (if known). As will

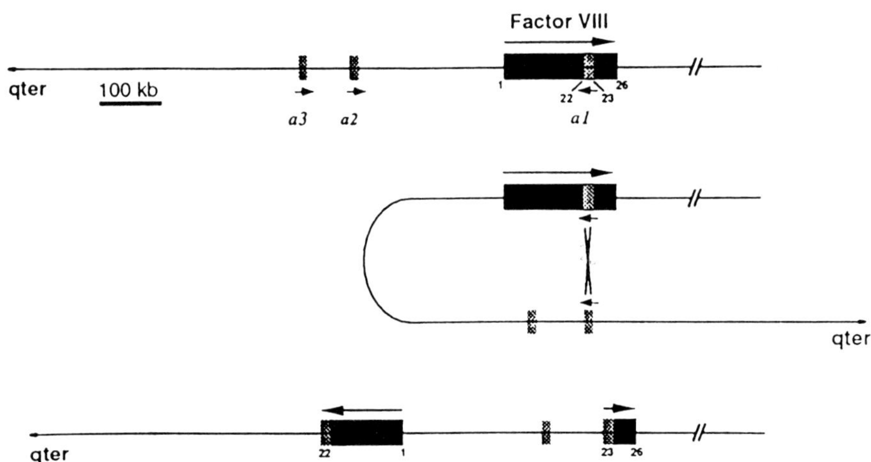

Fig. 3.4 Schematic representation of the mechanism of one type of the common inversion of the factor VIII gene due to intrachromosomal crossing-over between the homologous sequences *a1* and *a3*. The partial inversion includes exons 1–22 of the gene. (Figure reproduced with permission from Antonarakis *et al.*, 1995.)

Table 3.1 Single-base substitutions found in the factor VIII (FVIII) gene of patients with hemophilia A

Exon/ intron	Codon*	Nucleotide change†	Codon change	FVIII:C (u/dl)‡	FVIII:Ag (u/dl)§	Severity**	Inhibitor††	Comments
Exon 1	19	ATG-ATA(1)	Met-Ile	<1	?	Severe	No	Start codon
Exon 1	−5	CGA-TGA (3)	Arg-Stop	<1	<1	Severe	No	Signal peptide
Exon 1	7	CTG-CGG (1)	Leu-Arg	<1	?	Severe	No	
Exon 1	11	GAA-GTA (1)	Glu-Val	?	?	Mild	No	
Exon 1	22	GGT-TGT (1)	Gly-Cys	<1	?	Severe	No	
Exon 1	29	AGA-AAA (1)	Arg-Cys	<1	?	Severe	No	−1 IVS 1 acceptor splice site
Intron 2	–	cga-tga (1)	–	<1	?	Severe	No	Probably a neutral change ~300 bp 3′ to exon 2
Exon 2	56	GAT-GAA (1)	Asp-Glu	3	?	Moderate	No	
Exon 3	70	GGT-GAT (1)	Gly-Asp	<1	?	Severe	No	−1 IVS 2 donor splice site
Exon 3	73	GGT-GTT (1)	Gly-Val	?	?	Mild	?	
Exon 3	80	GTT-GAT (1)	Val-Asp	<1	?	Severe	No	
Exon 3	85	GTC-GAC (1)	Val-Asp	?	?	Mild	?	
Exon 3	89	AAG-ACG (1)	Lys-Thr	?	?	Mild	?	
Exon 3	91	ATG-GTG (1)	Met-Val	?	?	Mild	?	
Exon 3	98	CTT-CGT (1)	Leu-Arg	<1	?	Severe	No	
Exon 3	111	GGT-CGT (1)	Gly-Arg	<1	?	Severe	No	
Exon 3	113	GAA-GAC (1)	Glu-Asp	<1	?	Severe	Yes	
Exon 4	114	TAT-TGT (1)	Tyr-Cys	6.3	10.7	Mild	No	
Exon 4	116	GAT-GGT (1)	Asp-Gly	<1	?	Severe	No	
Exon 4	118	AGC-ATC (2)	Thr-Ile	2.1	10.7	Moderate	No	
Exon 4	139	GAG-TAG (1)	Gln-Stop	<1	?	Severe	No	
Exon 4	145	GGT-GTT (1)	Gly-Val	?	?	Mild	?	
Exon 4	146	CCA-TCA (1)	Pro-Ser	<1	?	Severe	No	
Exon 4	156	TAC-TAA (1)	Tyr-Stop	<1	?	Severe	No	
Exon 4	162	GTG-ATG (11)	Val-Met	5.3–9.0	3.7–14	Moderate/mild	No	
Exon 4	166	AAA-ACA (1)	Lys-Thr	8	9.8	Mild	No	
Exon 4	170	TCA-TTA (1)	Ser-Leu	3.5	8.7	Moderate	No	
Intron 4	–	cga-caa (1)	–	5–10	41	Mild	No	Proposed to activate cryptic splice site 1 kb 3′ to exon 4
Intron 4	–	ag/-gg/ (1)	–	1.7	1.3	Severe	No	−2 IVS4 acceptor splice site
Exon 5	203	GAT-GTT (1)	Asp-Val	2.0	8.5	Moderate	No	
Exon 5	205	G/gt..ag/GG-T/ gt..ag/GG (1)	Gly-Trp	3.2	?	Moderate	?	−1 IVS5 donor splice site
Intron 5	–	ag/-gg/ (1)	–	<1	?	Severe	No	−2 IVS 5 acceptor splice site
Intron 6	–	G/gta-G/gtg (1)	–	3	?	Moderate	No	+3 IVS 6 donor splice site
Intron 6	–	ag/-ac/ (1)	–	?	?	Severe	?	−1 IVS 6 acceptor splice site
Exon 7	247	GGA-GAA (1)	Gly-Glu	10	?	Mild	No	
Exon 7	255	TGG-TGA (1)	Trp-Stop	?	?	Severe	?	
Exon 7	259	GGA-AGA (1)	Gly-Arg	<1	?	Severe	No	
Exon 7	266	GTG-GGG (1)	Val-Gly	?	?	Mild	?	
Exon 7	272	GAA-GGA (1)	Glu-Gly	2	3.5	Moderate	No	
Exon 7	272	GAA-AAA (1)	Glu-Lys	6	?	Mild	?	
Exon 7	275	AGA-ATA (2)	Thr-Ile	4–5	20–40	Moderate	No	
Exon 7	280	AAC-ATC (1)	Asn-Ile	8–12	?	Mild	No	
Exon 7	282	CGC-CAC (4)	Arg-His	<1	18	Severe	No	
Exon 7	282	CGC-CTC (3)	Arg-Leu	<1, 20	?	Severe/mild	No	
Exon 7	289	TCG-TTG (1)	Ser-Leu	37	106	?	?	
Exon 7	293	TTC-TCC (1)	Phe-Ser	?	?	Mild	?	
Exon 7	295	ACT-GCT (5)	Thr-Ala	7–22	5–18	Moderate/mild	No	
Exon 7	308	CTG-CCG (1)	Leu-Pro	<1	?	Severe	No	
Exon 8	323	TAT-TAA (2)	Tyr-Stop	<1	?	Severe	No	
Exon 8	326	GTA-CTA (2)	Val-Leu	?	?	Severe	No	
Exon 8	329	TGT-TAT (2)	Cys-Tyr	<1	?	Severe	No	
Exon 8	329	TGT-CGT (1)	Cys-Arg	?	?	Severe	No	
Exon 8	329	TGT-TCT (1)	Cys-Ser	2.6	3.2	Moderate	No	
Exon 8	336	CGA-TGA (9)	Arg-Stop	<1	<1	Severe	No	Activated protein C cleavage site
Exon 8	372	CGC-CCC (1)	Arg-Pro	3	?	Severe	No	Thrombin activation site
Exon 8	372	CGC-CAC (4)	Arg-His	3–5	57–325	Severe/mild	No	Thrombin activation site
Exon 8	372	CGC-TGC (5)	Arg-Cys	<1–3	74–80	Severe/moderate	No	Thrombin activation site
Exon 8	373	TCA-TTA (1)	Ser-Leu	8	110	Mild	No	Thrombin activation site
Exon 8	373	TCA-TAA (1)	Ser-Stop	<1	<1	Severe	No	Thrombin activation site
Exon 8	373	TCA-CCA (1)	Ser-Pro	10	100	Mild	No	Thrombin activation site
Exon 8	386	ATT-AGT (1)	Ile-Ser	<1	?	Severe	No	
Exon 8	390	GAG-GGG (2)	Glu-Gly	<1/3.5	?	Severe/moderate	No	
Exon 9	412	TTG-TTT (2)	Leu-Phe	5–7	6.4	Moderate/mild	No	
Exon 9	425	AAA-AGA (1)	Lys-Arg	<1	5	Severe	No	

Table 3.1 (Continued)

Exon/ intron	Codon*	Nucleotide change†	Codon change	FVIII:C (u/dl)‡	FvIII:Ag (u/dl)§	Severity**	Inhibitor††	Comments
Exon 9	427	CGA-TGA (3)	Arg-Stop	<1	<1	Severe	Yes	
Exon 9	431	TAC-AAC (1)	Tyr-Asn	4	?	Moderate	No	
Exon 10	469	GCA-GGA (1)	Ala-Gly	2.3	45.3	Moderate	No	
Exon 10	473	TAT-CAT (1)	Tyr-His	?	?	Mild	No	
Exon 10	473	TAT-TGT (2)	Tyr-Cys	2.7/3.5	?	Moderate	No	
Exon 10	475	ATC-ACC (2)	Ile-Thr	5.5/7.0	6.9/8.8	Mild	No	
Exon 10	479	[C]GGA-AGA (3)	Gly-Arg	2–18	?/31.6	Moderate/mild	No	
Exon 11	504	CTG-CTT (4)	Leu-Leu	?	?	Mild	?	Potential new acceptor site
Exon 11	525	GAT-AAT (1)	Asp-Asn	6	61	Moderate	No	
Exon 11	527	CGG-TGG (11)	Arg-Trp	9.5–23	43–245	Mild	No	
Exon 11	531	CGC-GGC (1)	Arg-Gly	9.2	?	Moderate	No	
Exon 11	531	CGC-TGC (4)	Arg-Cys	4.2/6.7	?	Moderate	?	
Exon 11	531	CGC-CAC (2)	Arg-His	23.5/32	>20/33.2	Mild	No	
Exon 11	531	CGC-TGC (1)	Arg-Cys	6.5	8.3	Mild	No	
Exon 11	535	AGT-GGT (3)	Ser-Gly	?	?	Mild	No	
Exon 11	542	GAT-GGT (1)	Asp-Gly	<1	5	Severe	No	
Exon 11	557	GAA-TAA (1)	Glu-Stop	<1%	?	Moderate	No	
Exon 11	558	TCT-TTT (1)	Ser-Phe	21	175	?	?	
Exon 11	565	CAG/gt-AAG/gt (2)	Gln-Lys	?	?	Moderate/mild	No	−3 IVS 11 donor splice site
Exon 12	566	ATA-ACA (2)	Ile-Thr	4	200	Moderate	No	New N-glycosylation site N564
Exon 12	577	TCT-CCT (1)	Ser-Pro	?	?	?	?	
Exon 12	583	CGA-TGA (5)	Arg-Stop	<1	<1	Severe	No	
Exon 12	584	AGC-ATC (1)	Ser-Ile	?	?	?	?	Loss N-glycosylation site N582
Exon 12	585	TGG-TGC (1)	Trp-Cys	<1	?	Severe	No	
Exon 12	586	TAC-TCC (1)	Tyr-Ser	<1	?	Severe	No	
Exon 12	593	CGC-TGC (11)	Arg-Cys	7–15	?	Moderate/mild	No	
Exon 12	612	AAC-AGC (1)	Asn-Ser	?	?	?	?	
Intron 12	–	/gtgagt-gtgaat (1)	–	?	?	Mild	?	+5 1VS 12 donor splice site
Intron 12	–	g-a at -37 (1)	–	?	?	Moderate	?	Not proven to be pathologic
Exon 13	634	GTG-GCG (1)	Val-Ala	5	138	Mild	No	
Exon 13	634	GTG-ATG (1)	Val-Met	<1	175	Severe	No	
Exon 13	636	TAC-TAG (2)	Tyr-Stop	<1	?	Severe	Yes	
Exon 13	644	GCA-GTA (1)	Ala-Val	14	25	Moderate/mild	No	
Exon 13	658	TTC-CTC (1)	Phe-Leu	5.1	50.5	Moderate/mild	No	
Exon 14	698	CGG-TGG (1)	Arg-Trp	?	?	Mild	No	
Exon 14	701	GGC-GAC (1)	Gly-Asp	2	?	Moderate	Yes	Multicopper oxidase I site
Exon 14	704	[C]GCC-ACC (3)	Ala-Thr	4.5	5.5	Moderate/mild	No	
Exon 14	720	[C]GAG-AAG (2)	Glu-Lys	12.5/30	>20.0	Mild	No	
Exon 14	795	CGA-TGA (1)	Arg-Stop	<1	<1	Severe	No	
Exon 14	1038	GAG-AAG (1)	Glu-Lys	2.4	10–20	Moderate/mild	No	
Exon 14	1441	AAT-AAA (1)	Asn-Lys	6	7	?	?	
Exon 14	1462	CTG-CGG (1)	Leu-Pro	?	?	?	?	
Exon 14	1615	GAG-TAG (1)	Glu-Stop	<1	?	Severe	No	
Exon 14	1680	TAT-TTT (22)	Tyr-Phe	2–10	5.4–20	Moderate/mild	No	Sulfated Tyr/vWF binding
Exon 14	1680	TAT-TGT (1)	Tyr-Cys	?	?	Severe	No	Sulfated Tyr/vWF binding
Exon 14	1686	GAG-TAG (1)	Gln-Stop	<1	?	Severe	?	
Exon 14	1689	CGC-TGC (13)	Arg-Cys	<1–12	40–220	Severe/moderate/mild	No	Thrombin activation site
Exon 14	1689	CGC-CAC (2)	Arg-His	7/11	100/165	Mild	No	Thrombin activation site
Exon 14	1696	CGA-TGA (2)	Arg-Stop	<1	?	Severe	Yes	
Exon 14	1696	CGA-GGA (1)	Arg-Gly	17	?	Mild	No	
Exon 14	1698	CGC-TGC (1)	Arg-Cys	<1	?	Severe	?	
Exon 14	1704	GAG-AAG (1)	Glu-Lys	<1	?	Severe	No	
Exon 14	1709	TAT-TGT (1)	Tyr-Cys	18	?	Moderate	No	
Intron 14	–	ag/GTA-ag/GTG (1)	–	<1.0	<2.5	Severe	No	−3 IVS 14 acceptor splice site
Exon 15	1750	GGA-AGA (5)	Gly-Arg	20–26	21–27	Mild	No	
Exon 15	1756	TTG-GTG (1)	Leu-Val	5.0	1.5	Moderate/mild	No	
Exon 15	1756	TTG-TTC (1)	Leu-Phe	18.5	?	Mild	No	
Exon 15	1760	GGG-GAG (1)	Gly-Glu	<1	?	Severe	No	
Exon 15	1772	ATG-ACG (1)	Met-Thr	<1	72	Severe	No	New N-glcosylation site N1770
Exon 16	1781	CGT-CAT (4)	Arg-His	2.0–2.5	4.7–5.4	Moderate/mild	No	
Exon 16	1781	CGT-TGT (1)	Arg-Cys	4–7	?	Mild	No	
Exon 16	1781	CGT-GGT (1)	Arg-Gly	5.0	?	Moderate/mild	No	
Exon 16	1784	TCC-TAC (1)	Ser-Tyr	?	?	Severe	?	
Exon 16	1789	CTT-TTT (3)	Leu-Phe	7.2	?	Mild	No	
Exon 16	1796	GAG-TAG (1)	Gln-Stop	<1	?	Severe	Yes	
Exon 16	1823	ATG-ATA (1)	Met-Ile	4.6	?	Moderate	No	
Exon 16	1825	CCC-TCC (1)	Pro-Ser	15	?	Moderate	No	
Exon 16	1826	ACT-CCT (1)	Thr-Pro	?	?	Mild	No	

Table 3.1 (Continued)

Exon/intron	Codon*	Nucleotide change†	Codon change	FVIII:C (u/dl)‡	FvIII:Ag (u/dl)§	Severity**	Inhibitor††	Comments
Exon 16	1827	AAA-TAA (2)	Lys-Stop	<1	?	Severe	Yes	
Exon 16	1834	GCC-GTC (1)	Ala-Val	18	?	Mild	No	
Exon 16	1834	GCC-ACC (1)	Ala-Thr	<1	?	Severe	No	May not be sole mutation
Exon 16	1843	CTG/gt-CTA/gt (1)	Leu-Leu	9–18	?	Moderate	?	−1 IVS 16 donor splice site
Exon 17	1846	GAT-AAT (1)	Asp-Asn	<1	?	Severe	No	
Exon 17	1846	GAT-TAT (1)	Asp-Tyr	<1	?	Severe	No	
Exon 17	1848	CAC-CGC (1)	His-Arg	1–5	?	Moderate/mild	No	
Exon 17	1854	CCC-CGC (1)	Pro-Arg	<1	?	Severe	No	
Exon 17	1869	AGA-ATA (1)	Arg-Ile	<1	?	Severe	No	
Exon 17	1874	CAG-TAG (1)	Gln-Stop	<1	?	Severe	Yes	
Exon 17	1885	GAG-AAG (1)	Glu-Lys	<1	?	Severe	No	
Exon 18	1922	AAT-AGT (2)	Asn-Ser	?	?	Severe/moderate	?	
Exon 18	1922	AAT-GAT (2)	Asn-Asp	<1	?	Moderate	?	
Exon 18	1941	CGA-TGA (10)	Arg-Stop	<1	<0.1	Severe	Yes	
Exon 18	1941	CGA-CAA (6)	Arg-Gln	2–17	20	Moderate/mild	No	
Exon 18	1941	CGA-CTA (1)	Arg-Leu	7	?	Moderate	No	
Exon 18	1942	TGG-TAG (1)	Trp-Stop	<1	?	Severe	No	
Exon 18	1948	GGC-GAC (1)	Gly-Asp	7.4	48.7	Moderate	No	
Exon 18	1960	GGA-GTA (1)	Gly-Val	6.0	?	Mild	No	
Exon 18	1961	CAT-TAT (1)	His-Tyr	10.5	7.8	Mild	No	
Exon 18	1966	CGA-TGA (6)	Arg-Stop	<1	9.1	Severe	Yes	
Exon 18	1987	GAA-TAA (1)	Glu-Stop	<1	?	Severe	No	
Exon 19	1997	CGG-TGG (3)	Arg-Trp	<1–3.4	?	Severe	No	
Exon 19	2019	AAT-AGT (1)	Asn-Ser	5.0	3.3	Moderate/mild	No	
Exon 21	2046	TGG-CGG (1)	Trp-Arg	?	?	Moderate	No	
Exon 21	2069	TCT-TTT (1)	Ser-Phe	<1.0	?	Severe	No	
Exon 22	2074	GAT-GGT (3)	Asp-Gly	4.5–9.0	10–15.2	Mild	No	
Exon 22	2101	TTT-TTG (2)	Phe-Leu	7-11	5.3	Moderate/mild	No	
Exon 22	2105	TAT-TGT (1)	Tyr-Cys	14	?	Mild	No	
Exon 22	2116	CGA-TGA (8)	Arg-Stop	<1	?	Severe	No	
Exon 22	2116	CGA-CCA (1)	Arg-Pro	<1	?	Severe	?	
Exon 22	2119	TCC-TAC (2)	Ser-Tyr	3.5–8	9.2	Moderate/mild	No	
Exon 23	2147	CGA-TGA (7)	Arg-Stop	<1	>0.1	Severe	Yes	
Exon 23	2150	CGT-CAT (14)	Arg-His	<1–7	?	Severe/moderate/mild	No	
Exon 22	2153	CGA-CAA (1)	Pro-Gln	3.0	5.6	Moderate	No	
Exon 23	2154	ACT-ATT (1)	Thr-Ile	6	?	Mild	No	
Exon 23	2159	CGC-TGC (13)	Arg-Cys	6–19	6–15.7	Moderate/mild	No	
Exon 23	2159	CGC-CTC (2)	Arg-Leu	12/25	14.8/?	Mild	No	
Exon 23	2159	CGC-CAC (1)	Arg-His	22.0	11.9	Mild	No	
Exon 23	2163	CGC-CAC (1)	Arg-His	?	?	Moderate	?	
Exon 23	2163	CGC-TGC (1)	Arg-Cys	1	<10	Moderate	No	
Exon 23	2166	GTT-GCT (1)	Leu-Ser	<1	?	Severe	No	
Exon 24	2192	GCT-CCT (1)	Ala-Pro	1	?	Moderate	No	
Exon 24	2209	CGA-CAA (12)	Arg-Gln	<1–7	?/4–130	Severe/moderate/mild	Yes	
Exon 24	2209	CGA-CTA (1)	Arg-Leu	3	2.5	Moderate	No	
Exon 24	2209	CGA-TGA (12)	Arg-Stop	<1	?	Severe	Yes	
Exon 24	2209	CGA-GGA (1)	Arg-Gly	<1	?	Severe	No	
Exon 25	2223	ag/GTG-ag/ATG (1)	Val-Met	?	?	?	?	+1 Intron 24 acceptor splice site
Exon 25	2229	TGG-TGT (2)	Trp-Cys	3	?	Moderate/mild	Yes	
Exon 25	2246	CAG-CGG (2)	Gln-Arg	40–4.5	<1/1.1	Moderate	No	
Exon 25	2270	CAG-TAG (1)	Gln-Stop	<1	?	Severe	No	
Intron 25	–	caa-cga (1)	–	<1	?	Severe	No	Probably a neutral change ~1.9 kb 5′ to exon 26
Exon 26	2300	CCG-CTG (1)	Pro-Leu	7.5	?	Mild	?	
Exon 26	2300	CCG-TCG (1)	Pro-Ser	16	?	Mild	No	
Exon 26	2304	CGC-CAC (1)	Arg-His	10.0	?	Mild	No	
Exon 26	2304	CGC-TGC (2)	Arg-Cys	1	<10	Moderate	No	
Exon 26	2307	CGA-TGA (10)	Arg-Stop	<1	?	Severe	Yes	
Exon 26	2307	CGA-CAA (4)	Arg-Gln	2–10	6	Moderate/mild	No	
Exon 26	2307	CGA-CTA (6)	Arg-Leu	<1–2	4	Severe/moderate/mild	No	

All values labeled ? were unreported in the original communications.

*Codons numbered after scheme of Vehar *et al.* (1984), i.e. starts at mature N-terminus and 19 signal peptide residues numbered negatively.

†Numbers in parentheses indicate number of separate reports (in unrelated kindreds) of the missense mutation in the database.

§,‡Where multiple instances occur in the database, FVIII:C and FVIII:Ag values are shown as a range of the available data: many reports have incomplete data and the full database should be consulted for details.

**Where multiple instances occur a single level of clinical severity is quoted if all reports agree, otherwise the range is given.

††Where multiple instances occur inhibitor status is given as 'yes' if at least one of the studies found an inhibitor: 'no' indicates that all the reports were negative.

Table 3.2A Large deletions in the factor VIII (FVIII) gene

Exon (s) deleted	Size of deletion (kb)	Patient/ family	FVIII:C (u/dl)	FVIII:Ag (u/dl)	Severity	Inhibitors	References
1–26	>210	?	?	?	Severe	No	Casarino et al. (1986)
1–26	>210	H1	?	?	Severe	Yes	Casula et al. (1990)
1–6	>55	H328	<1	?	Severe	Yes	Millar et al. (1990)
1–5	>35	484	<1	?	Severe	No	Higuchi et al. (1989)
1	?	1	<1	?	Severe	No	Reiner and Thompson (1992)
1	>2	JH13	<1	<1	Severe	No	Youssofian et al. (1988d)
1	>1	H309	<1	?	Severe	No	Millar et al. (1990)
1	?	JH145	?	?	Severe	?	Higuchi et al. (1991b)
Exon 1/intron 1	13	HD7	<1	?	Severe	No	Schwaab et al. (1993)
Intron 1*	7	1067	?	?	Severe	No	Levinson et al. (1990)
2–4	?	TWN11	<1	?	Severe	Yes	Lin et al. (1993)
2–3	9–12	JH21	<1	<1	Severe	No	Youssoufian et al. (1988d)
							Cutting et al. (1988)
							Woods-Samuels et al. (1991)
3–13	60	JH22	C1	<|	Severe	Yes	Youssoufian et al. (1988d)
							Cutting et al. (1988)
3–5	11.7	H151	<1	?	Severe	No	Millar et al. (1990)
3	1.7–2.0	656	<1	?	Severe	No	Higuchi et al. (1988, 1989)
4–25	133–145	JH23	<1	<1	Severe	No	Youssoufian et al. (1988d)
							Cutting et al. (1988)
4–10	?	TWN27,112	<1	?	Severe	Yes	Lin et al. (1993)
5–13	57	H571	<1	?	Severe	Yes	Millar et al. (1990)
5,6	?	?	?	?	Severe	?	Gitschier et al. (1989)
5,6	2.5–10	2253	?	?	Severe	Yes	Levinson et al. (1990)
5	2	H275	?	?	Severe	No	Broecker-Vriends et al. (1990)
5 or 6	2	?	?	?	Severe	?	Broecker-Vriends et al. (1988)
5,6	?	OX 26	<1	?	Severe	No	Naylor et al. (1993a)
6	10	1059	?	?	Severe	No	Levinson et al. (1990)
6	7	JH6	<1	<1	Severe	No	Youssoufian et al. (1987b)
6	3–6	2213	?	?	Severe	No	Levinson et al. (1990)
6	?	TWN108	<1	?	Severe	Yes	Lin et al. (1993)
6	<6	HD8	<1	?	Severe	No	Schwaab et al. (1993)
6	8–13	HD9	<1	?	Severe	No	Schwaab et al. (1993)
7–22	110	H2	?	?	Severe	Yes	Casula et al. (1990)
7–14	40–56	JH24	<1	<1	Severe	No	Youssoufian et al. (1988d)
7–9	15–20	505	<1	?	Severe	Yes	Higachi et al. (1989)
10	4.8	149	<1	?	Severe	No	Krepelovi et al. (1992a)
11–22	60	JH1	?	?	Severe	Yes	Antonarakis et al. (1985)
							Cutting et al. (1988)
							Woods-Samuels et al. (1991)
14–22	>36	H20	?	?	Severe	Yes	Nafa et al. (1990)
14–22	?	?	?	?	Severe	Yes	Lillicrap (unpublished results)
14–21	50	H229	<1	?	Severe	Yes	Millar et al. (1990)
Intron 13/exon 14 6.1		15‡	<1	?	Severe	No	Krepelova et al. (1992a)
Intron 13/exon 14 6.1		311‡	<1	?	Severe	Yes	Krepelova et al. (1992a)
Intron 13/exon 14 4.6		112	<1	?	Severe	Yes	Krepelova et al. (1992a)
14	12-16	194/513	<1	?	Severe	Yes	Higuchi et al. (1989)
14	6	?	<1	<0.1	Severe	Yes	Mikani et al. (1988b)
14	2.3–3.0	580	<1	?	Severe	No	Higuchi et al. (1989)
14	2.5	JH7	<1	<1	Severe	No	Youssoufian et al. (1987b)
							Woods-Samuels et al. (1991)
14	2.5	JH37	?	?	Severe	?	Woods-Samuels et al. (1991)
15–22	~50	5	<1	?	Severe	Yes	Reiner and Thompson (1992)
15–22	>15	H157	<1	<1	Severe	No	Michaelides et al. (unpublished results)
15–22	>19	RP308	<1	?	Severe	Yes	Figuerido et al. (unpublished results)
15–21	?	JH141	?	?	Severe	?	Higuchi et al. (1991b)
15–18	13	?	?	?	Severe	Yes	Camerino et al. (1986)
							Bardoni et al. (1988)
15	?	JH29	?	?	Severe	?	Antonarakis et al. (unpublished results)
16	>0.2	GLA11	1	?	Severe	No	Bidichandani et al. (unpublished results)
16–26	>95	?	<1	?	Severe	Yes	Figueiredo et al. (1992)
Intron 15/exon 16 0.304		HD10	<1	?	Severe	No	Schwaab et al. (1993)
17–19	?	1	?	?	Severe	No	Wehnert et al. (1989)
18,19†?	?	5	?	?	Severe	?	Grover et al. (1987)
19	1.9	OX27	<1	?	Severe	No	Naylor et al. (1993a)
19–21	47	H58	<1	?	Severe	Yes	Millar et al. (1990)
22	5.5	JH10	2-5	?	Moderate	No	Youssoufian et al. (1987b)
Intron 22†	?	2	?	?	Severe	No	Wehnert et al. (1989)

Table 3.2A Continued

Exon (s) deleted	See of deletion (kb)	Patient/ family	FVIII:C (u/dl)	FVIII:Ag (u/dl)	Severity	Inhibitors	References
Intron 22†	?	3	?	?	Moderate	No	Wehnert *et al.* (1989)
23–26	?	?	?	?	Severe	Yes	Din *et al.* (1986)
23–26	?	HA664	?	?	Severe	Yes	Lavergne *et al.* (1992)
23–25	>16	JH9	<1	<1	Severe	No	Youssoufian *et al.* (1987b)
23–25	39	H96	<1	?	Severe	Yes	Gitschier *et al.* (1985)
23–24	?	HA711	?	?	Moderate	No	Lavergne *et al.* (1992)
24–25	>3.4	JH8	<1	<1	Severe	No	Youssoufian *et al.* (1987b)
26	22	H51	<1	?	Severe	No	Gitschier *et al.* (1985)
26	>18	277	<1	?	Severe	No	Higuchi *et al.* (1989)
26	14	JH26	<1	<1	Severe	No	Youssoufian *et al.* (1988d)
26	8.7	?	?	?	Severe	?	Bernardi *et al.* (1989)
26	>2	H73	?	?	Severe	No	Nafa *et al.* (1990)
26	>2	?	?	?	Severe	No	Youssoufian *et al.* (1987c)
26	>2	H8	?	?	Severe	?	Bernardi *et al.* (1989a)
26	?	JH12	?	?	Severe	?	Antonarakis *et al.* (unpublished results)
26	?	HA364	?	?	Severe	No	Lavergne *et al.* (1992)
26	?	HA544	?	?	Severe	No	Lavergne *et al.* (1992)
26	?	HA599	?	?	Severe	No	Lavergne *et al.* (1992)
26	<10.5	RI620	<1	?	Severe	No	Figuerido *et al.* (1994)
26	?	HD12	<1	?	Severe	No	Schwaab *et al.* (1993)
part 26	?	HD11	<1	?	Severe	No	Schwaab *et al.* (1993)

*Not proven to be cause of disease phenotype, although segregates with disease allele.
†Precise extent unknown but includes at least region indicated
‡Patients related.

be seen, many defects (e.g. Val 162 → Met) occur in multiple reports: for the purposes of this summary any available data have been pooled from such reports to provide a summary entry. The online database should be consulted for details of individual cases, together with appropriate references.

SEQUENCE DELETIONS

FVIII gene deletions have been divided arbitrarily into large (>100 bp) and small (<100 bp), and are listed in Table 3.2A and Table 3.2B respectively. Full references may be found in the online database.

Large deletions

There are 80 unique large deletions reported in the database (Table 3.2A), from less than 1 kb up to more than 210 kb deleting the entire gene. The mechanism in most of these is probably non-homologous recombination (Woods-Samuels, Kazazian and Antonarakis, 1991), and is responsible for about 5% of severe hemophilia A cases. As might be expected, large deletions in the FVIII gene almost invariably give rise to clinically severe disease with no FVIII activity measurable in plasma samples and no antigen detected (where assays have been performed). Truncated proteins, if produced, are likely to be poorly expressed, inactive and/or rapidly cleared from the circulation. There are three reports of clinically merely moderate disease associated with deletions involving exons 22 (Youssoufian *et al.*, 1987) and exons 23–24 (Wehnert, Herrmann and Wulff, 1989; Lavergne *et al.*,

1992) and these may result from inframe splicing of mRNA to delete exon 22 or both 23 and 24 with subsequent secretion of hypoactive FVIII lacking 52 or 98 amino acids respectively. However, FVIII activity levels were measured in only one case (2–5%, deletion of exon 22; Youssoufian *et al.*, 1987) and FVIII:Ag levels were not reported.

There is a highly significant level of development of FVIII inhibitors in this group of patients (26 of 71 tested, 37%), although there is no obvious correlation between size of deletion and inhibitor status.

Small deletions

There are reports of 35 unique small (<100 bp) deletions in the database, varying in size from 1 to 86 bp: they are distributed fairly evenly through the exons and almost all are associated with severe disease. However, there are only two reports of FVIII inhibitors from 31 patients tested (6%) – a much lower proportion than that found in the large-deletion subgroup.

Most of these small deletions produce frameshifts and consequent abolition of FVIII expression, but there are a small number of interesting inframe deletions. Deletion of Phe652 by removal of a triplet of bases gives rise to reduced expression/stability of a hypofunctional FVIII molecule with severe bleeding (Lin, Lin and Shen, 1993), unfortunately this is the only inframe deletion where activity and antigen levels have been reported. Thus, deletion of 12 bases giving rise to removal of a 4-residue peptide sequence (339–342) causes severe disease, but whether from defective expression or

Table 3.2B   Small deletions in the factor VIII (FVIII) gene

Exon/ intron	Codons	Size in bp (nucleotides deleted)	Patient/ family	FVIII:C (u/dl)	FVIII:Ag (u/dl)	Severity	Inhibitors	Comments	References
Exon 1/Intron 1	14–29	86	RP451	<1	?	Severe	No	Includes IVSI donor splice site	Figueiredo *et al.* (1994)
Exon 2	48	2 (AA)	TWN49	<1	?	Severe	No	Frameshift	Lin *et al.* (1993)
Exon 2	50–51	4(GTTT)or(TTTG)	HD12	<1	?	Severe	No	Frameshift	Seehafer *et al.* (unpublished results)
Exon 3/Intron 3	104–111	23	JH72	?	?	Severe	?	Includes IVS3 donor splice site	Higuchi *et al.* (1991b)
Exon 3	103	2(GT)	HD13	<1	?	Severe	No	Frameshift	Seehafer *et al.* (unpublished results)
Exon 4	154–156	5(TACCT)	?	<1	?	Severe	?	Frameshift	Bidichandani *et al.* (1994b)
Exon 6	210–211	2 (AG)	TWN73	<1	?	Severe	No	Frameshift	Lin *et al.* (1993)
Exon 7	264	1 (T)	HD14	<1	?	Severe	No	Frameshift	Seehafer *et al.* (unpublished results)
Exon 7	283	1 (G)	HD15	<1	?	Severe	?	Frameshift	Seehafer *et al.* (unpublished results)
Exon 8	339–342	12(AATAATGAAGAA)	?	?	?	Severe	?	Deletes Asn Asn Glu Glu	Gitschier *et al.* (unpublished results)
Exon 8	339–342	12(AATAATGAAGAA)	?	?	?	Severe	?	Deletes Asn Asn Glu Glu	Kazazian *et al.* (unpublished results)
Exon 8	340–341	4(AATG)	H23	?	?	Severe	No	Frameshift	Kogan and Gitschier (1990)
Exon 8	341	2(GA)	JH31	?	?	Severe	?	Frameshift	Antonarakis *et al.* (unpublished results)
Exon 8	381–382	2(TT)	HD16	<1	?	Severe	No	Frameshift	Seehafer *et al.* (unpublished results)
Exon 9	412	1 (G)	TWN85	<1	?	Severe	No	Frameshift	Lin *et al.* (1993)
Exon 10	483–487	11(CCGTCCTTTGT)	TWN99	<1	?	Severe	No	Frameshift	Lin *et al.* (1993)
Exon 13	652/653	3(TTC)	JH155	1.4	12	Severe	No	Deletes Phe 652	Lin *et al.* (1993)
Exon 14	969	2 (AG)	TWN89	<1	?	Severe	No	Frameshift	Lin *et al.* (1993)
Exon 14	1164	2 (AA)	TWN79	<1	?	Severe	No	Frameshift	Lin *et al.* (1993)
Exon 14	1194	1 (A)	TWN40,51	<1	?	Severe	No	Frameshift	Lin *et al.* (1993)
Exon 14	1194	1 (A)	TWN107	<1	?	Severe	No	Frameshift	Lin *et al.* (1993)
Exon 14	1212	1 (C)	OX 11	<1	?	Severe	No	Frameshift	Naylor *et al.* (1993b)
Exon 14	1355–1356	4 (TAGA)	TWN90	<1	?	Severe	No	Frameshift	Lin *et al.* (1993)
Exon 14	1412–1414	5 (CTCTT)	Guine Bisao	1.0	?	Severe	No	Frameshift	David *et al.* (unpublished results)
Exon 14	1422–5	4(AAGA)	OX21	<1	?	Severe	No	Frameshift	Naylor *et al.* (1993b)
Exon 14	1439	1(A)	JH142	?	?	Severe	?	A8 → A7, Frameshift	Antonarakis *et al.* (unpublished results)
Exon 14	1439	1 (A)	OX32	<1	?	Severe	No	Frameshift	Naylor *et al.* (1993b)
Exon 14	1535–6	2(GA)	JH80	?	?	Severe	?	Frameshift	Higuchi *et al.* (1991b)
Exon 14	1601	1 (C)	TWN63	<1	?	Severe	No	Frameshift	Lin *et al.* (1993)
Exon 17	1880	1(C)	GLA6	<1	?	Severe	Yes	Frameshift	Bidichandani *et al.* (unpublished results)
Exon 18	1967–1968	1 (A)	HD17	<1	?	Severe	No	Frameshift	Seehafer *et al.* (unpublished results)
Exon 18	1967–1968	1(A)	HD18	<1	?	Severe	No	Frameshift	Seehafer *et al.* (unpublished results)
Exon 19	1998	1(G)	HD19	<1	?	Severe	Yes	Frameshift	Seehafer *et al.* (unpublished results)
Exon 23	2119	2	JH 148	?	?	?	?	Frameshift	Kazazian *et al.* (unpublished results)
Exon 23	2136	2 (AA)	JH69	?	?	Severe	?	A4 → A2, Frameshift	Antonarakis *et al.* (unpublished results)
Exon 24	2205	3 (CTC)	JH90	?	?	Moderate	No	Deletes Pro 2205	Economou *et al.* (1992)
Exon 24	2205	3(CTC)	JH91	?	?	Moderate	No	Deletes Pro 2205	Economou *et al.* (1992)
Exon 24	2205	3(CTC)	TWN104	<1	?	Severe	No	Deletes Pro 2205	Lin *et al.* (1993)
Exon 24	2214	1 (G)	HD20	<1	?	Severe	No	Frameshift	Seehafer *et al.* (unpublished results)
Exon 25	2246	2 (AG)	TWN23	<1	?	Severe	No	Frameshift	Lin *et al.* (1993)
Exon 26	2285–2287	5(AAATC)	HD21	<1	?	Severe	No	Frameshift	Seehafer *et al.* (unpublished results)

Table 3.3 Insertions in the factor VIII gene causing hemophilia A

Exon	Nature of insertion	Patient	FVIII:C	FVIII:Ag	Severity	Inhibitors	Reference
2	10 bp (TTCCATTCAA at codon 38)	TWN3,80,52,96	<1	?	Severe	?	Lin *et al.* (1993)
11	1 bp (G at codon 513)	JH100	?	?	Severe	?	Economou *et al.* (unpublished results)
12	3 bp (ATC at codon 613)	H775	<1	?	Severe	No	Lavergne *et al.* (unpublished results)
13	1 bp (A at codon 669)	HP50	<1	?	Severe	No	Seehafer *et al.* (unpublished results)
14	3.8 Kb LINE element	JH27	?	?	Severe	?	Kazazian *et al.* (1988)
14	2.1 Kb LINE element	JH28	?	?	Severe	Yes	Kazazian *et al.* (1988)
14	2 bp (AA at codon 1324)	TWN94	<1	?	Severe	?	Lin *et al.* (1993)
14	1 bp (A at codon 961)	OX 19	<1		Severe	No	Naylor *et al.* (1993b)
14	1 bp (TCA → TCAA at codon 1395)	JH77	<1	?	Severe	?	Higuchi *et al.* (1991b)
14	1 bp (A in stretch of 8 A residues at codons 1439-1441)	JH81	<1	?	Severe	?	Higuchi *et al.* (1991b)
14	1 bp (A in stretch of 8 A residues at codons 1439-1441)	Porto3	1.4	1.0	Severe	No	David *et al.* (1994)
14	1 bp (A at codon 1590)	TWN60	<1	?	Severe	?	Lin *et al.* (1993)
17	1 bp (T at codon 1855)	HP	<1	?	Severe	No	Schwaab *et al.* (unpublished results)
17	1 bp (A in stretch of 4 A residues in codon 1888)	JH129	?	?	Severe	?	Higuchi *et al.* (1991b)

function in coagulation is not known (Gitschier *et al.*, personal communication; Kazazian *et al.*, personal communication). Deletion of Pro2205 is associated in two cases with moderate hemophilia (Economou, Kazazian and Antonarakis, 1992) but in a third with severe disease (Lin, Lin and Shen, 1993), and in this last patient's plasma the FVIII activity was undetectable – the reason for this discrepancy in clinical phenotype is unknown.

SEQUENCE INSERTIONS

The hemophilia A database lists just 13 different insertions (Table 3.3) varying in size from 1 bp up to 2.1 kb and 3.8 Kb LINE elements (retrotransposon sequences found distributed throughout the genome in approximately 105 copies; Kazazian *et al.*, 1988). Most insertions are of 1 bp, often an A in a stretch of A residues. There are two cases reported of a single A insertion in such a stretch of 8 As (Higuchi *et al.*, 1991; David *et al.*, 1994) where a single A deletion has also been described (codons 1439–1441; Antonarakis *et al.*, personal communication). A 10 bp insertion in exon 2 was found to be a tandem duplication of existing sequence (Lin, Lin and Shen, 1993). All insertions are associated with severe disease and are either gross insertions or predicted frameshifts, save a 3 bp insertion at codon 613 in a patient with an unmeasurable FVIII: C level (Lavergne *et al.*, personal communication): unfortunately, no FVIII:Ag level was reported so it is not known whether this predicted variant protein is underexpressed or is inactive. Full references may be found in the online database.

Table 3.4 Hemophilia A – summary of different mutations reported

Exon	Point mutations			Deletions		
	Missense*	Nonsense	Splicing†	Small	Large	Insertions
1	5	1	1	1	–	–
2	1	–	–	2	–	1
3	9	–	1	2	–	–
4	8	2	1	1	–	–
5	2	–	2	–	–	–
6	–	–	2	1	–	–
7	13	1	1	2	–	–
8	11	3	–	4	–	–
9	3	1	–	1	–	–
10	5	–	–	1	–	–
11	10	1	2	–	–	1
12	7	1	1	–	–	1
13	4	1	–	1	–	1
14	15	4	–	10	–	7
15	5	–	1	–	–	–
16	10	2	1	–	–	–
17	6	1	–	1	–	2
18	7	4	–	1	–	–
19	2	–	–	1	–	–
20	–	–	–	–	–	–
21	2	–	–	–	–	–
22	5	1	–	–	–	–
23	9	1	–	2	–	–
24	4	1	–	2	–	–
25	3	1	1	1	–	–
26	6	1	–	1	–	–
Total	155	27	14	35	80	13

*Including 5 missense mutations which are predicted to affect splice junctions.

†In the case of intronic substutions, donor splice mutations are referred to the preceding exon while acceptor mutations are referred to the exon following.

DETECTION OF FVIII MUTATIONS

The introduction of the PCR (Saiki *et al.*, 1988) for the specific amplification *in vitro* of short stretches of DNA has revolutionized analysis of patient DNA for mutations (see Table 3.4). Genomic DNA may be derived from a hemophilic subject, for example by extraction from white blood cells, then all the exons including splice junctions may be amplified by use of sequence-specific DNA primers. The amplified stretches can then be directly sequenced to indicate the presence of any of the defects described above. There are however two problems with this approach when analyzing the FVIII gene: first, the large size of the coding region – 26 exons with over 9 kb of coding sequence to be searched, and second, this strategy may not detect gene rearrangements where the exonic sequence is unaltered (see above). These and other considerations have led to the adoption of other strategies which, while still dependent on PCR, give faster and easier identification of the defects. For missense/polymorphism detection, a variety of gel-based prescreening methods have been used to target a particular exon for sequencing (for a detailed review, see Michaelides *et al.*, 1995), while non-deletional rearrangements may be detected by Southern blotting using a probe corresponding to the *F8A* region of intron 22 (Lakich *et al.*, 1993).

Structure–function relationships of altered FVIII molecules in CRM+ve hemophilia A

In the case of predicted single amino-acid substitutions, two broad categories of phenotype are found:

1. Cases (CRM-reduced or CRM–ve) in which plasma FVIII antigen is reduced concomitantly with activity, presumably as a result of a coagulation-normal protein being either poorly expressed or more rapidly cleared from the circulation than normal: the ways in which the substitutions produce this phenotype are unknown in all cases.
2. Approximately normal circulating levels of FVIII antigen with reduced or absent FVIII:C activity (CRM+ve). From the standpoint of an understanding of the structure–function relationships of the molecule in coagulation, it is primarily this latter CRM+ve group that is of interest. Unfortunately, the CRM status is only reported in 72 of the 155 single amino-acid substitutions in the database, and of these, the majority are found to be CRM–ve. Of the remainder, the defect is broadly understood in a small number only. Mutations at or after critical Arg residues at thrombin cleavage sites (residues 372/373 and 1689/1690) have been shown to render the molecule resistant to thrombin activation resulting in reduced coagulant activity (Shima *et al.*, 1989; Gitschier *et al.*,

1988; Pattinson *et al.*, 1990; Higuchi *et al.*, 1990; Schwaab *et al.*, 1991; Arai *et al.*, 1989, 1990; O'Brien, Pattinson and Tuddenham, 1990; O'Brien and Tuddenham, 1989; Johnson *et al.*, 1994); mutation of a Tyr residue at 1680 (to Phe) which when sulfated forms part of a binding site for carrier vWf is a frequently reported defect resulting in low plasma FVIII antigen levels with even lower activity (e.g. Higuchi *et al.*, 1991); and there are two predicted new N-glycosylation sites created by mutations I566T and M1772T which result in normal circulating antigen levels with grossly reduced or absent activity (Aly *et al.*, 1992; Tuddenham *et al.*, personal communication); deglycosylation of the plasma FVIII restored some coagulant activity.

Detailed understanding on a molecular level of how substitutions result in dysfunctional FVIII will have to remain in abeyance until a three-dimensional molecular structure is available. It would be expected that in some cases defective interaction with one of the ligands of FVIII (factor IXa, phospholipid membrane, divalent cations) will be responsible for reduced functional activity.

References

Aly, A.M., Higuchi, M., Kasper, C.K., Kazazian, H.H., Jr., Antonarakis, S.E. and Hoyer, L.W. (1992) Hemophilia A due to mutations that create new N-glycosylation sites. *Proc. Natl. Acad. Sci. USA* **89**, 4933–4937.

Antonarakis, S.E., Kazazian, H.H., Jr. and Tuddenham, E.G.D. (1995) Molecular etiology of factor VIII deficiency in hemophilia A. *Hum. Mutat.* **5**, 1–22.

Arai, M., Inaba, H., Higuchi, M., Antonarakis, S.E., Kazazian, H.H., Jr., Fujimaki, M. and Hoyer, L.W. (1989) Direct characterization of factor VIII in plasma: detection of a mutation altering a thrombin cleavage site (arginine-372 → histidine). *Proc. Natl. Acad. Sci. USA* **86**, 4277–4281.

Arai, M., Higuchi, M., Antonarakis, S.E., Kazazian, H.H., Jr., Phillips, J.A., Janco, R.L. and Hoyer, L.W. (1990) Characterization of a thrombin cleavage site mutation (Arg 1689 to Cys) in the factor VIII gene of two unrelated patients with cross-reacting material-positive hemophilia A. *Blood* **75**, 384–389.

Bontempo, F.A., Lewis, J.H., Gorenc, T.J., Spero, J.A., Ragni, M.V., Scott, J.P. and Starzl, T.E. (1987) Liver transplantation in hemophilia A. *Blood* **69**, 1721–1724.

Curtis, J.E., Helgerson, S.L., Parker, E.T. and Lollar, P. (1994) Isolation and characterization of thrombin-activated human factor VIII. *J. Biol. Chem.* **269**, 6246–6251.

David, D., Moreira, I., Lalloz, M.R., Rosa, H.A., Schwaab, R., Morais, S., Diniz, M.J., de Deus, G., Campos, M., Lavinha, J., Johnson, D. and Tuddenham, E.G.D. (1994) Analysis of the essential sequences of the factor VIII gene in twelve hemophilia A patients by single-stranded conformation polymorphism. *Blood Coagul. Fibrinolysis* **5**, 257–264.

Dorner, A.J., Bole, D.G. and Kaufman, R.J. (1987) The relationship of N-linked glycosylation and heavy chain-binding protein association with the secretion of glycoproteins. *J. Cell Biol.* **105**, 2665–2674.

Eaton, D., Rodriguez, H. and Vehar, G.A. (1986) Proteolytic processing of human factor VIII. Correlation of specific cleavages by thrombin, factor Xa, and activated protein C with activation and inactivation of factor VIII coagulant activity. *Biochemistry* **25**, 505–512.

Economou, E.P., Kazazian, H.H., Jr. and Antonarakis, S.E. (1992) Detection of mutations in the factor VIII gene using single-stranded conformational polymorphism (SSCP). *Genomics* **13**, 909–911.

Fay, P.J., Haidaris, P.J. and Huggins, C.F. (1993) Role of the COOH-terminal acidic region of A1 subunit in A2 subunit retention in human factor VIIIa. *J. Biol. Chem.* **268**, 17861–17866.

Freije, D. and Schlessinger, D. (1992) A 1.6-Mb contig of yeast artificial chromosomes around the human factor VIII gene reveals three regions homologous to probes for the DXS115 locus and two for the DXYS64 locus. *Am. J. Hum. Genet.* **51**, 66–80.

Gitschier, J., Wood, W.I., Goralka, T.M., Wion, K.L., Chen, E.Y., Eaton, D.H., Vehar, G.A., Capon, D.J. and Lawn, R.M. (1984) Characterization of the human factor VIII gene. *Nature* **312**, 326–330.

Gitschier, J., Kogan, S., Levinson, B. and Tuddenham, E.G. (1988) Mutations of factor VIII cleavage sites in hemophilia A. *Blood* **72**, 1022–1028.

Higuchi, M., Wong, C., Kochhan, L., Olek, K., Aronis, S., Kasper, C.K., Kazazian, H.H., Jr. and Antonarakis, S.E. (1990) Characterization of mutations in the factor VIII gene by direct sequencing of amplified genomic DNA. *Genomics* **6**, 65–71.

Higuchi, M., Kazazian, H.H., Jr., Kasch, L., Warren, T.C., McGinniss, M.J., Phillips, J.A., Kasper, C., Janco, R. and Antonarakis, S.E. (1991) Molecular characterization of severe hemophilia A suggests that about half the mutations are not within the coding regions and splice junctions of the factor VIII gene. *Proc. Natl. Acad. Sci. USA* **88**, 7405–7409.

Hill-Eubanks, D.C., Parker, C.G. and Lollar, P. (1989) Differential proteolytic activation of factor VIII-von Willebrand factor complex by thrombin. *Proc. Natl. Acad. Sci. USA* **86**, 6508–6512.

Johnson, D.J., Pemberton, S., Acquila, M., Mori, P.G., Tuddenham, E.G. and O'Brien, D.P. (1994) Factor VIII S373L: mutation at P1' site confers thrombin cleavage resistance, causing mild hemophilia A. *Thromb. Hemost.* **71**, 428–433.

Johnson, J.D., Edman, J.C. and Rutter, W.J. (1993) A receptor tyrosine kinase found in breast carcinoma cells has an extracellular discoidin I-like domain [published erratum appears in *Proc Natl. Acad. Sci USA* 1993 Nov. 15; 90(22):10891]. *Proc. Natl. Acad. Sci. USA* **90**, 5677–5681.

Kane, W.H. and Davie, E.W. (1986) Cloning of a cDNA coding for human factor V, a blood coagulation factor homologous to factor VIII and ceruloplasmin. *Proc. Natl. Acad. Sci. USA* **83**, 6800–6804.

Kaufman, R.J., Wasley, L.C. and Dorner, A.J. (1988) Synthesis, processing, and secretion of recombinant human factor VIII expressed in mammalian cells. *J. Biol. Chem.* **263**, 6352–6362.

Kazazian, H.H., Jr., Wong, C., Youssoufian, H., Scott, A.F., Phillips, D.G. and Antonarakis, S.E. (1988) Hemophilia A resulting from de novo insertion of L1 sequences represents a novel mechanism for mutation in man. *Nature* **332**, 164–166.

Kazazian, H.H., Jr., Tuddenham, E.G.D. and Antonarakis, S.E. (1995) Hemophilia A and parahemophilia: deficiencies of coagulation factors VIII and V. In *The Metabolic and Molecular Bases of Inherited Disease* (VIIth Edition, Eds. Scriver, Beaudet, Sly and Valle), McGraw-Hill, New York, pp. 3241–3267.

Koeberl, D.D., Halbert, C.L., Krumm, A. and Miller, A.D. (1995) Sequences within the coding regions of clotting factor VIII and CFTR block transcriptional elongation. *Hum. Gen. Ther.* **6**, 469–479.

Koschinsky, M.L., Funk, W.D., van Oost, B.A. and MacGillivray, R.T. (1986) Complete cDNA sequence of human preceruloplasmin. *Proc. Natl. Acad. Sci. USA* **83**, 5086–5090.

Lakich, D., Kazazian, H.H., Jr., Antonarakis, S.E. and Gitschier, J. (1993) Inversions disrupting the factor VIII gene are a common cause of severe hemophilia A. *Nat. Genet.* **5**, 236–241.

Lavergne, J.M., Bahnak, B.R., Vidaud, M., Laurian, Y. and Meyer, D. (1992) A directed search for mutations in hemophilia A using restriction enzyme analysis and denaturing gradient gel electrophoresis. A study of seven exons in the factor VIII gene of 170 cases. *Nouv. Rev. Fr. Hematol.* **34**, 85–91.

Levinson, B., Kenwrick, S., Lakich, D., Hammonds, G., Jr. and Gitschier, J. (1990) A transcribed gene in an intron of the human factor VIII gene. *Genomics* **7**, 1–11.

Levinson, B., Kenwrick S., Gamel, P., Fisher, K. and Gitschier, J. (1992) Evidence for a third transcript from the human factor VIII gene. *Genomics* **14**, 585–589.

Leyte, A., van Schijndel, H.B., Niehrs, C., Huttner, W.B., Verbeet, M.P., Mertens, K. and van Mourik, J.A. (1991) Sulfation of Tyr1680 of human blood coagulation factor VIII is essential for the interaction of factor VIII with von Willebrand factor. *J. Biol. Chem.* **266**, 740–746.

Lin, S.W., Lin, S.R. and Shen, M.C. (1993) Characterization of genetic defects of hemophilia A in patients of Chinese origin. *Genomics* **18**, 496–504.

Mann, K.G., Nesheim, M.E., Church, W.R., Haley, P. and Krishnaswamy, S. (1990) Surface-dependent reactions of the vitamin K-dependent enzyme complexes. *Blood* **76**, 1–16.

Marquette, K.A., Pittman, D.D. and Kaufman, R.J. (1995) A 110-amino acid region within the A1-domain of coagulation factor VIII inhibits secretion from mammalian cells. *J. Biol. Chem.* **270**, 10297–10303.

Michaelides, K., Schwaab, R., Lalloz, M.R.A., Schmidt, W. and Tuddenham, E.G.D. (1995) Mutational analysis: new mutations. In *PCR II – A Practical Approach* (IRL Press, Oxford. Chap. 13) pp. 255–288.

Munro, S. and Pelham, H.R. (1986) An Hsp70-like protein in the ER: identity with the 78 kd glucose-regulated protein and immunoglobulin heavy chain binding protein. *Cell* **46**, 291–300.

Naylor, J.A., Green, P.M., Rizza, C.R. and Giannelli, F. (1992) Factor VIII gene explains all cases of hemophilia A. *Lancet* **340**, 1066–1067.

Naylor, J.A., Brinke, A., Hassock, S., Green, P.M. and Giannelli, F. (1993) Characteristic mRNA abnormality found in half the patients with severe hemophilia A is due to large DNA inversions. *Hum. Mol. Genet.* **2**, 1773–1778.

O'Brien, D.P., Pattinson, J.K. and Tuddenham, E.G. (1990) Purification and characterization of factor VIII 372-Cys: a hypofunctional cofactor from a patient with moderately severe hemophilia A. *Blood* **75**, 1664–1672.

O'Brien, D.P., Johnson, D., Byfield, P. and Tuddenham, E.G. (1992) Inactivation of factor VIII by factor IXa. *Biochemistry* **31**, 2805–2812.

O'Brien, D.P. and Tuddenham, E.G. (1989) Purification and characterization of factor VIII 1,689-Cys: a nonfunctional cofactor occurring in a patient with severe hemophilia A. *Blood* **73**, 2117–2122.

Pattinson, J.K., Millar, D.S., McVey, J.H., Grundy, C.B., Wieland, K., Mibashan, R.S., Martinowitz, U., Tan Un, K., Vidaud, M., Goossens, M., Sampietro, M., Mannucci, P.M., Krawczak M., Reiss, J., Zoll, B., Whitmore, D., Bowcock S., Wensley, R., Ajani, A., Mitchell, V., Rizza, C., Maia, R., Winter, P., Mayne, E.E., Schwartz, M., Green, P.J., Kakkar, V.V., Tuddenham, E.G.D. and Cooper, D.N. (1990) The molecular genetic analysis of hemophilia A: a directed search strategy for the detection of point mutations in the human factor VIII gene. *Blood* **76**, 2242–2248.

Pittman, D.D., Wang, J.H. and Kaufman, R.J. (1992) Identification and functional importance of tyrosine sulfate residues within recombinant factor VIII. *Biochemistry* **31**, 3315–3325.

Pittman, D.D. and Kaufman, R.J. (1988) Proteolytic requirements for thrombin activation of anti-hemophilic factor (factor VIII). *Proc. Natl. Acad. Sci. USA* **85**, 2429–2433.

Poustka, A., Dietrich, A., Langenstein, G., Toniolo, D., Warren, S.T. and Lehrach, H. (1991) Physical map of human Xq27-qter: localizing the region of the fragile X mutation. *Proc. Natl. Acad. Sci. USA* **88**, 8302–8306.

Rossiter, J.P., Young, M., Kimberland, M.L., Hutter, P., Ketterling, R.P., Gitschier, J., Horst, J., Morris, M.A., Schaid, D.J., de Moerloose, P., Sommer, S.S., Kazazian, H.H. and Antonarakis, S.E. (1994) Factor VIII gene inversions causing severe hemophilia A originate almost exclusively in male germ cells. *Hum. Mol. Genet.* **3**, 1035–1039.

Rotblat, F., Goodall, A.H., O'Brien, D.P., Rawlings, E., Middleton, S. and Tuddenham, E.G.D. (1983) Monoclonal antibodies to human procoagulant factor VIII. *J. Lab. Clin. Med.* **101**, 736–746.

Saiki, R.K., Gelfand, D.H., Stoffel, S., Scharf, S.J., Higuchi, R., Horn, G.T., Mullis, K.B. and Erlich, H.A. (1988) Primer-directed enzymatic amplification of DNA with a thermostable DNA polymerase. *Science* **239**, 487–491.

Schwaab, R., Ludwig, M., Kochhan, L., Oldenburg, J., McVey, J.H., Egli, H., Brackmann, H.H. and Olek K. (1991) Detection and characterisation of two missense mutations at a cleavage site in the factor VIII light chain. *Thromb. Res.* **61**, 225–234.

Shima, M., Ware, J., Yoshioka, A., Fukui, H. and Fulcher, C.A. (1989) An arginine to cysteine amino acid substitution at a critical thrombin cleavage site in a dysfunctional factor VIII molecule. *Blood* **74**, 1612–1617.

Stubbs, J.D., Lekutis, C., Singer, K.L., Bui, A., Yuzuki, D., Srinivasan, U. and Parry, G. (1990) cDNA cloning of a mouse mammary epithelial cell surface protein reveals the existence of epidermal growth factor-like domains linked to factor VIII-like sequences. *Proc. Natl. Acad. Sci. USA* **87**, 8417–8421.

Tuddenham, E.G., Schwaab, R., Seehafer, J., Millar, D.S., Gitschier, J., Higuchi, M., Bidichandani, S., Connor, J.M., Hoyer, L.W., Yoshioka, A., Peake, I.R., Olek, K., Kazazian, H.H., Lavergne, J.-M., Giannelli, F., Antonarakis, S.E. and Cooper, D.N. (1994) Hemophilia A: database of nucleotide substitutions, deletions, insertions and rearrangements of the factor VIII gene, second edition. *Nucleic. Acids. Res.* **22**, 4851–4868.

van Dieijen, G., Tans, G., Rosing, J. and Hemker, H.C. (1981) The role of phospholipid and factor VIIIa in the activation of bovine factor X. *J. Biol. Chem.* **256**, 3433–3442.

Vehar, G.A., Keyt, B., Eaton, D., Rodriguez, H., O'Brien, D.P., Rotblat, F., Oppermann, H., Keck R., Wood, W.I., Harkins, R.N., Tuddenham, E.G.D., Lawn, R.M. and Capon, D.J. (1984) Structure of human factor VIII. *Nature* **312**, 337–342.

Walker, F.J., Chavin, S.I. and Fay, P.J. (1987) Inactivation of factor VIII by activated protein C and protein S. *Arch. Biochem. Biophys.* **252**, 322–328.

Wehnert, M., Herrmann, F.H. and Wulff, K. (1989) Partial deletions of factor VIII gene as molecular diagnostic markers in hemophilia A. *Dis. Markers* **7**, 113–117.

Wion, K.L., Kelly, D., Summerfield, J.A., Tuddenham, E.G.D. and Lawn, R.M. (1985) Distribution of factor VIII mRNA and antigen in human liver and other tissues. *Nature* **317**, 726–729.

Woods-Samuels, P., Kazazian, H.H., Jr. and Antonarakis, S.E. (1991) Non-homologous recombination in the human genome: deletions in the human factor VIII gene. *Genomics* **10**, 94–101.

Youssoufian, H., Antonarakis, S.E., Aronis, S., Tsiftis, G., Phillips, D.G. and Kazazian, H.H. (1987) Characterization of five partial deletions of the factor VIII gene. *Proc. Natl. Acad. Sci. USA* **84**, 3772–3776.

Zelechowska, M.G., van Mourik J.A. and Brodniewicz-Proba, T. (1985) Ultrastructural localization of factor VIII procoagulant antigen in human liver hepatocytes. *Nature* **317**, 729–731.

4 THE MOLECULAR BIOLOGY OF HEMOPHILIA B

H. R. Roberts and D. K. Liles

The blood-clotting protein, factor IX, was first described in 1952, at which time virtually nothing was known about the factor IX gene nor the genetic defects in the protein that led to hemophilia B (Aggeler *et al.*, 1952; Biggs *et al.*, 1952). Since that time, however, there has been incredible progress in our understanding of the molecular biology of all the blood coagulation proteins, but in particular the molecular biology of factor IX and the molecular defects that lead to hemophilia B. In the recent hemophilia B database, 476 unique molecular events are recorded and these do not include large deletions and insertions (Giannelli *et al.*, 1994). The purpose of this chapter is to review first, the basic organization of the factor IX gene; second, the gene product and its function; and third, the genetic defects in each region of the gene and how these defects result in hemophilia B of varying degrees of severity. At the end of the chapter, an abbreviated list of the known molecular defects in hemophilia B will be listed so as to give the reader an idea of the enormous genetic diversity that leads to the limited phenotypic expression of this hereditary bleeding disorder.

The gene

The factor IX gene is located on the long arm of the X chromosome at position 27.1, as shown in Figure 4.1 (Chance *et al.*, 1983; Kurachi *et al.*, 1993). The location of other genes such as the factor VIII and fragile X site are also depicted (Purrello *et al.*, 1985). The factor IX gene is comprised of 33 kb arranged into 8 exons and 7 intervening sequences (introns; Anson, Choo and Rees, 1984; Yoshitake *et al.*, 1985). The entire gene, including the introns, has been sequenced and several polymorphisms have been described. These are listed in Table 4.1 and have been helpful in family studies and carrier detection of hemophilia B (McGraw *et al.*, 1985; Hay *et*

al., 1986; Winship *et al.*, 1984; Driscoll *et al.*, 1988; Winship, Rees and Alkan, 1989). The alanine–threonine polymorphism at position 148 of the factor IX protein was the first one to be described and was later referred to as the Malmo mutation (Wallmark *et al.*, 1991).

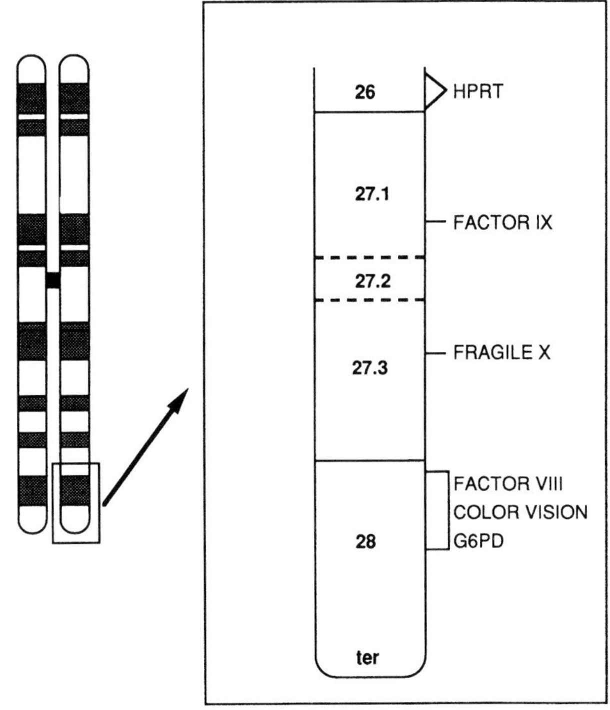

Fig. 4.1 Schematic representation of the X chromosome. The gene for factor IX is located on the long arm at position 27.1. The location of the fragile X gene and the factor VIII gene are shown for the purpose of orientation. Hypoxanthine-guanine phosphoribosyl transferase (HPRT) = G6PD = glucose-6-phosphate dehydrogenase. From Roberts, H.R. (1993) Molecular biology of hemophilia B. *Thrombosis and Haemostasis*, 70, 1–9, and reproduced with permission.

Hemophilia. Edited by C.D. Forbes, L. Aledort and R. Madhok. Published in 1997 by Chapman & Hall, London. ISBN 0 412 63820 7

Table 4.1   Polymorphisms in or near the human factor IX gene

Polymorphism	Location	Gene frequency of minor allele	
		In Caucasian population	In American black population
Ala/Thr dimorphism in activation peptide	Amino acid 148 in mature protein	0.33	0.03–0.15
Taq I	Intron D	0.29–0.35	0.14
Xmn I	Intron C	0.29	0.12
Hinf I/Dde I	Intron A	0.24	0.36
Hha I	8 kb 3′ to exon 8	0.39	
Msp I	Intron D	0.22	0.39
5′ Bam HI	5′ flanking sequence	0.06	0.48
Bam HI	Intron B	0	0.13

Updated and modified from High, A.K. and Roberts, H.R. (eds) (1995) *Molecular Basis of Thrombosis and Hemostasis*, Marcel Dekker, New York, p. 222, reprinted with permission.

A schematic representation of the factor IX gene, the messenger RNA (mRNA) and the resulting gene product is shown in Figure 4.2. The gene contains a promoter region, and regions that encode the signal peptide and propeptide as well as regions that encode the various domains of the protein product, namely a domain that contains 12 γ-carboxyglutamic acid residues (the Gla domain characteristic of all vitamin K-dependent clotting factors), two epidermal growth factor-like domains (EGF-1 and EGF-2), an activation peptide, and a catalytic domain that contains the catalytic triad of histidine[221], aspartic acid[269] and serine[365]. Figure 4.2 depicts the relative positions of the domain structures and the arginyl residues at positions 145 and 180 that define the activation peptide. The amino-terminal amino acid of the mature protein is tyrosine, while the carboxy-terminal

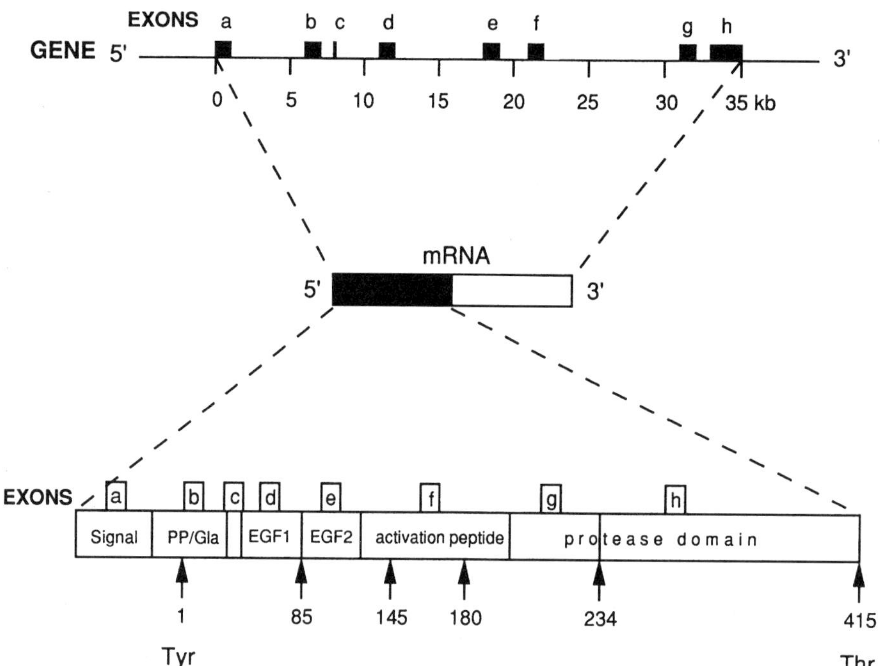

Fig. 4.2 The factor IX gene, messenger RNA and resulting protein product. Note that the exons roughly encode a particular domain, such that exon a encodes the signal peptide, exon b encodes the propeptide and Gla domains, exon c encodes the aromatic stack region connecting the Gla and the epidermal growth factor-like (EGF-1) domains, exon d encodes the first EGF domain, exon e encodes the second EGF domain, exon f encodes the activation peptide, and exon g and h together encode the catalytic (protease) domain. From Roberts, H.R. (1993) Molecular biology of hemophilia B. *Thrombosis and Haemostasis*, **70**, 1–9, and reproduced with permission.

amino acid is threonine. Notice that each exon roughly codes the domains described above (Fig. 4.2).

The molecular defects

Identification of the molecular defects responsible for hemophilia B did not begin until 1983 when Noyes and colleagues reported the defect in factor IX Chapel Hill (Noyes *et al.*, 1983) This variant has a histidine substitution for arginine at position 145. The amino acid bond between the Arg145 and the Ala146 is cleaved in normal factor IX during activation by factor XIa. The histidine substitution at position 145 prevents this cleavage and results in a mild form of hemophilia B.

Since 1983 there has been a rapid increase in the number of mutations that lead to factor IX deficiency. In the 1994 database, more than 476 distinct molecular defects have been reported to result in hemophilia B (Giannelli *et al.*, 1994). There have now been reports of mutations in all regions of the factor IX gene. Many of the mutations have been noted to occur at CG doublets, resulting in a C → T or a G → A transition (Koeberl *et al.*, 1989). This occurs because the cytosine is often methylated, making it unstable and susceptible to deamination. With deamination, the methylated cytosine is converted to thymine. Since thymidme is a normal nucleotide it is not repaired and a mutation results. CG doublets appear to be 'hotspots' for mutations and this may explain the high number of sporadic mutations that account for about one-third of the cases of hemophilia B. Some of the more frequent repeat mutations do not involve CG doublets but are due to a founder effect (Sommer, 1992; Thompson *et al.*, 1990).

The factor IX promoter region

THE NORMAL PROMOTER REGION

Figure 4.3 depicts the promoter region of the factor IX gene. Promoters are regions of the gene which bind RNA polymerase and are therefore near the start site of transcription. Regulation of transcription occurs in the promoter region. Regulation can be mediated by *cis*-acting agents, which are endogenous DNA sequences, or by *trans*-acting elements. *Trans*-acting elements are exogenous factors which bind to the promoter region and regulate transcription (Gill and Tijian, 1992). In the factor IX promoter, several *trans*-acting factors have been identified, including hepatic nuclear factor 4 (HNF-4), the CCAAT/enhancer binding protein (C/EBP), an unidentified protein (??), the D-site binding protein (DBP), and the nuclear factor 1-liver (NF-1L).

MUTATIONS IN THE PROMOTER REGION

Table 4.2 contains a list of representative mutations in the promoter region with the typical phenotypic characteristics. Substitutions in the promoter region of factor IX have classically resulted in the factor IX Leyden phenotype. This phenotype was first described in 1970 by Veltkamp and colleagues. Subsequently, 15 distinct mutations have been reported in this area (Giannelli *et al.*, 1994). Most patients with this phenotype have a severe hemorrhagic disorder and lack factor IX antigen and activity at birth. At puberty, however, there is a gradual increase in factor IX levels at a rate of 4–5% per year until the patient reaches about age 20 (Briet *et al.*, 1982). The increase in circulating factor IX is coincident with alleviation of the hemophilic condition.

The Leyden phenotype has been attributed to a number of mutations, involving many of the *trans*-acting elements mentioned previously (Crossley and Brownlee, 1990; Picketts, Lillicrap and Mueller, 1993; Reijnen *et al.*, 1992). In 1986, Briet and colleagues were able to induce factor IX expression in a prepubertal boy by the use of exogenous steroids, including testosterone (Briet, Wijnands and Veltkamp, 1986). Since then, Crossley and colleagues (1992) have suggested the existence of a so-called androgen-responsive element in the promoter

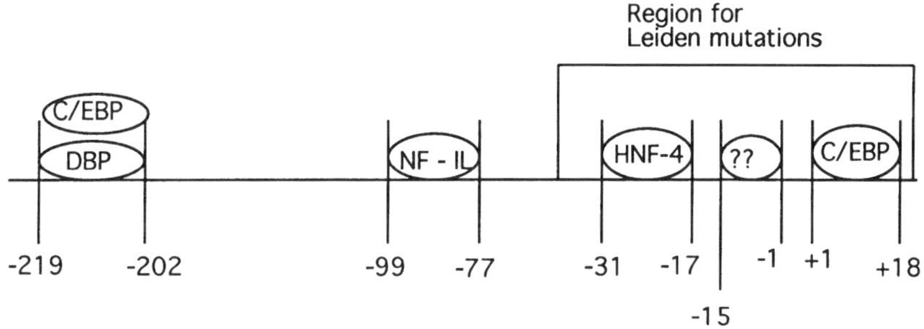

Fig. 4.3 Schematic representation of the factor IX promoter region. The region in which mutations result in the Leiden (Leyden) phenotype of hemophilia B is shown. This region binds *trans*-acting agents, including the hepatic nuclear factor-4 (HNF-4), the CCAAT/enhancer-binding protein (C/EBP), and an unknown protein (??) DBP = D-site binding protein; NF–1L = nuclear factor 1-liver. Updated and modified from High, K.H. and Roberts, H.R. (1995) Factor IX, in: *Molecular Basis of Thrombosis and Hemostasis* (eds K.H. High and H.R. Roberts), Marcel Dekker, New York, and reproduced with permission.

Table 4.2   Mutations in the promoter region of the factor IX gene

Nucleotide substitution	Nucleotide change	FIX%	FIX antigen	Comments
−26	G→C	<1	<1	Mutation in androgen-responsive element and HNF-4 site. FIX activity **fails** to rise after puberty*
−21	T→G	<1-70		Disruption of HNF-4-binding site; FIX activity increases after puberty
−20	T→A	<1−>60	<1−>60	FIX activity increases after puberty
−20	T→C	9		FIX activity increases after puberty
−6	G→A	13–70		FIX activity increases after puberty
−5	A→T	3		FIX activity increases after puberty
−6	T→A	<2−>20		FIX activity increases after puberty
8	T→C	1–32		C/EBP binding site; FIX clotting activity increases after puberty
13	A→G	<1−>60	<1−>60	C/EBP binding site; FIX clotting activity increases after puberty
13	Delete 1	<1−>60	<1−>60	C/EBP binding site; FIX clotting activity increases after puberty
13	A→C	<1		C/EBP binding site

HNF-4 = Hepatic nuclear factor 4; FIX = factor IX; C/EBP = CCAAT/enhancer-binding protein.
*Disrupts binding of both HNF-4 and an unidentified protein-binding site that overlaps the HNF-4 site.
Updated and modified from Roberts, H.R. (1993) Molecular biology of hemophilia B. *Thrombosis and Haemostasis*, **70**, 1–9, and reprinted with permission.

region corresponding to a region in the vicinity of the HNF-4-binding site. This would include the mutations at −20 and −21. However, there is a mutation at −26 which does not result in the Leyden phenotype, in that there is no change in the hemophilic condition after puberty. This mutation probably disrupts an androgen-responsive element close to the HNF-4-binding site, as well as the binding site of an as yet unidentified protein which overlaps the HNF-4 region. Although there have been several hypotheses explaining the Leyden phenotype, none of them can adequately explain how changes at puberty interact with the promoter region to induce an increase in factor IX clotting and antigenic activity.

The signal peptide

THE NORMAL SIGNAL PEPTIDE

The signal peptide serves to guide the protein through the endoplasmic reticulum for proper processing, including glycosylation and protein folding. The exact length of the signal peptide is still unknown since there are three potential start sites for transcription in the factor IX gene. These potential start sites are located at positions −46, −41, and −39 relative to the start site of the mature factor IX protein. In the endoplasmic reticulum the signal peptide is cleaved from the immature protein by the signal peptidase between the Cys[19] and the Thre[18].

MUTATIONS IN THE SIGNAL PEPTIDE

Five distinct mutations have presently been documented in the signal peptide, not including frameshift mutations,

as shown in Figure 4.4 (Giannelli *et al.*, 1994). Table 4.3 lists representative mutations in the signal peptide of factor IX. Notice that most of these result in severe hemophilia B with a marked decrease in factor IX antigen. It is likely that mutations in this region result in an unstable protein that is not expressed. One exception is the substitution of an arginyl for a cysteine residue at position −19, which results in a mild phenotype with a factor IX activity of 20% (Bottema *et al.*, 1991).

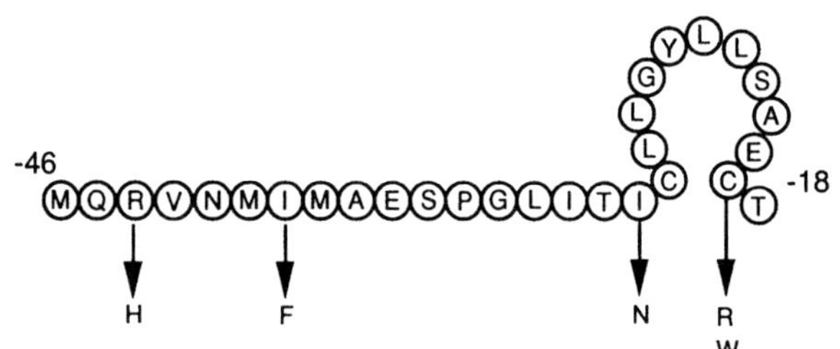

Fig. 4.4 The normal signal peptide, including amino acids −46 to −19. The mutations resulting in amino acid substitutions are represented by the arrows. Mutations resulting from gross gene deletions or insertions and frameshift mutations are not depicted. Mutations have been described at the −19 cysteine residue, which is the location of cleavage site of the signal peptidase. In these and subsequent figures, amino acids are designated by a single letter. A = Alanine; C = Cysteine; D = Aspartic acid; E = Glutamic acid; F = Phenylalanine; G = Glycine; H = Histidine; I = Isoleucine; K = Lysine; L = Leucine; M = Methionine; N = Asparagine; P = Proline; Q = Glutamine; R = Arginine; S = Serine; T = Threonine; V = Valine; W = Tryptophan; Y = Tyrosine. Updated and modified from Roberts, H.R. (1993) Molecular biology of hemophilia B. *Thrombosis and Haemostasis*, **70**, 1–9, and reproduced with permission.

Table 4.3 Mutations in the signal peptide region of the factor IX

Nucleotide substitution	Amino acid change	FIX%	FIX antigen
79: T→A	−30: I → N	2	<1
111: T→C	−19: C → R	20	
112: Delete 1	−19: Frameshift	<1	
113: T→G	−19: C → W	<5	<10

FIX = Factor IX.
Reprinted from Roberts, H.R. (1993) Molecular biology of hemophilia B, *Thrombosis and Haemostasis*, **70**, with permission.

The propeptide region

THE NORMAL PROPEPTIDE REGION

The propeptide, including amino acid residues −18 to −1, is necessary for intracellular recognition of the nascent factor IX protein by the vitamin K-dependent carboxylase recently isolated and characterized by Wu and colleagues (Wu, Morris and Stafford, 1991; Wu *et al.*, 1991). This intracellular reaction results in posttranslational modification of 12 amino-terminal glutamyl residues, resulting in the formation of γ-carboxyglutamic acid (Gla) residues. The exact mechanism by which the propeptide interacts with the carboxylase enzyme is not yet understood, although residues at positions −18, −17, −16, −15 and −10 in the propeptide are essential for post-translational modification (Foster *et al.*, 1987; Jorgensen *et al.*, 1987; Huber *et al.*, 1990; Morris *et al.*, 1993; Rabiet *et al.*, 1987). These residues are apparently critical for the necessary conformation of the molecule at the intracellular site of carboxylation. The propeptide is cleaved from the protein prior to secretion of the mature molecule into the circulation. If the propeptide is not cleaved, the protein cannot be activated and does not bind to membrane surfaces (Bristol *et al.*, 1994).

MUTATIONS OF THE PROPEPTIDE REGION

A schematic representation of the mutations affecting the propeptide is shown in Figure 4.5. Table 4.4 lists some of the common mutations in this region. The most frequently affected residue in this region is the −4 arginine, which has three documented different amino acid substitutions in more than 50 patients reported in the database (Giannelli *et al.*, 1994). At least two variants, one with a −4 arginine to glutamine substitution and the other with a −1 arginine to serine substitution, have a factor IX antigen which circulates with the propeptide still attached (Bentley *et al.*, 1986; Diuguid *et al.*, 1986; Ware *et al.*, 1989). This results in severe hemophilia B, probably because the propeptide induces an altered conformation in the factor IX molecule that interferes with activation or exposure of the active site. Even though one would

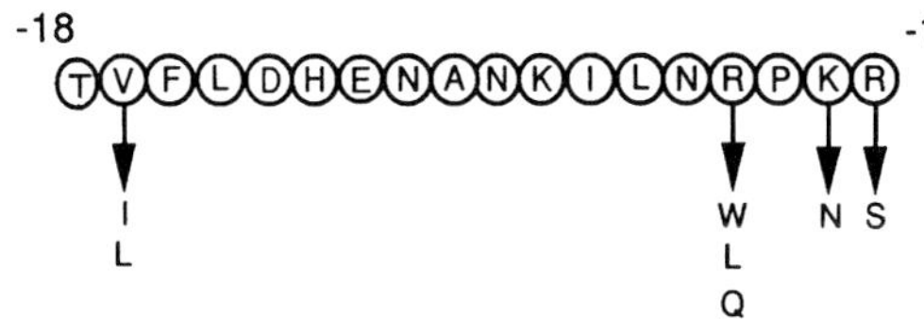

Fig. 4.5 Schematic representation of the normal propeptide. The normal propeptide spans a region from amino acid −18 to −1. The mutations which result in amino acid substitutions are depicted by the arrows. Updated and modified from Roberts, H.R. (1993), Molecular biology of hemophilia B. *Thrombosis and Haemostasis*, **70**, 1–9, and reproduced with permission.

Table 4.4   Representative mutations in the propeptide region

Nucleotide substitution	Amino acid change	FIX%	FIX antigen
114 insert AT	Premature stop after AA-18	<1	<1
117 G→A	−17: V→I	<1	2
6364: C→T	−4: R→W	4	36
6364: C→T	−4: R→W	<1	40
6365: G→A	−4: R→Q	<1	38
6372: G→T	−2: K→N	<1	37
6375: G→C or T	−1: R→S	<1	80

FIX = Factor IX.
Updated and modified from Roberts, H.R. (1993) Molecular biology of hemophilia B. *Thrombosis and Haemostasis*, **70**, and reprinted with permission.

expect that mutations in the propeptide would result in a molecule that is undercarboxylated, this does not seem to be the case, as shown by Wu and colleagues (1990). They have shown that a 59-amino-acid recombinant peptide containing mutations at the −1 (R → Q) and −4 (R → S) positions undergoes normal carboxylation in the presence of carboxylase and vitamin K. This suggests that the undercarboxylation reported in some of the factor IX molecules isolated from patients with a mutation at the −4 position may not be correct.

The γ-carboxyglutamic acid domain

THE NORMAL GLA REGION

The first 46 amino acids of the mature factor IX molecule comprise the Gla domain. Twelve Gla residues are present, and occur in pairs. They are necessary for calcium-dependent binding of factor IXa to activated platelets, and probably account for the low-affinity calcium binding sites (Bajaj, 1982). The exact mechanism by which this region binds the platelet membrane has not been completely elucidated. The Gla domain also contains a binding site for endothelial cells that may be different from the binding site for platelets (Cheung *et al.*, 1992). In addition, there appears to be a calcium-dependent conformational interaction between the Gla domain and EGF-l (McCord *et al.*, 1990; Valcarce *et al.*, 1994)

MUTATIONS IN THE GLA DOMAIN

Mutations in the Gla domain are depicted schematically in Figure 4.6 with representative mutations and their phenotypic expression listed in Table 4.5. There are now more than 50 mutations reported in this domain (Giannelli *et al.*, 1994). Nine of the 12 Gla residues are reported to have undergone mutations, and most result in severe hemophilia B. The patients with mutations at Gla 7 (E → A) and Gla 8 (E → A) are moderately affected, however, and have 4% and 5% factor IX activity, respectively (Winship and Dragon, 1991; Saad *et al.*, 1994). These two Gla residues are paired. Thus, they would seem to be quite important to function. However, the substitution of an alanine at these positions may be less disruptive than other Gla substitutions such as with a lysine, as is seen with factor IX Seattle 3 (27 E → K; Chen *et al.*, 1989). Like the Gla 7 → alanine mutant, the lysine 27 substitution perturbs calcium binding but, in addition, also perturbs the net charge of the region. This probably contributes to an additional conformational alteration. This may explain why the Seattle 3 substitution results in more severe disease than that seen in the Ala substitutions for Gla 7 and 8 (Winship and Dragon, 1991).

Epidermal growth factor-like domains

THE NORMAL EPIDERMAL GROWTH FACTOR-LIKE DOMAINS

Amino acids 47 through 85 comprise EGF-1. The EGF-1 domain possesses a high-affinity calcium-binding site with a Kd in the range of 10–100 µmol/l. The EGF-1 domain also contains a β hydroxy aspartate at position 64 but, in contrast to other vitamin K-dependent proteins, the content of β hydroxy aspartate in factor IX is only

Table 4.5 Representative mutations in the Gla domain

Nucleotide substitution	Amino acid change	FIX%	FIX antigen
6392: Delete 1	Premature stop after AA6	<1	
6395: A→C	7: E→A (Gla mutant)	5	5
6398: A→G	8: E→G (Gla mutant)	2	45
6398: A→C	8: E→A (Gla mutant)	4	
6402: −6 Delete 5	Premature stop after AA9 frameshift	<1	<1
6424: G→A	17: E→K (Gla mutant)	<1	
6434: A→T	20: E→V (Gla mutant)	?	?
6436: G→A	21: E→K (Gla mutant)	<1	52
6451: G→C	26: E→Q (Gla mutant)	<1	42
6454: G→A	27: E→K (Gla mutant)	<1	30
6455: A→T	27: E→V (Gla mutant)	<1	3
6456: A→C	27: E→D (Gla mutant)	<1	90
6460: C→T	29: R→stop	<1	<1
6463: G→A	30: E→K (Gla mutant)	1	
6474: A→C	33: E→D	4	33

FIX = Factor IX.
Updated and modified from Roberts, H.R. (1993) Molecular biology of hemophilia B. *Thrombosis and Haemostasis, 70,* and reprinted with permission

about 0.26 mol per mol of protein (Fernland and Stenflo 1983). The function of this unique amino acid is unclear, although the aspartyl residue at this position appears to contribute a calcium coordinate for the high-affinity calcium-binding site (McCord *et al.*, 1990; Selander-Sunnerhagen *et al.*, 1992). This calcium ion binding site is important in stabilizing interactions between EGF-1 and the Gla domain (Valcarce, Holmgren and Stenflo, 1994). These interactions are required for the correct surface orientation of factor IX (McCord *et al.*, 1990). There is also mounting evidence that the EGF-1 domain plays some role in the interaction of factor IX with tissue factor and factor VIIa (Chang *et al.*, 1995; Zhong *et al.*, 1994).

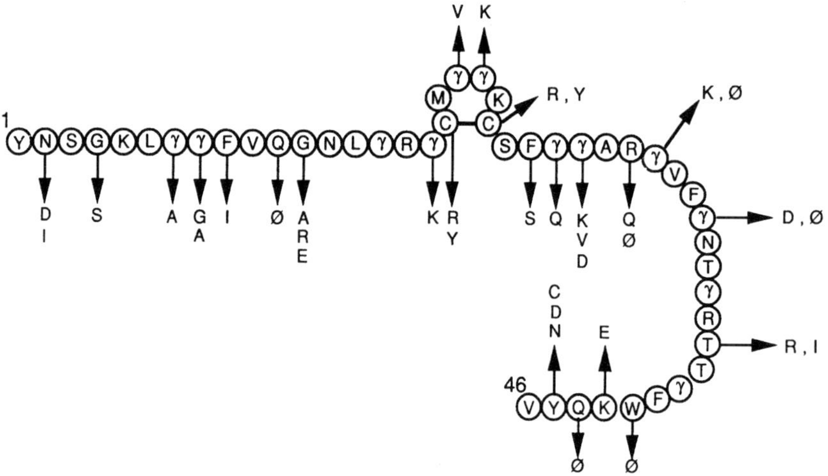

Fig. 4.6 The normal Gla domain. γ refers to γ-carboxyglutamic acid. Ø refers to a stop codon that substitutes for the one encoding for the normal amino acid at this position. This region contains 12 glutamyl residues that are modified by a vitamin K-dependent carboxylase. Mutations which result in amino acid changes or stop codons are depicted by the arrows. Note that mutations have been observed at nine of the 12 Gla residues. Updated and modified from Roberts, H.R. (1993) Molecular biology of hemophilia B. *Thrombosis and Haemostasis, 70,* 1–9, and reproduced with permission.

The second domain is comprised of residues 86–124. Hertzberg and colleagues have recently shown that the second EGF domain probably has a major role in incorporation of factor IXa into the tenase complex, although the precise interaction between factor IX and its cofactors and substrates has not been completely clarified (Hertzberg *et al.*, 1992).

MUTATIONS IN EGF-1 AND EGF-2

Over 20 distinct mutations, not including gross deletions or insertions have been reported in the EGF-1 domain (Giannelli *et al.*, 1994; Fig. 4.7). EGF-1 mutations result in hemophilia B of varying degrees of severity, ranging from very severe to mild disease (Table 4.6). Factor IX antigen levels range from undetectable to normal levels) as is evident from the table. Factor IX clotting activity ranges from <1% (severely affected) to about 20% (mildly affected). A well-characterized mutation, factor IX Alabama, results in a moderate bleeding tendency, presumably as a result of a conformational change in factor IX resulting from loss of a calcium coordinate for the high-affinity calcium-binding site (McCord *et al.*, 1990). This mutation also results in a diminished interaction with factor VIII, probably because of a distortion in the conformation between the Gla domain and EGF-1. Abnormalities in the activation of factor IX by factor XIa have also been reported to result from mutation in this region (Lozier *et al.*, 1990).

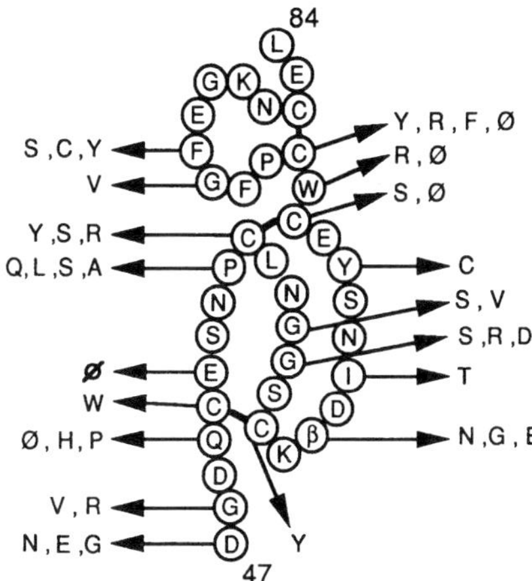

Fig. 4.7 A schematic of the first epidermal growth factor-like (EGF-1) domain. Ø refers to a stop codon that substitutes for the one encoding for the normal amino acid at this position. There is a β hydroxy aspartate at position 64. Amino acid substitutions and stop codons are depicted by the arrows. Mutations resulting from gross gene deletions or insertions and frameshifts are not shown. Updated and modified from Roberts, H.R. (1993), Molecular biology of hemophilia B. *Thrombosis and Haemostasis*, **70**, 1–9, and reproduced with permission.

Table 4.6 Representative mutations in the first epidermal growth factor-like domain

Nucleotide substitution	Amino acid change	FIX%	FIX antigen
10392: A→G	47: D→G (Alabama)	10	100
10393: T→A	47: D→E	1	80
10401: A→C	50: Q→P (New London)	<1	114
10415: C→T	55: P→S	12	52
10430: G→A*	60: G→S	14	
10442: G→A	64: D→N (β OH Asp)	3	117
10443: A→G	64: D→G (β OH Asp)	8	87
10444: T→G	64: D→E (β OH Asp)	12	46
10507-10:			
Delete 4	Donor splice site mutation		
17660-3:			
Delete 4	acceptor splice site mutation		20

FIX = Factor IX.
*27 patients with identical CG→CA mutations reported in database.
Updated and modified from Roberts, H.R. (1993) Molecular biology of hemophilia B. *Thrombosis and Haemostasis*, **70**, and reprinted with permission.

In excess of 30 unique mutations have been detected in the second EGF domain (Giannelli *et al.*, 1994; Fig. 4.8). Most of these result in severe hemophilia B with markedly decreased factor IX antigen (Table 4.7).

The activation peptide

THE NORMAL ACTIVATION PEPTIDE

The activation peptide begins with an arginyl residue at position 145 and ends with an arginyl residue at position 180. These residues are cleaved by the two activators of factor IX, factor XIa and factor VIIa/tissue factor. The activation of factor IX is shown schematically in Figure 4.9. Factor IXα and factor IXaα are transient intermediate forms resulting from different rates of proteolysis of the Arg[180] and Arg[145] bonds. Release of the activation peptide leads to the fully active mature enzyme factor IXaβ. Even though the activation peptide is not covalently

Table 4.7 Representative mutations in the second epidermal growth factor-like region

Nucleotide substitution	Amino acid change	FIX%	FIX antigen
17678: G→C	88: C→S	<1	
17727: Insert TT	Premature stop after AA 105	<1	<1
17738: T→C	108: V→A	20	120
17756: G→C	114: G→A	5	4
17761: C→T	116: R→stop	<1	3
20375: G→T	132: C→F	<1	<1

FIX = Factor IX.
Updated and modified from Roberts, H.R. (1993) Molecular biology of hemophilia B. *Thrombosis and Haemostasis*, **70**, and reprinted with permission.

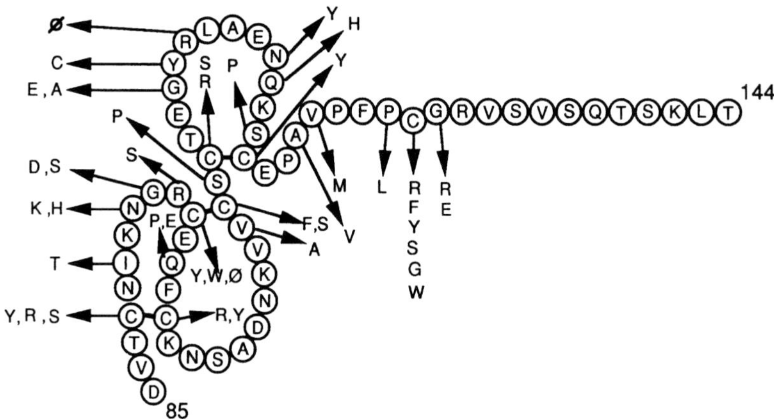

Fig. 4.8 An illustration of the second epidermal growth factor-like domain (EGF-2). The normal EGF-2 domain spans amino acids 85–144. Ø refers to a stop codon that substitutes for the one encoding for the normal amino acid at this position. The mutations which result in amino acid substitutions or stop codons are depicted by the arrows. Updated and modified from Roberts, H.R. (1993) Molecular biology of hemophilia B. *Thrombosis and Haemostasis*, **70**, 1–9, and reproduced with permission.

linked to factor IX after activation, there is suggestive evidence that the peptide remains associated with the active enzyme in a non-covalent manner.

MUTATIONS IN THE ACTIVATION PEPTIDE

Mutations in this region are shown schematically in Figure 4.10. The majority of those so far described occur at the amino- or carboxy-terminal arginyl residues (Giannelli *et al.*, 1994). A list of representative mutations is shown in Table 4.8. Substitution at the Arg^{145} position results in mild hemophilia, since a substitution here gives rise to a molecule similar to the normal factor IXaα, where the activation peptide remains covalently attached to the light chain and interferes with lipid binding. The first factor IX variant to be characterized on the molecular level, factor IX Chapel Hill, has a substitution of a histidine for the Arg^{145} (Braunstein *et al.*, 1981; Noyes *et al.*, 1983). Interestingly, mutations in the middle of the activation peptide away from the cleavage sites give rise to stop codons, resulting in a truncated molecule.

Some of the more interesting mutations occur at or near the Arg^{180} position since, when activated by either factor XIa or the factor VIIa–tissue factor complex, a form of the molecule resembling factor IXa is produced.

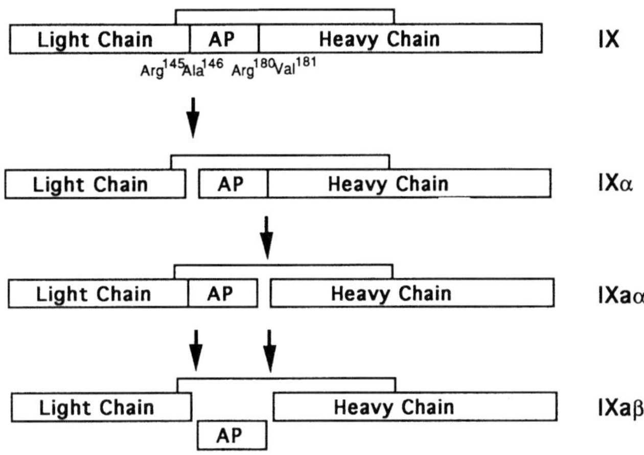

Fig. 4.9 A schematic illustration of the normal activation peptide (AP) of factor IX and its intermediates. When the Arg^{145}–Arg^{146} bond is cleaved, the intermediate factor IXα is formed. This intermediate is seen when there is a mutation involving the Arg^{180} residue and results in a variant referred to as hemophilia Bm. When the Arg^{180}–Val^{181} bond is cleaved, the intermediate factor IXaα is formed. This intermediate results from a mutation at the Arg^{145} residue. Factor IXaα can be generated from normal factor IX by Russell's viper venom. In normal factor IX both the Arg^{145} and the Arg^{180} bonds are cleaved, resulting in a fully active enzyme, referred to as factor IXaβ. From Roberts, H.R. (1993), Molecular biology of hemophilia B. *Thrombosis and Haemostasis*, **70**, 1–9, and reproduced with permission.

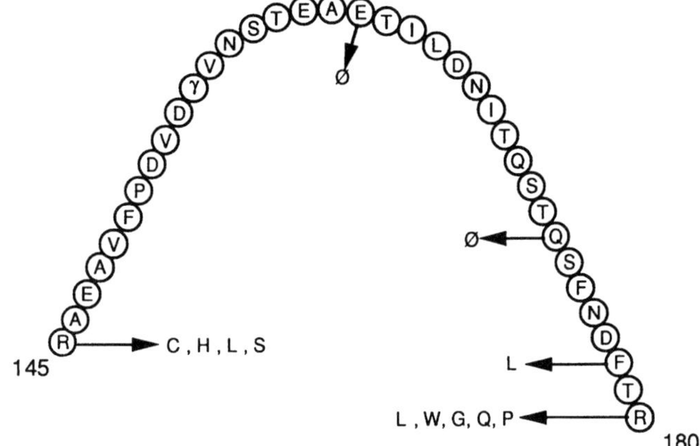

Fig. 4.10 Schematic diagram of the normal activation peptide. Mutations that result in amino acid substitutions and stop codons are depicted by the arrows. Ø refers to a stop codon that substitutes for the one encoding for the normal amino acid at this position. Updated and modified from Roberts, H.R. (1993), Molecular biology of hemophilia B. *Thrombosis and Haemostasis*, **70**, 1–9, and reproduced with permission.

Table 4.8 Representative mutations in the activation peptide region

Nucleotide substitution	Amino acid change	FIX%	FIX antigen
20413: C→T	145: R→C	2	
20414: G→A	145: R→H	8	100
20464: G→T	162: E→stop	<1	
20497: C→T	173: Q→stop	<1	
20501: delete 1	Premature stop after AA174	2	<1
20518: C→T	180: R→W (Deventer, Bm mutation)	<1	130
20519:G→A	180: R→Q (Hilo, Bm variant)	<1	120

FIX = Factor IX.
Updated and modified from Roberts, H.R. (1993) Molecular biology of hemophilia B. *Thrombosis and Haemostasis*, **70**, and reprinted with permission.

Table 4.9 Representative mutations in the catalytic domain

Nucleotide substitution	Amino acid change	FIX%	FIX antigen
20521: G→T	181: V→F (Bm mutation)	<1	130
20524: G→T	182: V→A (Bm mutation)	<1	120
20525: T→C	182: V→A (Bm mutation)	23	100
20531-3: Delete 3	184: Delete G	<1	92
20551: C→A	191: Q→K	<1	<1
20561: G→A	194: W→stop	<1	<1
30070: G→C	206: C→S*	<1	<1
30150: G→A	233: A→T	12	
30863: C→T	248: R→stop	<1	<1
31008: C→T	296: T→M	5	17
31041: T→C	307: V→A	15	40
31211: G→A	364: D→N (Bm mutation)	2	
31215: G→T	365: S→I†	<1	
31216: T→A	365: S→R†	1	90
31223: C→A	368: P→T (Bm mutation)	<1	156
31290: C→T	390: A→V (Bm mutation)	<1	100
31307: G→A	396: G→R (Bm mutation)	<1	90

FIX = Factor IX.
*Mutation of original patient with Christmas disease.
†Active site serine.
Updated and modified from Roberts, H.R. (1993) Molecular biology of hemophilia B. *Thrombosis and Haemostasis*, **70**, and reprinted with permission.

Here the activation peptide remains attached to the heavy chain. This molecule has no detectable activity and gives rise to a form of hemophilia B referred to as hemophilia Bm (Hougie and Twomey, 1967). Hemophilia Bm, originally described by Hougie and Twomey, was found in a family whose surname began with 'm' and whose plasma not only lacked factor IX clotting activity and exhibited a prolonged partial thromboplastin time, but also a remarkably prolonged ox-brain prothrombin time (Huang *et al.*, 1989; Bertina *et al.*, 1990). The prolongation of the prothrombin time apparently occurs because the abnormal factor IX molecule competes with factor VIIa for the substrate factor X. If one removes the abnormal factor IX from the patient's plasma by adsorption with an antifactor IX antibody, the ox-brain prothrombin time becomes normal (Lefkowitz *et al.*, 1993).

The catalytic domain

THE NORMAL CATALYTIC DOMAIN

The catalytic domain is the largest one in factor IX, stretching from amino acid 181 to 415. It is depicted schematically in Figure 4.11. This region contains the active site triad–histidine[221], serine[365] and aspartic acid[264] typical for serine protease enzymes.

MUTATIONS IN THE CATALYTIC DOMAIN

Over 200 unique molecular defects have been described in the catalytic domain (Giannelli *et al.*, 1994). Table 4.9 lists some of the representative mutations reported in this region. The original hemophilia B patient described by Biggs and colleagues in 1952 as Christmas disease has now been characterized on a molecular basis and found to have a mutation in the catalytic domain, at position 206 (C → S) (Biggs *et al.*, 1952; Taylor *et al.*, 1992). This form of hemophilia B is interesting for many reasons, not the least of which is historical. The 40 years between one of the first descriptions of hemophilia B and the identification of the specific genetic defect is illustrative of the enormous medical progress that was catalyzed by the introduction of molecular genetic technology.

Several of the mutations at the amino terminus (Val[181] and Val[182]) and carboxy terminus (Ala[390] and Gly[396]) of the catalytic domain result in hemophilia Bm variants like the variants noted around the Arg180 site in the activation peptide (Hamaguchi *et al.*, 1993). The Bm effect does not appear to be as great as with those around the activation peptide, although it does suggest an abnormal interaction between the heavy chain and the factor VIIa–tissue factor complex.

Factor IX Sauda, resulting from a substitution of an alanine for the valine[307] (A → V) in the heavy chain, is a good example of mild hemophilia B resulting from mutation in the catalytic domain (Monroe *et al.*, 1991). The patient is asymptomatic; the defect was discovered in a surgical work-up. This variant activates normally by cleavage at the Arg[145] and Arg[181] bonds but the activated form has markedly reduced activity. Interaction with factor VIIIa almost completely restores activity of factor IXa Sauda. Molecular modeling studies comparing this variant with norrnal factor IXa suggest that in the normal molecule the Val[181] interacts through van der Waals forces with the Val[307]. Val[181], which becomes the amino-terminus of the catalytic domain, forms an ion pair with Asp[364] that opens the active site and aligns the active site serine. In the mutant molecule, the Ala[307], which is smaller than the normal valine, causes malalignment of

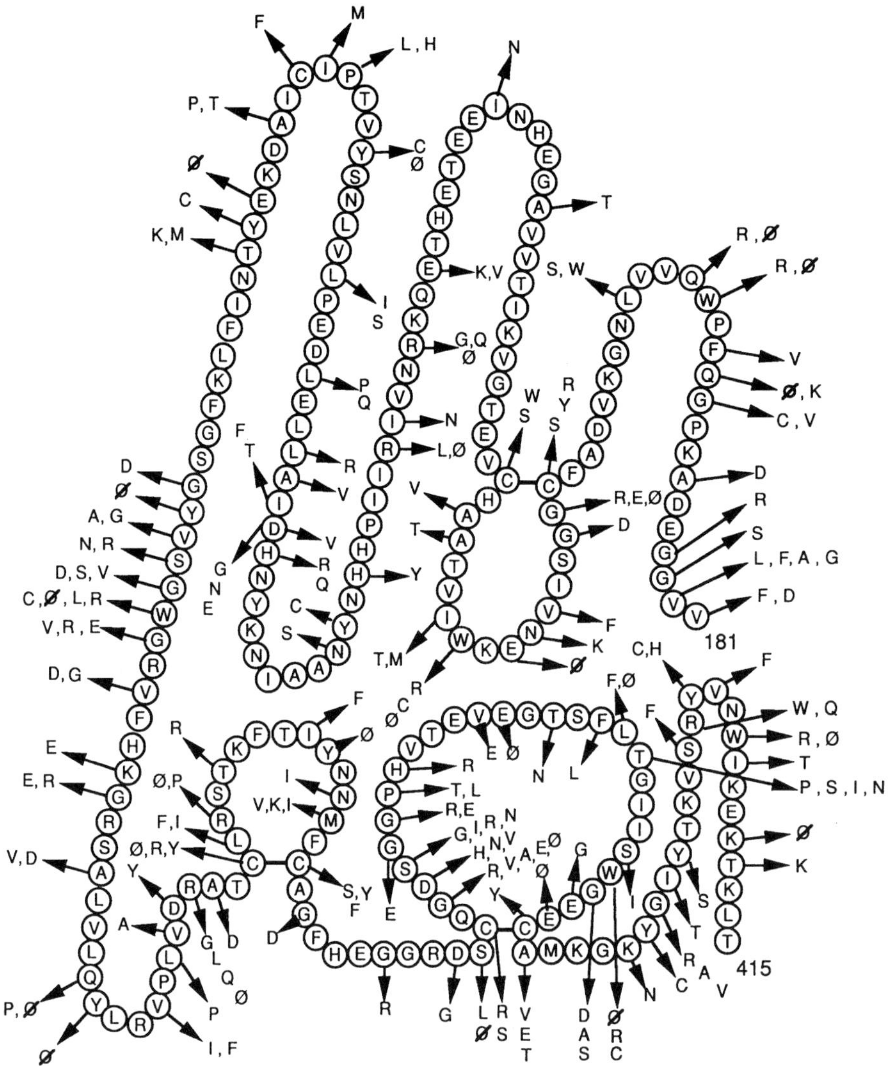

Fig. 4.11 The catalytic domain is depicted. The catalytic domain contains the active site triad characteristic of serine proteases. Updated and modified from Roberts, H.R. (1993) Molecular biology of hemophilia B. *Thrombosis and Haemostasis*, 70, 1–9, and reproduced with permission.

the ion pairing to Asp^{364}, thereby altering the position of the active site serine.

Many mutations in the catalytic domain probably result from a founder effect, since numerous patients with identical defects have been reported to the database. For example, there are numerous patients with mutations that occur at position 397 (397 I → T; 31 cases) and 248 (248 R → Stop; 27 cases, and 248 R → Q; 28 cases).

Gross gene deletions or insertions

Although the hemophilia B database is extensive, it does not include gross gene deletions or insertions involving more than 20 nucleotides. So far, Thompson (1991) has reported more than 30 cases of gross gene deletions or insertions, all of which lead to severe hemophilia B.

The first mutation in factor IX was described in 1983. Within 9 years, an additional 278 unique mutations were recorded, and by 1994, this number increased to 476 (Giannelli *et al.*, 1992; 1994). It is anticipated that even more genetic alterations will be found, as more patients with hemophilia B are studied. The huge number of distinct mutations that lead to a limited phenotypic expression of factor IX deficiency is impressive. To give the reader a better idea of the enormous genetic variation that can lead to a single clinical defect, we have included a shortened version of the 1994 hemophilia B database in the appendix.

Knowledge of the molecular defects causing hemophilia B has contributed much to our understanding of the structure and function of normal factor IX. The modern techniques of molecular biology and biochemistry should lead to further understanding of the interaction of factor IX with its cofactors and substrates and, in the foreseeable future, to gene therapy for factor IX deficiency.

Appendix: Mutations in the factor IX gene

Nucleotide position and mutation	Amino acid change	Clotting activity (% normal)	Antigen level (% normal)
−793, G → A	None	<1	<1
−26, G → C	None	<1	<1
−21, T → G	None	<1 → 10	<1 → 10
−20, T → A	None	<1 → 60	<1 → 60
−20, T → C	None	7 → 20	
−6, G → A*	None	13 → 70	
−6, G → C	None	1 → 30	1 → 30
−5, A → T	None	3	
−5, A → G	None	7	
6,7, or 8, Δ1	None	5	
6, T → A	None	<1 → 37	
8, T → C	None	1 → 32	
13, A → G	None	<1 → 60	<1 → 60
13, Δ1	None	<1 → 60	<1 → 60
13, A → C	None	<1	
37, G → A*	−44, Arg → His	<1	<1
48, A → T	−40, Ile → Phe	<1	<1
58, Δ1	−37	<6	<1
79, T → A	−30, Ile → Asn	2	<1
89, Δ1	−27	<1	
111, T → C	−19, Cys → Arg	20	
111–120, Δ10	−19		<1
112, Δ1	−19	<1	
113, T → G	−19, Cys → Trp	<5	<10
114, Ins AT	−18	<1	<1
116, A → G	−18, None		
117, G → A	−17, Val → Ile	<1	2
117, G → C	−17, Val → Leu	<1	
118, G → T	‡	2	
122, G → A	‡	3	2
6,320, T → G	§		
6,325, G → A	§	<1	
6,325, G → T	§	<1	
6,325, Δ2,Ins A	§	<1	
6,364, C → T*	−4, Arg → Trp	2	32
6,365, G → T	−4, Arg → Leu	<1	43
6,365, G → A*	−4, Arg → Gln	<1	54
6,370, Ins T	−2**	<1	
6,372, G → T	−2, Lys → Asn	<1	37
6,375, G → C/T	−1, Arg → Ser	<1	80
6,379, A → G	2, Asn → Asp	6	
6,379, Δ1	2, **	<1	<1
6,380, A → T	2, Asn → Ile	1	60
6,385, G → A	4, Gly → Ser	21	
6,390, A → G	‡	7	
6,392, Δ1	6, **	<1	
6,395, A → C	7, Glu → Ala	5	5
6,398-91†, Δ2	8, **	<1	<0.1
6,398, A → G	8, Glu → Gly	2	45
6,398, A → C	8, Glu → Ala	4	
6,400, T → A	9, Phe → Ile	14	118
6,401-10, Δ10	9, **	<1	<1
6,402-6, Δ5	9, **	<1	<l
6,406, C → T	11, Glu → Stop	<1	0.2
6,409, G → A	12, Gly → Arg	<1.13	46
6,410, G → C	12, Gly → Ala	3	97
6,410, G → A	12, Gly → Glu	<1	
6,411, Δ1	12, **	<1	<1
6,416-17, Δ2	14, **	4	4
6,420-5, Δ6	15, ΔArg, Glu	<1	
6,424, G → A	17, Glu → Lys	<1	58
6,427†,T → C	18, Cys → Arg	<1	100
6,428, G → A	18, Cys → Tyr	1.5	27
6,434, A → T	20, Glu → Val		
6,436, G → A	21, Glu → Lys	<1	52
6,441, Δ1	22, **	1	
6,442, T → C	23, Cys → Arg	<1	35
6,443, G → A	23, Cys → Tyr	<1	19
6,449, T → C	25, Phe → Ser	2	32
6,451, G → C	26, Glu → Gln	<1	42
6,454, G → A	27, Glu → Lys	<1	30
6,455, A → T	27, Glu → Val	<1	3
6,456, A → C	27, Glu → Asp	<1	90
6,460, C → T*	29, Arg → Stop	<1	<1
6,461†, G → A*	29, Arg → Gln	22	66
6,463, G → T	30, Glu → Stop	<1	
6,463, G → A	30, Glu → Lys	1	
6,466, Δ1	31, **	<1	<0.1
6,472, Ins GG	33, **		
6,472, G → T	33, Glu → Stop	<1	
6,474, A → C	33, Glu → Asp	4	
6,484–6, Δ3	37, ΔArg	<1	12
6,488, C → G	38, Thr → Arg	<1	
6,488, C → T	38, Thr → Ile	7	
6,491–4† or 6,492–5†, Δ4	‡(1 double)	<1	<1
6,492, G → C	‡	2	
6,494†, G → A	‡	<1	
6,495, T → C	‡	1	1
6,575, C → G	triple	<1	<1
6,666–75, Δ10	§	<1	0.2
6,677, G → C	§	5	
6,677, G → A	§	<1	
6,680–1, Δ2	39, **	<1	<1
6,684, Δ1	41, **	<1	
6,688, G → A	42, Trp → Stop	2	
6,690, A → G	43, Lys → Glu		14 96
6,693, C → T	44, Gln → Stop	<1	
6,696, T → A	45, Tyr → Asn	9	
6,696, T → G	45, Tyr → Asp	9	59
6.697, A → G	45, Tyr → Cys		
6,702, G → A	47, Asp → Asn	<1	<1
6,704, T → G	‡	0.5	0.4
6,704*,T → C	‡	1	<1
6,707, G → C	‡	5	
6,707, G → A	‡	1.3	
10,389, A → G	§	<1	27
10,390, A → T	§	<1	
10,391, G → A	§	3	
10,392, A → G	47, Asp → Gly	10	100
10,393†,T → A	47, Asp → Glu	7	85
10,394, G → A	48, Gly → Arg	28	101
10,395, G → T	48, Gly → Val	19	108
10,397-9, Δ3, Ins A	49,**	1	
10,400, C → T	50, Gln → Stop	<1	
10,401, A → C	50, Gln → Pro	<1	114
10,402, G → C	50, Gln → His	24	
10,405†,T → G	51, Cys → Trp	<1	<1
10,406, G → T	52, Glu → Stop	<1	20
10,415†,C → G	55, Pro → Ala	10	46
10,415, C → T	55, Pro → Ser	12	52
10,416, C → T	55, Pro → Leu	26	
10,416, C → A	55, Pro → Gln	6	34
10,418, T → C	56, Cys → Arg	<1	
10,418, T → A	56, Cys → Ser	1	2
10,419, G → C	56, Cys → Ser	<1	<1
10,419, G → A	56, Cys → Tyr	1	2

Nucleotide position and mutation	Amino acid change	Clotting activity (% normal)	Antigen level (% normal)
10,427, G → A	59, Gly → Ser	18	
10,428, G → T	59, Gly → Val	2	
10,430†, G → A*	60, Gly → Ser	13	28
10,430, G → C	60, Gly → Arg	<1	6
10,431, G → A	60, Gly → Asp	1	2
10,434-5, Δ2	61, **		
10,437, G → A	62, Cys → Tyr		
10,442, G → A	64, Asp → Asn	3	117
10,443, A → G	64, Asp → Gly	8	87
10,444, T → G	64, Asp → Glu	12	46
10,449† T → C	66, Ile → Thr	18	91
10,458†, A → G	69, Tyr → Cys	<1	
10,463, T → A	71, Cys → Ser		
10,464, G → C	71, Cys → Ser		
10,465, T → A	71, Cys → Stop	6	
10,466†, T → A	72, Trp → Arg		
10,468, G → A	72, Trp → Stop	<1	
10,469, T → C	73, Cys → Arg	1	1
10,470, G → A	73, Cys → Tyr	<1	
10,470, G → T	73, Cys → Phe	<1	
10,471, T → A	73, Cys → Stop	<1	
10,479, G → T	76, Gly → Val	6	12
10,482, T → G	77, Phe → Tyr		
10,482, T → C	77, Phe → Ser	12	66
10,506–9 or 10–13, Δ4	‡	5	15
10,507, T → A	‡		
10,507–10, Δ4	‡		
10,512†, A → G	2 double, 1 triple	1	1
17,660–3, Δ4	§	20	
17,667, A → G	§	3	3
17,667, A → C	§	3	4
17,668, G → C	§	<1	<1
17,669, Δ1	85, **	<1	<1
17,669–75, Δ7	85, **	2	2
17,677, T → C	88, Cys → Arg	<2	
17,678, G → C	88, Cys → Ser	<1	
17,678, G → A	88, Cys → Tyr	<1	9
17,684, T → C	90, Ile → Thr	15	
17,689, A → C	92, Asn → His	2	66
17,691†, T → A	92, Asn → Lys	<1	86
17,692, G → A	93, Gly → Ser	3	22
17,693, G → A	93, Gly → Asp	2	30
17,696, Ins A	94, **	1	
17,697, A → T	94, Arg → Ser	1	84
17,699†, G → A	95, Cys → Tyr	2	6
17,700, C → A	95, Cys → Stop	<1	
17,700, C → G	95, Cys → Trp	<1	2
17,704, C → G	97, Gln → Glu	<1	<1
17,705, A → C	97, Gln → Pro		
17,706, Δ1	97, **	<1	<13
17,710, T → C	99, Cys → Arg	<1	
17,711, G → A	99, Cys → Tyr	<1	
17,713–8, Ins A	101, **	<1	
17,717, Ins A	101, **	<1	
17,718, Ins A	101, **	<1	
17,727, Ins TT	105, **	<1	<1
17,736†,G → A	107, None	18	21
17,738, T → C	107, Val → Ala	20	120
17,740, G → C	109, Cys → Ser	<1	
17,741, G → T	109, Cys → Phe	<1	
17,743, T → C	110, Ser → Pro	7	<1
17,746, T → C	111, Cys → Arg	<1	<6
17,746, Ins 26	111, **	<1	<1
17,747, G → C	111, Cys → Ser	<1	
17,754, 5 or 6Δ1	114 or 115	<1	
17,756†, G → C	114, Gly → Ala	9	4
17,756, G → A	114, Gly → Glu		
17,759†, A → G	115, Tyr → Cys	1	1
17,761†, C → T*	116, Arg → Stop	<1	<1
17,761, C → A	116, None	5	5
17,764, Ins C	117, **	<1	
17,773, A → T	120, Asn → Tyr	<1	0.4
17,778†, G → T	121, Gln → His		
17,782, T → C	123, Ser → Pro	<1	
17,786, G → A	124, Cys → Tyr	2	
17,795, C → T	127, Ala → Val	<1	<6
17,796, A → T	127, None		
17,796, A → C	127, None		
17,796, A → G	127, None		
17,797, G → A	128, Val → Met	1	
17,798†, G → T	‡	<1	<1
17,799, T → G	‡	<1	
17,799, T → C	‡	<1	
17,799, T → A	‡		
17,810, A → G	‡	7	6
20,372, C → T	131, Pro → Leu		
20,374†, T → C	132, Cys → Arg	<1	<1
20,374, T → G	132, Cys → Gly		
20,375†, G → T	132, Cys → Phe	<1	<0.1
20,375†, G → A	132, Cys → Tyr	<1	<6
20,375, G → C	132, Cy → Ser	<1	
20,376, T → G	132, Cys → Trp	<1	
20,377, G → A	133, Gly → Arg	4	4
20,378, G → A	133, Gly → Glu	<1	<1
20,380–1, Δ2	134**	<1	
20,387–8†, Δ2	136**	<1	<1
20,398, Δ1	140**		
20,413†, C → T*	145, Arg → Cys	3	43
20,413, C → G	145, Arg → Leu	2	40
20,413, C → A	145, Arg → Ser		
20,414†, G → A	145, Arg → His	7	106
20,414, G → T	145, Arg → Leu	7	60
20,464, G → T	162, Glu → Stop	<1	
20,466–78, Δ13	162, **	<1	
20,497, C → T	173, Glu → Stop	<1	
20,501, Δ1	174, **	2	<1
20,510, Δ1	177, **	<1	0.5
20,512, T → C	178, Phe → Leu	<1	85
20,518†, C → T*	180, Arg → Trp	<1	88
20,518†, C → G	180, Arg → Gly	<1	80
20,519†, G → A*	180, Arg → Gln	<1	112
20,519, G → T	180, Arg → Leu	<1	73
20,519, G → C	180, Arg → Pro	<2	
20,521, G → T	181, Val → Phe	<1	130
20,522, T → A	181, Val → Asp		
20,524†, G → C	182, Val → Leu	10	132
20,524, G → T	182, Val → Phe	<1	120
20,525, T → C	182, Val → Ala	23	100
20,525, T → G	182, Val → Gly	2	72
20,527-9, Δ3	183, ΔGly	<1	97
20,527, G → A	183, Gly → Ser	13	
20,530, G → A	184, Gly → Arg	<1	100
20,530-2	184, ΔGly	1	
20,531-3, Δ3	184, ΔGly	<1	92
20,540, C → A	187, Ala → Asp	<1	
20,548, G → T	190, Gly → Cys	1	
20,549, G → T	190, Gly → Val	<1	36
20,551, C → T	191, Gln → Stop	<1	<1
20,551, C → A	191, Gln → Lys	<1	<1

Nucleotide position and mutation	Amino acid change	Clotting activity (% normal)	Antigen level (% normal)
20,553, A → G	191, None	3	2
20,554, T → G	192, Phe → Val	2	<6
20,560†, T → C	194, Trp → Arg	4	4
20,560, T → A	194, Trp → Arg	<1	1
20,561†, G → A	194, Trp → Stop	<1	<1
20,562, G → A	194, Trp → Stop	<1	
20,563, C → T	195, Gln → Stop	<1	<1
20,564, A → G	195, Gln → Arg	<1	<1
20,565, G → A	195, None	<1	<1
20,566, G → T	‡	<0.5	0.3
20,566, G → A	‡	<1	<1
20,567, T → C	‡	<1	
30,038, G → A	§	<1	
30,038†, G → C	§	<1	<1
30,046, T → G	198, Leu → Trp	2	
30,046, T → C	198, Leu → Ser	<1	<1
30,050, Δ1	199, **	<1	
30,058, Δ4	202, **		
30,069†, T → C	206, Cys → Arg	<1	
30,070†, G → C	206, Cys → Ser	<1	<1
30,070†, G → A	206, Cys → Tyr	<1	
30,072†, G → A	207, Gly → Arg	<1	
30,072, G → T	207, Gly → Stop	<1	<1
30,073, G → A	207, Gly → Glu	<1	56
30,076, G → A	208, Gly → Asp		1
30,084†, G → T	211, Val → Phe	6	
30,089, T → G	212, Asn → Lys	16	
30,090, G → T	213, Glu → Stop	<1	<1
30,096†, T → C	215, Trp → Arg	1	<1
30,097, G → A	215, Trp → Stop	<1	0.1
30,098, G → T	215, Trp → Cys	<1	<6
30,100†, T → C	216, Ile → Thr	5	4
30,101, T → G	216, Ile → Met	15	4
30,107, G → A	219, Ala → Thr		
30,112†, C → T	220, Ala → Val	5	9
30,117, T → A	222, Cys → Ser	2	
30,119, T → G	222, Cys → Trp	1	
30,134†, T → C	None		
30,150†, G → A*	233, Ala → Thr	13	12
30,152, Ins A	233, **	<1	<1
30,154, G → A	‡	1	1
30,800†, Ins A	None		
30,821†, G → A	§	<1	<1
30,834, T → A	238, Ile → Asn	20	
30,839–41, Δ3	240, ΔGlu	<1	
30,845, Δ1	242	<1	22
30,854, G → A	245, Glu → Lys	2	74
30,855, A → T	245, Glu → Val	3	39
30,857, Δ1	246, **	<1	3
30,863†, C → T	248, Arg → Stop	<1	<1
30,863, C → G	248, Arg → Gly	<1	
30,864†, G → A*	248, Arg → Gln	4	4
30,873, T → A	251, Ile → Asn	<1	
30,875†, C → T*	252, Arg → Stop	<1	<1
30,876, G → T	252, Arg → Leu	13	
30,890, C → T	257, His → Tyr	<1	<0.1
30,890, Δ1	257, **	<1	<8
30,897, A → G	259, Tyr → Cys	<1	<1
30,900†, A → G	260, Asn → Ser	16	
30,924, A → G	268, His → Arg	7	
30,925, T → G	268, His → Gln	8	2
30,926, G → A	269, Asp → Asn	1.5	
30,927, A → T	269, Asp → Val	<1	
30,927†, A → G	269, Asp → Gly	<1	
30,928, C → A	269, Asp → Glu	<1	5
30,929, A → T	270, Ile → Phe	1	1
30,930†, T → C	270, Ile → Thr	<1	<1
30,933†, C → T	271, Ala → Val	12	4
30,936, T → G	272, Leu → Arg	<1	2
30,942, Δ1	274, **		
30,945†, T → C	275, Leu → Pro	<1	7
30,945, T → A	275, Leu → Gln	<1	
30,950-7, Δ8	277, **	<1	<0.1
30,956, T → A	279, Leu → Ile	13	13
30,957, T → C	279, Leu → Ser	<1	
30,972, A → G	284, Tyr → Cys		
30,973, C → A	284, Tyr → Stop	<1	1
30,981, C → T	287, Pro → Leu	<1	<1
30,981, C → A	287, Pro → His		
30,985, T → G	288, Ile → Met	<1	<1
30,987, G → T	289, Cys → Phe	2	
30,992, G → C	291, Ala → Pro	2	3
30,992†, G → A	291, Ala → Thr	8	13
31,001, G → T	294, Glu → Stop	<1	<1
31,004, Ins CA	295, **	<1	
31,005, A → G	295, Tyr → Cys	<1	
31,007, Δ1	296, **		
31,008†, C → T*	296, Thr → Met	5	8
31,008, C → A	296, Thr → Lys		
31,012, C → T	None		
31,035, G → A	305, Gly → Asp	<1	0.3
31,039, T → A	306, Tyr → Stop	<1	<1
31,041†, T → C	307, Val → Ala	16	45
31,041, T → G	307, Val → Gly	3	4
31,043, A → C	308, Ser → Arg	2	
31,044, G → A	308, Ser → Asn	5	26
31,045, T → G	308, Ser → Arg	<1	
31,046, G → A	309, Gly → Ser	<1	65
31,047, G → T	309, Gly → Val	<1	58
31,047, G → A	309, Gly → Asp	<1	
31,049, T → C	310, Trp → Arg	<1	86
31,050, G → T	310, Trp → Leu	4	
31,051†, G → A	310, Trp → Stop	<1	<1
31,051†, G → C	310, Trp → Cys	1	5
31,051, G → T	310, Trp → Cys	<1	
31,052†, G → A	311, Gly → Arg	3	100
31,053, G → A	311, Gly → Glu	<1	100
31,053, G → T	311, Gly → Val	<1	
31,059, T → G	313, Val → Gly	<1	100
31,059, T → A	313, Val → Asp	2.5	100
31,059-60, Δ2	313, **	<1	<2
31,067, A → G	316, Lys → Glu		
31,070, G → C	317, Gly → Arg	<1	
31,071, G → A	317, Gly → Glu		
31,080†, C → A	320, Ala → Asp	2	90
31,080, C → T	320, Ala → Val		
31,084-90, Δ7	321, **	<1	<1
31,091, C → T	324, Gln → Stop	4	4
31,092, A → C	324, Gln → Pro	<1	<6
31,096, C → G	325, Tyr → Stop	4	
31,096, C → A	325, Tyr → Stop	<1	<1
31,103†, G → T	328, Val → Phe	4	4
31,103, G → A	328, Val → Ile	1	<1
31,110, T → C	330, Leu → Pro	7	
31,110–12†, Δ3††	331, ΔVal	<1	<1
31,113, T → C	331, Val → Ala	7	96
31,115†, G → T	332, Asp → Tyr	4	
31,118†, C → T*	333, Arg → Stop	<1	<1
31,118†, C → G	333, Arg → Gly	6	66
31,119, G → T	333, Arg → Leu	2	150

Nucleotide position and mutation	Amino acid change	Clotting activity (% normal)	Antigen level (% normal)
31,119†, G → A*	333, Ar → Gln	2	93
31,122†, C → A	334, Ala → Asp	18	100
31,127†, T → C	336, Cys → Arg	1	3
31,128, G → A	336, Cys → Tyr	<1	<1
31,129, T → A	336, Cys → Stop	<1	
31,130, C → A	337, Leu → Ile	4	120
31,130, C → T	337, Leu → Phe		72
31,133†, C → T*	338, Arg → Stop	<1	<1
31,134, G → C	338 Arg → Pro	13	27
31,140, C → G	340, Thr → Arg	<1	
31,141, 2 or 3 Ins AA	340 or 341		
31,149–51, Δ3 31,158–62, Δ5 31,158, Ins G	343, **	<1	<1
31,151, A → T	344, Ile → Phe	1	87
31,156, T → A	345, Tyr → Stop		
31,157†, 8 or 9 Ins AA	346, **	<1	<1
31,157–9 or 31,160–2, Δ3	346 or 347 ΔAsn		
31,161, A → T	347, Asn → Ile	<1	2
31,163, A → G348, Met → Val		3	103
31,164, T → A	348, Met → Lys	<1	12
31,165, G → A	348, Met → Ile	<1	71
31,166 or 7, Δ1	349, **	<1	
31,170, G → C	350, Cys → Ser	<1	45
31,170†, G → A	350, Cys → Tyr	<1	<1
31,170, G → T	350, Cys → Phe	1	5
31,176, G → A	352, Gly → Asn		
31,187, G → A	356, Gly → Arg	4	
31,194–5, Δ2	358, **	<1	
31,197, A → G	359, Asp → Gly	1.5	
31,200†, C → T	360, Ser → Leu	1	130
31,200†, C → G	360, Ser → Stop	<1	
31,202, T → A	361, Cys → Ser	<1	
31,202, T → C	361, Cys → Arg	<1	<1
31,208, G → T	363, Gly → Stop	<1	
31,208, G → A	363, Gly → Arg	<1	110
31,209†, G → T	363, Gly → Val	1-5	100
31,209, G → C	363, Gly → Ala	3	100
31,209†, G → A	363, Gly → Glu	1	53
31,210–13, Ins AGAT	364, **	<1	<1
31,211†, G → C	364, Asp → His	1	97
31,211, G → A	364, Asp → Asn	1	
31,212, A → T	364, Asp → Val	<1	130
31,213–14, TA → CG	365, Ser → Gly	<1	89
31,214, A → G	365, Ser → Gly		
31,215†, G → T	365, Ser → Ile	<1	
31,215, G → A	365, Ser → Asn	2	
31,216, T → A	365, Ser → Arg	1	90
31,216, T → G	365, Ser → Arg	<1	100
31,218†, G → A	366, Gly → Glu	3	32
31,220†, G → A	367, Gly → Arg	<1	14
31,221, G → A	367, Gly → Glu	<1	
31,223†, C → A	368, Pro → Thr	2	156
31,224†, C → T	368, Pro → Leu	2	62
31,227, A → G	369, His → Arg	<1	<1
31,239, T → A	273, Val → Glu	1	1
31,241, G → T	374, Glu → Stop	1	1
31,248, C → A	376, Thr → Asn	15	13
31,253, T → C	378, Phe → Leu	<1	<1
31,257, T → G	379, Leu → Stop	<1	
31,258, A → C	379, Leu → Phe	8	
31,259, A → C	380, Thr → Pro	<1	
31,260, C → G	380, Thr → Ser	7	<10
31,260, C → T	380, Thr → Ile	<1	1
31,260, C → A	380, Thr → Asn	1.4	
31,261, Δ1	380, **	<1	<10
31,270, Ins T	383, **	<1	
31,272, G → T	384, Ser → Ile	1.8	
31,274, T → A	385, Tyr → Arg		
31,274, T → C	385, Tyr → Arg	<1	
31,276, G → A	385, Tyr → Stop	<1	
31,276, G → T	385, Tyr → Cys	1	
31,277, G → A	386, Gly → Ser		
31,278, G → C	386, Gly → Ala	<1	
31,278, G → A	386, 61y → Asp	2	120
31,281, A → G	387, Glu → Gly	2	95
31,283, G → T	388, Glu → Stop		
31,286–7, Δ2	389, **	<1	
31,287†, G → A	389, Cys → Tyr	3	2
31,289, G → A	390, Ala → Thr	3	40
31,290†, C → T	390, Ala → Val	1	90
31,290†, C → A	390, Ala → Glu	2	30
31,303, A → C	394, Lys → Asn		
31,305, A → G	395, Tyr → Cys	<1	
31,307†, G → A	396, Gly → Arg	<1	100
31,307–20, Δ14	396, **	<1	
31,308, G → C	396, Gly → Ala	1	112
31,308, G → T	396, Gly → Val		
31,311†, T → C	397, Ile → Thr	3	73
31,314, A → C	398, Tyr → Ser		
31,318, Ins ATATATACC	399, In frame	2	
31,326, C → T	402, Ser → Phe	8	
31,327–8, Δ2 InsAAGGTACCAA	402, **	3	9
31,321–8, Δ8	400, **	<1	
31,328†, C → T*	403, Arg → Trp		
31,329, G → A*	403, Arg → Gln	24	60
31,329, Δ1	403, **	<1	
31,331, T → C	404, Tyr → His	4	
31,332, A → G	404, Tyr → Cys		
31,334, G → T	405, Val → Phe	23	26
31,340, T → C	407, Trp → Arg	<1	2
31,342, G → A	407, Trp → Stop	<1	<1
31,344, T → C	408, Ile → Thr	1	1
31,344 or 5, Δ1	408, **	<1	0.2
31,346, Ins GATT	408, **	<1	
31,352, A → T	411, Lys → Stop	<1	<1
31,350–5, Δ1	410-412	<1	<1
31,356, C → A	412, Thr → Lys	3	1
32,528, A → G	3' UTR	1.5	<1

Δ = deletion. Ins = insertion.
*Mutation of a CG to either TG or CA.
†Two or more similar mutations have been reported at this site.
‡ = donor splice.
§Acceptor splice.
**Frameshift.
††31,111-3, or 31,112-4, or 31,113-5.
Updated and modified from Roberts, H.R. and Hoffman, M. (1995) Hemophilia and related conditions – inherited deficiencies of prothrombin (factor II), factor VII, factor V, and factors VII to XII, in *William's Hematology*, 5th edn (eds E. Beutler, M.A. Lichtman, B.S. Coller and T.J. Kipps), McGraw-Hill, New York, pp. 1413–1438, and reprinted with permission.

References

Aggeler, P., White, S., Glendenning, M. *et al.* (1952) Plasma thromboplastin component (PTC) deficiency: a new disease resembling hemophilia. *Proc Soc Exp Biol Med*, **79**, 692–694.

Anson, D., Choo, K. and Rees, D. (1984) The gene structure of human anti-hemophilic factor IX. *EMBO J*, **3**, 1053–1060.

Bajaj, S. (1982) Co-operative Ca^{2+}-binding to human factor IX. *J Biol Chem*, **257**, 4127–44132.

Bentley, A., Rees, D., Riza, C. and Brownlee, G. (1986) Defective propeptide processing of blood clotting factor IX caused by mutations of arginine to glutamine at position –4. *Cell*, **45**, 343–348.

Bertina, R., van der Linden, I., Mannucci, P. *et al.* (1990) Mutations in hemophilia Bm occur at the Arg 180-Val-181 activation site or in the catalytic domain of factor IX. *J Biol Chem*, **265**, 10876–10883.

Biggs, R, Douglas, A., McFarlane, R. *et al.* (1952) Christmas disease: a condition previously mistaken for hemophilia. *Br Med J*, **2**, 1378–1382.

Bottema, C., Bottema, M., Ketterling, R. *et al.* (1991) Why does the human factor IX gene have a G + C content of 40%? *Am J Hum Genet*, **49**, 839–850.

Braunstein, K., Noyes, C., Griffith, M. *et al.* (1981) Characterization of factor IX Chapel Hill. *J Clin Invest*, **68**, 1420–1426.

Briet, E., Bertina, R., Van Tilburg, N. and Veltkamp, J. (1982) Haemophilia B Leyden: a sex-linked hereditary disorder that improves after puberty. *N Engl J Med*, **306**, 788–790.

Briet, E., Wijnands, M. and Veltkamp, J. (1986) The prophylactic treatment of haemophilia B Leyden with anabolic steroids. *Ann Intern Med*, **103**, 225–226.

Bristol, J. A., Freedman, S. J., Furie, B. C. and Furie, B. (1994) Profactor IX: the propeptide inhibits binding to membrane surfaces and activation by factor XIa. *Biochemistry*, **33**, 14136–14143.

Chance, P., Dyer, K., Kurachi, K. *et al.* (1983) Regional localization of human factor IX gene by molecular hybridization. *Hum Genet*, **65**, 207–208.

Chang, J.-Y., Monroe, D. M., Stafford, D. W. and Roberts, H. (1995) Replacing the first epidermal growth factor like domain of factor IX with that of factor VII enhances clotting activity. *Thromb Haemostas*.

Chen, S., Thompson, A., Zhang, M. and Scott, C. (1989) Three point mutations in the factor IX genes of five hemophilia B patients. *J Clin Invest*, **84**, 113–118.

Cheung, W.-F., Hamaguchi, N., Smith, K. and Stafford, D. (1992) The binding of human factor IX to endothelial cells is mediated by residues 3-11. *J Biol Chem*, **267**, 20529–20531.

Crossley, M. and Brownlee, G. (1990) Disruption of a C/EBP binding site in the factor IX promoter is associated with haemophilia B. *Nature*, **345**, 444–446.

Crossley, M., Ludwig, M., Stowell, K. *et al.* (1992) Recovery from hemophilia B Leyden: an androgen-responsive element in the factor IX promoter. *Science*, **257**, 377–379.

Diuguid, D., Rabiet, M.-J., Furie, B. *et al.* (1986) Molecular basis of hemophilia B: a defective enzyme due to an unprocessed propeptide caused by a point mutation in the factor IX precursor. *Proc Natl Acad Sci USA*, **83**, 5803–5807.

Driscoll, M., Dispenzieri, A., Tobias, E., Miller, C. and Aledort, L. (1988) A second BamHI DNA polymorphism and haplotype association in the factor IX gene. *Blood*, **72**, 61–65.

Fernland, P. and Stenflo, J. (1983) β Hydroxyaspartic acid in vitamin K-dependent proteins. *J Biol Chem*, **258**, 12509–12512.

Foster, D., Rudinski, M., Schach, B. *et al.* (1987) Propeptide of human protein C is necessary for gamma-carboxylation. *Biochemistry*, **26**, 7003–7011.

Giannelli, F., Green, P., High, K. *et al.* (1992) Haemophilia B: database of point mutations and short additions and deletions – third edition, 1992. *Nucl Acids Res*, **20**, 2027–2063.

Giannelli, F., Green, P., Sommer, S. *et al.* (1994) Haemophilia B: database of point mutations and short additions and deletions – fifth edition. *Nucl Acids Res*, **22**, 3534–3546.

Gill, G. and Tijian, R. (1992) Eukaryotic coactivators associated with the TATA box binding protein. *Curr Opin Genet Dev*, **2**, 236–242.

Hamaguchi, N., Roberts, H. and Stafford, D. (1993) Mutations in the catalytic domain of factor IX that are related to the subclass hemophilia Bm. *Biochemistry*, **32**, 6324–6329.

Hay, C., Robertson, K., Yong, S. *et al.* (1986) Use of a BamHI polymorphism in the factor IX gene for the determination of hemophilia B carrier status. *Blood*, **67**, 1508–1511.

Hertzberg, M., Ben-Tal, O., Furie, B. and Furie, B. (1992) Construction, expression, and characterization of a chimera of factor IX and factor X. The role of the second epidermal growth factor domain and serine protease domain in factor Va binding. *J Biol Chem*, **267**, 14759–14766.

Hougie, C. and Twomey, J. (1967) Haemophilia Bm: a new type of factor IX deficiency. *Lancet*, 698–700.

Huang, M.-N., Kasper, C., Roberts, H., Stafford, D. and High, K. (1989) Molecular defect in factor IX Hilo, a hemophilia Bm variant: Arg → Gln at the carboxyterminal cleavage site of the activation peptide. *Blood*, **73**, 718–721.

Huber, P., Schmitz, T., Griffin, J. *et al.* (1990) Identification of amino acids in the γ carboxylation recognition site on the propeptide of prothrombin. *J Biol Chem*, **265**, 12467–12473.

Jorgensen, M., Cantor, A., Furie, B. *et al.* (1987) Recognition site directing vitamin K-dependent gamma carboxylation residues on the propeptide of factor IX. *Cell*, **48**, 185–191.

Koeberl, D., Bottema, C., Berstedde, J. and Sommer, S. (1989) Functionally important regions of the factor IX gene have a low rate of polymorphisms and a high rate of mutations in the dinucleotide CpG. *Am J Hum Genet*, **45**, 448–457.

Kurachi, K., Kurachi, S., Furukawa, M. and Yao, S.-N. (1993) Biology of factor IX. *Blood Coagul Fibrinolysis*, **4**, 953–974.

Lefkowitz, J., Monroe, D., Kasper, C. and Roberts, H. (1993) Comparison of the behavior of normal factor IX and the factor IX Bm variant Hilo in the prothrombin time test using tissue factors from bovine, human and rabbit sources. *Am J Hematol*, **43**, 177–182.

Lozier, J. N., Monroe, D. M., Stanfield-Oakley, S. *et al.* (1990) Factor IX New London: substitution of proline for glutamine atposition 50 causes severe hemophilia B. *Blood*, **75**, 1097–1104.

McCord, D. M., Monroe, D. M., Smith, K. J. *et al.* (1990) Characterization of the functional defect in factor IX Alabama: evidence for a conformational change due to high-affinity calcium binding in the first epidermal growth factor domain. *J Biol Chem*, **265**, 10250–10254.

McGraw, R., Davis, L., Noyes, C. *et al.* (1985) Evidence for a prevalent dimorphism in the activation peptide of human coagulation factor IX. *Proc Natl Acad Sci USA*, **82**, 2847–2851.

Monroe, D., Lefkowitz, J., Stormorken, H., High, K. and Roberts, H. (1991) Functional consequences of a Valine 307 to Alanine mutation in factor IX Sauda. *Blood*, **65**, 712.

Morris, D., Soute, B., Vermeer, C. and Stafford, D. (1993) Characterization of the purified vitamin K-dependent gamma-glutamyl carboxylase. *J Biol Chem*, **268**, 8735–8742.

Noyes, C. M., Griffith, M. J., Roberts, H. R. and Lundblad, R. L. (1983) Identification of the molecular defect in factor IX Chapel Hill substitution of histidine for arginine at position 145. *Proc Natl Acad Sci*. **80**, 4200–4202.

Picketts, D., Lillicrap, D. and Mueller, C. (1993) Synergy between transcription factors DBP and C/EBP compensates for a hemophilia B Leyden factor IX mutation. *Nature Genet*, **3**, 175–179.

Purrello, M., Alhadeff, B., Esposito, D. *et al.* (1985) The human genes for hemophilia A and hemophilia B flank the X chromosome fragile site at Xq27.3. *EMBO J*, **4**, 725–729.

Rabiet, M.-J., Jorgensen, M., Furie, B. and Furie, B. (1987) Effect of propeptide mutations on posttranslational processing of factor IX: evidence that β-hydroxylation and γ-carboxylation are independent events. *J Biol Chem*, **262**, 14895–14898.

Reijnen, M., Sladek, F., Bertina, R. and Reitsma, P. (1992) Disruption of a binding site for hepatocyte nuclear factor 4 results in hemophilia B Leyden. *Proc Natl Acad Sci*, **89**, 6300–6303.

Saad, S., Rowley, G., Tagiavacca, L., Green, P. and Giannelli, F. (1994) First report on UK database of haemophilia B mutations and pedigrees. UK haemophilia centres. *Thromb Haemost*, **71**, 563–570.

Selander-Sunnerhagen, M., Ullner, M., Persson, E. *et al.* (1992) How an Epidermal Growth Factor (EGF) like domain binds calcium. *J Biol Chem*, **267**, 19642–19649.

Sommer, S. (1992) Assessment of the underlying pattern of human germline mutations: lessons from the factor IX gene. *FASEB J*, **6**, 2767–2774.

Taylor, S., Duffin, J., Cameron, C. *et al.* (1992) Characterization of the original Christmas disease mutation (cysteine 206 → serine) from clinical recognition to molecular pathogenesis. *Thromb Haemostas*, **67**, 63–65.

Thompson, A. (1991) Molecular biology of the hemophilias. *Prog Hemostas Thromb*, **10**, 175–214.

Thompson, A., Bajaj, S., Chen, S. and MacGillivray, R. (1990) 'Founder' effect in different families with haemophilia B mutation. *Lancet*, **335**, 418.

Valcarce, C., Holmgren, A. and Stenflo, J. (1994) Calcium-dependent interaction between gamma carboxyglutamic acid-containing and *N*-terminal epidermal growth factor-like modules in factor X. *J Biol Chem*, **269**, 26011–26016.

Veltkamp, J., Meilof, J., Remmelts, H. *et al.* (1970) Another genetic variant of haemophilia B: haemophilia B Leyden. *Scand J Haematol*, **7**, 82–90.

Wallmark, A., Kunkel, G., Mouhli, H. *et al.* (1991) Population genetics of the Malmo polymorphism of coagulation factor IX. *Hum Hered*, **41**, 391–396.

Ware, J., Diuguid, Q., Liebman, H. *et al.* (1989) Factor IX San Dimas: substitution of a glutamine for Arg-4 in the propeptide leads to incomplete carboxylation and altered phospholipid binding properties. *J Biol Chem*, **264**, 11401–11406.

Winship, P., Anson, D., Rizza, C. and Brownlee, G. (1984) Carrier detection in haemophilia B using two further intragenic restriction fragment length polymorphisms. *Nucl Acids Res*, **12**, 8861–8872.

Winship, P. R. and Dragon, A. C. (1991) Identification of haemophilia B patients with mutations in the two calcium binding domains of factor IX: importance of a β-OH Asp 64 → Asn change. *Br J Haematol*, **77**, 102–109.

Winship, P., Rees, D. and Alkan, M. (1989) Detection of polymorphism at cytosine phosphoguanidine dinucleotides and diagnosis of haemophilia B carriers. *Lancet*, **1**, 631–634.

Wu, S., Cheung, W., Frazier, D. and Stafford, D. (199l) Cloning and expression of the cDNA for human gamma-glutamyl carboxylase. *Science*, **254**, 1634–1636.

Wu, S., Morris, D. and Stafford, D. (1991) Identification and purification to near homogeneity of the vitamin K-dependent carboxylase. *Proc Natl Acad Sci*, **88**, 2236–2240.

Wu, S.-M., Soute, B., Vermeer, C. and Stafford, D. (1990) *In vitro* gamma carboxylation of a 59-residue recombinant peptide including the propeptide and gamma-carboxyglutamic acid domain of coagulation factor IX. *J Biol Chem*, **265**, 13124–13129.

Yoshitake, S., Schach, B., Foster, D. *et al*. (1985) Nucleotide sequence of the gene for human factor IX (antihemophilic factor B). *Biochemistry*, **24**, 3736–3750.

Zhong, D., Smith, K. J., Birktoft, J. J. and Bajaj, S. P. (1994) First epidermal growth factor-like domain of human blood coagulation factor IX is required for its activation by factor VIIa/tissue factor but not by factor XIa. *Proc Natl Acad Sci*, **91**, 3574–3578.

PART TWO

Clinical Features

DIED]—In Frederick county (Virginia) Mr. Isaac Zoll, aged 19. His death was occafioned by a flight cut in one of his feet, with an ax. From the time of his receiving the wound, till he expired, no method could be devifed to ftop the bleeding : if the wound was bound up, the blood gufhed out at his mouth or noftrils.— Five brothers to the above perfon have bled to death, at different periods, from the following accidents : One received a prick with a thorn— another, a fcratch with a comb—a third, a prick with a needle—a fourth bruifed his cheek againft a ftove—and the fifth received a cut in one of his thumbs. The father of the above perfons has had two wives, and by each, feveral child- ren ; thofe who died in this fingular manner were all of the firft wife.————At Charlefton,

5 THE DIAGNOSIS OF HEMOPHILIA A AND B AND VON WILLEBRAND'S DISEASE

K.A. Rickard

Clinical presentation of bleeding associated with the diagnosis of the hemophilias and von Willebrand's disease

The diagnosis of hemophilia is frequently made in childhood and quite often in early childhood. Severe von Willebrand's disease is frequently diagnosed in childhood, while the milder forms of hemophilia and von Willebrand's disease may not be diagnosed until late childhood or early adulthood.

CHILDHOOD PRESENTATIONS OF BLEEDING

A review of pediatric experiences leading to the diagnosis of hemophilia or von Willebrand's disease indicates that they can generally be separated into families who have a recognized history of hemophilia or von Willebrand's disease and those families who do not.

A family history

If there is a family history, parents will generally request testing at or soon after birth. This may frequently be done on cord blood and then a low factor VIIIc or IXc on cord blood should be confirmed as soon as possible in a venous sample from the baby. Even in the presence of a family history, there is often misunderstanding on the part of parents, nurses and physicians about the sex-linked genetic nature of hemophilia. Such fundamental knowledge that the daughter of a person with hemophilia must be a carrier and hence may have sons with hemophilia needs to be appreciated, while the possible 50/50 probability of the carrier status of female relatives of the person with hemophilia also needs general and medical recognition. Accordingly, every effort should be made to organize education of families and the extended family members with these conditions about the sex-linked nature of the inheritance of hemophilia.

Absent family history

Experiences over a 25-year period at our children's hospital in Sydney when parents are unsuspecting of the possibilities of hemophilia relate such initial problems in the child with hemophilia as bleeding around the mouth, tongue or frenulum after minor trauma or dental trauma, excessive bleeding at circumcision, scalp and intracranial bleeding with trauma and excessive bruising with minor trauma, particularly as the child becomes mobile. Also seen are bleeding and extensive bruising after intramuscular injections and attempted or successful venipuncture, iron-deficiency anemia from gastrointestinal bleeding and bleeding after such surgical procedures as hernia repair or tonsillectomy. It is now suggested that some 30% of people with hemophilia do not have a family history and a genetic mutation is the cause of this situation (World Health Organization (WHO), 1991). In our pediatric experiences, the majority of the memorable presentations of bleeding in young children with hemophilia have been in families without a prior history. Accordingly, clinicians must have a strong index of suspicion of such conditions as hemophilia or von Willebrand's disease when untoward bleeding occurs in childhood. This state of mind is not readily achieved, since in the total medical scene, the hemophilias are, after all, relatively uncommon conditions.

The congenital coagulation disorders are uncommon, with an overall incidence of about 10–20 for 100 000 of the population. Hemophilia A occurs in about 5–10 per 100 000 while the incidence of hemophilia B is about one-fifth that of hemophilia A.

Hemophilia. Edited by C.D. Forbes, L. Aledort and R. Madhok. Published in 1997 by Chapman & Hall, London. ISBN 0 412 63820 7

Presentation in adulthood

If hemophilia or von Willebrand's disease is not diagnosed until early adulthood then it is probably so-called mild in nature. In the adult, such problems as excessive bleeding following surgery, dentistry or trauma may occasion the diagnosis or the diagnosis may be a completely incidental finding. In young adult females, von Willebrand's disease may present with menorrhagia and here the gynecologist or physician requests hemostatic assessment and the diagnosis is disclosed. Unfortunately, some families try to avoid the reality of hemophilia and mild hemophilia may go undeclared – even to the extent of responsible family members not warning a suspected adult of the likelihood of the hemophilia status prior to surgery or intervention, with near disastrous consequences.

Clinical steps in diagnosis

THE REFERRAL

A common situation will be for the parents to attend their local medical officer or for the doctor to refer the child to a pediatric physician or hematologist because of the presence of easy bruising or bleeding. It is important to sit down with the parents and patient and elicit a careful and full medical history, including the nature of bleeding, its relation to other events such as trauma or surgery and whether medications are being taken. Study of the family history in relation to bleeding and construction of a comprehensive family tree as can best be recalled by the parents or older patient is extremely valuable. A careful and thorough physical examination of the patient must be done. Here one must be conscious of the extent and nature of bruising or bleeding, the musculoskeletal development and a search should be made for evidence of current or recent hemarthroses and muscle or other hematomas.

Following the history and examination, the physician must request the relevant laboratory examinations, and if necessary can seek advice from the pathologist responsible for the performance of the various relevant tests. For pathologists who may have referred patients suspected of having a bleeding disorder, it is important that they see and assess the patient and family in a face-to-face situation so that they can be sure the appropriate tests are requested and performed.

COLLECTION OF BLOOD SAMPLES

When the laboratory study of the hemostatic mechanisms is to be undertaken, it is vital that relevant samples – preferably venous rather than capillary – are efficiently and cleanly collected into the appropriate containers for coagulation testing. Containers containing 0.105 mol/l sodium citrate as anticoagulant are recommended, with a ratio of one part of citrate to nine parts of blood.

Samples should be quickly despatched to the laboratory if assays of labile coagulation factors, especially factor V and factor VIII, are requested. These assays are best done on fresh specimens with a minimum of delay. Ideally, it is best for the samples for coagulation testing and assays to be collected from the patient on the same site as the laboratory rather than to have the specimens despatched over long distances. Thus, it is often more efficient to request the patient to attend the hematology department or laboratory facility in person. If personal attendance is not possible and samples need to be despatched, they should be refrigerated and those for assays must be spun down, plasma-separated, despatched and maintained in a frozen state until the test laboratory is reached. Unless collected blood samples are dealt with in this manner, then equivocal or misleading results may be obtained.

TESTING FOR HEMOPHILIA A, B OR VON WILLEBRAND'S DISEASE

The clinician's approach to the request for various laboratory tests will to some extent again be determined by the presence or absence of a family history and a diagnosis of that family's bleeding tendency. Accordingly, if there is a maternal uncle with hemophilia, it is very important that the factor VIII or factor IX of the child or young man is ascertained as soon as possible. If on the other hand there is no known family history but a bleeding disorder is suspected, then broader brush strokes are required to cover the various contingencies of possible diagnoses in the tests being requested.

In the absence of a family history, it is important to obtain a general view of the hemostatic mechanism as well as to ascertain the general hematological, renal and hepatic status of the patient. Requests would therefore be for a full blood count to determine hemoglobin levels as well as white cell and platelet numbers. Tests of renal and hepatic function may also be requested. It is important to examine the blood film to exclude certain hematologic malignant abnormalities, which may be indicated by the blood count and blood film. Such entities as acute or chronic leukemia, thrombocytopenia or some congenital platelet anomalies may thus be detected. Beside platelet numbers, we must determine aspects of platelet function, and this can be done by assessing platelet aggregation patterns under the stimulus of adenosine diphosphate (ADP), collagen, adrenalin and ristocetin. Characteristic aggregation patterns are produced with the various agonists in the different platelet disorders (Born, 1962; O'Brien, 1962; Hutton and Ludlam, 1989). Some laboratories may also assess platelet adhesive properties by various techniques such as glass bead column stickiness (Bowie *et al.*, 1969; Bowie and Owen, 1973). Perhaps one of the best tests to assess platelet function is the Ivy skin bleeding time (Ivy *et al.*, 1935; Mielke *et al.*, 1969), which will be normal in the hemophilias and prolonged in von Willebrand's disease and thrombocytopenia. There has been considerable debate in the medical literature recently and at medical conferences about the absolute clinical value of the skin bleeding time (Yardumian, Mackie and Machin, 1986; Rogers and Levine, 1990, Editorial, 1991). One recent author suggests that the bleeding time does not predict surgical bleeding (Lind, 1991). Suffice to say, our laboratory still performs Ivy skin bleeding times but is wary of this test in young children because of its uncertain interpretation. Accordingly, we tend to avoid the bleeding time in very small children.

Having determined hematologic parameters and platelet numbers and function, the coagulation system must be tested. The screening tests of the coagulation system are the prothrombin time to assess the extrinsic clotting system, i.e., factors II, V, VII and X, whilst a one-stage screening test such as the partial thromboplastin with kaolin (PTTK) or activated partial thromboplastin time (APTT) is used to assess the intrinsic coagulation system and especially factors VIII, IX, XI and XII. In the hemophilias and von Willebrand's disease, the prothrombin time or prothrombin ratio, which is frequently expressed as an international normalized ratio (International Committee, 1985; Poller, 1985; Taskforce, 1991a), will be normal but the APTT or PTTK will be prolonged. Unfortunately, the extent of lengthening of the APTT (PTTK) outside the laboratory's normal range does not directly correlate with the level of the deficient clotting factor, other than to say that severe deficiency will probably provide marked lengthening of that screening test, APTT (PTTK).

In the presence of a prolonged APTT (PTTK), unless the family history is certain, the laboratory will then need to assess by assay the relevant clotting factors, namely factor VIIIc, IXc, V and XI or XII. Hemophilia A will have a reduced level of factor VIIIc, Hemophilia B will have a reduced level of factor IXc, whilst in von Willebrand's disease there is generally a reduced factor VIIIc level (Nilsson *et al.*, 1957; Biggs and Matthews, 1963; Cornu *et al.*, 1963). However, mildly affected patients and severely affected patients with variant forms of von Willebrand's disease may have normal plasma factor VIIIc levels (Montgomery and Coller, 1994).

Accordingly, the clinical pathologist responsible for the testing of the person suspected of having one of the congenital bleeding disorders must consider the possibility of von Willebrand's disease and arrange the appropriate tests. At this stage it might be mentioned that the clinical laboratory testing for von Willebrand's disease is by no means easy but by no means impossible. Unfortunately, however, the label of von Willebrand's disease is sometimes applied on minimal grounds and then it is very difficult to have this diagnosis removed from that unfortunate patient. Essential tests to be performed for the diagnosis of the von Willebrand's syndrome, beside the factor VIIIc level and the skin bleeding time, are measurement of plasma von Willebrand factor (vWf:Ag), von Willebrand factor activity as ristocetin cofactor activity (vWf:RCo) and a qualitative assessment of the von Willebrand factor multimers (Zimmerman *et al.*, 1975a,b; Meyer *et al.*, 1980; Ruggeri and Zimmerman, 1981).

It is only when all these parameters are carefully measured that the presence or absence of von Willebrand's disease can be determined. Having done all the above tests, the clinician or pathologist is now in a position to make a statement about the nature and severity of the underlying bleeding disorder, whether this be hemophilia A, hemophilia B or von Willebrand's disease.

In relation to the interpretation of results, this can only be legitimately done if the responsible laboratory meets recognized national or international standards of quality, quality control and assurance (Taskforce, General Hematology, 1991). All such laboratories offering these services must regularly relate their performance indices to outside standards and quality control measures. If this is not done and standards are not maintained, then results may be misleading. Part of such quality control is specimen reception, specimen identification and valid distribution of results. All this is important in the diagnosis of the hemophilias and von Willebrand's disease. In this area of good laboratory practice, it is fundamental that results are clearly documented, recorded and quickly and efficiently despatched to the relevant clinician by post, courier or computer access.

Relationship of severity of defect to clinical manifestations

The clinical severity of the hemophilias is directly related to the level of factor VIIIc or factor IXc and the clinical symptoms are generally proportional to the level of factor VIIIc in von Willebrand's disease (Rizza, 1981; Holmberg and Nilsson, 1985). But symptoms in von Willebrand's disease do vary. The clinical problems in severe von Willebrand's disease are obviously different from that in mild disease. There is also clinical variability depending upon the type; autosominal dominant type 1 may have mild symptoms while patients with type II variants may have severe bleeding (Holmberg and Nilsson, 1985). The degree of severity of hemophilia appears to be the same in affected family members or kindreds, which presumably is due to the inheritance of a common molecular defect in that family (Tuddenham, 1989).

The unit of activity of factor VIIIc is the amount of factor VIII coagulant activity in 1 ml of fresh normal plasma (Biggs and Matthews, 1966). Diagnostic laboratories now refer or compare to an international standard as distributed by the WHO (WHO/World Federation of Haemophilia (WFH), 1991). Many countries develop their own international standard based on the WHO reference values and the value assigned to a carefully prepared national standard may be the average value after independent assay by a number of reference laboratories in that country (Rizza and Rhymes, 1982). Normal values for factor VIIIc expressed in reference to average normal plasma range from 50 to 200 u/dl. Accordingly, levels less than 50 u/dl are regarded as abnormal. It also needs to be remembered that these biologic assays of factor VIIIc or factor IXc discussed below have an intrinsic error possibility and values assigned need to be considered in the context of the laboratory's normal ranges.

A frequent classification for hemophilia is to define the severity of the condition as severe, moderate or mild (Rizza, 1981; Brettler and Levine, 1994). This classification is certainly reasonable but it is important always to be aware of the 'core' diagnosis, which is hemophilia. To say that a person has mild hemophilia may give the misleading impression to less knowledgeable health care professionals who may then think there is little cause for concern because the individual only has mild hemophilia and hence mistakenly believe that teeth or an appendix may be removed without the administration of prophylactic factor VIII or factor IX. If such procedures are performed without the necessary factor replacement it is more often than not to the patient's discomfort and postoperative bleeding and complications even of a life-threatening nature can occur. Accordingly, when thinking about hemophilia and the classification of the grades of severity, it is important to remember the common denominator – that we are dealing with a person with hemophilia (Kasper and Dietrich, 1985). Many a medical officer has been embarrassed in the postoperative period by misinterpretating the diagnosis of so-called mild hemophilia.

Patients or families with severe hemophilia have factor VIIIc or factor IXc levels of 0–1 u/dl, moderately affected patients have levels in the 2–5 u/dl range, whilst mildly affected patients have levels greater than 5 u/dl. The clinical manifestations of the hemophilia relate directly to these levels (Rizza, 1981; Brettler and Levine, 1994). The person with severe hemophilia is most likely to experience frequent, spontaneous bleeds or hemarthroses unless on prophylactic treatment and these people often proceed to severe hemophilic arthropathy manifested by joint destruction and associated muscular atrophy leading to crippling deformities. One or two joints may be thus involved, but often there is multiple joint damage, especially affecting the weight bearing joints of ankles and knees; this is not infrequently associated with hemophilic arthropathy of the elbows. Hemophilic pseudocysts can also be seen in moderate or severe hemophilia.

The person with moderate hemophilia may occasionally experience spontaneous bleeds but more often bleeding follows minor trauma or interventive procedures. These people can have joint problems but with nowhere near the frequency of severe hemophilia. A troublesome joint in moderate hemophilia is often referred to as a target joint and this joint can certainly demonstrate the pathologic changes seen in severe hemophilia. Our local experience suggests that hemophilic pseudotumours may be seen in moderate and mild hemophilia.

The person with mild hemophilia rarely, if ever, experiences spontaneous bleeds but will bleed following trauma. Joint problems rarely, if ever, occur. Probably the biggest hazard to the person with mild hemophilia is the misguided medical or dental practitioner who thinks that because this person has mild hemophilia then procedures can be done without cover of factor VIII or factor IX infusions. Patient and family education about the nature and vagaries of hemophilia is most important. It is vital to the patient's own welfare that he understands the necessity for treatment if he believes that bleeding is about to occur or is actually happening, that he must receive treatment before and after surgical or dental procedures, and that he should, place himself in the care of a physician who really understands and has an excellent working knowledge of the care of people with hemophilia. This responsibility for the person with hemophilia not only applies to the physician but also to the relevant hospital or area health authority. The levels of service that hospitals can provide for persons with hemophilia do vary and accordingly it is better for the hemophilia service to be rationalized.

Laboratory diagnosis

THE LABORATORY

Inherent in the laboratory diagnosis of the hemophilias or von Willebrand's disease is the presence of an efficiently functioning hemostasis laboratory staffed by well-trained, experienced and competent medical laboratory scientists. For the hemostasis laboratory to maintain standards and accuracy it should not operate in a vacuum but be an active participant in various national and even international quality control and assessment programs. Participation in quality assurance programs enables the laboratory to be confident that its results are consistent with its peer group and that good and safe laboratory practice is maintained. It is ideal if such important diagnostic laboratories are periodically and independently assessed by outside reviewers, leading to a qualification for the laboratory of accreditation by a recognized national testing authority.

Tests for hemostasis

The hemostatic mechanism or normal control of bleeding involves the physiologic integration of platelet function, coagulation and fibrinolysis. Accordingly, if we are endeavoring to assess the hemostatic mechanisms in an individual we should be able to test each of these systems (Pitney, 1968; Owen *et al.*, 1975; Rickard, 1976; Brozovic, 1991).

Probably the only valid *in vivo* test of the hemostatic mechanism is the skin bleeding time, done under carefully controlled conditions. The other tests of the hemostatic mechanisms are all *in vitro* studies and it can only be assumed that their interaction is normal or abnormal in any one individual being tested based on their *in vitro* test procedures.

Hemostasis screening tests

The full blood count. A full blood count should be done to determine the basic parameters of hemoglobin level, white cell and platelet count. An expertly made and stained blood film should be examined to determine if there are underlying hematologic abnormalities present in the person who is essentially presenting with a bleeding or bruising tendency. Thus it is important to exclude at the outset such diagnoses as acute or chronic leukemia, while the presence of thrombocytopenia should also be apparent on the blood count and blood film and examination. Some of the rare congenital platelet abnormalities may also be detected by the expert on blood film examination.

Coagulation screening tests. A number of very simple, one-stage screening tests of the coagulation mechanism provide important information if they are correctly and expertly performed. The important tests here are the prothrombin time, APTT or the PTTK, the thrombin time and measurement of plasma fibrinogen. In addition, considerable information may be obtained by simple mixing tests. If a prolonged PTTK or APTT is corrected by a mixture of equal volumes of normal plasma and the abnormal plasma, this quickly suggests a coagulation factor deficiency and, depending on which system we are testing, a rapid assessment may be made of the possible factor or factors absent. This is indeed the basis of the previously popular thromboplastin generation test (Biggs and Douglas, 1953) but now most laboratories would quickly move to assay the possible clotting factors involved.

The prothrombin time. The one-stage prothrombin time, results of which may be expressed as an absolute time compared with control plasma, a prothrombin index (control plasma time being the numerator and test plasma time being the denominator) or a prothrombin ratio (test plasma time over control plasma time) or, indeed, as the international normalized ratio (INR = PR^{ISI}), where ISI is the sensitivity index of the thromboplastin being used (International Committee, 1985; Taskforce, General Haematology, 1991). However, the INR is more properly related to an expression of the prothrombin time ratio for patients taking oral anticoagulants and in the assessment of hemostasis it is probably more relevant to express the prothrombin time as a ratio or absolute time in seconds.

The one-stage prothrombin time is generally considered to evaluate the integrity of the so-called extrinsic coagulation system and as such, it rapidly assesses whether the factors II, V, VII and X are in the range of normality. A long prothrombin time suggests a deficiency of one or more of the above factors which may be seen in vitamin K deficiency, liver disease or with oral anticoagulant therapy. Prothrombin times will be normal in classical hemophilia, hemophilia B and von Willebrand's disease but will be prolonged with congenital factor V deficiency or parahemophilia and in congenital deficiencies of factor VII or factor X.

The partial thromboplastin time. The intrinsic system is evaluated by the one-stage screening test called a PTTK (Proctor and Rapaport, 1961) or APTT. The thromboplastin generation screening test can also be of value in the testing procedure (Hicks and Pitney, 1957). Laboratories may use one or other or indeed all of these tests to assess the intrinsic coagulation system. The PTTK test is tried and true but unfortunately is not readily accommodated to automated systems since the opacity of the kaolin system does not lend itself to instrumental detection of end-points. The APTT does, however, lend itself to instrumental use because of the transparency of the reagents and hence may be readily utilized for automated testing on the various laboratory coagulation monitors that are now available. The prolongation of the PTTK or APTT may suggest deficiencies of one or more of the clotting factors in the intrinsic coagulation system but especially factors VIII, IX, V, XI and XII. In this context if the prothrombin time is normal, then factor V deficiency is unlikely. In the hemophilias and von Willebrand's disease, characteristically the PTTK or APTT screening tests will be prolonged, hence the need to move to specific assays of the various coagulation factors. The isolated prolonged APTT or PTTK in the young boy or young man with a history of easy bruising or bleeding tendency is a typical warning or alert signal that we may be dealing with hemophilia A, B or von Willebrand's disease.

Unfortunately, it is not quite so straightforward since there are some other situations which may also cause a prolonged APTT or PTTK in the presence of a normal prothrombin time (Ewing and Kasper, 1982). Here, one should specially think of the presence of heparin or a lupus-like anticoagulant or a circulating antifactor VIII inhibitor (Exner *et al.*, 1978). Fortunately these situations are very rare indeed in young males, hence the relevance of a suspicion that the underlying diagnosis is, hemophilia A or B or von Willebrand's disease in the presence of a prolonged APTT. Here again, simple mixing tests may be of help since circulating anticoagulants or inhibitors will prolong the PTTK or APTT of the mixture rather than correct it and the strong lupus-like anticoagulants may do likewise. Mixing tests will usually correct the prolonged APTT or PTTK in the hemophilias.

The thrombin time. Another useful screening test is a simple thrombin time of the patient's plasma compared to normal plasma. Heparin will prolong the thrombin time and can be neutralized in the thrombin time by the simple addition of, toluidine blue. It is also useful to measure plasma fibrinogen. Congenital abnormalities of fibrinogen are extremely rare but fibrinogen levels may be diminished in liver disease and in the acute defibrination states.

The Echis *test.* The *Echis* clotting time is used in conjunction with the prothrombin time to differentiate between liver disease and vitamin K deficiency. Factors II, VII, IX and X are synthesized in the liver as precursor forms and vitamin K is necessary for their conversion to functional factors (Corrigan and Ernest, 1980).

The *Echis carinatus* venom activates both factor II precursor and factor II to form thrombin whereas thromboplastin can only activate factor II and not factor II precursor. In liver disease, factor II precursor and factor II are reduced, whereas in vitamin K deficiency, factor II precursor is present but functional factor II is reduced. Therefore, the *Echis* clotting time in liver disease would be abnormal, whereas in vitamin K deficiency and during warfarin therapy, the *Echis* clotting time would be normal. It can be seen that this is a useful simple test to differentiate between abnormalities due to intrinsic liver disease or abnormalities associated with vitamin K deficiency.

PLATELET FUNCTION TESTING

In the clinical laboratory platelet function testing most commonly relates to qualitative and quantitative studies of platelet aggregation done using a platelet aggregometer and the common platelet agonists ADP, collagen, adrenalin and ristocetin (Born, 1962; O'Brien, 1962). Some laboratories may also measure platelet adhesive properties by the passage of native or heparinized blood through glass bead columns and calculate the number of platelets sticking in the column, as a measure of platelet adhesion (Bowie and Owen, 1971). Finally, the skin bleeding time, if correctly performed under standardized conditions, is a useful non-discriminatory test of platelet function and also platelet number (Yardumian, Mackie and Machin, 1986; Rogers and Levine, 1990, 1992; Editorial, 1991). However, there is little point in the performance of the skin bleeding time if there is thrombocytopenia since the bleeding time will invariably be prolonged. In all tests of platelet function, it is important to exclude the possibility that the patient is taking medication, especially aspirin, which is known to have an adverse affect on all tests of platelet function (O'Brien, 1962; Yardumian, Mackie and Machin, 1986).

Platelet aggregation performed using an aggregometer quantitates and plots increasing light transmission in platelet-rich plasma as platelets progressively aggregate. The shape of the curves with the various agonists is typical, especially for ADP, where there is a primary and secondary wave of platelet aggregation due to added ADP and release of intrinsic ADP respectively. The slope and magnitude of the resulting curves may be quantified and used for comparative purposes (Yardumian, Mackie and Machin, 1986; Taskforce, 1991b). In the hemophilias, platelet aggregation patterns will be normal.

Another important agonist for measuring platelet aggregation is the antibiotic compound ristocetin which again produces typical aggregation curves, but ristocetin-induced platelet aggregation is generally abnormal in von Willebrand's disease (Howard, Sawers and Firkin, 1973; Meyer *et al.*, 1973). Platelet aggregation in the presence of other inducers can be normal. Modifications of ristocetin-induced platelet aggregation are used to measure the von Willebrand factor, ristocetin cofactor, vWf R:Co activity (Weiss *et al.*, 1973; Meyer *et al.*, 1974). This will be reduced in von Willebrand's disease but normal in the hemophilias.

TESTING THE FIBRINOLYTIC SYSTEM

It is unusual for primary abnormalities of the fibrinolytic system to be a cause of bleeding or bruising, especially in children or young adults. Certainly, in older adults with significant liver disease, fibrinolytic enhancement may be a factor in the bleeding propensity. A reasonable screening test for the fibrinolytic system is the euglobulin clot lysis time (Von Kaulla, 1963); in the presence of enhanced plasminogen activator activity, euglobulin clot lysis will occur more quickly than normal. This is a non-discriminatory test and assays of plasminogen, plasmin and antiplasmins are necessary to try and obtain some assessment of fibrinolytic activity. In the diagnosis of hemophilia and von Willebrand's disease these tests are not particularly relevant nor diagnostic.

ASSESSMENT OF THE FACTOR VIII MOLECULAR COMPLEX

Assay of factor VIIIC

The factor VIII molecular complex comprises factor VIII coagulant (FVIIIc) and von Willebrand factor (Marder *et al.*, 1985). Factor VIIIc can be adequately assessed by a one-stage PTTK bioassay. This may be conveniently done by the use of the manual one-stage PTTK parallel line bioassays with coagulation assayed reference plasma as the standard (Hardisty and MacPherson, 1962; Rizza and Rhymes, 1982).

The various moieties of the von Willebrand factor also need to be assayed in relation to the differential diagnosis of hemophilia A and von Willebrand's disease (Hoyer *et al.*, 1983). Accordingly, it is necessary to measure von Willebrand factor antigen (vWf:Ag), von Willebrand factor activity (ristocetin cofactor activity, vWf:RCo) and von Willebrand factor multimers (Marder *et al.*, 1985). vWf:Ag is measured by immunoassay, frequently performed by quantitative immunoelectrophoresis, with the amount of von Willebrand factor being proportional to the height of the resulting rocket in agarose gels containing anti vWf antibody – the so-called Laurell immunoelectrophoresis technique (Laurell, 1966; Zimmerman *et al.*, 1975a,b). Alternatively, an enzyme-linked immunoabsorbent assay (ELISA) can be used to measure vWf:Ag (Ruggeri *et al.*, 1976; Ness and Perkins, 1979). The ratio of factor VIIIc to vWf:Ag is a useful parameter. In normal persons, the ratio of factor VIIIc to vWf:Ag is close to 1; in people with hemophilia and obligatory carriers of hemophilia, the ratio is usually less than 1, perhaps in the range of 0.5–0.6, whilst possible carriers of hemophilia A may also have values less than 1 (Rickard, 1976; WHO, 1992). In von Willebrand' s disease both parameters are reduced and so the ratio may be non-discriminatory. Generally in von Willebrand's disease vWf:Ag is more reduced than the FVIIIc level.

The von Willebrand factor multimers

In many ways this is a definitive test for the presence of von Willebrand's disease, since the major types of von Willebrand's disease, types I–III have characteristic variations m their multimeric pattern when compared with normal controls (Rugger and Zimmerman, 1981; Holmberg and Nilsson, 1992).

The von Willebrand factor multimers are a qualitative measure of the structure of the von Willebrand molecule and the function of von Willebrand's factor is frequently abnormal because the larger von Willebrand's factor multimers are missing. As a type of screening procedure, electrophoresis to von Willebrand multimers may be done in the first instance using low-resolution gels but more definitive studies of multimeric pattern will generally require the use of high-resolution gels (Ciavarella and Antonucchi, 1985). The various types of von Willebrand's disease exhibit different multimeric patterns – in type I there is a qualitative decrease in all the multimers; in type II the high-molecular-weight multimers are absent; in type IIb and platelet von Willebrand's disease some of the high-molecular-weight multimers are absent, whilst in Type III all multimers are absent (Holmberg and Nilsson, 1992).

Ristocetin cofactor assays

The von Willebrand factor is essential for normal platelet function, particularly aggregation and adhesion (Weiss, Truitto and Baumgartner, 1978). vWf:RCo is a laboratory measure of this von Willebrand factor activity (Weiss *et al.*, 1973). Assessment is made by quantitative measurement of fixed washed normal platelet aggregation in the presence of dilutions of normal plasma for the derivation of a standard curve and this is compared to the degree of platelet aggregation supported by the test plasma, which may be deficient in von Willebrand factor activity (Brozovic and Mackie, 1991). A well maintained and efficiently functioning platelet aggregometer with chart recorder is necessary for these experiments.

THE VON WILLEBRAND FACTOR ACTIVITY ASSAY AND AN ELISA SYSTEM

In the ELISA system, a monoclonal antibody is used to detect the von Willebrand factor or more particularly, an epitope of the von Willebrand factor which is responsible for the binding of the von Willebrand factor to glycoprotein 1B on platelets (Ruggeri *et al.*, 1972; De Marco, 1985). The von Willebrand factor monoclonal antibody complexes are then detected by an anti-von Willebrand factor polyclonal antibody conjugated to a detectable marker such as horseradish peroxidase (Ruggeri *et al.*, 1976). This is a reproducible assay and has advantages over the more tedious bioassay based on ristocetin induced aggregation of fixed platelets.

ASSAY OF FACTOR IX

One-stage bioassays of factor IXc based on the PTTK system may be performed in a similar manner to those for factor VIIIc. The degree of correction of clotting times in the PTTK system on factor IX-deficient plasma is compared using dilutions of test plasma and a coagulation-assayed reference plasma (Biggs, 1972; Brozovic and Mackie, 1991). Clotting times are plotted on log–log graph paper. The percentage of factor IX is plotted on the x axis and the clotting time is seconds on the y axis. Parallel lines should be obtained and from these the factor IX level is derived as a percentage or u/dl.

ASSAYS FOR FACTOR II, V, VII AND X

These factors are assessed in the prothrombin time system and their individual assays are dependent on the application of this test (Brozovic and Mackie, 1991). Accordingly, the assay of each factor consists of performing the prothrombin time with varying dilutions of patient plasma and a specific factor-deficient substrate. The corrective effect of test plasma prothrombin time is compared to that of a standard reference plasma.

Using log–log graph paper, the per cent factor is plotted on the x axis and the clotting times on the y axis. The assayed reference plasma is plotted according to its reference value. From the parallel lines of best fit, the percentage of factor level in the test plasma can be calculated.

CLOTTING FACTOR ASSAYS AND CHROMOGENIC SUBSTRATES

These synthetic peptides utilize the concept that the bond split by a protease is an amide bond and p-nitroaniline (pNA) is released by the amidolytic activity of the enzymes. The release of pNA which is proportional to the activity of the enzyme can then be measured spectrophotometrically. Good chromogenic substrates are now readily available and may be classified as substrates for proenzymes, enzymes or activators and inhibitors of blood coagulation. The use of chromogenic substrates can be automated using spectrophotometric and centrifugal analyzers. Accordingly, there is a wide clinical application for the use and expansion of chromogenic substrates for population assays of clotting factors. Assay of the antihemophilia factors, factor VIIIc and factor IXc can be done using chromogenic substrates. Here assay of factor IX is regarded as a proenzyme and factor VIII as a cofactor.

Differential diagnosis

At the bedside, the differential diagnosis of the hemophilias and von Willebrand's disease is from multiple other causes of bleeding disorders. However, the clinical context and circumstances of the hemophilias will certainly reduce the range of these possibilities. In hemophilia we are frequently thinking about a male baby, a young boy or a young man who may have joint-related symptoms at presentation such as hemarthroses or joint swelling, in addition to easy bruising and a bleeding tendency. This should certainly alert the clinician to the possibility of hemophilia. The person with von Willebrand's disease may be either male or a female with menorrhagia, and it would be rather uncommon but not impossible, for this person to have joint problems. The clinical presentation is thus all important when one thinks of differential diagnosis.

It will not be possible to differentiate on clinical grounds alone the presence of hemophilia A or B or perhaps even von Willebrand's disease. Results of laboratory tests are essential to separate these conditions – low factor VIIIc in hemophilia A, low factor IXc in hemophilia B and the long bleeding time, reduced factor VIIIc and abnormal platelet function in von Willebrand's disease (Table 5.1).

If one wishes to pursue the question of differential diagnosis of the younger person presenting with a bleeding tendency, then such conditions as platelet disorders like thrombocytopenia or platelet function disorders of a congenital or acquired nature need consideration. The cause of a thrombocytopenia might be apparent such as drug-induced thrombocytopenia or thrombocytopenia associated with a hematologic malignancy like acute or chronic leukemia. Acquired platelet function disorders are not all that uncommon, especially those associated with aspirin injestion, renal disease or paraproteinnaemias (Castaldi, Rosenberg and Stewart, 1966; Perkins, McKenzie and Fudenberg, 1970; Roth and Majerus, 1975). Congenital platelet function disorders are relatively uncommon and those that might spring to mind are Bernard–Soulier syndrome, Glanzmann's thrombasthenia, storage pool disorders or platelet-type von Willebrand's disease (Lusher and Barnhart, 1977). Joint problems are rare in these unusual platelet conditions and laboratory

Table 5.1 Differential diagnosis of hemophilia A, B and von Willebrand's disease: laboratory studies

	INR	PTTK (APTT)	FVIIIc	FIXc	vWf: Ag	vWf: RCo	vWf Multimers	Platelet aggregation				
								ADP	Collagen	Ristocetin	Platelet adhesion	
HA	N	P	R	N	N	N	N	N	N	N	N	
HB	N	P	N	R	N	N	N	N	N	N	N	
Para H	P	P	N	N	N	N	N	N	N	N	N	FV R
vWd	N	P	R	N	R	R	R	N	N	R	R	
FXI	N	P	N	N	N	N	N	N	N	N	N	FXI R

INR = International normalized ratio; PTTK = partial thromboplastin time with kaolin; APTT = activated partial thromboplastin time; FVIIIc = factor IXc; vWF: Ag = von Willebrand and factor antigen; vWF: RCO = von Willebrand factor ristocetin cofactor; ADP = adenosine diphosphate; HA = hemophilia A; HB = hemophilia B; Para H = factor V deficiency; vWD = von Willebrand's disease; FXI = factor XI deficiency; N = normal; R = reduced or abnormal.

tests, particularly those of platelet function and assays of factor VIIIc and factor IXc, should quickly differentiate between these conditions.

Severe liver disease may also have clinical features of a bleeding tendency, but it is more than likely that this underlying disorder will have been previously recognized, the patient may be jaundiced and have hepatomegaly or hepatosplenomegaly and other stigmata of chronic liver disease. Acute liver disease will usually present as a fulminating illness. Another condition that might be mentioned, although rarely seen in a young child or young adult, is a circulating inhibitor of a spontaneous nature that is an autoantibody to factor VIII or, rarely, to factor IX. Finally, for the sake of completion, the other congenital coagulation factor deficiencies be mentioned – factor V deficiency or parahemophilia and congenital deficiencies of factor XI, VII or X – the latter two being very uncommon. Factor XI deficiency may present with spontaneous bleeding and perhaps with bleeding after surgery or interventive procedures. This condition occurs mainly in people with Jewish background and is well described in the Ashkenazai Jews in Israel (Seligsohn, 1993).

Combined deficiencies

COMBINED DEFICIENCIES OF THE VITAMIN K-DEPENDENT FACTORS

All the vitamin K-dependent coagulation factors and are synthesized in the liver. Their synthesis is dependent upon the activity of vitamin K for the post-translational carboxylation of the gamma-glutamyl residues and all these factors have similar biochemical characteristics. Factor IX like factor VIII is a sex-linked characteristic while the other three display an autosomal pattern of inheritance. Some inherited combined deficiencies have been reported such as those of factor VII and factor IX and factor VII and factor X (Bloom and Thomas, 1981).

COMBINED DEFICIENCIES OF FACTOR V AND FACTOR VIII

Although rare, combined deficiencies of these factors have been reported in certain families with a suggestion that the deficiencies are transmitted together. Factor V/VIII deficiency has been reported in Jews of Oriental or Sephardic extraction (Bloom and Thomas, 1981). These two factors have similar biochemical characteristics and both act with phospholipids as coenzymes in the coagulation sequence. One postulate is that the combined deficiency is due to a common defect of a regulatory or structural gene affecting the systems of both factor V and factor VIII. Clinically the condition is similar to isolated factor V deficiency and exhibits an automsomal inheritance (Bloom and Thomas, 1981).

References

Biggs, R. (1972) *Human Blood Coagulation, Haemostasis and Thrombosis*, Blackwell Scientific Publications, Oxford, UK.

Biggs, R. and Douglas, A.S. (1953) The thromboplastin generation test. *Journal of Clinical Pathology*, **6**, 615–619.

Biggs, R. and Matthews, J.M. (1963) The treatment of haemorrhage in von Willebrand's disease and the blood level of factor VIII (AHG). *British Journal of Haematology*, **9**, 203–207.

Biggs, R. and Matthews, J.M. (1966) The plasma concentration of factor VIII in the treatment of haemophilia, in *The Treatment of Haemophilia and Other Coagulation Disorders* (eds R. Biggs and R.G. MacFarlane), Blackwell Scientific Publications, Oxford.

Bloom, A.L. and Thomas, D.P. (eds) (1981) Inherited disorders of blood coagulation, in *Haemostasis and Thrombosis*, Churchill Livingstone, Edinburgh.

Born, G.V.R. (1962) Aggregation of blood platelets by adenosine diphosphate and its reversal. *Nature*, **194**, 927–929.

Bowie, E.J.W. and Owen, C.A. (1971) The value of measuring platelet 'adhesiveness' in the diagnosis of bleeding diseases. *American Journal of Clinical Pathology*, **60**, 302–307.

Bowie, E.J.W., Owen, C.A., Thompson, J.H. and Didisheim, P. (1969) Platelet 'adhesiveness' in von Willebrand's disease. *American Journal of Clinical Pathology*, **52**, 69–74.

Bowie, E.J.W. and Owen, C.A. (1971) The value of measuring platelet 'adhesiveness' in the diagnosis of bleeding diseases. *American Journal of Clinical Pathology*, **60**, 302–307.

Brettler, D. and Levine, P. (1994) Clinical manifestations and therapy of inherited coagulation factor deficiencies, in *Haemostasis and Thrombosis: Basic Principles and Clinical Practice*, 3rd edn (eds R.W. Colman, J. Hirsh, V.J. Marder and E. Salzman), J.B. Lippincott, Philadelphia.

Brozovic, M. (1991) Investigation of haemostasis, in *Practical Haematology*, 7th edn (eds J.V. Dacie and S.M. Lewis), J. and A. Churchill, London.

Brozovic, M. and Mackie, I. (1991) Investigation of a bleeding tendency, in *Practical Haematology*, 7th edn (eds J.V. Dacie and S.M. Lewis), J. and A. Churchill, London.

Castaldi, P.A. and Rosenberg, M.C. and Stewart, J.H. (1966) The bleeding disorder of uremia. *Lancet*, **ii**, 66–68.

Ciavarella, G. and Antonucchi, S. (1985) High resolution analysis of von Willebrand factor multimeric composition defines a new variant of type I von Willebrand's disease with aberrant structure but presence of all size multimers. *Blood*, **66**, 1423–1429.

Cornu, P., Larrieu, M.J., Caen, J. and Bernard, J. (1963) Transfusion studies in von Willebrand's disease. Effect on bleeding time and factor VIII. *British Journal of Haematology*, **9**, 189–192.

Corrigan, J.J. and Ernest, E.L. (1980) Factor II antigen in liver disease and warfarin induced vitamin K deficiency. *American Journal of Hematology*, **8**, 249–253.

DeMarco, L., Grolami, A., Russell, S. and Ruggeri, Z.M. (1985) Interaction of asialo vWf with glycoprotein 1b induces fibrinogen binding to the glycoprotein IIb/IIIa complexes and mediates platelet aggregation. *Journal of Clinical Investigation*, **75**, 1198–1205.

Editorial (1991) The bleeding time. *Lancet*, **337**, 1447.

Ewing, N.P. and Kasper, C.K. (1982) *In vitro* detection of mild inhibitors to factor VIII in hemophilia. *American Journal of Clinical Pathology*, **77**, 749–753.

Exner, T., Rickard, K.A. and Kronenberg, H. (1978) A sensitive test demonstrating the lupus anticoagulant and its behavioural patterns. *British Journal of Haematology*, **40**, 143–151.

Hardisty, R.M. and MacPherson, J.C. (1962) A one stage factor VIII anti haemophilic globulin assay and its use on venous and capillary blood. *Thrombosis Diathesis Haemorrhagica*, **7**, 215–218.

Hicks, N.D. and Pitney, W.R. (1957) A rapid screening test for disorders of thromboplastin degeneration. *British Journal of Haematology*, **3**, 227–233.

Holmberg, L. and Nilsson, I.M. (1985) Von Willebrand's disease, in *Clinics in Haematology. Coagulation Disorders*, vol. 14 (ed. Z. Ruggeri), W.B. Saunders, London, pp. 461–488.

Holmberg, L. and Nilsson, I.M. (1992) Von Willebrand's disease. *European Journal of Haematology*, **48**, 127–141.

Howard, M.A., Sawers, R.J. and Firkin, B.J. (1973) Rostocetin: a means of differentiating von Willebrand's disease into two groups. *Blood*, **41**, 687–692.

Hoyer, L.N., Rizza, C.R., Tuddenham, E.G.D. *et al.* (1983) von Willebrand factor multimer patterns in von Willebrand's disease. *British Journal of Haematology*, **55**, 493–507.

Hutton, R.A. and Ludlam, C.A. (1989) Platelet function testing. *Journal of Clinical Pathology*, **42**, 858–864.

International Committee for Standardisation in Haematology, International Committee on Thrombosis and Haemostasis (1985) ICTH recommendations for reporting prothrombin time in oral anticoagulant control. *Thrombosis and Haemostasis*, **53**, 155–156.

Ivy, A.C., Shapiro, P.F. and Melnick, P. (1935) The bleeding tendency in jaundice. *Surgery Gynecology and Obstetrics*, **67**, 781–784.

Kasper, C. and Dietrich, S. (1985) Comprehensive management of haemophilia, in *Clinics in Haematology*, vol. 14 (ed. Z. Ruggeri), W.B. Saunders, London, pp. 489–512.

Laurell, C.B. (1966) Quantitative estimation of proteins by electrophoresis in agarose gel containing antibodies. *Analytical Biochemistry*, **15**, 45–53.

Lind, S. (1991) The bleeding time does not predict surgical bleeding. *Blood*, **77**, 2547–2552.

Lusher, J.M. and Barnhart, M.I. (1977) Congenital disorders affecting platelets. *Seminars in Thrombosis and Haemostasis*, **4**, 123–138.

Marder, V.J., Mannucci, P.M., Firkin, B.J. *et al.* (1985) Standard nomenclature for factor VIII and von Willebrand factor. A recommendation by the International Committee on Thrombosis and Haemostasis. *Thrombosis and Haemostasis*, **54**, 871–872.

Meyer, D., Jenkins, C.S.P., Dreyfus, M.D. and Larrieu, M.J. (1973) Experimental model for von Willebrand's disease. *Nature*, **243**, 293–294.

Meyer, D., Jenkins, C.S.P., Dreyfus, M.D. *et al.* (1974) Willebrand factor and ristocetin II. Relation between Willebrand factor, Willebrand antigen and factor VIII activity. *British Journal of Haematology*, **28**, 579–593.

Meyer, D., Obert, B., Pietu, G. *et al.* (1980) Multimeric structure of factor VIII/vWf in von Willebrand's disease. *Journal of Laboratory and Clinical Medicine*, **95**, 590–597.

Mielke, C.H., Kaneshiro, M.M., Maher, I.A. *et al.* (1969) The standardised normal ivy bleeding time and its prolongation by aspirin. *Blood*, **34**, 204–209.

Montgomery, R.B., Coller, B.S. (1994) von Willebrand's disease, in *Haemostasis and Thrombosis. Basic Principles and Clinical Practice*, 3rd edn (ed. R.W. Coleman, J. Hirsh, V.J. Marder and E. Salzman), J.B. Lippincott, Philadelphia, USA.

Ness, P.M. and Perkins, H.A. (1979) A simple amino assay (EIA) test for factor VIII related antigen. *Thrombosis and Haemostasis*, **42**, 848–852.

Nilsson, I.M., Blomback, M., Jorpes, E.J., Blomack, B. and Johansson, S. (1957) von Willebrand's disease and its connection with human plasma fraction 1-0. *Acta Medica Scandinavica*, **159**, 157–161.

O'Brien, J.R. (1962) Platelet aggregation. ii. Some results from a new method of study. *Journal of Clinical Pathology*, **15**, 452–457.

Owen, C.A., Bowie, E.J.W. and Thompson, J. (1975) *Testing of Hemostasis and Blood Coagulation. Diagnosis of Bleeding Disorders*. Little, Brown, Boston, Massachusetts.

Perkins, H.A., McKenzie, M.R. and Fudenberg, H.H. (1970) Haemostatic defects in dysproteinemias. *Blood*, **35**, 695–701.

Pitney, W.R. (1968) Investigation of the haemorrhagic disorders, in *Practical Haematology*, 4th edn (eds J.V. Dacie and S.M. Lewis), A. Churchill, London, UK.

Proctor, P.R. and Rapaport, S.I. (1961) The partial thromboplastin time with kaolin. A simple screening test for first stage plasma clotting factor deficiency. *American Journal of Pathology*, **36**, 212–215.

Poller, L. (1985) Therapeutic ranges in anticoagulant administration. *British Medical Journal*, **290**, 1683–1686.

Rickard, K.A. (1976) Specific diagnostic tests in the management of the haemophilias, in *Proceedings of the XI Congress of World Federation of Haemophilia* (Eds Editorial Board of the World Federation of Haemophilia), Academia Press, Tokyo, Japan, pp. 93–99.

Rickard, K.A. and Power, P. (1976) Haemophilia carrier detection. The Royal Prince Alfred Experience. *Australian and New Zealand Journal of Medicine*, **46**, 215.

Rizza, C.R. (1981) Management of patients with inherited blood coagulation defects, in *Haemostasis and Thrombosis* (eds A.L. Bloom and D.P. Thomas), Churchill Livingstone, Edinburgh.

Rizza, C.R. and Rhymes, I.L. (1982) Coagulation assays of factor VIIIc and IXc, in *The Haemophilias* (ed. A.L. Bloom), Churchill Livingstone, Edinburgh.

Rogers, R.P.C. and Levine, J. (1990) A critical reappraisal of the bleeding time. *Seminars in Thrombosis and Haemostasis*, **16**, 1–68.

Rogers, R.P.C. and Levine, J. (1992) Bleeding time revisited. *Blood*, **79**, 2495–2496.

Roth, C.J. and Majerus, P.W. (1975) The mechanism of the effect of aspirin on human platelets. *Journal of Clinical Investigation*, **56**, 624–630.

Ruggeri, Z.M. and Zimmerman, T.S. (1981) The complex multimeric composition of factor VIII/vWf. *Blood*, **57**, 1140–1146.

Ruggeri, Z.M., De Marco, L., Gatti, L. *et al* (1972) Platelets have more than one binding site for vWf. *Journal of Clinical Investigation*, **72**, 1–14.

Ruggeri, Z.M., Mannucci, P.M., Jeffcoate, S.L. and Ingram, G.I.C. (1976) Immunoradiometric assays of factor VIII related antigen with observations in 32 patients with von Willebrand's disease. *British Journal of Haematology*, **33**, 221–230.

Seligsohn, U. (1993) Factor XI deficiency. *Thrombosis and Haemostasis*, **70**, 168–170.

Taskforce, General Haematology (1991) Code for good laboratory practice in haematology laboratories, in *Standard Haematology Practice* (ed. B. Roberts), Blackwell Scientific Publications, Oxford, UK.

Taskforce, Haemostasis and Thrombosis (1991a) Oral anticoagulants, in *Standard Haematology Practice* (ed. B. Roberts), Blackwell Scientific Publications, Oxford, UK.

Taskforce, Haemostasis and Thrombosis (1991b) Platelet function testing, in *Standard Haematology Practice* (ed. B. Roberts), Blackwell Scientific Publications, Oxford, UK.

Tuddenham, E.G.J. (1989) Factor VIII and hemophilia A, in *Clinical Haematology. The Molecular Biology of Coagulation* (ed. E.G.D. Tuddenham) Baillière, London, UK.

Von Kaulla, K.N. (1963) *Chemistry of Thrombolysis: Human Fibrinolytic Enzymes*. Thomas, Springfield, Illinois, USA.

Weiss, H.J., Hoyer, L.N., Rickles, F.R. *et al.* (1973) Quantitative assay of a plasma factor deficient in von Willebrand's disease that is necessary for platelet aggregation. Relationship to factor VIII procoagulant activity and antigen content. *Journal of Clinical Investigation*, **52**, 2708–2719.

Weiss, H.J., Truitto, V.T. and Baumgartner, H.R. (1978) Effect of sheer rate in platelet interaction with subendothelium in citrated and native blood, i. Sheer dependent decrease of adherence in von Willebrand's disease and the Bernard Soulier syndrome. *Journal of Laboratory and Clinical Medicine*, **92**, 750–764.

WHO, WFH Memorandum (1991) Prevention and control of haemophilia. *Bulletin of the World Health Organisation, Geneva*, **69**, 17–26.

WHO, WFH Memorandum (1992) Carrier detection and prenatal diagnosis. *Bulletin of the World Health Organisation, Geneva*, **4**, 1–79.

Yardumian, D.A., Mackie, I.J. and Machin, S.J. (1986) Laboratory investigation of platelet function. Review of methodology. *Journal of Clinical Pathology*, **39**, 701–711.

Zimmerman, T.S., Hoyer, L.W., Dickson, L. and Edgington, T.S. (1975) Determination of the von Willebrand's disease antigen (factor VIII related antigen) in plasma by quantitative immunoelectrophoresis. *Journal of Laboratory and Clinical Medicine*, **86**, 152–158.

Zimmerman, T.S., Roberts, J. and Edgington, T.S. (1975) Factor VIII related antigen. Multiple molecular forms in human plasma. *Proceedings of National Academy of Science, USA* **75**, 5121–5124.

6 DIAGNOSIS OF HEMOPHILIA A AND B CARRIERS AND PRENATAL DIAGNOSIS

A.C. Goodeve and I.R. Peake

Hemophilia A and B are X-linked diseases where precise carrier detection and prenatal diagnosis are increasingly an integral part of care of the patient and family. Carrier assessment can be made in several ways:

1. Clinical diagnosis based on an individual's bleeding history in a family where hemophilia has been diagnosed.
2. Diagnosis within a family with hemophilia based upon a detailed family tree where no uncertainties (e.g. questions of paternity) are present.
3. Diagnosis based on reduced levels of plasma factor VIII (FVIII) or factor IX (FIX).
4. Genetic diagnosis by analysis of the FVIII or FIX genes within families either by polymorphism-based gene tracking (linkage analysis) or mutation detection.

The last two procedures may also be performed for prenatal diagnosis of hemophilia.

In this chapter the procedures outlined above will be elaborated and the relative merits of each discussed.

Clinical and phenotypic diagnosis of carrier status

Female carriers of hemophilia A or B have generally inherited their abnormal FVIII or FIX gene from one of their parents, together with a normal gene. Thus, on average, carriers of severe disease, where affected males have very low or undetectable levels of FVIII or FIX, will have plasma levels around 50% of normal. Carriers of milder conditions will tend to have levels greater than 50%, since the defective gene will be able to produce some clotting factor.

Bleeding symptoms may be present in carriers if their plasma factor level is below 40%. This generally occurs as a result of extreme lyonization, although other rare possibilities, including homozygosity, Turner's syndrome and co-inheritance of von Willebrand's disease should be considered.

The starting point for any family study in hemophilia must be an accurate family tree, showing the precise relationship between affected and non-affected family members. The nature of the inherited condition (hemophilia A or B) must be certain and the ethnic background of the family may also be important (see below).

With good family data it may be immediately possible to exclude or include carrier status in certain females. Thus, carriership can be excluded for a female if hemophilia only occurs in her paternal family and her father is not a hemophiliac. Alternately, a female may be diagnosed as a obligate carrier if her father has hemophilia or she has more than one hemophilic son or she has one affected son and her family includes a well-documented hemophiliac on her maternal side.

The remaining females within a hemophilic family should be considered to be possible carriers, particularly in families where the individual concerned has one hemophilic son and no family history of the disease (isolated cases). The assignment to a possible carrier of a probability of carriership is the essence of carrier detection and is only absolute when the precise genetic defect within the FVIII or FIX gene has been identified within her family and herself. Conversely, the absence of the mutation confers the status of non-carrier (see below). However, the procedures necessary for such diagnoses are unavailable to the majority of the world's hemophilic families at present and phenotypic methods are still widely used in carrier analysis.

The assessment of carrier status based on a family tree is calculated using anterior and descendent pedigree information to calculate an overall probability or odds of carriership. Thus, the daughter of a hemophiliac will have

Hemophilia. Edited by C.D. Forbes, L. Aledort and R. Madhok. Published in 1997 by Chapman & Hall, London. ISBN 0 412 63820 7

a probability of carriership of 1.0 (obligate carrier), and her daughters a probability of 0.5. Her granddaughters will have a probability of 0.25 (0.5 × 0.5). These procedures are described in detail in the recent 'Report of a joint WHO/WFH meeting on the control of hemophilia: carrier detection and prenatal diagnosis' (Peake *et al.*, 1993) and the reader is strongly advised to refer to this document for further examples and information both in regard to family tree-based calculations and to phenotypic assessment (see below).

Phenotypic assessment of carrier status, which is subsequently combined with the assessment from the pedigree data, is based on the lower levels of FVIII and FIX generally seen in obligate carriers (see above). These procedures require accurate measurement of clotting factors (FVIII, FIX and von Willebrand factor; vWf) and the use of national and international plasma standards in order to standardize locally obtained normal plasma pools used in these assays is strongly recommended.

Carriers of hemophilia A will on average have 50% of the normal plasma level of FVIII, measured either as FVIII clotting activity (FVIII:C) or immunologically (FVIII:Ag). Since there is no clear advantage in either measurement, the FVIII:C assay is invariably used. Based on the FVIII:C assay alone, no more than 80% of obligate carriers will have a level below the normal range because of the considerable overlap between the range of normal and carrier levels. This figure can be improved by measurement of the level of vWf:Ag since vWf and FVIII circulate in plasma as a complex with a fixed stoichiometric relationship and vWf:Ag levels are, of course, normal in hemophiliacs and carriers. Thus, if the ratio of FVIII to vWf:Ag in normal plasma is 1.0, then in an obligate carrier of hemophilia A it will be 0.5. This ratio has been shown to be a better discriminant of carrier status than the level of FVIII alone and can be used to provide a probability which may then be combined with that obtained from the pedigree data. Currently, however, the preferred method for carrier probability assessment from laboratory data in hemophilia A is bivariate linear discriminant analysis, based on levels of FVIII:C and vWf:Ag and accommodating the effects of age and ABO blood group on the levels (for details, see Peake *et al.*, 1993). The calculations outlined above for hemophilia A can be simplified using a universal discriminant which obviates the need for a reference group of known carriers (Green *et al.*, 1986).

For hemophilia B univariate linear discriminant analysis is recommended, using FIX:C measurements and applying a correction for the use of oral contraceptives (Peake *et al.*, 1993). The routine estimation of FIX:Ag levels is not justified, except in cases where significant levels are present in the affected relative (i.e. cross-reacting material-positive (CRM+) hemophilia B).

The final stage in this process is to combine pedigree and laboratory data to give an overall probability or odds of carriership. Although these methods can give useful information in many cases and be of considerable help to the proband and her family, absolute diagnosis is not possible because of the vagaries of lyonization and the large range of factor levels seen in both normal and carrier populations. Only genetic analysis, discussed below, can provide an absolute diagnosis of carrier or non-carrier status.

Genetic screening for hemophilia A and B

The carrier status of females with hemophilia can be determined by one of two forms of genetic analysis. The affected FVIII or FIX gene can be tracked indirectly through the family using polymorphism-based linkage analysis. This is the most widely used procedure. Alternatively, the causative mutation can be identified in the hemophiliac using a mutation screening procedure followed by DNA sequencing, and then sought in his female relatives. Apart from the FVIII gene inversion, the mutation detection techniques are technically demanding and expensive and only available in a small number of specialized laboratories.

DIRECTION MUTATION DETECTION

Hemophilia A

The FVIII gene inversion mutation (Lakich *et al.*, 1993; Naylor *et al.*, 1993; Goodeve *et al.*, 1994a) is the cause of hemophilia in approximately 42% of patients with severe hemophilia A (Antonarakis *et al.*, 1995). Patients with severe disease account for about 40% of hemophilia A cases, so the inversion is seen in 20–25% of all hemophilia A patients.

Analysis for the presence of the FVIII gene inversion should be performed as part of the diagnosis of carrier state in all families with severe hemophilia A. The detection of this mutation in the hemophiliac defines the cause of his disease and facilitates determination of female carrier status. In families where no hemophiliac is available for analysis, females who carry the inversion mutation on one X chromosome can be readily identified as carriers by Southern blotting (Chapter 3). Many laboratories which do not perform analysis of other FVIII mutations do offer detection of the inversion mutation.

The remaining 75–80% of patients with hemophilia A will have other mutations (discussed in detail in Chapter 3; Wacey *et al.*, 1996) and a large proportion of these mutations will be due to single nucleotide changes. As the FVIII gene is large, a mutation screening procedure is used prior to DNA sequencing to identify any mutations. For effective analysis, the 5′, entire coding region of the gene, intron–exon boundaries and 3′ region (approximately 10 kb in total) should be analyzed by a method which will detect close to 100% of mutations.

The procedures most commonly utilized are chemical cleavage mismatch detection (Naylor *et al.*, 1991), denaturing gradient gel electrophoresis (Higuchi *et al.*, 1991) and single strand conformation polymorphism (SSCP) (David *et al.*, 1994). Genomic DNA or FVIII messenger RNA obtained as an illegitimate transcript from peripheral blood lymphocytes is used. Once a mutation has been identified in an affected male, its presence can readily be ascertained in any female relatives by specific restriction enzyme analysis, SSCP or DNA sequencing, enabling their carrier status to be confirmed or excluded, and similarly used to determine fetal hemophilia status at prenatal diagnosis.

Hemophilia B

Hemophilia B may be caused by a large number of different mutations which occur throughout the FIX gene. The majority of these are single nucleotide changes. There are no common mutations, although repeat observations of mutations do occur, particularly at CpG dinucleotides.

The FIX gene is relatively small, spanning only 34 kb, of which the entire sequence is known. As for the FVIII gene, mutation detection for FIX requires the complete 5′, coding, intron–exon boundaries and 3′ regions to be analyzed. This entails analysis of less than 3 kb of sequence; mismatch detection methods and rapid direct sequencing of polymerase chain reaction (PCR)-amplified DNA enable this to be achieved. National databases listing the molecular defects in each individual with hemophilia B are being established in the UK (Saad *et al.*, 1994), Sweden and New Zealand and an international database has also been established (Giannelli *et al.*, 1996). Their use will facilitate rapid and accurate carrier diagnosis in female relatives.

POLYMORPHISM-BASED GENE TRACKING (LINKAGE ANALYSIS)

In order to track FVIII or FIX genes through a family affected by hemophilia, a means of differentiating normal from defective copies of the gene is required. Neutral polymorphic variations in DNA sequence are used to enable this discrimination to be made. DNA polymorphisms occur between and within individuals at a given genetic locus. The forms of variation most commonly employed in carrier analysis for hemophilia are nucleotide substitution polymorphisms, which are detected by restriction enzyme analysis (restriction fragment length polymorphism; RFLP), allele-specific oligonucleotide (ASO) hybridization or similar techniques. For RFLPs, two forms or alleles are possible; one is recognized and

cleaved by the restriction enzyme (+) and the other is not recognized or cut (−). An example of an RFLP is shown in Fig. 6.1. As only two alleles exist a maximum of 50% of females can be heterozygous for a given RFLP.

Variable number tandem repeat (VNTR) polymorphisms consist of a difference in the number of a tandemly repeated motif in a DNA sequence, e.g. (CA)n, (AG)n, (CAG)n, (ATCT)n. Of these repetitive units, (CA)n is the most common and exists at approximately 50 000 locations throughout the human genome. A large proportion of these are polymorphic; the number of repeats varies between alleles. A significant number of VNTRs have greater than 10 alleles and thus a high proportion of individuals may be heterozygous, making these polymorphisms extremely useful in gene tracking. VNTR polymorphisms may also be referred to as short tandem repeats (STR) or microsatelites. An example of a VNTR is shown in Fig. 6.2.

For accurate diagnosis, the polymorphism used in gene tracking should be within the gene being followed. The greater the genetic distance between the loci of a polymorphic marker and the mutation, the higher the probability of meiotic recombination occurring between the two loci. This approximates to a risk of recombination of 1% (1 cM genetic distance) per 1000 kb distance between two loci. The FVIII gene spans 186 kb, and FIX only 34 kb. The risk of recombination separating an intragenic polymorphism from the mutation is thus very low for both genes, generally being stated as <1 %, and to date no case of such a recombination event has been reported for either FVIII or FIX genes.

The genomic location of DNA polymorphisms identified in the factor VIII and IX genes is illustrated in Figs 6.3 and 6.4 and listed in Tables 6.1–6.3, along with their utility (female heterozygosity) in different population groups. Two VNTR sequences have been identified in FVIII but none in FIX. The majority of the RFLPs shown can be amplified by PCR and analyzed following restriction enzyme digestion (Peake *et al.*, 1993).

The use of FVIII gene polymorphisms to track the defective FVIII gene in families with hemophilia A is demonstrated in Figures 6.5 and 6.6.

COMPARISON OF LINKAGE ANALYSIS WITH MUTATION DETECTION

The relative merits of direct mutation detection and linkage analysis are summarized in Table 6.4. Detection of the causative mutation has the advantages of yielding information on the cause of hemophilia in a particular individual and adding to the knowledge of FVIII or FIX function. There is a very low risk of error when the presence of a mutation is confirmed or refuted in an at risk female and further family members are not required for the analysis. Mutation detection is, however, technically

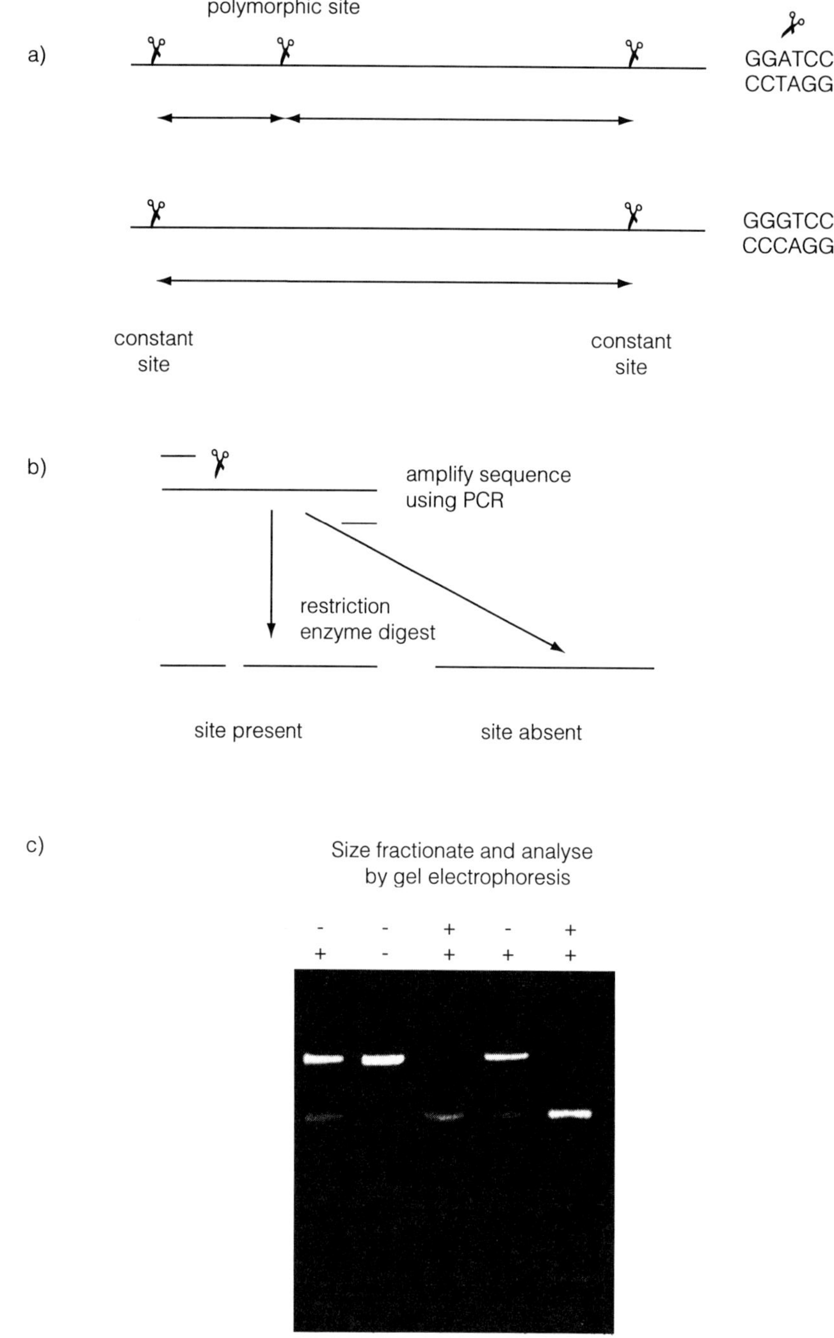

Fig. 6.1 Restriction fragment length polymorphism (RFLP). (a) The two horizontal lines represent stretches of DNA having (top) or lacking (bottom) the palindromic recognition and cutting site for a restriction enzyme (indicated by scissors). Constant sites exist throughout the human genome for each restriction enzyme. A small proportion of sites recognized by each enzyme are polymorphic, present on some but not all chromosomes at a given genetic locus. (b) To determine the polymorphic allele(s) present in an individual, polymerase chain reaction (PCR) amplification can be performed using oligonucleotide primers designed asymmetrically adjacent to the site. Following amplification, restriction enzyme digestion is performed. If the enzyme cuts, two smaller fragments of DNA are produced (+); if not, the original fragment remains (–). The restriction fragment length polymorphism can then be observed. (c) Polyacrylamide gel electrophoresis followed by ethidium bromide staining demonstrates the factor VIII BcII RFLP in five different females. + and – represent the two alleles.

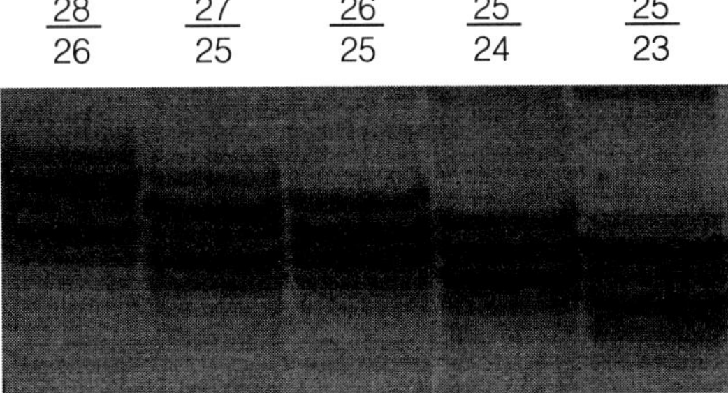

Fig. 6.2 Variable number tandem repeat (VNTR). (a) The top line represents the nucleotide sequence of a stretch of DNA having a $(CA)_n$ dinucleotide repeat. The number of repeats varies between chromosomes and can be referred to as a VNTR. (b) To determine the polymorphic allele(s) present in an individual, polymerase chain reaction (PCR) amplification is performed using oligonucleotide primers complementary to the unique DNA sequence flanking the repeat. Following amplification, PCR product is size-fractionated by polyacrylamide gel electrophoresis to determine allele repeat number. (c) Polyacrylamide gel electrophoresis followed by silver staining demonstrates the factor VIII intron 22 dinucleotide repeat in five heterozygous females. Number of repeat units is indicated for each individual.

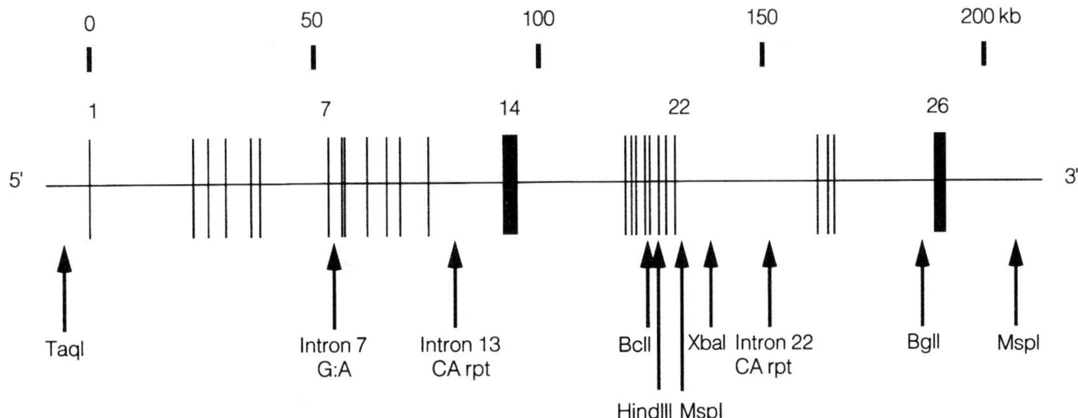

Fig. 6.3 Line diagram of the factor VIII gene. Vertical bars represent exons: the horizontal line indicates the entire 186 kb gene. Arrows indicate the position to 10 intragenic and flanking polymorphisms.

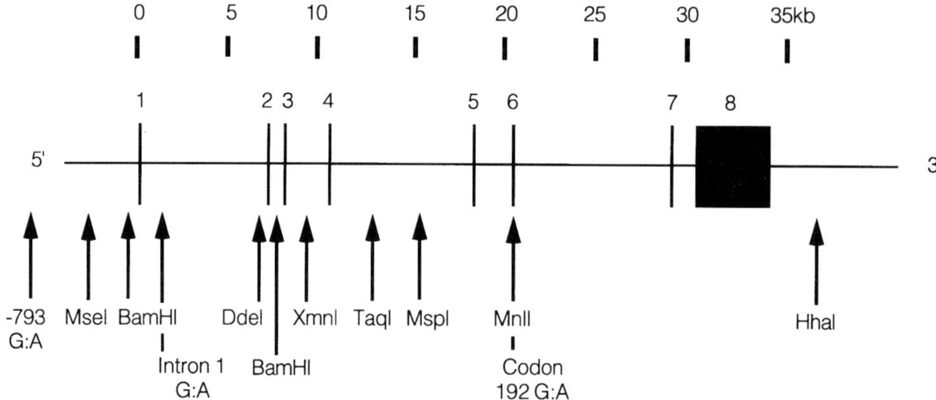

Fig. 6.4 Line diagram of the FIX gene. Vertical bars represent exons: the horizontal line indicates the entire 34 kb gene. Arrows indicate the position of 12 intragenic and flanking polymorphisms.

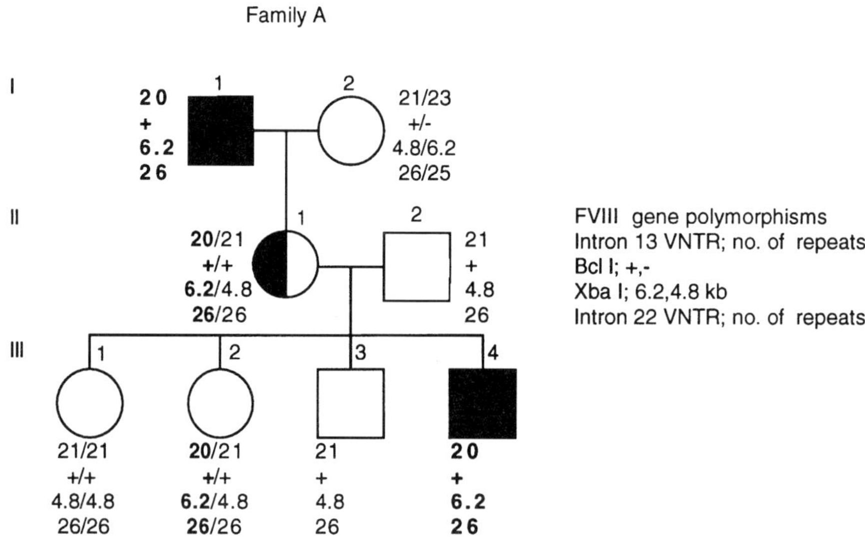

Fig. 6.5 Example of the use of factor VIII intragenic polymorphisms in determining female carrier status. The pedigree of family A demonstrates the utility of DNA polymorphisms in gene tracking by linkage analysis. In this example, where there is a family history of hemophilia A, female II-I, an obligate carrier of hemophilia A is heterozygous (or informative) for the intron 13 and XbaI polymorphisms, but not informative for those at BclI or in intron 22. The alleles seen in the males with hemophilia (I-1 and III-4) are those in phase with hemophilia in this family and form a haplotype (array of polymorphic markers on one chromosome). Inheritance of the same maternal haplotype indicates that III-2 is a carrier of hemophilia, whereas III-1, who has inherited the normal maternal alleles (also seen in unaffected son III-3), can be excluded from being a carrier. III-2 is informative for intron 13 and XbaI polymorphisms. Both can therefore be used in her children (at prenatal or later diagnosis) in the same manner.

demanding; highly trained personnel are required to perform analysis which may be costly in time and materials.

Linkage analysis is technically much simpler and quicker but does have several limitations to its usefulness. The lack of key family members, if they are deceased, uninterested or have lost contact with the family, is a frequent problem. In families with sporadic hemophilia, its usefulness is limited to excluding females from being carriers where they have not inherited with allele in phase with hemophilia. Mutation detection is required to determine carrier status in the remaining females in sporadic families.

SOURCE OF DNA

High-molecular-weight DNA for use in all the above genetic analyses is generally obtained from peripheral blood leukocytes in samples of whole anticoagulated blood. Traditionally this involves treatment with proteinase K followed by phenol chloroform extraction and, more recently, techniques involving salting out or the use of a silica matrix in DNA purification. Sodium citrate or ethylenediaminetetraacetic acid is the preferred anticoagulant for blood. 10 ml of blood will yield approximately 250 µg of DNA, sufficient for family studies and

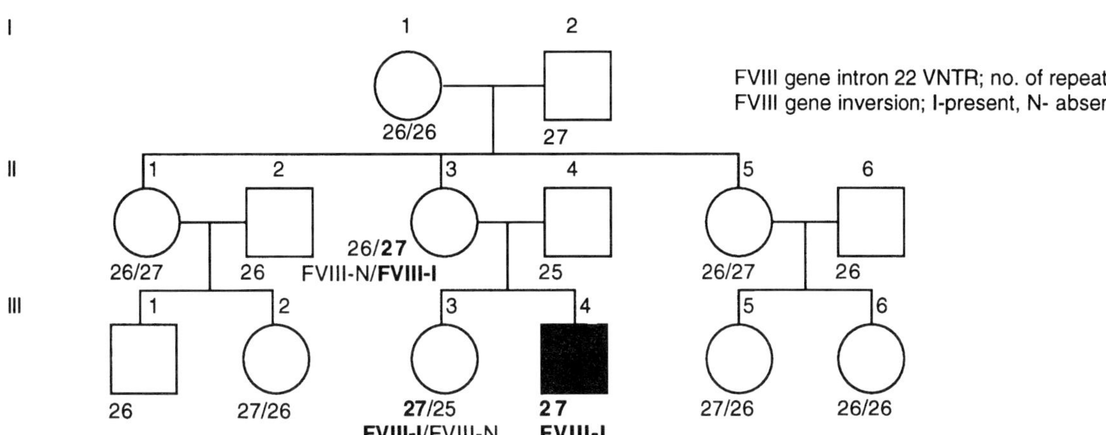

Fig. 6.6 Example of the use of direct mutation detection in determining female carrier status. Family B has sporadic severe hemophilia where there is a single case of severe hemophilia A (III-4). The intron 22 polymorphism, informative in this family, demonstrates that the normal maternal grandfather of the hemophiliac is the source of the affected allele which is in phase with the 27 dinucleotide repeat. All of his daughters inherit the same allele from him. Use of linkage analysis alone does not enable carrier status to be excluded from his daughters, II-1 and II-3, or their daughters, III-2 and III-5, all of whom have inherited the 27 repeat allele. The presence of the factor VIII gene inversion mutation in the patient III-4, his sister III-3 and his mother II-2 enables their carrier status to be unequivocally determined, however. All other at-risk females lack the inversion and are therefore excluded from carriership.

Table 6.1 Diallelic DNA polymorphisms within or flanking the human factor VIII gene

Restriction enzyme	Location	Detection method	Heterozygosity			
			Caucasian	Asian	Chinese	American Black
TaqI	5′	Probe	0.40	u	u	u
G/A	Intron 7	PCR	0.33	0.16*	u	u
BclI	Intron 18	PCR	0.39	0.43	0.33	0.31
HindIII	Intron 19	PCR	0.38	0.41	0.37	0.34
MspI†	Intron 22	Probe	0.01	0.13	u	0.01
XbaI	Intron 22	Probe	0.49	0.48‡	0.49	u
BglI	Intron 25	Probe	0.25	0.11	0.0	0.38
MspI	3′	Probe	0.43	u	u	u

u = Unknown; PCR = polymerase and chain reaction.
*Turkish Asian (Çaglayan, Gökmen and Kirdev, 1995).
†Inaba *et al.* (1990).
‡Thai: Goodeve *et al.* (1994).
Data from Peake *et al.* (1993).

storage for future needs. If PCR alone (without Southern blotting) is to be performed, there is no necessity for extraction of purified DNA. Many amplification protocols use whole blood or rapidly extracted impure DNA preparations.

Whole blood suitable for DNA extraction and extracted DNA are both stable for many years at −20°C. The World Health Organization (WHO) recommends that DNA (or blood where DNA extraction facilities are unavailable) should be stored from all individuals with hemophilia for future analysis in their families.

STRATEGY FOR CARRIER ANALYSIS: HEMOPHILIA A

For analysis of families with hemophilia A, the FVIII gene inversion (Chapter 3) should first be sought in those with severe disease where this analysis is available. If this is not present, polymorphism-based gene tracking is generally undertaken. The two dinucleotide repeat polymorphisms in introns 13 and 22, which can be analyzed together as a multiplex PCR, will together be informative in 70% of families. Xba I (analyzed by Southern blotting) and BclI

Table 6.2 Frequencies (%*) of dinucleotide repeats in intron 13 and intron 22 of the factor VIII gene in different populations

	International: Lalloz et al. (1991)	Canadian: Windsor, Taylor and Lillicrap (1994)	Hong Kong Chinese: Yip, Chan and Chan (1994)	German Kochhan et al. (1994)	Russian Slavs: Aseev et al. (1994)	Uzbekians: Aseev et al. (1994)	Taiwan Chinese: Lin et al. (1995)	Thai: Goodeve et al. unpublished	Italian: Goodeve et al. unpublished
(a) Intron 13									
No. of (CA)n									
28			1						
27			3						
26			32						
25			53						
24	1	1	9	2		1		3	
23	5	13	1	9	10	3		6	
22	11	48	1	9	11	3	2	9	3
21	29	25		23	19	14	24	11	22
20	45	7		47	56	80	69	59	61
19	7	4		7	3		3	21	6
18	1	1		2					
17		2		1					
16	1								

	International: Lalloz et al. (1991)	Canadian: Windsor, Taylor and Lillicrap (1994)	Hong Kong Chinese: Yip, Chan and Chan (1994)	Taiwan Chinese: Lin et al (1995)	Thai: Goodeve et al. unpublished	Italian: Goodeve et al. unpublished
(b) Intron 22						
No. of (GT)n (AG)n						
29				1		
28	1			1		
27		2	7	5	4	5
26	67	3	63	75	66	65
25	31	35	29	18	30	23
24		53				5
23	1	6				2
20			1			

will be informative in a further 15%. The figures given for Caucasians will vary in other ethnic groups but these four polymorphisms have been shown to be useful in all populations examined (Tables 6.1 and 6.2). In addition to the intron 22 XbaI polymorphism, the + allele of two extragenic XbaI polymorphisms located in the other copies of the intron 22 homologous region (Chapter 3) may be observed on XbaI Southern blots. As the further copies of the intron 22 homologous region lie only approximately 400 kb and 5′ to the FVIII gene, the risk of cross-over at each meiosis between the polymorphic loci and the FVIII gene should be less than 1%. The polymorphisms may therefore be useful in linkage analysis, particularly in Chinese people, where the rate of heterozygosity is higher than in Caucasians. Extragenic polymorphisms at loci St14 (60 bp multiallelic repeat) and DX13 (BglII RFLP) are occasionally used when intragenic markers prove uninformative. As these markers are some distance from the FVIII gene, a ≤5% meiotic recombination risk exists and caution should be exercised in their use.

Other FVIII gene polymorphisms are in allelic association (linkage disequilibrium) with Bcl1 in Caucasians, notably HindIII and BglI. In other populations, the extent of association may be different. The FVIII flanking markers TaqI and MspI are infrequently used due to both their linkage disequilibrium with BcI and as Southern blotting is required for their analysis. The intron 7 G/A polymorphism is useful in females who are uninformative but −/− for the BcI marker (Kogan and Gitschier, 1990). In cases where the FVIII inversion is not present and no intragenic polymorphisms are informative, mutation screening of the rest of the FVIII gene is the only possibility remaining to enable accurate carrier diagnosis to be made.

Table 6.3 DNA polymorphisms within or flanking the human factor IX gene

Restriction enzyme	Location	Detection method	Heterozygosity			
			Caucasian	Asian	Chinese	American Black
(A/G)	5' nucleotide 793	PCR	0.49*	u	0.50†	
MseI	5'	PCR	0.44	0.50	u	0.48‡
BamHI	5'	PCR	0.04	0.46	0.02	0.24
(A/G)	Intron 1 nucleotide 192	PCR	u	u	0.24§	u
DdeI**	Intron 1	PCR	0.36	u	0.0	0.46
BamHI	Intron 2	PCR	0.11	u	0.04	0.22
XmnI	Intron 3	PCR	0.41	0.07	0.02	0.21
TaqI	Intron 4	PCR	0.45	0.07	0.02	0.24
MspI	Intron 4	PCR	0.32	u	u	0.47
Mnl	Codon 148	PCR	0.44	0.07	0.06	0.20
(A/G)	Codon 192	PCR	0.01	0.11	0.39	0.01
HhaI	3'	PCR	0.48	0.43	0.28	0.49

u = unknown; PCR = Polymerase chain reaction;
*Rai and Winship (1996).
†Japanese; Toyozumi *et al.* (1995).
‡Weinmann, Reiner and Thompson (1993).
§Chen, Wang and Schoof (1992).
**Deletion/insertion: two major forms differ by 50 bp.
Data from Peake *et al.* (1993).

Table 6.4 Comparison of the advantages and disadvantages of linkage analysis and mutation detection in the determination of hemophilia carrier status

Parameter	Linkage analysis	Mutation detection
Ease of analysis	Technically simple	Technically demanding*
DNA samples required	From several family members	From hemophiliac and female under investigation
Family history of hemophilia	Where none, females can only be excluded for carriership	Carrier status can be determined regardless of prior history
Informative	In approximately 85% of families	In nearly 100% of families
Non-paternity	May result in incorrect carrier diagnosis	Carrier status can be determined regardless of paternity

*Unless the factor VIII gene inversion is present in cases of severe hemophilia A.

STRATEGY FOR CARRIER ANALYSIS: HEMOPHILIA B

Several nucleotide substitution polymorphisms, most of which can be detected as RFLPs and one insertion/deletion polymorphism (DdeI, intron 1), have been described in the FIX gene (Fig. 6.4; Table 6.3). In a white Caucasian population, the combined use of the 5' MseI RFLP, the 3' HhaI RFLP and the DdeI insertion/deletion polymorphism results in an overall heterozygosity rate of up to 81% as there is little linkage disequilibrium between these markers. Inclusion of the remaining polymorphisms increases the rate to above 90% (Winship *et al.*, 1993). In other ethnic groups, notably Asians, there is a lack of informative polymorphisms. However the 5' MseI is heterozygous in approximately 44% of females (Goodeve *et al.*, 1994b) and some polymorphisms have been identified which are particularly useful in oriental groups. Toyozumi *et al.* (1995) found that combined analysis by PCR of A/G at −793, A/G at codon 192 and HhaI was informative in 80% of Japanese females. For each ethnic group, therefore, a selected combination of FIX gene polymorphisms should be used for effective carrier and prenatal analysis.

Details of further ethnic variation and primers for PCR amplification are given in Peake *et al.* (1993).

MOSAICISM

Mutation events early in embryogenesis may lead to individuals who are germline and/or somatic mosaics for a heritable disorder. Such individuals have two populations of cells, one with and one lacking a particular mutation. Recurrence risk for offspring depends on the proportion of mutated germ cells, but the relative proportion of cells cannot be estimated.

At least one-third of all patients with hemophilia have no affected male relatives and are cases of sporadic hemophilia. The risk of their female relatives being carriers of hemophilia may therefore differ from those families where there is a history of disease. The probability of female relatives being carriers depends on the origin of the mutation; this is determined by the relative mutation frequency in males

A high proportion of mothers of isolated cases will be carriers if mutations occur predominantly in males. A study by Bröcker-Vriends *et al.* (l991) prior to recognition of the FVIII gene inversion estimated that the male:female mutation rate for all cases of hemophilia A to be at least 5.2, and possibly much higher. This ratio would result in 86% of mothers of isolated hemophilia A patients being true carriers of the disorder. The remaining 14% may be mosaics for the mutation, at risk of transmitting the affected allele to more than one child.

Studies by Rossiter *et al.* (1994) and Antonarakis *et al.* (1995) have examined the occurrence of the FVIII gene inversion in mothers of such patients. For all patients, 98% of mothers were found to have the mutation in their somatic cells. In those families with sporadic hemophilia, this proportion was reduced to 96% of mothers.

Rossiter *et al.* (1994) estimated absolute mutation rates for the inversion mutation to be 4.2×10^{-6} per male meiosis and 1.4×10^{-8} per female meiosis – the rate of occurrence in males is 302-fold higher than in females. Therefore the origin of the inversion is predominantly in male germ cell meiosis. The analysis of mutations in mothers of sporadic cases of non-inversion hemophilia A will enable more accurate estimation of mutation and carriership rates to be made and to examine how this differs from families with the inversion.

For hemophilia B, Montandon *et al.* (1992) estimated for a group of Swedish patients in which the mutations were ascertained that the mutation rate was 1.88×10^{-6} per generation in female meioses and 2.07×10^{-5} for males. The male-to-female mutation rate was estimated to be 11.0, implying that 96% of mothers of sporadic hemophilia B cases were carriers of the disorder. Other studies have indicated more equal male and female mutation rates, reducing this proportion.

Thus, due to the higher mutation rate in the FVIII and IX genes in males, a high proportion of mothers of sporadic cases of hemophilia are carriers. Their status as carriers can be confirmed by direct detection of the causative mutation, genetic analysis of remaining female family members is straightforward. However, in families where linkage analysis is used, females can be excluded but not included as carriers (Fig. 6.6).

Prenatal diagnosis of hemophilia

Prenatal diagnosis of hemophilia is generally restricted to those situations where the fetus is at risk of severe disease and invasive procedures should ideally only take place when the fetus is known to be male. However, although ultrasonography at 16–20 weeks will give a reliable diagnosis of fetal sex, chorion villus sampling (CVS) or early amniocentesis (Byrne *et al.*, 1991) can produce fetal material for analysis some 4–6 weeks earlier and in general it is this material that is used for both sex determination and hemophilia diagnosis, both based on DNA analysis. In addition, karyotype analysis may be performed if appropriate.

The first successful prenatal diagnoses of hemophilia A and B were performed in the late 1970s and utilized fetal blood obtained using fetoscopy and sampling from the blood vessels on the chorionic plate or umbilical cord (Mibashan *et al.*, 1980). Sample processing was meticulous and accurate levels of FVIII:C (and FVIII:Ag) and FIX:C were obtained. Diagnosis was based on a comparison of these levels with normal fetal blood levels for the particular gestational age (generally from 18 to 22 weeks). Using these procedures a fetal death rate of 2–5% was seen and the lateness of the diagnosis was held to be a discouragement to the proband. These procedures, including the more recent ultrasound guided cordocentesis, are now restricted for use in hemophilia only when a sample of fetal tissue for DNA analysis is not available.

Amniocentesis is traditionally performed from 16 weeks and will provide enough fetal cells to allow for rapid DNA analysis using the procedures given above, generally without prior culture to increase cell numbers. It is now possible however to obtain amniotic fluid at 10–14 weeks, with sufficient cellular material for PCR-based DNA analysis (Byrne *et al.*, 1991).

CVS can provide the earliest sample of fetal tissue, but it is clear that, if performed before 10 weeks, some fetal limb abnormalities can result (Firth *et al.*, 1991). CVS after 10 weeks is now the commonest procedure used in prenatal diagnosis of hemophilia and can generally provide sufficient DNA for both PCR and Southern blot-based analysis, the latter technique being particularly important in diagnosing the FVIII gene inversion seen in severe hemophilia A. If this is not possible then a polymorphic allele in phase with the mutation can frequently be found and used, or in some cases other previously identified mutations sought.

If requested, prenatal diagnosis can be offered to a carrier of hemophilia from 10 to 20 weeks' gestation. The particular technique used will depend to some extent on circumstances and available expertise. However, a confirmed carrier diagnosis is an important prerequisite and it is recommended that all possible carriers of childbearing age should be tested prior to pregnancy. The requirement of a blood sample from the affected family member for many of these diagnoses, especially if based on polymorphism analysis and because of increased mortality amongst hemophiliacs due in many cases to blood-borne virus infection, strongly reinforces the recommendation by WHO that blood and/or DNA samples should be stored from all persons with hemophilia.

Female hemophilia

LYONIZATION

The extent of phenotypic variation in female carriers of hemophilia is partly the result of X chromosome inactivation or lyonization. The process whereby one of the two female X chromosomes is almost completely inactivated early in embryonic life occurs randomly and results in all male and female cells having only a single functional X chromosome (as occurs naturally in males). The progeny of each cell maintain the same pattern of X inactivation; carriers of hemophilia are therefore somatic mosaics and have two different populations of cells. One population has the normal and the other the abnormal X chromosome functioning. If X inactivation has occurred randomly, carriers will produce half of the normal level of FVIII or FIX. Skewed X inactivation can lead to carriers having clotting factor levels varying from those in the mild hemophilia range to levels which are completely normal, rendering phenotypic determinations inaccurate.

In some instances X inactivation is non-random. Some other factor influences inactivation of the normal X chromosome – the one lacking the hemophilia mutation. Other causes can be that the female has a 45, X karyotype (Turner syndrome) or that there is a deletion elsewhere on the X chromosome which lacks a FVIII or FIX defect leading to its inactivation. Non-random X inactivation can be tested for by analysis of DNA methylation patterns in hemophilic females. Another cause of hemophilia in females is where they are the offspring of an affected male and carrier female. This situation may be unwittingly promoted by socializing between affected families. Females may then inherit affected paternal and maternal X chromosomes. In the case of consanguineous partners, affected females would be true homozygotes, but in most families females would bear two different mutations, the severity of their hemophilia being the result both of the two mutations inherited and the bias of lyonization.

Summary

For families with hemophilia A and B, effective female carrier analysis can be performed by accurate phenotype testing, or preferably by genetic analysis. Whereas direct detection of the causative mutation in the hemophiliac and its confirmation or exclusion in female relatives is to be preferred, the availability of this analysis is limited.

Polymorphism-based gene tracking, although having several limitations, is much simpler and more widely available than mutation detection. Its use permits accurate and rapid determination of female carrier status and prenatal diagnosis in a large proportion of families analyzed. For females determined genetically to be carriers, the reproductive options taken will depend to an extent on the counseling they receive and the overall care for the hemophiliac available in that country – whether sufficient good-quality clotting factor concentrate is available for effective treatment, and the quality of life and life expectancy of patients with hemophilia. Where treatment options are poor, carrier analysis and prenatal diagnosis can be an important part of the overall care of the hemophiliac and his family.

References

Antonarakis, S.E., Rossiter, J.P., Young, Y. *et al.* (1995) Factor VIII gene inversions in severe hemophilia A: Results of an international consortium study. *Blood*, 86, 2206–2212.

Aseev, M., Surin, V. Baboev, N. *et al.* (1994) Allele frequencies and molecular diagnosis in hemophilia A and B patients from Russia and from some Asian Republics of the former USSR. *Prenatal Diagnosis*, 14, 513–522.

Bröcker-Vriends, A.J.H.T., Briët, E., Dreesen, J.C.F.M. *et al.* (1990) Somatic origin of inherited hemophilia A. *Human Genetics*, 85, 288–292.

Bröcker-Vriends, A.J.H.T., Rosendaal, F.R., van Houwelingen, J.G. *et al.* (1991) Sex ratio of the mutation frequencies in hemophilia A: coagulation assays and RFLP analysis. *Journal of Medical Genetics*, 28, 672–680.

Byrne, D., Marks, K., Azar, G. *et al.* (1991) Randomized study of early amniocentesis versus chorionic villus sampling at 10–13 weeks gestation. Technical and cytogenetic comparison of 650 patients. *Ultrasound Obstetrics and Gynaecology*, 1, 235–240.

Çaglayan, S.H., Gokmen, Y. and Kirdev, B. (1995) Polymorphisms associated with the FVIII and FIX genes in the Turkish population. *Haemophilia*, 1, 184–189.

Chen, S,H., Wang, N.S. and Schoof, J. (1992) Haplotype analysis and polymorphic frequency data at two factor IX loci (F9-192 and F9-Hha1) in a Chinese population. *Humanity and Heredity*, 42, 204–205.

David, D., Moreira, I., Lalloz, M.A.R. *et al.* (1994) Analysis of the essential sequences of the factor VIII gene in 12 haemophilia A patients by single-stranded conformation polymorphism. *Blood Coagulation and Fibrinolysis*, 5, 257–264.

Firth, H.V., Boyd, P.A., Chamberlain, P. *et al.* (1991) Severe limb abnormalities after chorion villus sampling at 55–66 days gestation. *Lancet*, 337, 762–763.

Giannelli, F., Green, P.M., Sommer, S.S. *et al.* (1996) Hemophilia B (sixth edition): a database of point mutations and short additions and deletions. *Nucleic Acids Research*, 24, 103–118.

Goodeve, A.C., Preston, F.E and Peake, I.R. (1994a) Factor VIII gene rearrangements in patients with severe hemophilia A. *Lancet*, 343, 329–330.

Goodeve, A.C., Chuansumrit, A., Sasanakul, E. *et al.* (1994b) A comparison of the allelic frequencies of 10 DNA polymorphisms associated with factor VIII and factor IX genes in Thai and Western European population. *Blood Coagulation and Fibrinolysis*, 5, 29–35.

Green, P.P., Mannucci, P.M., Briët, E. *et al.* (1986) Carrier detection in hemophilia A: a cooperative international study. II. The efficacy of a universal discriminant. *Blood*, 67, 1560–1567.

Higuchi, M., Antonarakis, S.E., Kasch, L. *et al.* (1991) Molecular characterization of mild-to-moderate hemophilia A: detection of the mutation in 25 of 29 patients by denaturing gradient gel electrophoresis. *Proceedings of the National Academy of Sciences USA*, **88**, 8307–8311.

Inaba, H., Fujimaka, M., Kazazian, H.H. *et al.* (1990) MspI polymorphic site in intron 22 of the factor VIII gene in the Japanese population. *Human Genetics*, **84**, 214–215.

Kochhan, I., Lalloz, M.R.A., Oldenburg, J. *et al.* (1994) Hemophilia A diagnosed by automated fluorescent DNA detection of 10 factor VIII intron 13 dinucleotide repeat alleles. *Blood Coagulation and Fibrinolysis*, **5**, 497–501.

Kogan, S.C. and Gitschier, J. (1990) Genetic prediction of hemophilia A, in *PCR Protocols: A Guide to Methods and Applications* (eds M.A. Innis, D.H. Gelfand, J. J. Sninsky, J.J. White), Academic Press, San Diego, pp. 288–299.

Lakich, D., Kazazian, H., Antonarakis, S.E. *et al.* (1993) Inversions disrupting the factor VIII gene as a common cause of severe hemophilia A. *Nature Genetics*, **5**, 236–241.

Lalloz, M.R.A., McVey, J.H., Pattinson, J.K. *et al.* (1991) Hemophilia A diagnosis by analysis of a hypervariable dinucleotide repeat within the human factor VIII gene. *Lancet*, **338**, 207–211.

Lalloz, M.R.A., Schwaab, R., McVey, J.H. *et al.* (1994) Hemophilia A diagnosis by simultaneous analysis of two variable dinucleotide tandem repeats within the factor VIII gene. *British Journal of Haematology*, **86**, 804–809.

Lin, S.R., Chang, S.C., Lee, C.C. *et al.* (1995) Genetic diagnosis of hemophilia A of Chinese origin. *British Journal of Haematology*, **91**, 722–727.

Mibashan, R.S., Peake, I.R., Rodeck, C.H. *et al.* (1980) Dual diagnosis of prenatal hemophilia A by measurement of fetal factor VIIIC and VIIIC antigen (VIIICAg). *Lancet*, **2**, 994–997.

Montandon, A.J., Green, P.M., Bentley, D.R. *et al* (1992) Direct estimate of the hemophilia B (factor IX deficiency) mutation rate and of the ratio of the sex specific mutation rates in Sweden. *Human Genetics*, **89**, 319–322.

Naylor, J.A., Green, P.M., Montandon, A.J. *et al.* (1991) Detection of three novel mutations in two hemophilia A patients by rapid screening of whole essential region of factor VIII gene. *Lancet*, **337**, 635–639.

Naylor, J.A., Brinke, A., Hassock, S. *et al.* (1993) Characteristic mRNA abnormality found in half the patients with severe hemophilia A is due to large DNA inversions. *Human Molecular Genetics*, **2**, 1773–1778.

Peake, I.R., Lillicrap, D.P., Boulyjenkov, V. *et al.* (1993) Report of a joint WHO/WFH meeting on the control of hemophilia: carrier detection and prenatal diagnosis. *Blood Coagulation and Fibrinolysis*, **4**, 313–344.

Rai, H.K. and Winship, P.R. (1995) A −793 G to A transition in the factor IX gene promoter is polymorphic in the Caucasian population. *British Journal of Haematology*, **92**, 501–503.

Rossiter, J.P., Young, M., Kimberland, M.L. *et al.* (1994) Factor VIII gene inversions causing severe hemophilia A originate almost exclusively in male germ cells. *Human Molecular Genetics*, **3**, 1035–1039.

Saad, S., Rowley, G., Tagliavacca, L. *et al.* (1994) First report on UK database of hemophilia B mutations and pedigrees. *Thrombosis and Haemostasis*, **71**, 563–570.

Toyozumi, H., Kojima, T., Katsumi, A. *et al.* (1995) Valuable hemophilia B carrier diagnosis by use of two novel nucleotide polymorphisms (FIX 192 and FIX-793) and HhaI RFLP of the factor IX gene in Japanese subjects. *Thrombosis and Haemostasis*, **73**, 1223.

Wacey, A.I., Kemball-Cook, G., Kazazian, H.H. *et al.* (1996) The hemophilia A mutation search test and resource site, home page of the factor VIII mutation database: HAMSTeRS. *Nucleic Acids Research*, **24**, 100–102.

Weinmann, A.F., Reiner, A.P. and Thompson, A.R. (1993) A polymorphic MseI site 5′ to the factor IX gene varies among ethnic groups. *Human Molecular Genetics*, **2**, 486.

Windsor, S., Taylor, S.A.M. and Lillicrap, D. (1994) Multiplex analysis of two intragenic microsatellite repeat polymorphisms in the genetic diagnosis of hemophilia A. *British Journal of Haematology*, **84**, 804–809.

Winship, P.R., Nichols, C.E., Chuansumrit, A. and Peake, I.R. (1993) An MseI RFLP in the 5′ flanking region of the factor IX gene: its use for hemophilia B carrier detection in Caucasian and Thai populations. *British Journal of Haematology*, **84**, 101–105.

Yip, B., Chan, V. and Chan, T.K. (1994) Intragenic dinucleotide repeats in factor VIII gene for the diagnosis of hemophilia A. *British Journal of Haematology*, **88**, 889–891.

7 GENETIC COUNSELING IN HEMOPHILIA

D.E. Wilcox and J.M. Connor

The aims of this chapter are to:

1. Describe the process of genetic counseling in the hemophilias. This is illustrated by following a family through the various stages of the counseling process.
2. Describe the current methods of genetic diagnosis and illustrate how the results should be interpreted, avoiding pitfalls that are peculiar to the hemophilias and X-linked recessive inheritance.

Introduction

Genetic counseling is a complex process by which a physician seeks to advise and educate a patient and his or her family about a disease and to give specific risks of recurrence of the disease (either in a currently healthy individual or in a future generation) and how this recurrence may be treated or avoided. The aim of counseling is to give the patient and family understandable information, in a non-directive way, which will allow them to make informed decisions about genetic tests and reproductive options.

Before counseling can be given, the diagnosis in the affected individual must be established or confirmed. Accurate diagnosis in the proband (or affected individual) is the foundation of genetic counseling. The position of relatives in the family tree can then be used to estimate their risks and genetic testing can be offered where appropriate. A final role of the counselor is to offer long-term support to the individual and the family. The specialty has now been established long enough for three generations of some families to have received genetic counseling.

The genetic counselor must have clinical diagnostic skills together with an understanding of the appropriate laboratory tests. The counselor should understand how patterns of inheritance can be combined with test results using mathematical methods and be aware of those genetic mechanisms which can cause misinterpretation of test results. Finally, the counselor should be a good communicator and be sensitive to the psychologic stresses which exist within a family with genetic disease.

With respect to the X-linked hemophilias, the geneticist's main role is to help detect which females in the family are carriers and inform them about reproductive options. Currently carrier detection is not straightforward and is based on four different methods:

1. Pedigree analysis assesses a woman's risk from her position in the family tree using a knowledge of X-linked recessive inheritance.
2. Phenotypic testing compares a potential carrier's clotting activity with those of known carriers and controls. The results need to be interpreted together with other information from the pedigree.
3. Direct genotypic tests are able to detect the mutation in some families.
4. Indirect genotypic tests can track the chromosome believed to contain the mutation through several generations in most families.

With the exception of tests which directly detect the mutation, the results of these tests will produce a carrier risk rather than a definitive statement of carrier or non-carrier status. These risks should be combined using Bayes theorem to produce a final carrier risk.

Genetic counseling

THE REFERRAL

Patients are referred to genetic clinics from many sources, including hospital specialists such as hematologists and

Hemophilia. Edited by C.D. Forbes, L. Aledort and R. Madhok. Published in 1997 by Chapman & Hall, London. ISBN 0 412 63820 7

obstetricians, general practitioners, other health professionals and social workers, patient support groups and on many occasions patients will self-refer and contact the genetics department directly. If the referring doctor is able to enclose a brief family tree together with the names of affected individuals. the geneticist will be able to check and see if part of the family have already been seen and confirm the diagnosis in those named individuals.

THE APPOINTMENT

Many patients will have no clear idea of what genetic counseling entails. It is therefore helpful to enclose a brief letter with the appointment card explaining who the family will see and asking them to bring a note of affected relatives' addresses and dates of birth, together with the names of any doctors or hospitals attended. In hemophilia and other X-linked disorders it is worthwhile asking for a note of female relatives' married and maiden names as this may allow the geneticist to work back and link the family to an already known family whose names are recorded in the genetic register.

The appointment letter should be addressed to both parents and should indicate whether any others, such as affected relatives or children, should attend. About 40 minutes should be allocated for each new appointment to allow adequate time for history taking, examination, testing and preliminary counseling.

Genetic counseling clinics are held both in the regional genetic centers where the laboratory services are based and also at peripheral hospitals. These peripatetic clinics are important as the expense for an extended family making a trip to a regional center may be considerable. Non-attendance is not a major problem at genetic clinics.

THE CLINIC

The clinic should have easy access and suitable toilet facilities as many genetic disorders are associated with disability, e.g. hemophilia patients with arthropathy. The rooms should be quiet and free from disturbances such as telephones. They should be large enough to accommodate both an examination couch and sufficient seating for a large family. A less intimidating atmosphere can be created if the counselor's desk is placed against the wall with patients' seating to the side. It is very helpful to have a supervised play area nearby so that children can leave after examination and allow parents freedom for open discussion during counseling.

THE CONSULTATION

The history

After an introduction the counselor should identify each member of the family who has attended and make sure

that addresses and names of each individual's general practitioners are noted. This can lead into the taking of the family history and construction of the family tree. If the family are able to watch as the tree is drawn they can often clarify the exact relationship of more distant uncles and cousins. The process also allows the counselor to establish a rapport with the family which can be helpful when discussing difficult issues during the later counseling stage.

Although the hemophilias and von Willebrand's disease are inherited from only one side of the family, a family tree is drawn for both sides of the family, as this helps to allay feelings of guilt and avoids missing an equally important disorder on the other side of the family. The medical histories of each affected individual in the family are then noted, together with names of their doctors and hospitals attended. Their medical records should always be checked to confirm the diagnosis.

The family in Fig. 7.1 recently attended a genetic counseling clinic after Brian Robertson, III:3 the proband, had been diagnosed as having hemophilia A. The haematologist had already sent a DNA sample from Brian to the DNA laboratory and an inversion mutation was found in his hemophilia A gene. The hematologist then referred Steve and Julie Robertson for genetic counseling but she asked if her brother and sister and their families could also attend. The family tree was drawn (the spouses' families have been omitted for clarity) and Brian's grandfather, Brian Andrews, was noted to have died from a cerebral hemorrhage after falling downstairs. Because the referral letter had mentioned Mr Andrews, the geneticist had already confirmed from the hospital records that he also had hemophilia A.

The family structure is typical of X-linked recessive inheritance, with affected males in separate generations linked through a phenotypically normal female, Julie Robertson. She can be identified as being an obligate carrier not only because she has had an affected son but because in this family the hemophilia has been inherited from her father. As males only have one X chromosome, an affected male will pass the hemophilia gene to all his daughters but to none of his sons, who will receive his Y chromosome.

Mary Brown had brought her children along to be tested. She said that Graham was not Anna's natural father; she had no contact with Anna's natural father. Mary, by definition, is also an obligate carrier as her father was affected. This assumes that Brian Andrews was her biological father and, while non-paternity is not common, it can greatly distort genetic risks calculated from the pedigree or from a DNA family study.

Women of Katherine Andrews's generation are likely to be less open about paternity than their daughters, but if it is clearly explained how their daughters' risks have been calculated, a woman whose daughter has a differ-

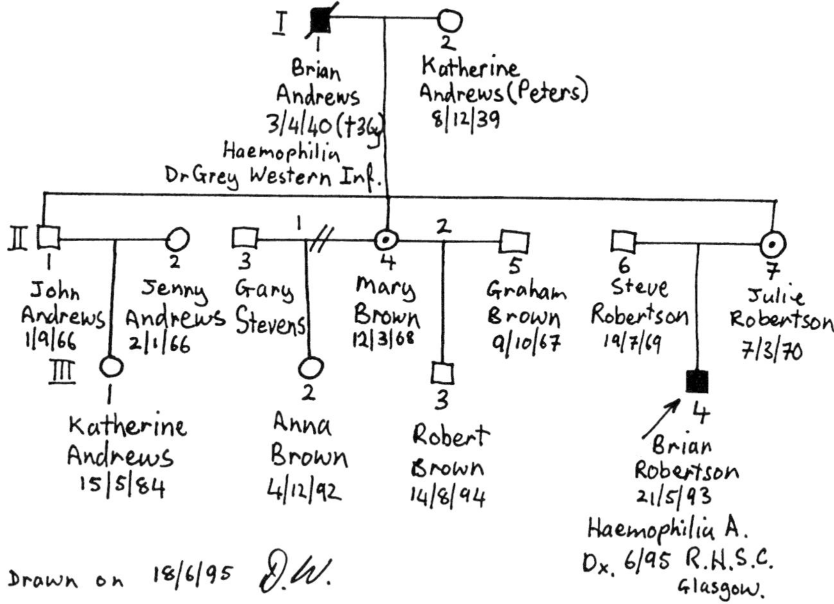

Fig. 7.1 Example of hemophilia A family seen for genetic counseling.

ent father may contact the counselor at a later time with confidential information. This is more likely to happen if the geneticist has been able to establish a rapport with the family.

At this point, after the family tree has been drawn, the counselor usually offers to see each couple separately but in this case the family were happy to be counseled together. The Browns said that their family was complete and Mary had chosen to be sterilized after Robert's birth. Julie Robertson said she would like to have at least one more child but was now very worried about hemophilia.

The examination

This is generally a most important part of a genetic consultation, particularly when the proband has a dysmorphic syndrome and identification of subtle clinical features can greatly aid diagnosis. In the hemophilias, the examination is of less importance and in this case the affected boy, Brian Robertson, was noted to have two large bruises on his legs and his cousin, Robert Brown, was normal.

GENETIC COUNSELING AND TESTING OF ADULTS

Counseling those at low risk

Patients may be assigned a low risk either because of their position in the pedigree or after they have had genetic testing. John Andrews was not at risk of inheriting hemophilia from his father and he and his wife were informed of this. Surprisingly, despite the relief of discovering their personal risk is low, some patients may have difficulty in coming to terms with this because of feelings of guilt. This is particularly so when others have been found to be at high risk. Other patients may have lived with an uncertain risk for so many years that it is almost part of their personality and they may take a long time to appreciate fully their low-risk status.

Counseling carriers

Mary Brown was told she was an obligate carrier and no further genetic tests would be necessary. It was emphasized that she should feel no guilt because everyone carries mutations which can be passed on to our children. At this point, the counselor will often explain to the spouse of a carrier for an X-linked recessive disorder such as hemophilia that he will also be a carrier for several different mutations. This is because many men find it difficult to accept that their son has inherited a disease and because it has come from the wife's side of the family can cause them to apportion blame unfairly. This can lead to additional discord in a marriage which is already under strain because of the diagnosis of an affected son.

GENETIC TESTING OF CHILDREN

Presymptomatic testing

Mary Brown was already aware that Robert was at risk and, with the aid of a diagram, it was explained that he had a 50% risk of having inherited the hemophilia mutation. Since hemophilia has childhood onset and is a treatable condition, presymptomatic genetic testing does not have major ethical constraints, as would be the case in testing a child with a 50% risk of developing an adult-onset untreatable disorder such as Huntington disease. In this situation childhood presymptomatic testing would be inappropriate.

A blood sample was taken from Robert for hematologic testing and for screening for the inversion mutation and arrangements were made for Graham and Mary to return to the clinic together to receive the result. If there is a high risk of an unfavorable test result both parents are always requested to attend. This saves one parent being further upset by having to give the result to the other. Bad news is always given in person and never over the telephone.

Carrier testing

Mary was very keen for her daughter Anna's carrier status to be determined. It was explained to Mary that as a small proportion of carriers may have bleeding problems in situations such as surgery, her factor VIII activity should be measured. It was emphasized that this would be done to determine her blood-clotting status and not to determine if she was a gene carrier.

It was explained that gene carrier status would only affect Anna in adult life when she chose to have a family. Since a proportion of adults decide not to have carrier tests, this should be a decision for Anna herself to make once she has reached the age of legal consent. At that time she would be offered a diagnostic test for her brother's mutation. Anna's details were recorded in the genetic register for future review and both the family and the general practitioner were informed of the need to offer Anna genetic counseling at the appropriate age.

BLOOD SAMPLING

Accurate labeling

If a large number of patients in a family are to be sampled together, extreme care should be exercised to avoid mixing the samples, which could seriously impair any future genetic analysis of the family. Good practice is to put the blood from the patient into unlabeled tubes and then immediately write the patient's full name and date of birth on the tube, as this avoids putting the sample into the wrong prelabeled tube. The counselor will be aware that several individuals in a family may share a name and thus the date of birth on the sample bottle is an essential safeguard.

High risk samples

The hematologist will have alerted the lab about all affected males who have received treatment from blood products. These samples should have DNA extracted in a laboratory with suitable containment facilities because of the risk of human immunodeficiency virus (HIV) and hepatitis infection.

Samples from other relatives

Because carrier detection by direct mutation analysis is possible in this family, it is not necessary to sample Anna's father Gary Stevens. If the mutation was not detectable then carrier detection would depend on an indirect, linked genetic marker family study. This would require a sample from Gary and, even although it will be many years before Anna is tested, it would be best to try to contact Gary now as tracing separated relatives becomes increasingly difficult with time. Contact can be made by letter asking the patient, if willing, to make an appointment to see his general practitioner to have blood taken. An accompanying sample bottle can be sent in a stout cardboard box inside a padded postal bag, together with a note of explanation asking for the general practitioner's assistance. In northern Europe temperatures are rarely high enough for the sample to deteriorate in transit using normal first-class postal services.

Samples by post

Sampling by post should be reserved for those relatives whose sample is needed only to counsel others. If the sample is going to be used to give genetic advice to the patient, he or she should receive appropriate counseling beforehand

REPRODUCTIVE OPTIONS FOR CARRIERS

Julie Robertson was already aware that she must be a carrier and it was explained that she had an overall 1 in 4 risk of having an affected male in each pregnancy and that if a boy rather than a girl was born, his risk would be 1 in 2. The Robertsons were very keen to have more children but both were determined that they would only do so if they could be assured that any pregnancy was normal.

All the reproductive options available to the Robertsons were discussed, as follows.

Accept the risk and start a pregnancy

Many couples from families where the hemophilia is relatively mild are happy to accept even a high risk of recurrence. In contrast, some families are relieved to hear that the recurrence risk for a carrier's son is 50% and not 100%!

Contraception

For many couples who have yet to decide about their future, contraception is a sensible choice. Even when they indicate that they do not wish to have any further children and seek sterilization, a period using safe contraception allows time for reflection and after the initial upset after the diagnosis of an affected son, many will change their minds.

Sterilisation

This is a good choice for those who decide that their family is complete or those who decide not to risk a further pregnancy because of the recurrence risk which the geneticist has given them. The couple should be carefully counseled beforehand and advised that it should be considered as irreversible. At first sight it would appear to be more sensible for the woman to be sterilized, but in practice many choose vasectomy, often at the insistence of the wife!

Adoption

Some couples wish to adopt a child, although some adoption agencies are reluctant to place a child in a family where there is already a child with a physically or mentally disabling disorder. It is also becoming increasingly difficult to adopt babies. The waiting list for adoption may be so long that by the time their turn comes, some older couples may not be eligible for adoption on age grounds.

Prenatal diagnosis

General considerations. Prenatal diagnosis is usually only performed when a couple wish to terminate a pregnancy which is at high risk. It follows that termination of pregnancy should be a legal option in the country of practice. There must be an accurate test available to the family. This would ideally be a test which detects the mutation directly but indirect, linked DNA markers are now accurate enough for most couples. The severity of hemophilia in the family should be enough to warrant termination of pregnancy. The couple are often well-placed to make a judgement if there is an older affected relative. However, they may have been unduly influenced if a mildly affected relative had contracted HIV from blood products and gone on to develop acquired immuno-deficiency syndrome (AIDS). In a newly diagnosed sporadic case it is very important for the family to be given as complete a picture as possible before they make their decision. If the mutation has been detected, it can be helpful to give some idea of the severity seen in other families with that molecular pathology. After counseling, the couple should have enough knowledge to make an informed decision.

Methods of prenatal diagnosis. In this case the family already knew the severity of the hemophilia and the treatment options. The advantages and disadvantages of prenatal sexing and diagnosis using ultrasound in the second trimester, chorionic villus sampling in the first trimester, amniocentesis and fetal blood sampling in the second trimester were discussed and, like many patients, Julie expressed an interest in chorionic villus sampling at 12 weeks with rapid polymerase chain reaction (PCR)-based sexing of the fetus followed by a mutation screen in a male fetus. Most women prefer the option of a first trimester termination and those who have experienced a second-trimester termination usually opt for first-trimester diagnosis and, if necessary, termination in a subsequent pregnancy. The hematologist had already found Julie's factor VIII activity to be normal and so an invasive test was not contraindicated.

Prepregnancy clinic. Julie was referred to the prepregnancy clinic at the regional obstetric unit offering chorionic villus sampling for further counseling about obstetric aspects of prenatal diagnosis. Here she would also meet a member of staff who would be able to offer counseling following a termination of pregnancy if this was necessary.

SUMMARY LETTERS

After an opportunity for final questions, the counseling session was concluded with a review of the discussion and the family were told that each couple would be sent a letter summarizing the advice they had been given. Copies of this letter would be sent to their general practitioners, together with a separate medical letter to the referring doctor. Just as the language used in the counseling session should be appropriate to the patient's understanding, so too should be the language used in the letter. The counselor also needs to be aware that some patients will have reading difficulties.

These letters are an important record of what was said to a patient and geneticists are now seeing patients who bring with them letters which were written 20 or 30 years ago to their parents or grandparents. These genetic letters are viewed as important family documents and are often kept together with such documents as insurance policies.

RECORD KEEPING AND CONFIDENTIALITY

The family tree and all individual patient records are stored together in one case note which is allocated a pedigree number by which each individual member of the family can be traced and linked together. Because of this, it is important that each person is aware that the information stored in his or her section is confidential and will not be available to other members of the family. It is the counselor's responsibility not to let any confidential information about another relative slip out during counseling.

For example, it would be very upsetting when discussing prenatal diagnosis to suggest that a woman asks her older sister about her experience, if the sister had chosen not to tell anyone about her test. If a family tree is being updated for a new branch of the family, the patient must not be able to see any confidential information such as carrier status of relatives on the original pedigree.

Genetic methods of carrier detection

PEDIGREE ANALYSIS

Familial cases

An accurate family tree is drawn. If there is more than one affected male in the family, the hemophilia is considered to be familial and a number of women may be identified as being obligate carriers from their position in the family tree. They require no further testing except where analysis of their DNA could contribute to carrier tests for their daughters. A woman may be said to be an obligate carrier if:

1. She is the daughter of an affected male.
2. She has two or more affected boys (excluding identical twins) or carrier daughters.
3. She has one affected boy or carrier daughter and another affected male on her mother's side of the family.

Sporadic cases

If only one male is affected, there are a number of possibilities for the mutation's origin:

1. His mother is a carrier and he has inherited it.
2. The mutation occurred after his mother's conception and she is a mosaic with the mutation in her ovaries.
3. The mutation has happened at his conception.
4. The mutation has happened after his conception and he is a mosaic.

In the case of mosaicism, recurrence risk depends on the proportion of gonadal tissue carrying the mutation. Table 7.1 shows the genetic risks to an affected male's relatives in each of these situations.

In hemophilia the mutation rate has been found to be higher in spermatogenesis than in oogenesis. The male to female mutation rates, v/μ have been found to be 9.6/1

in hemophilia A (Rosendaal *et al.*, 1990) and 11/1 in hemophilia B (Montandon *et al.*, 1992). In practice, the mother of a sporadic male is most likely to be a carrier. The mutation is more likely to have arisen in the affected male's grandfather's sperm than in his mother's egg.

BAYES THEOREM

Once a carrier is identified, her daughters can be given a 50% carrier risk, which is the risk that her X chromosome with the hemophilia will be passed on rather than her healthy X chromosome. This is sometimes known as the daughter's prior risk. If the daughter has a large number of healthy sons, it is more likely that she will be a non-carrier than a carrier. This probability can be estimated as a conditional risk and combined with her prior risk and other conditional risks from laboratory tests using Bayes theorem to produce a final carrier risk.

Carrier risks

A major advantage of pedigree analysis using Bayes theorem is that it is very low-tech and can be used where hematologic and genetic investigations are unavailable. A disadvantage is that a consultand can never be given a zero carrier risk; instead, she will be given a risk figure such as 20% or 1 in 5. She will also be given a recurrence risk of an affected male for her next pregnancy, which will be 1/4 of her carrier risk, which in this example would be 5% or 1 in 20.

Geneticists usually consider a low risk to be below 1 in 20 and a high risk to be above 1 in 10; but the consultand's perception of the risk will depend on her exposure to hemophilia; whether she is closely related, how severe the hemophilia is in the family and if there are any complicating factors such as HIV infection.

Example of Bayes theorem

Figure 7.2 shows a family with hemophilia B. Agnes McDonald must be a carrier because her two sons are affected. Mary Robb, Anna Harvey and Jean Mclaren all wish to know their carrier status. Before they had any family of their own, they each had a 50% carrier risk which was based on their prior risk of inheriting the affected allele from the mother's pair of hemophilia alleles.

Table 7.1 Genetic risks in the family of a sporadic affected male

Origin of the mutation	Her mother's carrier risk	His sisters' carrier risks	His daughter's carrier risks	His brothers' affected risks
Mother is a carrier	Up to 100% risk	50% risk	100% risk	50% risk
Mother is a mosaic	Not at risk	Up to 50% risk	100% risk	Up to 50% risk
Son is new mutation	Not at risk	Not at risk	100% risk	Not at risk
Son is a mosaic	Not at risk	Not at risk	Up to 100% risk	Not at risk

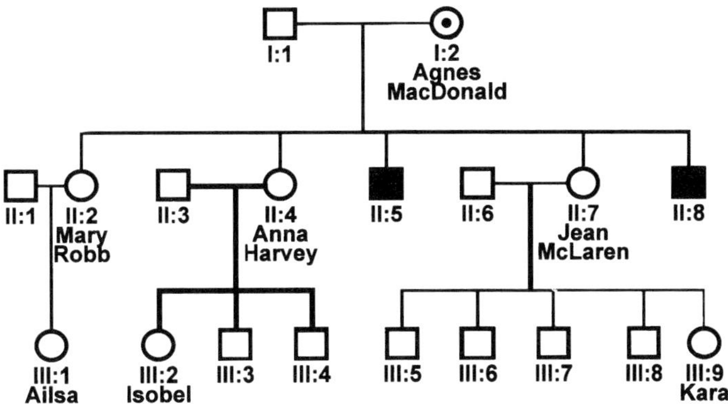

Figure 7.2 Example of a family with hemophilia B for risk calculation using Bayes theorem.

Since Jean has four healthy sons we would expect her to have a lower chance of being a carrier than Mary, who has no sons and whose carrier risk remains at 50%. The degree of risk reduction due to healthy sons (or grandsons) can be quantified using Bayes theorem (Emery, 1976). This method considers two possibilities – either that the consultand is a carrier or that she is a non-carrier.

Prior risk

Table 7.2 shows the calculation for Anna. Her prior risk of inheriting the hemophilia allele from her mother and being a carrier is 1/2. Her prior risk of being a non-carrier is also 1/2. We then consider her conditional risks which are created by her two healthy sons. The risk, if she is a carrier, that she will have a healthy son is 1/2. If she is a non-carrier, the risk that she will have a healthy son is 1. These risks are entered in the table for each son.

Joint risk

The joint risk is calculated by multiplying the prior and conditional risks in each column. This produces a joint risk in the carrier column of 1/8 and in the non-carrier column of 1/2, which is converted to 4/8 to give a

Table 7.2 Risk calculation for Ann Harvey (Fig. 7.2)

	Carrier	*Non-carrier*
Prior pedigree risk	1/2	1/2
Conditional risks		
Health son III:3	1/2	1
Healthy son III:4	1/2	1
Joint risk	1/8	1/2 = 4/8
Final risk	$\dfrac{1/8}{(1/8+4/8)}$	$\dfrac{4/8}{(1/8+4/8)}$
	$=1/5$	$=4/5$

common denominator which facilitates the later stage of the calculation.

Final risk

The final carrier risk is calculated by dividing the joint carrier risk by the sum of the joint carrier risk and the joint non-carrier risk. Figure 7.3 shows this in diagrammatic form. By canceling the common denominator, it can be seen that the final carrier risk is 1/5. Conversely, the final non-carrier risk is 4/5.

A similar calculation for Jean shows her final carrier risk to be 1/17. The carrier risks for Ailsa, Isobel and Kara are based on their prior risks which are half their mother's risks, there being no additional conditional information.

PHENOTYPIC TESTS

Various tests detect the activity of the factor VIII and factor IX gene products and have been recently reviewed (Peake *et al.*, 1993) and are discussed in detail in Chapter 9. Because these tests are not direct tests of the gene itself but are tests of gene expression, any factor which affects expression can influence the test results. In females the expression of X-linked recessive genes is affected by X chromosome inactivation. This is a random process and, depending on the relative proportions of healthy and hemophilia chromosomes which are inactivated, a carrier may have normal or abnormal clotting activity.

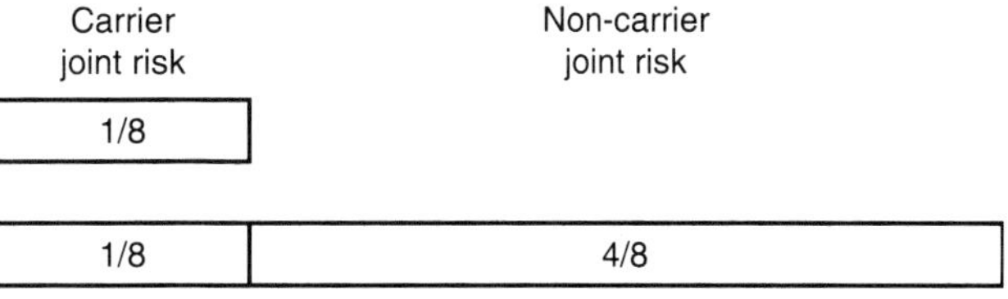

Fig. 7.3 Diagrammatic representation of how Anna Harvey's final carrier risk is calculated.

In practice, about 50% of carriers have clotting activities which fall below normal levels, while the other 50% have levels which overlap with normal. Consultands who have clotting activities within the normal range can have a carrier/non-carrier risk calculated by comparing their value with values obtained from obligate carriers and normal controls. There are various methods of doing this (Peake *et al.*, 1993), but all produce a result in the form of a carrier/non-carrier ratio.

An advantage of phenotypic tests of clotting activity is that they can detect carriers in families where the mutation is not detectable using direct genotypic tests (see below). This is particularly useful where the hemophilia is sporadic and the affected male may or may not be a new mutation. In such families indirect genotypic tests (see below) which track chromosomes through several generations cannot detect carriers. Once a carrier is detected, the geneticist knows the male is not a new mutation and other females in the family are at risk.

Example of Bayes calculation incorporating clotting activity risk ratios

Ailsa and Kara in Figure 7.2 both have clotting activity carrier/non-carrier ratios of 1:2. These results although, identical do not mean that they have the same carrier risks. The information needs to be interpreted in the context of the other information available from the pedigree. The prior risk for each is half of their mother's risk as calculated above. The calculations are shown in Tables 7.3 and 7.4 and show that Ailsa's carrier risk is 1/7 and Kara's risk is 1/67.

Table 7.3 Consultand Ailsa Robb (Fig. 7.2)

	Carrier	Non-carrier
Prior pedigree risk	1/4	3/4
Conditional risks: clotting activity	1	2
Joint risk	1/4	6/4
Final risk	$\dfrac{1/4}{1/4+6/4}$	$\dfrac{6/4}{1/4+6/4}$
	$=1/7$	$=6/7$

Table 7.4 Consultand Kara McLaren (Fig. 7.2)

	Carrier	Non-carrier
Prior pedigree risk	1/34	33/34
Conditional risks: clotting activity	1	2
Joint risk	1/34	66/34
Final risk	$\dfrac{1/34}{1/34+66/34}$	$\dfrac{6/4}{1/4+66/34}$
	$=1/67$	$=66/67$

GENOTYPIC TESTS

There are two types of genotypic tests; direct and indirect.

Direct genotypic tests

Direct tests are able to identify the mutation causing the hemophilia. Unfortunately, there are many mutations which cause hemophilia and it is not yet possible to detect the mutation in every family. DNA from an affected male in each family should be screened for mutations and, if none are found, a sample should be stored in the DNA bank of the regional genetics center for analysis in the future. The results of mutation screening in each family should be recorded in the genetic register.

These tests are the most satisfactory because, once a mutation is detected in an affected individual, all other at-risk relatives can be offered an accurate genetic test even if intervening relatives are unavailable for testing. An example would be the detection of the inversion involving exons 1–22 which causes 45% of serious cases of hemophilia A (Lakich *et al.*, 1993).

Example of direct mutation detection. Figure 7.4 shows a family in which III:1 has hemophilia A. His cousins III:3 and III:4 wish carrier testing but none of the individuals in generations I and II were available for testing. The diagram below the pedigree represents the results of a test which detects the mutation. The smaller DNA fragments migrate further down the electrophoresis gel than the larger fragments. The normal situation is shown in III:2 who is healthy and has bands 1,4 and 5. The mutation in the affected male causes the replacement of bands 1 and 4 with bands 2 and 3. III:4 must be a carrier

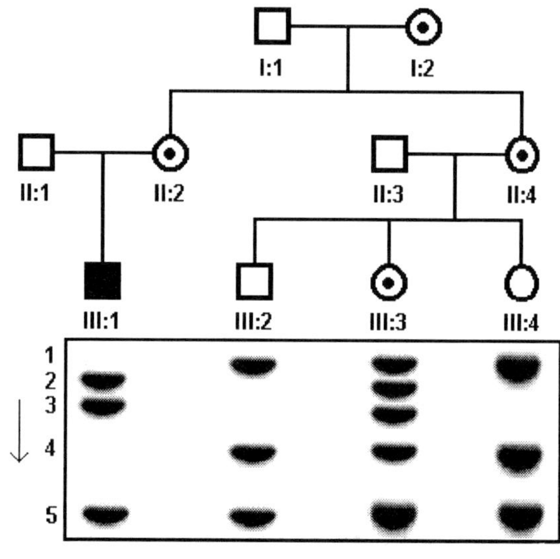

Fig. 7.4 Family with hemophilia A showing direct mutation detection.

because she is a heterozygote. Her healthy hemophilia gene is represented by bands 1, 4 and 5 and her affected hemophilia gene shows bands 2, 3 and 5. Band 5 appears greater in density because it is produced by both alleles.

Confidentiality when relatives' genotypes can be inferred. Although II:2, I:2 and II:4 in Figure 7.4 have not been tested, they can be identified as being obligate carriers because III:3 is a carrier. If these women were not tested because they did not wish to know their carrier status then III:3 should be advised to keep her test result to herself.

Mosaicism. At first sight it would appear that a genotypic test, which directly detects the mutation, can be interpreted in isolation of the woman's position in the pedigree and other test results. While this is true for sisters, aunts and granddaughters of an affected male, it is not true for the mother who has no previous family history but has an affected son. If DNA testing shows she does not have her son's mutation it is not safe to assume that he is the result of a new mutation.

If the hemophilia mutation arose after her conception, during embryogenesis, she could be a mosaic of normal and hemophilia cells. The genotype of her sampled cells may, therefore, not be representative of the gonadal cells. In practice the mother of a sporadic case who does not have his mutation in her somatic cells should be given a recurrence risk. Data from hemophilia families are not yet available but data from Duchenne X-linked muscular dystrophy suggests a recurrence risk of 5% in such circumstances (van Essen *et al.*, 1992).

Figure 7.5 shows an example of mosaicism. II:1 has been diagnosed as having hemophilia A and the inversion

mutation has been detected. His mother I:2 is homozygous for the normal hemophilia allele in DNA obtained from a blood sample and at first sight appears to be a non-carrier. In this example her daughter has been tested and is found to be a carrier because she is heterozygous for the normal and mutated hemophilia alleles. This must mean that some or all of I:2's ovarian cells carry the mutation and the recurrence risk of an affected male could be as high as 25% if all gonadal tissue carries the mutation.

Isolating the mutation in a branch of the family. Once a mutation is detected in a family the geneticist will try to isolate it to a branch of a family by screening the mothers and sisters of affected males or obligate carriers and the granddaughters of affected males. In Figure 7.4 the mother and sister of I:2 should be offered carrier tests, as should the daughters of III:3. The descendants of III:4 do not require testing as she has been shown not to carry the mutation. In Figure 7.5 the mother and sisters of I:2 do not require testing as the mutation has been shown to have occurred after her conception because she is a mosaic. The daughters of II:2 should be offered testing.

Indirect genotypic tests

When the mutation causing hemophilia has not been detected, indirect genotypic tests may be employed to predict the genotype in other members of a hemophilia family. These tests do not detect the mutation directly but track the region of the chromosome adjacent to or linked to the mutation. Gene tracking only works in familial cases where there are two or more affected males or there is one affected male and one or more carriers. Ideally three generations should be available for testing.

Gene tracking depends on identifying normal genetic variations or polymorphisms in the region of the gene. The key carrier female who wishes prenatal diagnosis or whose daughters seek carrier detection should carry two forms of the polymorphism, i.e. she should be heterozygous or informative for the marker. By studying her normal and hemophiliac male relatives it should be possible to determine which of the marker alleles is segregating with the hemophilia allele.

Inaccuracy caused by genetic recombination. Unfortunately, genetic recombination (or exchange of genetic material which takes place between chromosome pairs at meiosis) can cause the marker which was segregating with the hemophilia allele to switch to the other chromosome, resulting in a false genetic prediction. The closer the marker is to the mutation, there is less chance that a recombination will occur and the genetic prediction will be more accurate.

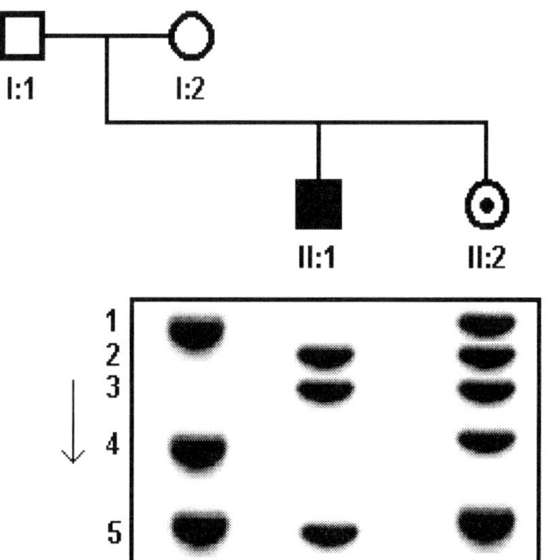

Fig. 7.5 Family with hemophilia A showing evidence of gonadal mosaicism.

Intragenic markers. If the marker is within the hemophilia gene (intragenic), then the chance of a recombination occurring will be 1% or less. This degree of accuracy is sufficient for most families and no other tests would be necessary. Using widely available intragenic markers, 95% of key females in a hemophilia A family are informative and, in hemophilia B, 85% of carriers are informative (Peake *et al.*, 1993). Families who are non-informative for intragenic markers may be further studied using extragenic markers.

Extragenic markers. If the marker is extragenic then the chance of recombination rises, for example, the linked marker ST14 (DXS52) shows 5% recombination with hemophilia A. This introduces a significant error into any genetic prediction using the marker alone but results from extragenic linked markers may be used as an additional conditional risk and can be combined with pedigree risks and clotting factor risks in a Bayes calculation to produce a satisfactory combined or final risk.

A major drawback of indirect genetic linkage studies is that all stated relationships in the pedigree have to be correct. Undisclosed non-paternity can lead to serious misinterpretation of this type of test.

Example of indirect gene tracking using a linked marker. Figure 7.6 shows a family with hemophilia A in which III:1 wishes to have carrier detection. Her mother is an obligate carrier and is thus the key female in this analysis. Her brother's DNA has no detectable mutation and her mother was homozygous or non-informative for the available intragenic genetic markers. She is heterozygous for a linked extragenic marker which in this family recognizes two alleles – an F allele which migrates quickly through an electrophoresis gel and an S allele which travels more slowly. The marker shows 5% recombination with the hemophilia gene.

A diagram of the electrophoresis gel is shown below the pedigree. The DNA fragments are migrating from top to bottom. The parental origins of each child's bands are shown by the thin connecting lines which are superimposed on the gel. Above the gel are bars representing the region of the X chromosome containing the hemophilia gene (allele H is affected, allele + is normal) and the marker (alleles F and S).

Both the healthy son, III:2 and the affected son have inherited the marker F allele and so one must be a recombinant. If I:1's DNA was not available for analysis it would not be possible to decide in which son the recombination took place. However, I:1 has the marker S and the hemophilia mutation. Since he only has one X chromosome, this must have been passed to II:2 unaltered by recombination. This allows us to assign the phase of the marker alleles with the hemophilia alleles in II:2. S and H must have been inherited from I:1, while F and + must have come from her mother, I:2. This now allows us to say that the recombination must have taken place in III:3 who is F and H. The F marker allele originated in his healthy grandmother while the affected H hemophilia allele came from his affected grandfather.

The S and the F alleles are common in the population and have no causative effect with hemophilia. Although in I:1 the S is associated with the hemophilia-affected allele, this is not the case for all individuals who carry the S allele. This is clearly illustrated by II:1, who is related to the family only by marriage. Although his marker allele is S his hemophilia allele is the normal +. The consultand, III:1, is also heterozygous for the marker having both the F and the S alleles. The S must have come from her father, together with a healthy hemophilia allele +. The F must have come from her mother and, if no recombination has occurred, the test predicts that she will

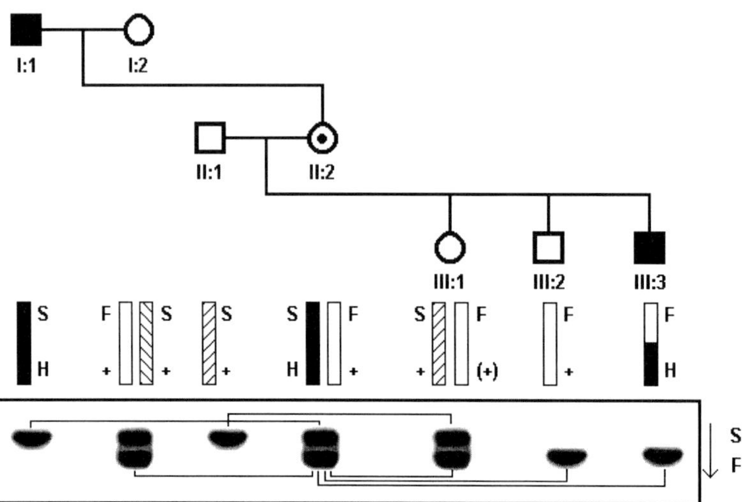

Fig. 7.6 Family with hemophilia A analyzed with an extragenic marker.

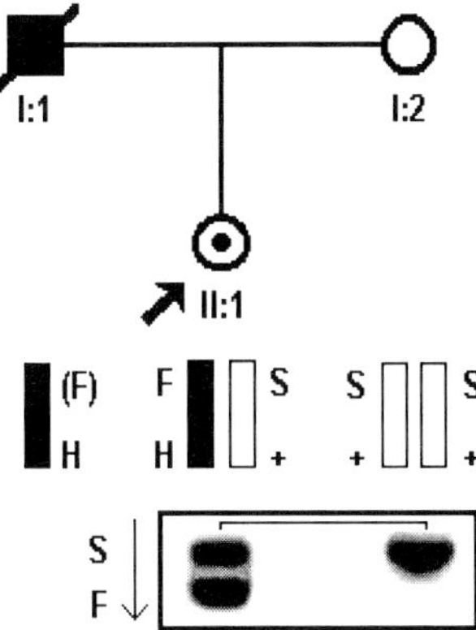

Fig. 7.7 Example of using marker results to infer genotype in an unavailable relative in order to identify the hemophilia chromosome.

Table 7.5 Consultand III:1 (Fig. 7.6)

	Carrier	Non-carrier
Prior pedigree risk	1/2	1/2
Conditional risks:		
clotting activity	1	3
low risk F allele	1/20	19.20
Joint risk	1/40	57/40
Final risk	$\dfrac{1/40}{1/40+57/40}$	$\dfrac{57/40}{1/40+57/40}$
	$=1/58$	$=57/58$

have inherited her mother's healthy + allele along with it. With 5% recombination, the accuracy of the prediction that she is a non-carrier will be 95%. With a 5% error rate this result should be included with pedigree and clotting factor risks in a Bayes calculation.

Example using extragenic marker results in Bayes calculation. III:1 in Figure 7.6 has a prior pedigree risk of 1/2 and her carrier/non carrier ratio calculated from clotting activity is 1:3. The Bayes calculation is shown in Table 7. If III:1 really is a carrier, we would expect her to inherit the low-risk allele F only if a recombination has occurred, i.e. in 1/20 (5%) of occasions. If III:1 is really a non-carrier, we would expect her to inherit the low-risk allele F if no recombination has occurred, i.e. in 19/20 (95%) of occasions. III:1's final carrier risk is 1/58, which means that her chance of having an affected male in her first pregnancy is 1/4 of this – 1/232.

Inferring genotypes when key relatives are unavailable for testing. In the above example all relatives were available for testing but it is often possible to infer the genotype of DNA markers in key relatives who are deceased or unavailable. Figure 7.7 shows a pedigree where II:1 wishes prenatal diagnosis but her father is dead. To offer prenatal diagnosis the geneticist needs to find a

marker for which she is heterozygous and some way of assigning which marker allele is associated with the affected hemophilia allele. This can most easily be done if her mother is homozygous for a probe for which II:1 is heterozygous.

II:1 must have received an X chromosome containing the marker allele S and the healthy hemophilia allele + from her mother. The marker F allele must have come from her father, together with the affected hemophilia allele H. II:1 could be offered prenatal diagnosis on the basis that if a male fetus inherited F it would be affected (subject to recombination). This assumes that I:1 was her biological father and that II:1 is therefore an obligate carrier.

References

Emery, A.E.H. (1976) *Methodology in Medical Genetics, An Introduction to Statistical Methods*, Churchill Livingstone, Edinburgh.

Lakich, D., Kazazian, H.H., Stylianos, E. *et al.* (1993) Inversions disrupting the factor VIII gene are a common cause of severe haemophilia A. *Nature Genetics*, 5, 236–241.

Montandon, A.J., Green, P.M., Bentley, D.R. *et al.* (1992) Direct estimate of the haemophilia B (factor IX deficiency) mutation rate and of the ratio of the sex-specific mutation rates in Sweden. *Human Genetics*, 89, 319–322.

Peake, I.R., Lillicrap, D.P., Boulyjenkov, V. *et al.* (1993) Report of a joint WHO/WFH meeting on control of haemophilia: carrier detection and prenatal diagnosis. *Blood Coagulation and Fibrinolysis*, 4, 313–344.

Rosendaal, F.R., Bröcker-Vriends, A.H.J.T., van Houwelingen, J.C. *et al.* (1990) Sex ratio of mutation rates in haemophilia A: estimation and meta-analysis. *Human Genetics*, 86, 139–146.

van Essen, A.J., Abbs, S., Baiget, M. *et al.* (1992) Parental origin and germline mosaicism of deletions and duplications of the dystrophin gene: a European study. *Human Genetics*, 88, 249–257.

8 CENTRAL AND PERIPHERAL NERVOUS SYSTEM BLEEDING

J.P. Hanley and C.A. Ludlam

Hemorrhage affecting the nervous system is a relatively common problem and results in considerable mortality and morbidity for those with hemophilia. Damage may follow bleeding into the brain or spinal cord or indirectly from pressure on peripheral nerves, usually from bleeding into adjacent structures such as muscle or joints. Prior to human immunodeficiency virus (HIV) infection, intracranial hemorrhage (ICH) was the commonest cause of death amongst severe hemophiliacs and, in those who survived this complication, there is considerable neurologic impairment.

Peripheral nerve damage, while less dramatic than intracranial bleeding, is responsible for both acute and chronic morbidity which may increase the degree of disability in those with arthropathy.

We will discuss historic aspects as well as the contemporary incidence, diagnosis and management of nervous system bleeding in hemophiliacs. In addition we will outline how the development of modern treatment methods and the introduction of new imaging techniques have changed the management of nervous system bleeding in recent years.

Intracranial hemorrhage in hemophilia

HISTORIC REVIEW

Prior to the development of coagulation factor replacement therapy, invasive investigations were rarely performed on hemophiliacs presenting with symptoms and signs suggesting ICH. In most cases the diagnosis of ICH was based on either clinical features or postmortem findings. As a result of diagnostic uncertainty, early authors tended to report the incidence of fatal intracranial bleeding and there was considerable difficulty obtaining accurate information concerning the incidence of non-fatal ICH. With the availability of cryoprecipitate and subsequently coagulation factor concentrates, it became possible to attempt invasive diagnostic techniques as well as neurosurgical operations. More recently, non-invasive methods such as computed tomographic (CT) and magnetic resonance imaging (MRI) scanning have proved an invaluable diagnostic tool and the contemporary approach to the investigation and management of ICH is discussed later in the chapter. It is of some interest to review the historic aspects of central nervous system (CNS) bleeding in hemophilia as the advances in coagulation factor therapy have profoundly influenced both investigation and management.

It has been recognized for many years that both posttraumatic, often after minor injury, and apparently spontaneous intracranial bleeding may occur in hemophiliacs. In the first account of blood transfusion used in hemophilia Lane (1840) reviews cases in the literature and refers to the death of two brothers from a family of bleeders: 'They died from falls, in which they received blows on the head not sufficiently severe to have produced much mischief in a sound state of the system, but which in them was followed by extravasation of blood within the cranium'. Prince Leopold, hemophiliac son of Queen Victoria, was advised to 'abstain from violent exertion of any kind' (Anonymous, 1868). Despite following this advice he was reported to have died following a minor head injury: 'The weakness of the knee seems to have caused the fall, but the nature of the intracranial complication is obscure' (Anonymous, 1884). Another account from the early part of this century outlines 19 cases of spontaneous lesions in the nervous system, mainly intracranial, in individuals with a strong personal or family history of bleeding (Bulloch and Fildes, 1911). A series from 1930 reported 29 hospitalizations of individuals with a strong bleeding tendency and of these, only

Hemophilia. Edited by C.D. Forbes, L. Aledort and R. Madhok. Published in 1997 by Chapman & Hall, London. ISBN 0 412 63820 7

2 were classified as 'haemorrhages causing nervous lesions' and both were, in fact, peripheral nerve lesions. On the basis of the lack of observed cases, the author concluded that intracranial bleeding was extremely rare (Seddons, 1930). A comprehensive review of the literature was published in 1944 which systematically classified 45 reported cases of bleeding affecting the nervous system (Aggeler and Lucia, 1944).

In an attempt to tackle some of the diagnostic difficulties and calculate a more accurate incidence of ICH, a study in 1960 included only 25 individuals from the literature with laboratory evidence of hemophilia and an additional 6 individuals described by the author. Cases were classified as 'proved ICH' if bleeding was confirmed by objective methods (postmortem, surgery, blood in subdural or cerebrospinal fluid (CSF) aspirates) or 'probable ICH' if bleeding was suspected on clinical grounds only (Silverstein, 1960). This study concluded the overall incidence of ICH to be 6.3% with a mortality of 70%. There was some speculation as to whether, with the availability of improved therapy to control bleeding at other sites, the incidence of ICH in hemophiliacs was likely to decrease.

Some support for this prediction was provided by a study a few years later which assessed 109 hemophiliacs attending a single center. Over a 5-year period 15 (13.8%) experienced a total of 19 episodes of ICH (Kerr, 1964). On 9 occasions there was direct evidence to confirm the diagnosis of ICH (CSF examination, operative or necroscopy findings) but in 10 the diagnosis was based solely on clinical grounds with abnormal electroencephalogram (EEG) tracings in 7 cases. A slightly lower incidence of 4.3% was reported in a small series in 1966 (Davies *et al.*, 1966) and there was also some debate at this time as to whether the incidence of intracranial bleeding may be influenced by aspirin ingestion taken for headache (Quick, 1971).

Turning to the historic aspects of the treatment of ICH in hemophiliacs, in the past there were considerable difficulties in performing invasive diagnostic techniques as well as surgery in hemophiliacs with suspected hemorrhage. Despite occasional neurosurgical partial success (Jamieson, 1954; Fuerth, Teng and Goldenberg, 1961), the following statement summarizes the previously generally accepted approach: 'angiography and operation should be avoided unless absolutely necessary and then, only the minimum operation performed which is likely to save life' (Potter, 1965). It soon became apparent that conservative management with the use of plasma infusions in hemophiliacs with headache or neurologic signs was extremely valuable and 'once the patient has improved there is no justification for any other diagnostic or therapeutic surgical procedure' (Fessey and Meynell, 1966). By the late 1960s, however, reports of increasingly successful surgical intervention in

hemophiliacs, who failed to improve with conservative therapy, began to appear with operations performed after replacement therapy with cryoprecipitate of factor VIII concentrates (Simpson and Robson, 1960; Brown *et al.*, 1967; Prentice *et al.*, 1967; Carrea *et al.*, 1968; Moody and Mullan, 1968; Ferguson, Barton and Drake, 1968; Olsen, 1969; Myles, Harris and Hansebout, 1971; Friedman, Guerry and Wilkins, 1971; Matsuda *et al.*, 1977; Bennett and Sills, 1978) and the safer use of invasive diagnostic procedures (Curless and Corrigan, 1976). Subsequently a combined approach to the management of intracranial bleeding in hemophiliacs involving close cooperation between hematologists and neurosurgeons (Seeler and Imana, 1973) has become established in many centers and is discussed in more detail below.

INCIDENCE AND SITES OF ICH

Over the past 30 years many of the diagnostic difficulties discussed above have been overcome and much more accurate data concerning the incidence of ICH in hemophilia have become available from surveys of patients attending individual hemophilia centers and nationally collected mortality data.

All studies agree that the risk of ICH is strongly related to the severity of hemophilia, with the majority of bleeding episodes occurring in severe hemophiliacs (factor VIII/IX level <2%).

A retrospective survey of 201 patients attending one institution revealed CNS bleeding in 14.9% over a 13-year period (Gendelman, 1977) and a larger study of an estimated hemophiliac population, of all severities, identified 2500 episodes of CNS bleeding in 71 individuals (2.7% for hemophilia A and 3.6% for hemophilia B patients) during an 11-year period (1965–1976); (Eyster *et al.*, 1978). Another group reported 154 episodes of ICH in 106 hemophiliacs from a population of 1410 between 1960 and 1991. This study suggested an incidence of 7.5% or 1 in 13 patients (de Tezanos Pinto, Fernandez and Perez Bianco, 1992). This contrasts with a report from Israel which found only 8 episodes of ICH in 7 patients from a hemophiliac population of 288 between 1972 and 1982. The annual incidence of ICH was calculated to be only 0.27% (Martinowitz *et al.*, 1986).

As the collection of data concerning mortality in hemophiliacs has become more accurate, the incidence of fatal ICH has been well documented and is remarkably consistent between reports from different geographic locations. ICH was the commonest cause of death in UK hemophiliacs, accounting for 16 of 62 (26%) deaths between 1967 and 1974 (Biggs, 1977) and 26 of 89 (29%) between 1976 and 1980 (Rizza and Spooner, 1983). A similar picture was seen in Sweden, with ICH being the main cause in 37 of 118 (31%) deaths between

1957 and 1980 (Larsson and Wiechel, 1983) and it accounted for 35% of deaths in Danish hemophiliacs between 1949 and 1978 (Bacher, 1980). In the USA, between 1968 and 1979, intracerebral bleeding was thought to be the commonest cause of death (Aronson, 1988). Mortality data from developing nations are scanty but a short report which suggested that ICH was extremely common in Nigerian hemophiliacs has not been confirmed by any subsequent published material (Essien and Adeloye, 1972).

The studies mentioned above also provide information concerning the frequency of ICH at different anatomical sites. There would appear to be no particular site where bleeding, either apparently spontaneous or posttraumatic, occurs more frequently. Allowing for minor variations between reports, ICH is divided into three equal groups according to site of bleeding, with approximately one-third of patients with each of subdural, subarachnoid and intracerebral bleeding. Additionally, a minority have evidence of hemorrhage at more than one site.

In summary, there has been debate concerning the precise incidence of intracranial hemorrhage in hemophiliacs, with considerable variation in the reported incidence between studies. There is agreement that severe hemophiliacs are most at risk and there is no predilection for a particular site of ICH. Mortality data shows that, prior to the acquired immunodeficiency syndrome (AIDS) epidemic, ICH was consistently the commonest cause of death. With the development of modern methods of diagnosis and treatment, the overall incidence appears to be less than previously, although larger contemporary studies to confirm this suggestion are awaited. If the incidence is indeed falling it is likely to represent prevention of posttraumatic ICH by the prompt use of coagulation factor replacement, as discussed below, as well as the more widespread use of routine prophylaxis.

HEAD TRAUMA AND ICH

Before discussing the features and management of established ICH in hemophiliacs, it is useful to consider the assessment of head trauma and the use of coagulation factor replacement therapy to prevent ICH following head trauma.

Relationship between head trauma and ICH

The precise role of head trauma in causing ICH in hemophiliacs is an area of some controversy. Retrospective studies have suggested that only approximately half of cases of ICH are precipitated by head trauma (Eyster *et al.* 1978; Visconti and Hilgartner, 1980). Others argue, however, that minor trauma which is not recalled by the patient may often be important in apparently 'spontaneous' ICH (Hirsch *et al.*, 1983). Most studies agree that

there is often an appreciable delay between trauma and the development of symptoms, leading to an over-diagnosis of spontaneous ICH. The mechanisms of this delay are uncertain but minor trauma may damage small blood vessels, leading to a slowly developing hematoma, giving rise to late symptoms. This delay between trauma and presentation, however, was not observed in a recent series (Dietrich *et al.*, 1994). It is important therefore to recognize that the possibility of ICH should not be discounted on the basis of an absence of a history of trauma.

In an attempt to clarify some of the issues, a prospective study of head trauma in hemophilia was performed, aiming to establish the proportion leading to ICH (Andes, Wulff and Smith, 1984). All patients registered at a single centre ($n = 140$) were instructed to report all episodes of head trauma during a 2-year period. In total, there were 47 episodes of head trauma reported but only 6 of these led to intracranial bleeding. In addition there was 1 case of spontaneous intracranial bleeding during the study period, giving an overall incidence of 12%. There was a significant association between delay in coagulation factor replacement after head trauma and the development of hemorrhage confirmed on CT scan. In the 27 cases who received treatment within 6 h of injury, there were no cases of subsequent intracranial bleeding.

Role of CT scan in hemophiliacs with head trauma

In order to address the question as to when a CT scan should be considered after episodes of head injury in hemophiliacs, retrospective studies have reviewed a CT scan performed following trauma. In an analysis of 28 episodes of head injury which were defined as minor in 12, moderate in 12 and severe in 4, a CT scan detected hemorrhage in 3 cases and was normal in 25 (Hennes *et al*, 1987). All three instances of bleeding occurred in individuals who had sustained severe head trauma on the basis of altered mental status or symptoms/signs of having raised intracranial pressure (persistent headache, vomiting or focal neurologic deficit).

Another study assessed the value of CT scanning in the management of hemophiliac children with head trauma over a 7-year period. There were 109 episodes of head trauma, resulting in only 5 cases of intracranial hemorrhage confirmed on CT scan (Dietrich *et al.*, 1994). The symptoms and signs at presentation were correlated with the decision to perform an urgent CT scan as well as the CT findings. The episodes were divided into three groups: first, on 43 occasions a CT scan was not performed (factor replacement therapy was given in 42 cases). In this group there was no alteration in mental status (as assessed by Glasgow Coma Scale) or neurologic deficit but headache was present in 5 cases and vomiting reported in 1. Second, in 61 cases a CT scan was performed, which proved to be normal. In this group again there was no neurologic deficit but altered mental status in two, vomiting in four and headache in 15 cases. Finally, in the five cases of ICH confirmed on CT scan, there was both altered mental status and neurologic deficit in all cases as well as vomiting in five. Thus, to predict the likelihood of ICH after head injury, vomiting (80% versus 5%), altered mental status (100% versus 3%) and neurological deficit (100% versus 0%) were the most useful features. The authors suggested that all hemophiliac children with head trauma should receive coagulation factor replacement after head injury but an urgent CT scan is only indicated in the presence of headache, vomiting or neurologic deficit.

Although it is clear from such retrospective studies that CT scanning is only required in a minority of head injuries in hemophiliacs, there is a need for standard criteria for the assessment of severity of head injury to be devised and evaluated in prospective studies. Figure 8.1 outlines a scheme for the management of hemophiliacs with head trauma.

Coagulation factor replacement therapy after minor head injury

From the preceding discussion it is clear that particular symptoms and signs, when present following head trauma, are highly suggestive of ICH and warrant urgent investigation and treatment. At the other end of the spectrum, when should factor replacement be given after minor head injury – a frequent occurrence, particularly in children – in order to prevent subsequent ICH? Guidelines should probably err on the side of caution and advise that replacement therapy should be given in all cases of head trauma which involve anything more than an extremely trivial knock. Certainly, any trauma which results in even minor bruising should be considered sufficient to warrant replacement therapy.

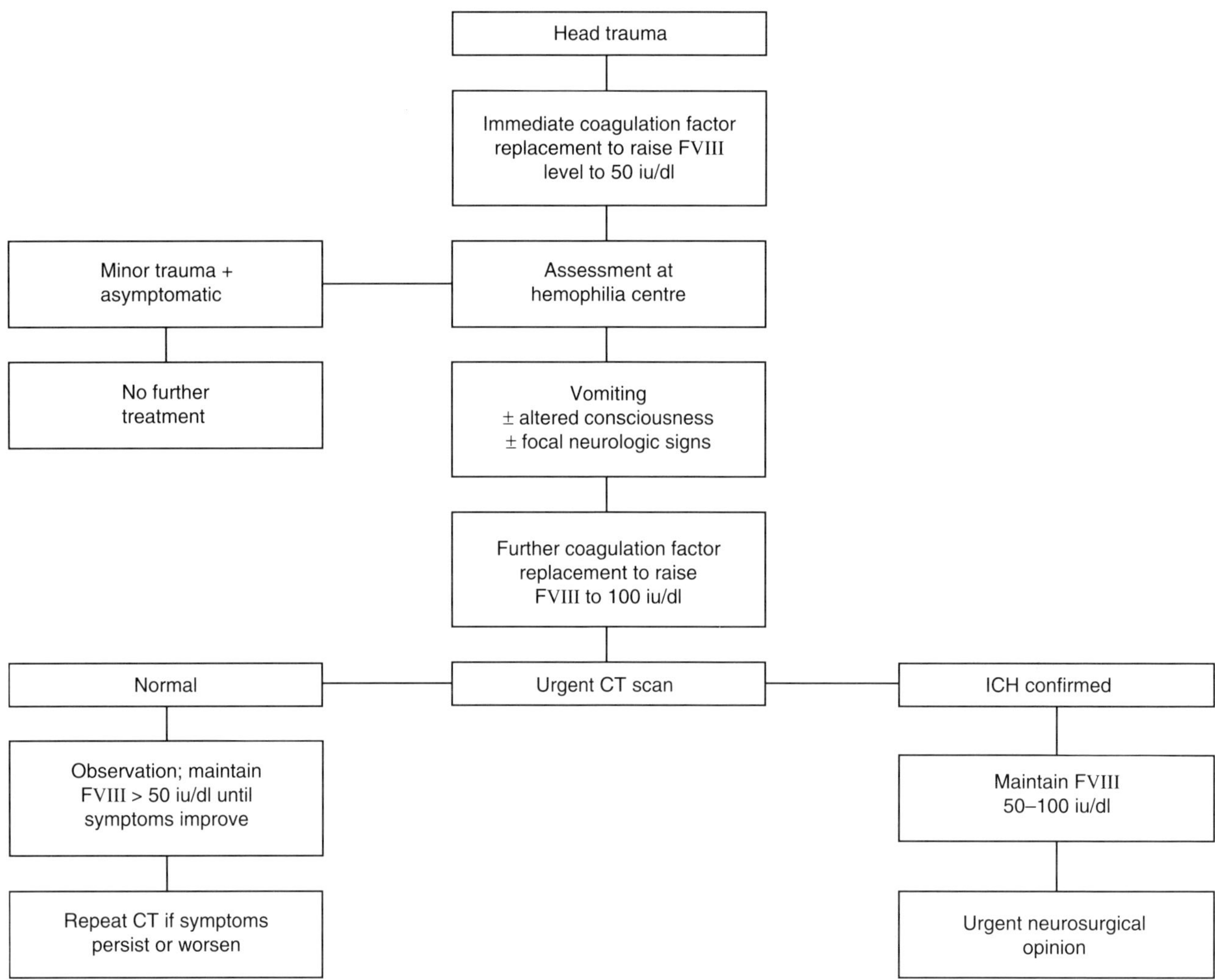

Fig. 8.1 Management of head trauma in hemophilia. FVIII = Factor VIII; CT = computed tomography; ICH = intracranial hemorrhage.

CLINICAL FEATURES AND INVESTIGATION OF ICH

The clinical features of ICH in hemophiliacs do not differ significantly from non-hemophiliacs, with headache, vomiting, convulsions, confusion, blurred vision or coma being the most common presenting features (Eyster *et al.*, 1978) with or without a history of preceding trauma.

CT scanning of the brain was applied to the investigation of hemophiliacs with suspected intracranial hemorrhage soon after the development of the technique (Kinney *et al.*, 1977) and has proved to be an invaluable non-invasive diagnostic investigation and currently the investigation of choice in suspected ICH (Fig. 8.2). More recently, MRI has emerged as an alternative to CT. The use of MRI in the assessment of hemophiliacs with intracranial bleeding is yet to be evaluated.

TREATMENT OF ESTABLISHED ICH

The management of head injury in an attempt to prevent bleeding after head trauma and the indications for performing CT scanning are discussed above. In this section the approaches to the care of hemophiliacs with established intracranial hemorrhage, either posttraumatic or apparently spontaneous and confirmed by CT scan, are discussed. Management guidelines have been suggested by some authors (Guthrie and Sacra, 1980; DeBehnke and Angelos, 1990). A summary of current treatment options is presented in Fig. 8.3.

The most important aspect of the management of intracranial bleeding in hemophiliacs is the prompt administration of coagulation factor replacement. This should be done immediately when there is clinical suspicion of ICH and prior to any confirmatory investigations.

Despite the widespread use of early coagulation factor therapy, the overall outcome reported in some studies in the 1970s and 1980s remained poor with a mortality of over 50% (Martinowitz *et al.*, 1986). Even in studies with a lower mortality, neurologic sequelae were present in around 50% of survivors (Eyster *et al.*, 1978; Visconti and Hilgartner, 1980). The precise reasons for this are unclear but may be related to a still inappropriate initial delay in the administration of factor concentrate followed by a reluctance to consider early neurosurgical intervention and an uncertainty as to whether early surgery would improve outcome.

The role of neurosurgical intervention was addressed in a small prospective study in hemophiliac boys which aimed to manage all cases of neurologic bleeding according to a uniform protocol (Yue and Mann, 1986). Over a 3-year period a CT scan was performed on all hemophiliacs presenting with neurologic signs or symptoms ($n = 7$). In addition all children presenting with ICH were screened for hemophilia which detected 2 additional patients with severe hemophilia A. Surgery was indicated on the basis of standard neurosurgical criteria in all 9 patients and was performed after aggressive factor VIII replacement with regular laboratory monitoring to ensure adequate levels. The outcome in this study was excellent with no subsequent neurologic deficit in eight of nine patients (one patient was already disabled prior to the intracranial event and was reported not to have suffered any additional deficit). Thus, with aggressive modern management and early neurosurgical intervention it would appear that the outcome after ICH may be

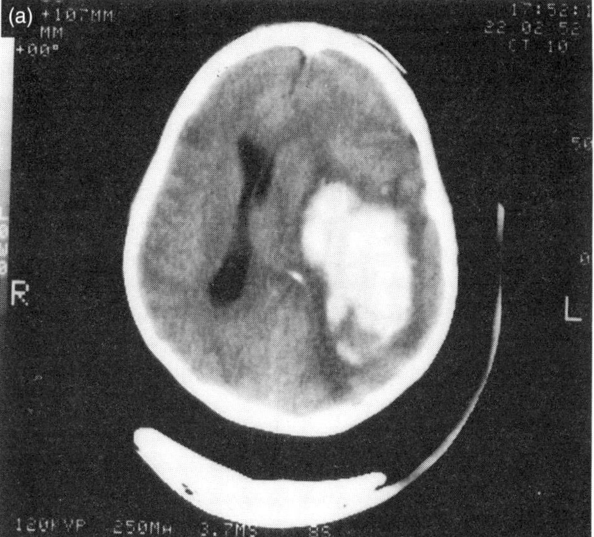
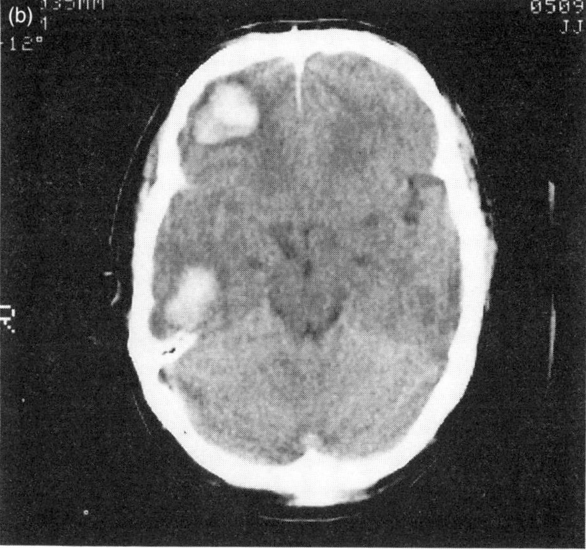

Fig. 8.2 (a) Computed tomographic (CT) scan of large spontaneous intracerebral bleed with associated cerebral edema and midline shift. (b) CT scan showing two sites of hemorrhage following head injury.

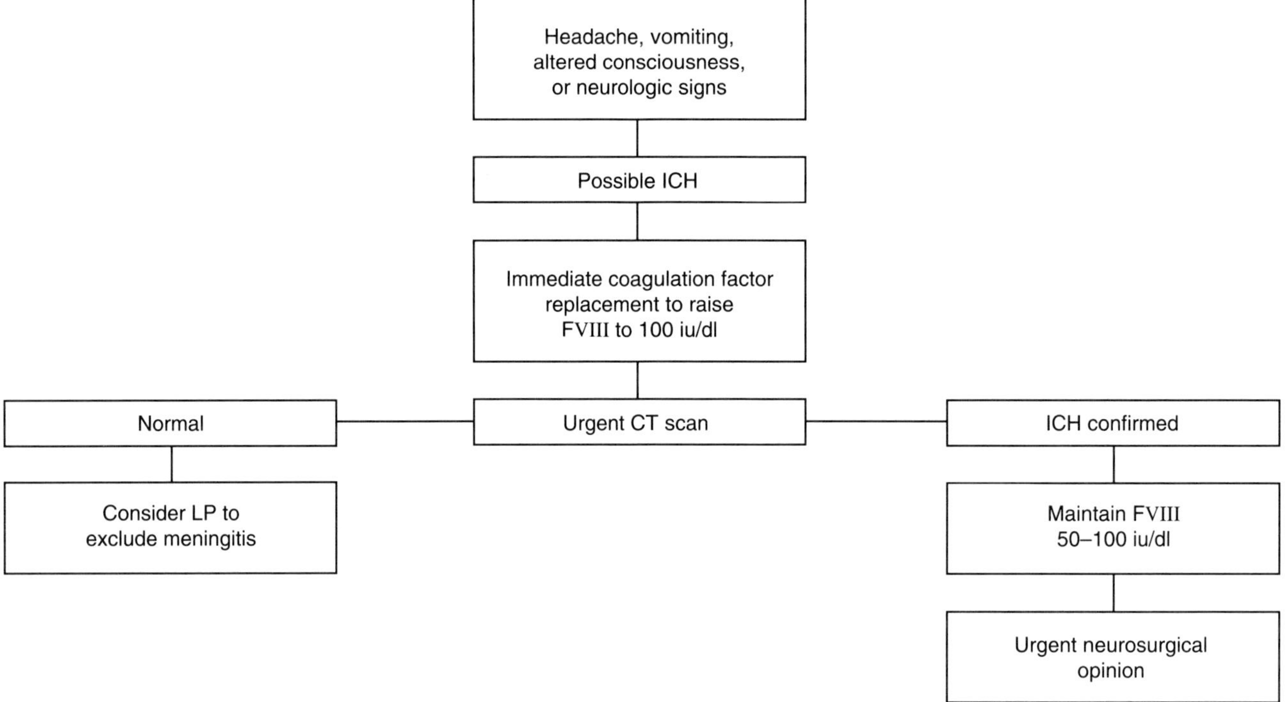

Fig. 8.3 Management of possible intracranial hemorrhage in hemophilia. ICH = Intracranial hemorrhage; LP = lumbar puncture.

much improved and a joint approach between hematologists and neurosurgeons is now widely applied to the management of ICH in hemophiliacs.

Apart from early neurosurgical intervention, when appropriate, there are several other aspects to management of ICH in hemophilia:

Coagulation factor replacement. It is clearly important to maintain adequate factor VIII/IX levels after surgery and therapy should be continued for at least 14 days. There has been recent interest in the use of continuous infusions of factor VIII to maintain the level in those with intracranial bleeds (Martinowitz *et al.*, 1992) or undergoing neurosurgery (Doughty *et al.*, 1995). In those with ICH who do not require surgery, coagulation factor replacement should continue at least until symptoms and signs have entirely resolved. Sequential CT scanning may be useful to document improvement in response to therapy and help in the decision as to duration of treatment with coagulation factor replacement (Gore *et al.*, 1981).

Antifibrinolytic therapy. Antifibrinolytic drugs such as tranexamic acid may have a role in the management of ICH (Martinowitz *et al.*, 1986). It is thought that the clot-stabilizing properties of these drugs may be useful in preventing rebleeding. There are no data available to support the routine use of antifibrinolytics but they may be useful in selected cases. Antifibrinolytics should not be used if the patient is also receiving prothrombin complex concentrates because of the risk of thrombosis.

Anticonvulsant therapy. Many authors have observed that convulsions appear to be extremely common in hemophiliacs with ICH (Lutschg and Vassella, 1981). There is the danger of seizures provoking further bleeding and some have recommended prophylactic anticonvulsants (Sakima *et al.*, 1983).

Management of intracranial hemorrhage in hemophiliacs with inhibitors or complex coagulaopathies. Surprisingly, the mortality of those with antifactor VIII antibodies is not reported to be higher than those without an inhibitor (Eyster *et al.*, 1978). High-dose factor VIII, porcine factor VIII, factor VIII inhibitor-bypassing activity (FEIBA) or recombinant activated factor VIIa (rVIIa) may be used successfully. In those who fail to respond to monotherapy, rapid immune tolerance induction or the use of multiple agents to control bleeding may be required. The successful use of continuous exchange transfusion, immunosuppression, antifibrinolytics and high doses of factor VIII has been reported in a hemophiliac with an anti-factor VIII antibody and a subdural hematoma (Edson *et al.*, 1973).

More recently, rVIIa has been used to treat a Jehovah's Witness with antifactor VIII antibodies who became unconscious due to a subdural hematoma. Interestingly, this patient recovered fully following treatment with rVIIa, without surgical intervention (Majundar and Savidge, 1993). rVIIa was used to treat successfully 5 episodes of ICH in 2 patients, with neurologic improvements within 3 days of therapy (Schmidt *et al.*, 1994).

On the 8th day of treatment in 1 patient, an episode of ataxia and nystagmus occurred which was thought to be a thrombotic brainstem event, possibly related to rVIIa treatment. An uneventful recovery followed. Further studies are required but it seems likely that rVIIa may emerge as the treatment of choice in hemophiliacs with inhibitors and ICH.

Chronic liver disease, usually due to hepatitis C infection, may lead to coagulation abnormalities in hemophiliacs. The best management of individuals with such complex coagulaopathies is unclear. A recent report of the management of a mild hemophiliac (factor VIII level 10%) who bled from an arteriovenous malformation is of interest (Andrews *et al.*, 1994). The case was complicated by hypodysfibrinogenemia and immune thrombocytopenia. He was successfully prepared for surgery by plasmapheresis and replacement with fresh frozen plasma. Such approaches may need to be considered in hemophiliacs with ICH in association with additional coagulation abnormalities.

LONG-TERM FOLLOW-UP OF ICH

Few studies have addressed the question of the long-term morbidity present in hemophiliacs who survive episodes of intracranial bleeding. In the past, there appears to have been significant neurologic sequelae in as many as 47% (Eyster *et al,*. 1978; Visconti and Hilgartner, 1980). In addition, the persistence of abnormal CT scan appearances does not correlate well with clinical findings (Pettersson, McClure and Fitz, 1984). As modern treatment has reduced the mortality associated with acute intracranial hemorrhage, it is likely that the long-term sequelae will likewise reduce.

The role of prophylactic therapy to prevent recurrent intracranial bleeding is unclear. In children, many will now receive prophylaxis to prevent arthropathy so the issue will not arise. Certainly, in cases of recurrent ICH prophylaxis has been used successfully (Miser *et al.*, 1984). In adults there may be strong arguments to recommend prophylaxis to prevent recurrence of bleeding, as this may occur in up to 26% (Eyster *et al.*, 1978).

SUBCLINICAL ICH

There has been considerable debate concerning the possibility that some hemophiliacs may experience subclinical intracranial bleeding leading to chronic, developmental, neurologic and/or psychiatric sequelae. This has been a difficult and controversial area of study as the reproducibility of findings has been called into question.

An interesting study of EEG patterns in children with hemophilia in the 1960s produced some startling results. The study group consisted of 50 patients aged between 18 months and 18 years. In the 38 cases in whom there was no clinical evidence of CNS hemorrhage, exactly half had an abnormal EEG pattern, with the other 50% having normal tracings. The 19 individuals with normal EEG patterns were considered to show the expected range of intelligence and emotional status. In contrast, 9 of the 19 with abnormal EEGs were graded as normal, with the remaining 10 impaired. The authors concluded that the EEG pattern provides a sharp discrimination between these two groups, suggesting that subtle intracerebral bleeding may occur more frequently than had been thought previously and 'may influence the ultimate intelligence and emotional qualities' (Denton and Gourdeau, 1970). These observations were not confirmed in another study which found abnormal EEG patterns in only 10% of a group of 30 haemophiliacs (Forbes and Renfrew, 1975).

More recently, MR has been used to study brain abnormalities in hemophiliacs. In a group of 124 HIV-negative patients (age 7–19 years), 22 individuals were found to have acquired lesions on MRI scanning (Wilson *et al.*, 1992). There was no clear association between a history of ICH and MRI abnormalities. Cerebral atrophy was present in 6 patients and in 14 individuals small, focal high-signal-intensity white-matter lesions were present. The significance of these was uncertain but they were thought unlikely to be hemorrhagic in origin. The authors speculated as to whether small-vessel infarction due to blood loss or hypercoagulability after coagulation factor replacement might have been seen. There was no attempt to correlate MRI findings with cognitive or emotional status in this study.

ICH IN NEONATES AND INFANTS

Despite the often considerable trauma associated with birth, serious bleeding is surprisingly uncommon in hemophiliacs during the perinatal period. The precise reasons for this are unclear. Previously it was thought that anti-hemophilic factors crossed the placenta, thereby protecting the baby from bleeding. In an elegant study as long ago as the 1960s, it was demonstrated by analysis of umbilical cord blood samples that there was no significant transplacental passage of maternal factor VIII (Baehner and Strauss, 1966). The nature of mechanisms which protect the newborn hemophiliac remains obscure but the observation that von Willebrand factor is elevated in normal neonates (Andrew *et al.*, 1987) may be relevant.

The precise incidence of neonatal intracranial bleeding is uncertain in both hemophiliac and normal full-term babies. Some studies suggest that clinically significant bleeding is relatively uncommon in both groups compared to the high risk of intracranial, particularly intraventricular, bleeding seen in premature neonates (McMenamin, Shackelford and Volpe, 1984). Interestingly, the risk of bleeding in such premature neonates is increased by the use of prothrombin complex concentrate (Waltl *et al.*, 1973) but may be reduced by the administration of factor XIII concentrate (Shirahata *et al.*, 1990).

In a large study performed on day 3 postpartum using ultrasonographic examination of the brains of 1000 clinically normal full-term neonates evidence of ICH was detected on ultrasound in a surprisingly high proportion (almost 10%). Only 4 infants, however, developed symptoms in the first year of life (Heibel *et al.*, 1993). Retrospective studies in hemophiliacs have reported a variable incidence of intracranial bleeding during the neonatal period with the lowest being less than 1% (Eyster *et al.*, 1978), contrasting with 3% (Ljung *et al.*, 1994) and 5.3% (Yoffe and Buchanan, 1988) in other studies. On the basis of these studies, the overall incidence of symptomatic neonatal ICH appears to be significantly higher in hemophiliacs compared to normal neonates. Table 8.1 summarizes the cases reported in the recent literature of perinatal bleeding in hemophilia A and B as well as other congenital coagulation disorders. As all these cases have been reported since 1960, they are well documented both in terms of the diagnosis of the bleeding disorder and the intracranial bleed. It can be seen that bleeding has been reported to occur at a variety of anatomic positions and is commonly at more than one site. Subgaleal hematomas (bleeding under the galea aponeurotica of the scalp), although not intracranial in site, are included as they may be associated with massive hemorrhage (Kozinin *et al.*, 1964; Kozinin, Ritz and Horowitz, 1965; Cohen, 1978; Royhans, Miser and Miser, 1982) and have been reported to be associated with vacuum extraction of hemophilic neonates (Ljung *et al.*, 1994). In a review of all causes of subgaleal bleeding, including hemophilia, the mortality was 22.8% (Plauche, 1980).

Symptoms and signs of intracranial bleeding in neonates vary considerably according to the size and site of the bleed. Dramatic symptoms such as convulsions, bradycardia, apneic episodes, altered body tone or bulging fontanelles are suggestive of ICH; stridor, due to vocal cord paralysis, is a rare presentation (Fah and Tan, 1994). Equally, symptoms may be much more subtle, such as poor feeding, reduced activity, irritability or jaundice. As these may mimic sepsis, it is very important to have a high degree of clinical suspicion for intracranial bleeding in the newborn (Black and Whitfield, 1991). It is particularly important to consider the possibility in the context of a congenital hemorrhagic disorder prior to the performance of invasive investigations such as lumbar puncture.

There has been some debate concerning the best mode of delivery of neonates known to be at risk of hemophilia. On the available evidence, management should be entirely dictated by obstetric circumstances. Vacuum extraction, however, should be avoided if possible because of the risk of subgaleal bleeding (Ljung *et al.*, 1994). It should be noted that apparently non-traumatic Cesarean section, performed for obstetric reasons, has been associated with neonatal ICH in hemophilia (Michaud, Rivard and Chessex, 1991) and Cesarean section does not always protect neonates at risk of ICH such as neonatal alloimmune thrombocytopenia (Sia *et al.*, 1985). In rare instances where antenatal diagnosis has confirmed the diagnosis of hemophilia and premature labor occurs, Cesarean section may be indicated to reduce the risk of intraventricular hemorrage (Baty *et al.*, 1985).

Following delivery the diagnosis of hemophilia is readily confirmed by performing the appropriate coagulation factor assays on umbilical cord blood samples. Once the diagnosis is established, it may be prudent to keep the baby under close observation and maintain a high clinical index of suspicion for possible ICH or undertake regular cranial ultrasound scans in the neonatal period to detect signs of ICH.

Neonatal ICH may be the first indication of a possible diagnosis of hemophilia. This is the situation in which there is often inappropriate delay in establishing the diagnosis of hemophilia and instituting appropriate treatment. This may occur for a variety of reasons. The lack of a positive family history may lead to the diagnosis not being considered. Coexisting abnormalities of hematological parameters and coagulation tests may cause confusion. In bleeding leading to hypovolemia, there may be disseminated intravascular coagulation with thrombocytopenia, hypofibrinogenemia and prolongation of the activated partial thromboplastin time (APTT) and prothrombin time (PT) and a possible diagnosis of hemophilia may be obscured (Schmidt and Zipursky, 1986). All cases of neonatal hemorrhage should, therefore, raise the possibility of a diagnosis of hemophilia until proven otherwise and appropriate coagulation testing performed. The detection of a prolonged APTT, even in the presence of coexisting coagulation abnormalities, should prompt the performance of specific factor assays. To avoid delay in treatment while these investigations are being performed, fresh frozen plasma (FFP) should be given to the neonate followed by coagulation factor replacement if appropriate (Kletzel *et al.*, 1989; Bray and Luban, 1987).

Once the diagnosis of intracranial hemorrhage in a neonate with hemophilia is established, management consists of coagulation factor replacement and consideration for neurosurgical intervention if there is not a rapid improvement in the clinical condition. There may be a problem of maintaining adequate factor levels without precipitating fluid overload. This may be successfully overcome by the use of exchange blood and plasma transfusions (Striegel and Edson, 1984) or by the use of high-potency products which require only a small volume for reconstitution.

The risk of bleeding in neonates with von Willebrand's disease appears extremely low (Chediak, Alban and Maxey, 1986) but antenatal detection by ultrasonography has been reported (Mullaart *et al.*, 1991). Intracranial bleeding *in utero* has also been reported in factor V deficiency (Whitelaw *et al.*, 1984) and factor X deficiency (De Sousa, Clark and Bradshaw, 1988). The detection of antenatal ICH should raise the possibility of a congenital bleeding disorder. Rarely acquired inhibitors to factor VIII may occur in association with pregnancy. Transplacental passage of such inhibitors leading to intracranial bleeding in the neonate has been reported (Ries, Wolfel and Maier-Brandt, 1995).

ICH IN HEMOPHILIACS WITH HIV INFECTION

There is some evidence that the incidence of intracranial bleeding is higher in hemophiliacs infected with HIV. In a comparative necroscopy study of neuropathology in 11 HIV-infected hemophiliacs and 31 non-hemophiliacs (Esiri *et al.*, 1989), evidence of fresh bleeding was found in 45% and old hemorrhage in 36% of the hemophiliac group. AIDS had been diagnosed prior to death in only 4 of the hemophiliacs compared to all but 1 of the non-hemophiliacs. In addition, pathologic evidence of cerebral opportunistic infections, whilst identified in some of the non-haemophiliacs, was not present in any of the hemophiliacs. Cirrhosis was present in 27% of the hemophiliacs. This study concluded that intracranial bleeding was a common cause of death in HIV-infected hemophiliacs even before the onset of clinical AIDS and may contribute to the excess mortality in this group observed in other studies (Darby *et al.*, 1989).

In another report, apparently spontaneous intracranial hemorrhage occurred in 4 of 18 patients with AIDS over a 5-year period (Andes and Wulff, 1990). A survey of mortality in hemophiliacs confirmed that, after correction for age and severity of hemophilia, the risk of fatal intracranial bleeding was 3.8 times higher in HIV-positive compared to HIV-negative individuals. Moreover, the risk was increased even in those with mild hemophilia (Koumbarelis *et al.*, 1994).

This apparent higher risk of ICH has several possible contributory factors. Thrombocytopenia, either immune-mediated or as a result of bone marrow suppression either by drugs or HIV itself, may occur and has been implicated in intracranial hemorrhagic deaths in hemophiliacs. In a study of 11 HIV-positive hemophiliacs with immune thrombocytopenic purpura (ITP), spontaneous intracranial bleeding occurred in 4 and was fatal in 3 cases (Ragni *et al.*, 1990). This contrasts with the relatively low risk of serious bleeding reported in non-hemophiliacs with HIV infection (Karpatkin, 1988) and suggests that HIV-positive hemophiliacs with ITP should receive treatment if the platelet count falls below $50 \times 10^9/l$, i.e. treatment should be considered at a higher platelet count than in non-hemophiliacs.

Coagulopathy associated with liver disease may also contribute to the risk of ICH and there is evidence that coinfection with HIV and hepatitis C virus accelerates the development of serious liver disease in hemophiliacs (Eyster *et al.*, 1994; Telfer *et al.*, 1994). There is also the possiblity that cognitive function may be impaired in individuals with AIDS, especially in the presence of AIDS dementia, leading to a delay in the recognition of the symptoms and signs associated with bleeding and subsequent administration of factor concentrates.

In view of the available evidence, individuals with HIV infection and those caring for them should be specifically counseled about the increased risk of spontaneous ICH and warned of the dangers of delay in treatment.

ICH IN OTHER CONGENITAL BLEEDING DISORDERS

Von Willebrand's disease (vWD) is a heterogeneous condition with a wide range of clinical bleeding problems. Historically, both postraumatic and spontaneous ICH has been considered to be rare in vWD compared to hemophilia (Buchanan and Leavell, 1956).

It is now recognized that vWD is a common bleeding disorder and asymptomatic cases are frequent. Case reports of posttraumatic ICH in vWD have appeared in the literature (Rice, 1982). One study discovered 4 cases of vWD during a prospective evaluation of 50 patients presenting with ICH. The authors made the point that vWD in this context may be underdiagnosed and suggested that bleeding time measurement should be performed on all individuals presenting with ICH (Almaani and Awidi, 1986). Further studies are required to evaluate the usefulness of screening for vWD in all cases of ICH. In traumatic cases, especially where the degree of trauma appears to provoke an inappropriate degree of bleeding, the diagnosis of vWD should be considered (Mizoi, Onuma and Mon, 1984).

Factor V deficiency has been associated with ICH (Seeler, 1972), including the neonatal period (Whitelaw *et al.*, 1984). Families with factor V deficiency with a number of siblings affected by ICH have been reported (Wadia *et al.*, 1992).

Factor X deficiency may present with ICH, particularly in the neonatal period (Table 8.1). Successful outcomes followed by prophylactic replacement therapy to prevent recurrence have been reported (El Kalla and Menon, 1991; Sandler and Gross, 1992).

Factor VII deficiency is reported to be associated with a particularly high incidence of intracranial bleeding (Matthay, Koerper and Ablin, 1979; Ragni *et al.*, 1981) and death in the early years of life. Successful treatment of individuals with factor VII deficiency and ICH has been described in both infants (Miano *et al.*, 1987) and adults (Hassan *et al.*, 1984). ICH has been reported in a

Table 8.1 Summary of reports of neonatal and early infanthood intracranial hemorrhage (ICH) in inherited coagulation disorders

Reference	Cases	Diagnosis	Mode of delivery	Bleeding site	Age at diagnosis of ICH	Delay in diagnosis of hemophilia	Management	Outcome
Silverstein (1960)	1	?	Not stated	Not stated	5 days	No	Conservative	Poor development
Kozinin et al. (1964)	1	A	Forceps	Subgaleal	1 day	Yes	Conservative	No sequelae
Kozinin, Ritz and Horowitz (1965)	2	A	Vaginal	Subgaleal	1 day	Yes	Conservative	No sequelae
		A	Vaginal	Subgaleal	1 day	No	Conservative	Initial good recovery, died 5 months
Baehner and Strauss (1966)	1	A	Not stated	Intracerebral	6 days	No	Not stated	Not stated
McCarthy and Coble (1973)	1	A	Vaginal	Subarachnoid	5 days	No	VP shunt	Mild developmental delay
Volpe et al. (1976)	1	A	Forceps	Subdural + intracerebral	20 h	Yes	Surgery	Impaired motor development
Eyster et al. (1978)	3	No individual details stated						
Cohen (1978)	1	A	Forceps	Subgaleal	12 h	Yes	Conservative	No sequelae
Machin et al. (1980)	1	X	Vaginal	Intracerebral	4 months	No	Not stated	Died
Royhans, Miser and Miser (1982)	2	A	Forceps	Subgaleal	1 day	No	Conservative	No sequelae
		A	Cesarean	Subgaleal	1 day	No	Conservative	No sequelae
Striegal and Edson (1984)	1	B	Not stated	Left temporal + occipital	5 weeks	Yes	Exchange transfusion	No sequelae
Petterson, McClute and Fitz (1984)	1	A	Not stated	Subdural	6 days	Not stated	Surgery	Mild right hemiparesis Speech difficulties
Whitelaw et al. (1984)	1	V	Cesarean	Periventricular	10 days	Yes	VA shunt	Not stated
Heldrich and Garg (1985)	1	A	Forceps	Subdural	6 days	No	Conservative	No sequelae
Olson et al. (1985)	1	A	Vaginal	Subdural + intracerebral	4 days	Not stated	Surgery VP shunt	Mild developmental delay
Sumer et al. (1986)	1	X	Vaginal	Subarachnoid	3 months	No	Conservative	Severe developmental delay, cortical blindness
Bray and Luban (1987)	2	A	Not stated	Cerebellum	5 weeks	Yes	Surgery	Hypotonia at 3 weeks
		A	Cesarean	Subdural	7 days	Yes	Surgery	Right-sided spasticity + focal seizures
De Sousa, Clark and Bradshaw (1988)	1	X	Cesarean	Subdural	35 weeks	No	Conservative + subdural taps	Initially neurologically intact; died at 7 months of ICH
Franze and Forrest (1988)	1	A	Vaginal	Sudural	2 days	Yes	Surgery	Not stated
Lognon et al (1988)	1	A	Vaginal	Subdural + intracerebral	6 days	No	Conservative	Died
Yoffe and Buchanan (1988)	8	A	Vaginal	Subdural + intracerebral	3 months	Yes	No individual information provided 7/8 required surgical intervention	
		A	Forceps	Subdural + intracerebral	2 months	No	5/8 significant chronic neurological problems	
		A	Vaginal	Subdural + subarachnoid	1 day	Yes		

		A	Vaginal	Subdural + subarachnoid	5 days	Yes		
		A	Vaginal	Intracerebral	1 month	Yes		
		A	Vaginal	Epidural	1 day	Yes		
		A	Forceps	ICH	1 day	Yes		
		B	Vaginal	Subdural	1 day	No		
Kletzel *et al*. (1989)	4	A	Forceps	Subdural	5 days	Yes	Surgery	Died 7 days
		A	Forceps	Ventricles	4 days	No	Conservative	Hydrocephalus VP shunt, normal development
		A	Vacuum	Subgaleal	2 days	No	Conservative	No sequelae
		B	Vaginal	Not identified	8 h	No	Conservative	No sequelae
Michaud, Rivard and Chessex (1991)	1	A	Elective CS	Left temporal	3 days	No	Conservative	No sequelae
Mullaart *et al*. (1991)	1	vWD	Vaginal	Periventricular	32 weeks†	No	Conservative	Mild left hemiparesis
El Kalla and Menon (1991)	2	X	Vaginal	Subarachnoid	3 days	No	Conservative	Recurrent bleed at 4 months, no sequelae
		X	Vaginal	Intracerebral	31 weeks†	No	Surgery VP shunt	Died at 4 months following ICH
Sandler and Gross (1992)	1	X	Vaginal	Subdural	6 weeks	No	Surgery	Recurrent bleeds at 11 and 24 weeks No sequelae
Fah and Tan (1993)	1	A	Vaginal	Right intracerebral	11 days	Yes	Surgery	Died. Aspiration pneumonia
Dietrich *et al*. (1994)	1	A	Forceps	Subarachnoid + subdural	< 1 day	No	Conservative	Hypotonia on hospital discharge
Chen *et al*. (1994)	1	A	Vacuum	Cerebellar	6 days	No	Conservative	No sequelae
Ljung *et al*. (1994)	4	Severe‡	1 CS (27 weeks' gestation), 1 Vacuum, 2 Vaginal		No individual details given			No major sequelae
	12		10 Vaccum, 1 Vaginal 1 Cesarean	Subgaleal	No individual details given			No sequelae

A = hemophilia A; B = hemophilia B; vWD = von Willebrand's disease; V = factor V deficiency; X = factor X deficiency.
*Ventricular dilation had been detected on antenatal ultrasound scan.
†Diagnosed *in utero* on routine ultrasound scan.
‡No stated if A or B.
VP = Ventriculoperitoneal; VA = ventriculoatrial; CS = Cesarean section.

patient with an acquired antifactor VII antibody (Delmer *et al.*, 1989); this was successfully managed with plasma exchange and immunosuppression.

Factor XIII deficiency is associated with a high risk of ICH which may be as high as 20–40% (Merchant *et al.*, 1992). In view of this risk it is recommended that individuals with severe factor XIII deficiency should receive regular lifelong prophylaxis with factor XIII concentrates which, because of the long half-life of factor XIII, may be administered every 3 or 4 weeks (Daly and Haddon, 1988)

Spinal bleeding in hemophilia

Hemorrhage in and around the spinal cord is much less common than either intracranial or peripheral nervous system bleeding but has been recognized for many years (Bulloch and Fildes, 1911; Seddons, 1930; Priest, 1935; Jones and Knighton, 1956). The precise incidence is not known but in a comprehensive review of the literature between 1850 and 1975, only 12 well-documented cases were found (Van Trotsenburg, 1975).

The signs and symptoms associated with spinal bleeding vary according to the anatomic structures affected and may be either posttraumatic or spontaneous. Spinal bleeding may be provoked by invasive procedures such as lumbar puncture. As with ICH, spinal bleeding should be considered an extremely urgent situation and prompt coagulation factor replacement therapy is mandatory.

Intraspinal bleeding, either epidural or extradural, usually presents with severe pain at the site of the hemorrhage and corresponding progressive motor and sensory loss below the level of the hematoma with or without sphincter disturbance. In infants the initial presentation may be with symptoms of irritability or refusal to walk (Cromwell, Kerber and Ferry, 1977). Bleeding in the cervical region causes pain in the neck and across the shoulders and may result in the development of a tetraparesis. In contrast to the acute symptoms associated with spinal cord bleeding, a hemophiliac pseudotumor of the spinal canal has been reported to cause spinal cord compression with slow progression of neurologic symptoms (Liu *et al.*, 1988).

The diagnosis of spinal bleeding may be confirmed with CT or MRI scan (Caldemeyer *et al.*, 1993) or myelography if these non-invasive methods are not available. Improvement may begin soon after appropriate coagulation factor replacement is given. Complete resolution of neurologic signs has been reported following intensive coagulation factor replacement therapy without the need for surgical decompression (Harvie *et al.*, 1977). If neurologic impairment fails to improve or worsens, then surgical decompression should be considered (Cromwell, Kerber and Ferry, 1977). Serial CT or MRI scans may be useful to document reolving hematoma in cases managed conservatively (Sheikh and Abildgaard, 1994).

Peripheral nervous system bleeding in hemophilia

Bleeding leading to lesions of the peripheral nervous system (PNS) has not received the same attention as intracranial bleeding. In a review in 1944, only 11 cases were found in the literature (Aggeler and Lucia, 1944). From subsequent studies, it has become clear that many hemophiliacs experience acute bleeding episodes affecting peripheral nerves and chronic dysfunction may result from recurrent bleeds. In individuals affected by severe arthropathy it may be difficult to distinguish loss of function, muscle atrophy and loss of tendon reflexes as a result of joint damage from peripheral nerve lesions (Van Trotsenburg, 1975). Peripheral nerves are usually damaged by compression due to adjacent intramuscular or intra-articular bleeding and controversy remains as to whether intraneural hemorrhage (bleeding within the nerve sheath) occurs. Whilst there is often recovery after an acute bleed, repeated episodes may lead to progressive and permanent loss of nerve function.

INCIDENCE OF PNS HEMORRHAGE

Early studies estimated the incidence of PNS dysfunction either on the basis of bleeding episodes resulting in hospital admission or surveys of non-bleeding patients. The diagnostic criteria used to establish peripheral nerve involvement may have been imprecise and there was often not a clear distinction between the incidence of acute and chronic PNS problems. In an attempt to avoid overdiagnosis of PNS lesions, some surveys included only patients with definite evidence of sensory loss. Of 206 patients admitted with acute bleeding episodes, 28 (13.6%) had evidence of peripheral neropathy (Silverstein, 1964). Femoral nerve lesions accounted for over half of these lesions.

Another longitudinal study of 234 hemophiliacs found 36 PNS lesions in 25 (10.8%); individuals (Ehrmann *et al.*, 1981). In a large survey of 1351 admissions to a single center between 1962 and 1986, 88 (6%) PNS lesions were observed in 54 patients. All studies agree that PNS lesions occur almost exclusively in individuals with severe hemophilia and the majority of these patients are aged between 10 and 30 (Katz *et al.*, 1991). PNS lesions appear to be unusual in infants.

GENERAL MANAGEMENT OF PERIPHERAL NERVE LESIONS IN HEMOPHILIACS

In common with all bleeding episodes in hemophiliacs, rapid recognition and administration of coagulation factor replacement are essential. Often intramuscular bleeds will respond to prompt treatment before the onset of peripheral nerve compression. In cases of established sensory or motor loss, immobilization and splinting should be performed along with adequate factor replacement. Once bleeding has resolved, vigorous physiotherapy should be used to maintain muscle bulk and prevent contractures (Duthie, 1994).

CLINICAL FEATURES OF BLEEDING AFFECTING SPECIFIC PERIPHERAL NERVES IN HEMOPHILIA

Table 8.2 outlines the relative frequency of peripheral nerve lesions in two of the largest published series.

Femoral nerve

Femoral nerve lesions were first reported in hemophiliacs in the early part of this century (Tallroth, 1939; Aggeler and Lucia, 1944). The femoral nerve is the commonest peripheral nerve affected in hemophiliacs (Table 8.2). It is particularly vulnerable to compression by bleeding into the iliopsoas muscle as it lies deep to the iliacus fascia and has also been reported as a result of massive pseudotumor of the ileum (Aggeler and Lucia, 1944). The constellation of signs and symptoms which result from iliopsoas bleeding is now well recognized (Brower and Wilde, 1966). Characteristically, a bleed presents with pain in the groin which may radiate to the lower back or thigh. Relief from pain may be achieved by flexing the hip and the patient assumes a characteristic position (Fig. 8.4). Forced extension is extremely painful but rotation of the hip, while flexed, is possible. Femoral nerve compression leads to

sensory loss over the anterior and medial aspects of the thigh, weakness of knee extension (quadriceps muscle, which may be paralyzed in severe cases) and loss of the patellar tendon reflex. In addition, a mass may be palpable in the iliac fossa and constipation and abdominal distension may occur.

The mechanism of compression of the femoral nerve was graphically demonstrated by experiments which involved the injection of saline into the psoas and iliacus muscles in fresh cadavers (Goodfellow, Fearn and Matthews, 1967). These experiments suggested that bleeding into the iliacus muscle was most likely to lead to femoral neuropathy.

The management of iliopsoas bleeds consists of prompt recognition and coagulation factor replacement. It is important to exclude other causes of pain in the iliac fossa, such as appendicitis. Ultrasound or CT scanning may demonstrate muscle hematoma in cases of diagnostic doubt and both methods may be useful to monitor the size of the hematoma. Coagulation factor replacement should be continued until there is complete resolution of the hematoma. The hip should be immobilized in the

Table 8.2 Frequency of peripheral nerve lesions in hemophiliacs from the two largest published reports

Nerve	Number of lesions	
	Katz et al. *(1991)*	*Ehrmann* et al. *(1981)*
Femoral	31	12
Median	10	6
Ulnar	7	4
Sciatic	4	5
Peroneal	0	3
Radial	3	2
Posterior interosseous	2	0
Lateral popliteal	1	0
Tibial	0	1
Lateral cutaneous of the thigh	0	1
Posterior tibialis	1	0
Sural	1	0
Thoracic	1	0
Maxillary	0	1
Obturator	0	1
Total	61	36

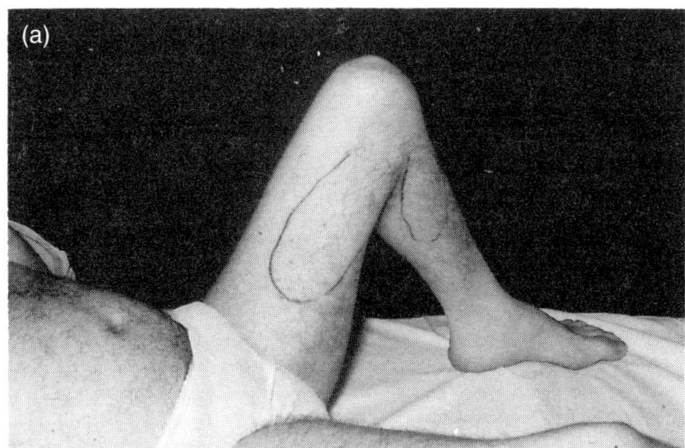

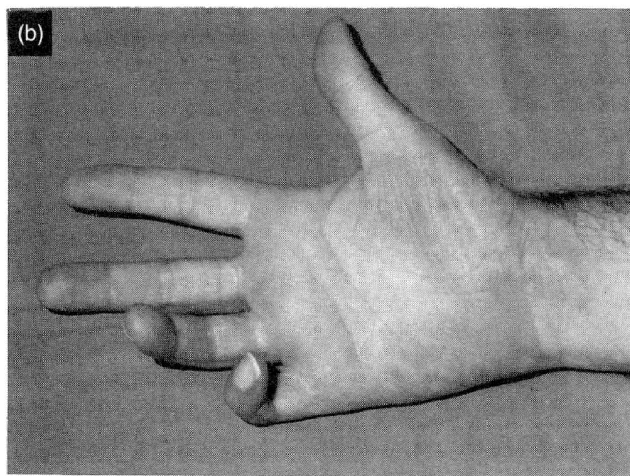

Fig. 8.4 (a) Iliopsoas bleed leading to the characteristic hip flexion and sensory loss (outlined by marker pen) due to femoral nerve compression. (b) Ulnar nerve compression due to elbow hemarthrosis.

most comfortable position and, following replacement therapy, there is usually rapid resolution of pain with gradual improvement in hip movement. The symptoms and signs of femoral nerve compression resolve slowly (mean duration 12 months). In one series of 31 lesions observed in 26 patients, 9 completely resolved, while 17 had complete return of motor function with a degree of residual sensory loss. The remaining 5 patients had permanent motor and sensory dysfunction (Katz *et al.*, 1991).

Median nerve

Bleeding in the forearm or wrist may cause compression of the median nerve (Lancourt, Gilbert and Posner, 1977). This may lead to the development of carpal tunnel syndrome (Khunadorn *et al.*, 1977; Molitor and Wimperis, 1990). The majority of cases can be managed successfully with rest, splinting and coagulation factor replacement. Acute carpal tunnel syndrome has been treated successfully by surgical decompression in cases that failed to respond to conservative treatment (Case, 1967). Such surgical intervention was only required in 1 of 10 cases of median nerve compression in another series and in all 10 recovery was complete on average after 7 months (range 3 weeks to 12 months, Katz *et al.*, 1991).

Ulnar nerve

The ulnar nerve is particularly susceptible to compression either due to direct trauma at the elbow or following elbow hemarthroses. In addition, bleeding in the forearm may affect the ulnar nerve and combined median and ulnar nerve palsies have been described. The prognosis for ulnar nerve lesions is variable, with 5 of 7 in one series recovering completely after an average time 7 months (range 3 days to 23 months, Katz *et al.*, 1991).

One of the few reports of intraneural hemorrhage was reported to affect the ulnar nerve. This followed minor trauma to the elbow in a boy with severe hemophilia A. Due to the development of a 'claw hand', surgical decompression was undertaken. At operation there was no free blood present but the ulnar nerve itself was discolored and hyperemic for 2–3 cm. Free blood escaped once the epineurium was divided. There was a rapid and complete clinical recovery following surgery (Cordingley and Crawford, 1984).

Autonomic neuropathy in hemophilia

There are only occasional reports of autonomic dysfunction in hemophiliacs (Berry, 1975) and it is unclear whether this is under reported. Interestingly, autonomic dysfunction may be detected in a significant number of patients with chronic liver disease (Hendrickse, Thulu-

vath and Triger, 1992). As liver disease is common in hemophiliacs, autonomic problems may become more frequent in the future.

References

Aggeler, P.M. and Lucia, S.P. (1944) The neurologic complications of hemophilia. *J Nerv Ment Dis*, **99**, 475–500.

Almaani, W.S. and Awidi, A.S. (1986) Spontaneous intracranial hemorrhage secondary to von Willebrand's disease. *Surg Neurol*, **26**, 457–460.

Andes, W.A. and Wulff, K. (1990) Intracranial hemorrhage in hemophiliacs with AIDS (letter). *Thromb Haemost*, **63**, 326.

Andes, W.A., Wulff, K. and Smith, W.B. (1984) Head trauma in hemophilia. A prospective study. *Arch Intern Med*, **144**, 1981–1983.

Andrew, M., Paes, B., Milner, R. *et al.* (1987) Development of the human coagulation system in the full-term infant. *Blood*, **70**, 165–172.

Andrews, B.T., Stricker, R.B., Kitt, D. *et al.* (1994) Case report: treatment of an intracranial arteriovenous malformation in a patient with complicated hemophilia. *Am J Med Sci*, **308**, 106–109.

Anonymous (1868) Prince Leopold. *Br Med J*, **1**, 148.

Anonymous (1884) The haemorrhagic diathesis. *Br Med J*, **686**.

Aronson, D.L. (1988) Cause of death in hemophilia A patients in the United States from 1968 to 1979. *Am J Hematol*, **27**, 7–12.

Bacher, T. (1980) Dodsfald blandt patienter med haemofil i Danmark i perioden 1949–1978. *Ugeskr Laeg*, **142**, 1600–1603.

Baehner, R.L. and Strauss, H.S. (1966) Haemophilia in the first year of life. *N Engl J Med*, **275**, 524–528.

Baty, B.J., Drayna, D., Leonard, C.O. and White, R. (1986) Prenatal diagnosis of factor VIII deficiency to help with the management of pregnancy and delivery (letter). *Lancet*, **1**, 207.

Bennett, M. and Sills, J. (1978) Cerebral haemorrhage in haemophilia. *Postgrad Med J*, **54**, 115–118.

Berry, P.R. (1975) Neurological complications of haemophilia. *NZ Med J*, **81**, 427–428.

Biggs, R. (1977) Haemophilia treatment in the United Kingdom from 1969 to 1974. *Br J Haematol*, **35**, 487–504.

Black, J.A. and Whitfield, M.F. (1991) Bleeding from one site, in *Neonatal Emergencies. Early Detection and Management*, 2nd edn, Butterworth-Heinemann, Oxford, pp. 94–101.

Bray, G.L. and Luban, N.L. (1987) Hemophilia presenting with intracranial hemorrhage. An approach to the infant with intracranial bleeding and coagulopathy. *Am J Dis Child*, **141**, 1215–1217.

Brower, T.D. and Wilde, A.H. (1966) Femoral neuropathy in hemophilia. *J Bone Joint Surg*, **48A**, 487–492.

Brown, D.L., Hardisty, R.M., Kosoy, M.H. and Bracken, C. (1967) Antihaemophilic globulin: preparation by an improved cryoprecipitation method and clinical use. *Br Med J*, **2**, 79–85.

Buchanan, J.C. and Leavell, B.S. (1956) Pseudohemophilia: report of 13 new cases and statistical review of previously reported cases. *Ann Intern Med*, **44**, 241–256.

Bulloch, W. and Fildes, P. (1911) Hemophilia: treasury of human inheritance, in *Francis Galton Laboratory Memoirs*, Cambridge University Press, London.

Caldemeyer, K.S., Mocharia, R., Moran, C.C. and Smith, R.R. (1993) Gadolinium enhancement in the center of a spinal epidural hematoma in a hemophiliac. *J Comput Assist Tomogr*, **17**, 321–323.

Carrea, R., Pavlovsky, A., Monges, J. *et al.* (1968) Medical and surgical management of intracranial bleeding in hemophilic children. *Acta Neurol Latinoamer*, **14**, 155–173.

Case, D.B. (1967) An acute carpal tunnel syndrome in a haemophiliac. *Br J Clin Pract* **21**, 254–255.

Chediak, J.R., Alban, G.M. and Maxey, B. (1986) Von Willebrand's disease and pregnancy: management during delivery and outcome of offspring. *Am J Obstet Gynecol*, **155**, 618–624.

Chen, S-H., Soong, W-J., Hsieh, Y-L. *et al.* (1994) Hemophilia A presenting with intracranial hemorrhage in a neonate: a case report. *Chin Med J (Taipei)*, **54**, 62–66.

Cohen, D. (1978) Neonatal subgaleal hemorrhage in hemophilia. *J Pediatr*, **93**, 1022–1023.

Cordingley, T. and Crawford, P.M. (1984) Ulnar nerve palsy in a haemophiliac due to intraneural haemorrahge. *Br Med J*, **289**, 18–19.

Cromwell, L.D., Kerber, C. and Ferry, P.C. (1977) Spinal cord compression and hematoma: an unusual complication in a hemophiliac infant. *Am J Roentgenol*, **128**, 847–849.

Curless, R.G. and Corrigan, J.J. (1976) Headache in classical hemophilia. *Child's Brain*, **2**, 187–194.

Daly, H.M. and Haddon, M.E. (1988) Clinical experience with a pasteurised human plasma concentrate in factor XIII deficiency. *Thromb Haemost*, **59**, 171–174.

Darby, S.C., Rizza, C.R., Doll, R. *et al.* (1989) Incidence of AIDS and excess of mortality associated with HIV in haemophiliacs in the United Kingdom: report on behalf of the directors of haemophilia centres in the United Kingdom. *Br Med J*, **298**, 1064–1068.

Davies, S.H., Turner, J.W., Cumming, R.A. *et al.* (1966) Management of intracranial haemorrhage in haemophilia. *Br Med J*, **2**, 1627–1630.

DeBehnke, D.J. and Angelos, M.G. (1990) Intracranial hemorrhage and hemophilia: case report and management guidelines. *J Emerg Med*, **8**, 423–427.

Delmer, A., Horellou, M.H., Andreu, G. *et al.* (1989) Life-threatening intracranial bleeding associated with the presence of an antifactor VII autoantibody. *Blood*, **74**, 229–232.

Denton, R.L. and Gourdeau, R. (1970) Electroencelphalographic patterns in hemophilia. *Bibl Haemat*, **34**, 135–138.

DeSousa, C., Clark, T. and Bradshaw, A. (1988) Antenatally diagnosed subdural haemorrhage in congenital factor X deficiency. *Arch Dis Child*, **63**, 1168–1174.

de Tezanos Pinto, M., Fernandez, J. and Perez Bianco, P.R. (1992) Update of 156 episodes of central nervous system bleeding in hemophiliacs. *Haemostasis*, **22**, 259–267.

Dietrich, A.M., James, C.D., King, D.R. *et al.* (1994) Head trauma in children with congenital coagulation disorders. *J Pediatr Surg*, **29**, 28–32.

Doughty, H.A., Coles, J., Parmar, K. *et al.* (1995) The successful removal of a bleeding intracranial tumour in a severe haemophiliac using an adjusted dose continuous infusion of monoclonal factor VIII. *Blood Coagul Fibrinolysis*, **6**, 31–34.

Duthie, R.B., Rizza, C.R., Giangrande, P.L.F. and Dodd, C.A.F. (1994) Peripheral nerve lesions, in *The Management of Musculoskeletal Problems in the Haemophilias*, 2nd edn, Oxford University Press, Oxford, pp. 118–128.

Edson, R.J., McArthur, J.R., Branda, R.F. *et al.* (1973) Successful management of a subdural hematoma in a hemophiliac with an anti-factor VIII antibody. *Blood*, **41**, 113–122.

Ehrmann, L., Lechner, K., Mamoli, B. *et al.* (1981) Peripheral nerve lesions in haemophilia. *J Neurol*, **225**, 175–182.

El Kalla, S. and Menon, N.S. (1991) Neonatal congenital factor X deficiency. *Pediatr Haematol Oncol*, **8**, 347–354.

Esiri, M.M., Scaravilli, F., Millard, P.R. and Harcourt-Webster, J.N. (1989) Neuropathology of HIV infection in haemophiliacs: comparitive necroscopy study. *Br Med J*, **299**, 1312–1315.

Essien, E.M. and Adeloye, A. (1972) Intracranial haemorrhage in haemophilia in Nigerians. *Trans R Soc Trop Med Hyg*, **66**, 255–257.

Eyster, E.M., Gill, F.M., Blatt, P.M. *et al.* (1978) Central nervous system bleeding in hemophiliacs. *Blood*, **51**, 1179–1188.

Eyster, M.E., Fried, M.W., Di, B. and Goedert, J.J. (1994) Increasing hepatitis C virus RNA levels in hemophiliacs: relationship to human immunodeficiency virus infection and liver disease. *Blood*, **84**, 1020–1023.

Fah, K.K. and Tan, H.K.K. (1994) An unusual cause of stridor in a neonate. *J Laryngol Otol*, **108**, 63–64.

Ferguson, G.G., Barton, W.B. and Drake, C.G. (1968) Subdural hematoma in hemophilia: successful treatment with cryoprecipitate. *J Neurosurg*, **29**, 524–528.

Fesset, B.M. and Meynell, M.J. (1966) Haemorrhage involving the central nervous system in haemophilia: account of the management of five cases. *Br Med J*, **2**, 211–212.

Forbes, C.D. and Renfrew, S. (1975) Electroencephalography in haemophilia and Christmas disease. *Haemostasis*, **4**, 36–39.

Franze, I. and Forrest, T.S. (1988) Sonographic diagnosis of a subdural hematoma as the initial manifestation of hemophilia in a newborn. *J Ultrasound Med*, **7**, 149–152.

Friedman, H., Guerry, R. and Wilkins, R.H. (1971) Intracerebral hematoma in a hemophiliac. Combined surgical and factor VIII treatment. *JAMA*, **215**, 791–792.

Fuerth, J.H., Teng, P. and Goldenberg, E. (1961) Surgery in a haemophiliac child with intracranial hemorrhage. *Pediatrics*, **28**, 800–804.

Gendelman, S. (1977) Hemophilia and the nervous system, *M Sinai J Med*, **3**, 402–408.

Goodfellow, J., Fearn, C.B.D'A. and Matthews, J.M. (1967) Iliacus haematoma. A common complication of haemophilia. *J Bone Joint Surg*, **49B**, 748–756.

Gore, R.M., Weinberg, P.E., Anandappa, E. *et al.* (1981) Intracranial complications of pediatric hematologic disorders: computed tomographic assessment. *Invest Radiol*, **16**, 175–180.

Guthrie, T.H., Jr. and Sacra, J.C. (1980) Emergency care of the hemophiliac patient. *Ann Emerg Med*, **9**, 476–479.

Harvie, A., Lowe, G.D.O., Forbes, C.D. *et al.* (1977) Intraspinal bleeding in haemophilia: treatment with factor VIII concentrate. *J Neurol, Neurosurg Psychiatry*, **40**, 1220–1223.

Hassan, H.J., Casalbore, P., De Laurenzi, A. *et al.* (1984) Hereditary factor VII deficiency: report of a case of intracranial hemorrhage. *Haemostasis*, **14**, 244–248.

Heibel, M., Heber, R., Bechinger, D. and Kornhuber, H.H. (1993) The early diagnosis of perinatal cerebral lesions in apparently normal full-term newborns by ultrasound of the brain. *Neuroradiology*, **35**, 85–91.

Heldrich, F. and Garg, P.P. (1985) Occult haemorrhage in a neonate with hemophilia A. *MMJ*, **34**, 351–354.

Hendrickse, M.T., Thuluvath, P.J. and Triger, D.R. (1992) Natural history of autonomic neuropathy in chronic liver disease. *Lancet*, **339**, 1462–1464.

Hennes, H., Losek, J.D., Sty, J.R. and Gill, J.C. (1987) Computerized tomography in hemophiliacs with head trauma. *Pediatr Emerg Care*, **3**, 147–149.

Hirsch, J.F., Zouaoui, A., Gazengel, C. *et al.* (1983) Intracranial hemorrhages in children with hemophilia: medical and surgical treatment. *Acta Neurol (Napoli)*, **5**, 456–460.

Jamieson, K.G. (1954) Extradural haematoma in a haemophilic child (complicated by diabetes insipidus). *Aust NZ J Surg*, **24**, 56–62.

Jones, R.K. and Knighton, R.S. (1956) Surgery in hemophiliacs with special reference to the central nervous system. *Ann Surg*, **144**, 1029–1034.

Karpatkin, S. (1988) Immunologic thrombocytopenic purpura in HIV-seropositive homosexuals, narcotic addicts and hemophiliacs. *Semin Hematol*, **25**, 219–229.

Katz, S.G., Nelson, I.W., Atkins, R.M. and Duthie, R.B. (1991) Peripheral nerve lesions in hemophilia. *J Bone Joint Surg*, **73**, 1016–1019.

Kerr, C.B. (1964) Intracranial haemorrhage in haemophilia. *J Neurol Neurosurg Psychiatry*, **27**, 166–173.

Khunadorn, N., Schlagenhauff, R.E., Tourbaf, K. and Papademetriou, T. (1977) Carpal tunnel syndrome in hemophilia. *NY State J Med*, **77**, 1314–1315.

Kinney, T.R., Zimmerman, R.A., Butler, R.B. and Gill, F.M. (1977) Computerized tomography in the management of intracranial bleeding in hemophilia. *J Pediatr*, **91**, 31-35.

Kletzel, M., Miller, C.H., Becton, D.L. *et al.* (1989) Postdelivery head bleeding in hemophilic neonates. Causes and management. *Am J Dis Child*, **143**, 1107–1110.

Koumbarelis, E., Rosendaal, F.R., Gialeraki, A. *et al.* (1994) Epidemiology of haemophilia in Greece: an overview. *Thromb Haemost*, **72**, 808–813.

Kozinn, P.J., Ritz, N.D. and Horowitz, A.W. (1965) Scalp hemorrhage as an emergency in the newborn. *JAMA*, **194**, 179–180.

Kozinn, P.J., Ritz, N.D., Moss, A.H. and Kaufman, A. (1964) Massive hemorrhage – scalps of newborn infants. *Am J Dis Child*, **108**, 413–417.

Lancourt, J.E., Gilbert, M.S. and Posner, M.A. (1977) Management of bleeding and associated complications of hemophilia in the hand and forearm. *J Bone Joint Surg*, **59A**, 451–460.

Lane, S. (1840) Successful transfusion of blood. *Lancet*, **i**, 185–188.

Larsson, S.A. and Wiechel, B. (1983) Deaths in Swedish hemophiliacs, 1957–1980. *Acta Med Scand*, **214**, 199–206.

Liu, S.S., White, W.L., Johnson, P.C. and Gauntt, C. (1988) Hemophilic pseudotumor of the spinal canal. *J Neurosurg*, **69**, 624–627.

Ljung, R., Lindgren, A.C., Petrini, P. and Tengborn, L. (1994) Normal vaginal delivery is to be recommended for haemophilia carrier gravidae. *Acta Paediatr*, **83**, 609–611.

Lognon, P., Bloc, D., Saliba, E. *et al.* (1988) Hematome intracranien neonatal chez un hemophilie A. *Arch Fr Pediatr*, **45**, 127–128.

Lutschg, J. and Vassella, F. (1981) Neurological complications in hemophilia. *Acta Paediatr Scand*, **70**, 235–241.

McCarthy, J.W. and Coble, L.L. (1973) Intracranial haemorrhage and subsequent communicating hydrocephalus in a neonate with classical haemophilia. *Pediatrics*, **51**, 122–124.

McMenamin, J.B., Shackelford, G.D. and Volpe, J.J. (1984) Outcome of neonatal intraventricular hemorrhage with periventricular echodense lesions. *Ann Neurol*, **15**, 285–290.

Machin, S.J., Winter, M.R., Davies, S.C. and Mackie, I.J. (1980) Factor X deficiency in the neonatal period. *Arch Dis Child*, **55**, 406–408.

Majumdar, G. and Savidge, G.F. (1993) Recombinant factor VIIa for intracranial haemorrhage in a Jehovah's Witness with severe haemophilia A and factor VIII inhibitors. *Blood Coag Fibrinolys*, **4**, 1031–1033.

Martinowitz, U., Heim, M., Tadmor, R. *et al.* (1986) Intracranial hemorrhage in patients with hemophilia. *Neurosurgery*, **18**, 538–541.

Martinowitz, U., Schulman, S., Gitel, S. *et al.* (1992) Adjusted dose continuous infusion of factor VIII in patients with haemophilia A. *Br J Haematol*, **82**, 729–734.

Matsuda, M., Handa, J., Asato, R. *et al.* (1977) Surgical treatment of intracranial hematoma and hydrocephalus in an infant with hemophilia A. *Surg Neurol*, **7**, 199–203.

Matthay, K.K., Koerper, M.A. and Ablin, A.R. (1979) Intracranial hemorrhage in congenital factor VII deficiency. *Journal of Pediatrics*, **94**, 413–415.

Merchant, R.H., Agarwal, B.R., Currimbhoy, Z. *et al.* (1992) Congenital factor XIII deficiency. *Indian Pediatr*, **29**, 831–836.

Miano, C., Rosati, D., Donfrancesco, A. *et al.* (1987) Recurrent intracranial hemorrhage in an infant with congenital factor VII deficiency. *Haematologica*, **72**, 188–189.

Michaud, J.L., Rivard, G.E. and Chessex, P. (1991) Intracranial hemorrhage in a newborn with hemophilia following elective cesarean section. *Am J Pediatr Hematol Oncol*, **13**, 473–475.

Miser, A.W., Roach, J.E., Harmel, R.P., Jr. *et al.* (1984) Insertion of a central venous catheter for long-term venous access in a child with severe hemophilia and recurrent intracranial hemorrhage. *Clin Pediatr*, **23**, 589.

Mizoi, K., Onuma, T. and Mori, K. (1984) Intracranial hemorrhage secondary to von Willebrand's disease and trauma. *Surg Neurol*, **22**, 495–498.

Molitor, P.J. and Wimperis, J.Z. (1990) Acute carpal tunnel syndrome in haemophiliacs. *Br J Clin Pathol*, **44**, 675–676.

Moody, R.A. and Mullan, S. (1968) Factor VIII in hemophilia. *J Neurol*, **29**, 520–523.

Mullaart, R.A., Van Dongen, P., Gabreels, F.J. and van Oostrom, C. (1991) Fetal periventricular hemorrhage in von Willebrand's disease: short review and first case presentation. *Am J Perinatol*, **8**, 190–192.

Myles, S.T., Harris, C.E.C. and Hansebout, R.R. (1971) Epidural hematoma in hemophilia: successful treatment. *CMAJ*, **104**, 51–52.

Olsen, E.R. (1969) Intracranial surgery in hemophiliacs. *Arch Neurol*, **21**, 401–412.

Olson, T.A., Alving, B.M., Cheshier, J.L. *et al.* (1985) Intracerebral and subdural haemorrhage in a neonate with hemophilia A. *Am J Pediatr Hematol Oncol*, **7**, 384–387.

Pettersson, H., McClure, P. and Fitz, C. (1984) Intracranial hemorrhage in hemophilic children. CT follow-up. *Acta Radiol*, **25**, 161–164.

Plauche, W.C. (1980) Subgaleal hematoma. A complication of instrumental delivery. *JAMA*, **244**, 1597–1598.

Potter, J.M. (1965) Head injury and haemophilia. *Acta Neurochir*, **13**, 380–387.

Prentice, C.R.M., Breckenridge, R.T., Forman, W.B. and Ratnoff, O.D. (1967) Treatment of haemophilia (factor VIII deficiency) with human antihaemophilic factor prepared by the cryoprecipitate process. *Lancet*, **i**, 457–460.

Priest, W.M. (1935) Epidural haemorrhage due to haemophilia causing compression of the spinal cord. *Lancet*, **ii**, 1289–1291.

Quick, A.J. (1971) Aspirin and bleeding. *JAMA*, **216**, 518.

Ragni, M.V., Lewis, J.H., Spero, J.A. and Hasiba, U. (1981) Factor VII deficiency. *Am J Hematol*, **10**, 79–88.

Ragni, M.V., Bontempo, F.A., Myers, D.J. *et al.* (1990) Hemorrhagic sequelae of immune thrombocytopenic purpura in human immunodeficiency virus-infected hemophiliacs. *Blood*, **75**, 1267–1272.

Rice, M.L. (1982) Acute subdural haematoma associated with von Willebrand's disease: a case report. *Aust NZ J Surg*, **52**, 86–88.

Ries, M., Wolfel, D. and Maier-Brandt, B. (1995) Severe intracranial hemorrhage in a newborn infant with transplacental transfer of an acquired factor VIII-C inhibitor. *J Pediatr*, **127**, 649–650.

Rizza, C.R. and Spooner, R.J. (1983) Treatment of haemophilia and related disorders in Britain and Northern Ireland during 1976–80: report on behalf of the directors of haemophilia centres in the United Kingdom. *Br Med J*, **286**, 929–933.

Royhans, J.A., Miser, A.W. and Miser, J.S. (1982) Subgaleal hemorrhage in infants with haemophilia: report of two cases and review of the literature. *Pediatrics*, **70**, 306–307.

Sakima, H.K., Kaplan, A.M., Baranko, P.V. *et al.* (1983) Nervous system complications of hemophilia. *Ariz Med*, **40**, 545–549.

Sandler, E. and Gross, S. (1992) Prevention of recurrent intracranial hemorrhage in a factor X-deficient infant. *Am J Pediatr Hematol Oncol*, **14**, 163–165.

Schmidt, B. and Zipursky, A. (1986) Disseminated intravascular coagulation masking neonatal hemophilia. *J Pediatr*, **109**, 886–888.

Schmidt, M.L., Gamerman, S., Smith, H.E. *et al.* (1994) Recombinant activated factor VII (rFVIIa) therapy for intracranial hemorrhage in hemophilia A patients with inhibitors. *Am J Hematol*, **47**, 36–40.

Seddons, H.J. (1930) Haemophilia as a cause of lesions in the nervous system. *Brain*, **53**, 306–310.

Seeler, R.A. (1972) Parahemophilia: factor V deficiency. *Med Clin North Am*, **56**, 119–125.

Seeler, R.A. and Imana, R.B. (1973) Intracranial hemorrhage in patients with hemophilia. *J Neurosurg*, **39**, 181–185.

Sheikh, A.A. and Abildgaard, C.F. (1994) Medical management of extensive spinal epidural hematoma in a child with factor IX deficiency. *Pediatr Emerg Care*, **10**, 26–29.

Shirahata, A., Nakamura, T., Shimono, M. *et al.* (1990) Blood coagulation findings and the efficacy of Factor XIII concentrate in premature infants with intracranial hemorrhages. *Thromb Res*, **57**, 755–763.

Sia, C.G., Amigo, N.C., Harper, R.G. *et al.* (1985) Failure of cesarean section to prevent intracranial hemorrhage in sibling with isoimmune neonatal thrombocytopenia. *Am J Obstet Gynecol*, **153**, 79–81.

Silverstein, A. (1960) Intracraial bleeding in haemophilia. *Arch Neurol*, **3**, 141–157.

Silverstein, A. (19640 Neuropathy in hemophilia. *JAMA*, **190**, 554–555.

Simpson, D.A. and Robson, H.N. (1960) Intracranial haemorrhage in disorders of blood coagulation. *Aust NZ J Surg*, **29**, 287–303.

Striegel, J.E. and Edson, J.R. (1984) Treatment of a spontaneous intracerebral hematoma with exchange transfusions in an infant with hemophilia B. *J Pediatr*, **105**, 278–280.

Sumer, T., Ahmad, M., Sumer, N.K. and Al-Mouzan, M.I. (1986) Severe congenital factor X deficiency with intracranial haemorrhage. *Eur J Pediatr*, **145**, 119–120.

Tallroth, A. (1939) Hemophilia with spontaneous hemorrhage in the iliopsoas muscle followed by injury to the femoral nerve. *Acta Chir Scand*, **84**, 1–10.

Telfer, P.T., Brown, D., Devereux, H. *et al.* (1994) HCV RNA levels and HIV infection: evidence for a viral interaction in haemophilic patients. *Br J Haematol*, **88**, 397–399.

Van Trotsenburg, L. (1975) Neurological complications of haemophilia, in *Handbook of Hemophilia* (eds K.M. and H.D. Hemker), American Elsevier, New York, pp. 389–404.

Visconti, E.B. and Hilgartner, M.W. (1980) Recognition and management of central nervous system hemorrhage in hemophilia. *Paediatrician*, **9**, 127–137.

Volpe, J.J., Manica, J.P., Land, V.J. and Coxe, W.S. (1976) Neonatal subdural hematoma associated with severe hemophilia A. *J Pediatr*, **88**, 1023–1025.

Wadis, R.S., Sangle, S.A., Kripalaney, S. *et al.* (1992) Familial intracranial haemorrhage due to factor V deficiency. *J. Neurol Neurosurg Psychiatry*, **55**, 227–228.

Walti, H., Kurz, R., Mitterstieler, G. *et al.* (1973) Intracranial haemorrhage in low-birth-weight infants and prophylactic administration of coagulation-factor concentrate. *Lancet*, **1**, 1284–1286.

Whitelaw, A., Haines, M.E., Bolsover, W. and Harris, E. (1984) Factor V deficiency and antenatal intraventricular haemorrhage. *Arch Dis Child*, **59**, 997–999.

Wilson, D.A., Nelson, M.D., Jr., Fenstermacher, M.J. *et al.* (1992) Brain abnormalities in male children and adolescents with hemophilia: detection with MR imaging. The hemophilia growth and development study group. *Radiology*, **185**, 553–558.

Yoffe, G. and Buchanan, G.R. (1988) Intracranial hemorrhage in newborn and young infants with hemophilia. *J Pediatr*, **113**, 333–336.

Yue, C.P. and Mann, K.S. (1986) The surgical management of intracranial hematomas in hemophiliac children. A prospective study. *Childs Nerv Syst*, **2**, 5–9.

9 ORAL BLEEDING

S. Sindet-Pedersen

Dental care in hemophilia – past and present

Dental care and, in particular, oral surgery has in the past produced tremendous therapeutic problems in the hemophilic patient; thus, it has previously been stated that such procedures should only be undertaken if the life of the patient was endangered (for review, see Atterbury, 1979). Fortunately, the comprehensive management of oral surgical procedures in the hemophilic patient has undergone changes in accordance with the changes in the hematologic approach to these patients.

TRANSFUSION WITH BLOOD AND PLASMA

After the introduction of transfusion with blood and/or plasma pre- and postoperatively, combined with various local hemostatic procedures, incidences of postoperative bleeding ranging from 78 to 100% were reported (Orr and Douglas, 1957; Wishart *et al.*, 1957; McIntyre *et al.*, 1959; Findlay and Nicholl, 1960; Johansen, 1969). Such high incidences of postoperative bleeding clearly demonstrate the inability of transfusions with blood and/or plasma alone combined with various local hemostatic procedures to secure hemostasis after oral surgery in the hemophilic patient.

REPLACEMENT THERAPY

After the introduction of specific replacement therapy with the missing coagulation factor more satisfactory results with respect to hemostasis postoperatively were achieved. Thus, incidences of postoperative bleeding ranging from 15% to 89% were reported when patients were substituted with factor VIII as the major source of substitution used in conjunction with different local hemostatic procedures (Bjørlin and Nilsson, 1963, 1965; Maycock *et al.*, 1963; Biggs *et al.*, 1965; Middleton *et al.*, 1965; Marder and Schulmann, 1966; Hausamen *et al.*, 1970). However, despite the fact that the incidence of postoperative bleeding was reduced by utilizing specific replacement therapy with factor VIII, some reports still included rather high incidences of bleeding following surgery, indicating that other variables than the level of factor VIII in plasma during and after surgery influenced hemostasis in the oral cavity. It is interesting to note that Biggs *et al.* (1965) did not find any correlation between the amount of replacement therapy administered and hemostatic effect following oral surgical procedures.

Within recent years the results following the use of relatively uniform levels of replacement therapy to approximately 30–50% of normal values preoperatively combined with various local hemostatic procedures have been reported. In these studies, the incidence of postoperative bleeding varied from 50 to 88% (Walsh *et al.*, 1971, 1975; Ramström and Blombäck, 1975). There are, however, big variations in the design of these studies, for which reason they are not directly comparable.

Steinberg, Levin and Bell (1984) reviewed the results in the literature of high-dosage replacement therapy administered in conjunction with oral surgery with respect to hemostatic effect; based on the data in the literature, these authors questioned the hemostatic effect of high-dosage substitution prior to oral surgery. In accordance with this, other authors have emphasized the contribution of local factors, in particular local fibrinolysis, and challenged the concept of the need to employ high-dosage substitution therapy (Ramström and Blombäck, 1975; Sindet-Pedersen and Stenbjerg, 1986; Sindet-Pedersen *et al.*, 1988a; Ramström *et al.*, 1989). On the other hand, there is no doubt that specific replacement therapy has reduced the number of fatal complications

Hemophilia. Edited by C.D. Forbes, L. Aledort and R. Madhok. Published in 1997 by Chapman & Hall, London. ISBN 0 412 63820 7

and major bleeding episodes in hemophilic patients exposed to oral surgery due to the fact that the replacement therapy results in improved fibrin formation at the site of surgery. However, the incidence of postoperative bleeding described in several of the studies, reporting results of high dosage replacement therapy, is so high that it cannot be stated that replacement therapy alone is sufficient to secure hemostasis postoperatively.

SYSTEMIC ANTIFIBRINOLYTIC TREATMENT

The introduction of antifibrinolytic drugs (for review, see Rizza, 1980; Ogston, 1984) constituted a new breakthrough in the management of hemophilic patients subjected to oral surgery. In the first clinical study of ε-aminocaproic acid (EACA, a pharmacologic inhibitor of fibrinolysis), Reid *et al.* (1964) described oral surgery performed in a total of 19 locations in 11 hemophilic patients; these patients were additionally treated with local hemostatics (oxydized cellulose soaked in thrombin) without any need for substitution therapy at all in any of the patients.

In a subsequent study by Cooksey, Perry and Raper (1966) the hemostatic effect of replacement therapy was compared with that of orally administered EACA in patients undergoing oral surgery. Findings from this study demonstrated that the antifibrinolytic drug produced more efficient hemostasis than did replacement therapy. The hemostatic effect of EACA has been documented in another clinical study where Tavenner (1968) found a reduced need for blood products administered in conjunction with oral surgery when hemophilic patients were treated with EACA compared to patients who did not receive EACA. These findings were confirmed in a double-blind study where reduction of transfusion requirements (from an average of 101.8 units per kg body weight to an average of 40.1 units per kg) as well as a reduction in the incidence of postoperative bleeding was observed when EACA was added to replacement therapy (Walsh *et al.*, 1971). These findings were supported by a subsequent survey conducted by Walsh *et al.* (1975). Similar findings – significant reduction of blood loss and transfusion requirements after oral surgery in patients with hemophilia A and B – were reported in a double-blind trial with the antifibrinolytic drug tranexamic acid, orally administered, by Forbes *et al.* (1972). Interestingly, Ramström and Blombäck (1975) observed a significant reduction of postoperative bleeding after replacement therapy to levels of only 5–10% of normal prior to surgery when combined with systemic tranexamic acid treatment; these authors also observed that no additional clinical effect with respect to postoperative bleeding could be obtained by higher replacement levels. There is thus ample evidence in the literature that systemic inhibitors of fibrinolysis can

reduce the incidence of bleeding and transfusion requirements in hemophilic patients undergoing oral surgery This modality of treatment must therefore be included when considering oral surgery in the hemophilic patient.

DDAVP IN CONJUNCTION WITH ORAL SURGERY

Mannucci and co-workers (1977) introduced DDAVP (desmopressin) as an alternative to replacement therapy in mild and moderately affected von Willebrand's and hemophilia A patients based on the fact that the drug induce a short-term rise in factor VIII and von Willebrand factor in the blood (Mannucci, 1986). The drug has also been evaluated for use in conjunction with oral surgery in patients with mild and moderate hemophilia A and von Willebrand's disease (e.g. Mannucci *et al.*, 1977; Wefers *et al.*, 1981; Wahl and Budde, 1982; Niessner and Kominger, 1983; Warrier and Lusher, 1983; Mariani *et al.*, 1984; De la Fuente *et al.*, 1985; Ghirardini *et al.*, 1988; Williamson and Eggleston, 1988; Berry and Berry, 1993; Rodeghiero *et al.*, 1993; Saulnier *et al.*, 1994). Summarizing the results of these studies, a large number of patients with mild or moderate hemophilia A and von Willebrand's disease have undergone oral surgery with sufficient hemostatic control after administration of DDAVP. However, due to the stimulatory effect of DDAVP on fibrinolysis treatment (Lowe and Small, 1988), DDAVP should always be combined with systemic antifibrinolytic therapy.

Tissue repair in the oral cavity

It has previously been demonstrated that the tissue thromboplastic activity as well as the fibrinolytic system are normal in patients with hemophilia (Astrup and Brakman, 1975). In addition, morphologic studies of the hemostatic plug have demonstrated that fibrin formation in hemophilic patients is limited to the deposition of thin strands of fibrin in the periphery of the wound, whereas the formation of fibrin in the central core of the wound is incomplete, caused by the low concentration of tissue thromboplastin and the missing reinforcement through the intrinsic system of coagulation (Sixma and van den Berg, 1984). Of course, fibrin formation in the oral cavity is governed by the same biologic principles as elsewhere in the body. However, the impaired fibrin is in a different biological situation when exposed to the oral cavity as compared to a fibrin clot somewhere in the tissues. This is due to the fact that fibrin even during its polymerization in the oral cavity, will be exposed not only to activators of fibrinolysis originating from the tissues but also those originating in the oral cavity (reviewed by Sindet-Pedersen, 1991).

There are two major sources of plasminogen activators in the oral environment – the mucosa and the saliva. The presence of plasminogen activators in oral mucosa has been demonstrated in several studies (Törteli, 1967; Bjørlin and Nilsson, 1968; Birn and Fejerskov, 1971; Wünschmann-Henderson and Astrup, 1972). Special attention has been drawn to the fact that plasminogen activators (tissue-type plasminogen activators; t-PA) are bound to epithelial cells (Southam, 1981; Southam and Moody, 1981; Birkedal-Hansen and Taylor, 1983; Sindet-Pedersen, Gram and Jespersen, 1987, 1990), indicating that epithelial cells may be participating actively in regulation of hemostasis in the oral cavity (for review, Sindet-Pedersen, 1991). Besides, saliva contains activators of fibrinolysis (Albrechtsen and Thaysen, 1955; Taylor, Doku and Romero, 1964; Schulte and Vorbauer, 1965; Gersel-Pedersen, 1982; Kjaeldgaard and Kjaeldgaard, 1987; Kjaeldgaard, Lagerlöf and Kjaeldgaard, 1989). It is interesting to note that it does not seem that glandular saliva is the source of salivary plasminogen activators. This is due to the fact that most of the fibrinolytic activity of whole saliva is recovered in the sediment (Ramström, 1975; Moody, 1982; Sindet-Pedersen, Gram and Jespersen, 1987). It is also interesting that the activator in saliva bound to epithelial cells has been identified as t-PA (Kjaeldgaard and Kjaeldgaard, 1986; Sindet-Pedersen, Gram and Jespersen, 1987; Schmid and Chambers, 1989). The presence of inhibitors of fibrinolysis in saliva has also recently been demonstrated (Kjaeldgaard, Kjaeldgaard and Gaffney, 1989a; Kinnby, Licander and Martinsson, 1991).

Summarizing the above-mentioned studies, there is ample evidence that activators of fibrinolysis are present in the environment of the oral cavity. The major sources of these activators of fibrinolysis are saliva and epithelial cells from the oral mucosa. This means that the clot in the oral cavity has to be resistant to tissue fibrinolysis as well as to the oral fibrinolysis in order to avoid premature degradation. It therefore seems relevant to focus on the possibilities of inhibiting fibrinolysis in the oral environment when treating hemophilic patients with oral bleeding problems.

Local hemostatics

LOCAL ANTIFIBRINOLYTIC TREATMENT

In the past, only a few papers have dealt with topical application of pharmacologic inhibitors of fibrinolysis in the oral cavity; data from these studies indicate a moderate hemostatic effect of local inhibition of fibrinolysis when EACA was administered topically only during surgery (Berry, Coster and Berry, 1977; Stajcic, 1985). However, a pharmacokinetic study has documented that one administration of 10 ml of a 5% solution of tran-

examic acid resulted in average concentrations of 7 mg of tranexamic acid per liter of saliva after 2h, and even 8h after local administration, the drug remained at detectable levels in the saliva (Sindet-Pedersen, 1987). Following these interesting findings, clinical studies were initiated to evaluate the hemostatic effect of tranexamic acid utilized as a mouthwash in hemophilic patients exposed to oral surgery; the first study documented a significant reduction of transfusion requirements as well as a reduced incidence of postoperative bleeding after administration of tranexamic acid as a mouthwash (10 ml 5% solution four times a day for 5 days; Sindet-Pedersen and Stenbjerg, 1986). The effect of topical application of tranexamic acid has also been evaluated among hemophilic patients with gingival hemorrhage and it was found that the demand for replacement therapy was significantly decreased in patients receiving systemic and local antifibrinolytic treatment with tranexamic acid compared to a group of patients receiving systemic antifibrinolytic treatment only (Sindet-Pedersen, Stenbjerg and Ingerslev, 1988). These results have since lent support in three double-blind studies, demonstrating that the incidence of bleeding complications after oral surgery among anticoagulant-treated patients, who also have impaired fibrin formation, can be significantly decreased when tranexamic acid is applied topically as a mouthwash during and after surgery (Sindet-Pedersen *et al.*, 1989; Ramström *et al.*, 1993; Borea *et al.*, 1993). The results of these studies together demonstrate the pathophysiologic role of oral fibrinolysis for development of bleeding among patients with impaired fibrin formation. Therefore, local antifibrinolytic treatment should be considered in the hemophilic patient who is to undergo procedures inducing bleeding in the oral cavity.

OTHER LOCAL HEMOSTATIC PROCEDURES

Several local hemostatic procedures have been recommended in the literature to reduce bleeding after oral surgery. These include the application of sponges of gelatin soaked in factor concentrate and thrombin (Johansen, 1969) and various types of splints or packs to compress the surgical site (e.g. Wörner, 1972; Pizzoni, Coitellaro and Mannucci, 1973; Kaneda *et al.*, 1981). A reduced incidence of postoperative bleeding and reduced amount of replacement therapy necessary to prevent bleeding were observed by Ramström and Blombäck (1975) and Ramström *et al.* (1989) after application of thrombin and oxidized cellulose in the dental alveolus combined with a splint covering the operated region. It has also been shown that oxidized cellulose soaked in a mixture of thrombin and EACA applied to the surgical site can reduce the incidence of postoperative bleeding (Vinckier and Vermylen, 1985), as can topical application of factor VIII at the dental extraction site (Nakajima *et al.*, 1978). Among other suggested local hemostatics in the literature, local infiltration of thrombin to the bone (Herfert, 1962), topically applied thrombin (Suzuki *et al*, 1983), microfibrillar collagen (Evans, 1977) and laser therapy of the bleeding wound (Grasser and Ackermann, 1977) should be mentioned.

Recently, the fibrin adhesion system was introduced; this consists of fibrinogen coagulated with thrombin containing aprotinin, which is an inhibitor of fibrinolysis and proteolysis; a number of reports have drawn attention to the ability of this hemostatic to improve hemostasis among patients with impaired fibrin formation, particularly when it is combined with antifibrinolytic drugs (e.g. Wutka, 1978; Wepner, Bukal and Beck-Mannogetta, 1979; Wepner, Fries and Platz, 1982; Baudo *et al.*, 1985; 1988; Rakocz *et al.*, 1993). Unfortunately, no controlled studies have been conducted with this material. Baudo *et al.* (1988) claimed a hemostatic effect of the fibrin adhesion system among hemophilic patients undergoing oral surgery; however, a careful perusal of the presented data revealed a significant reduction of the incidence among the patients who simultaneously received oral tranexamic acid (tablets) compared to those treated with the fibrin adhesion system alone (Sindet-Pedersen *et al.*, 1989a). These data thus suggest no particular effect of the fibrin adhesion as such, but further substantiate the pathophysiologic role of fibrinolysis in the oral environment.

Oral bleeding in the hemophilic patient with acquired inhibitors

The hemophilic patient with acquired inhibitors (approximately 15% of hemophilia A patients; Roberts and Cromartie, 1984) represents a very difficult patient population to manage. Most of the available literature on these patients is anecdotal, and only few studies dealing with rather small groups of patients undergoing oral procedures have been presented. In the past, the most frequently employed treatment has been a combination of replacement therapy with activated prothrombin complex concentrates (PCC) combined with systemic antifibrinolytic therapy with EACA or tranexamic acid (Preston *et al.*, 1977; Mannucci *et al.*, 1979; Agrestini *et al.* 1981; Hanna *et al.*, 1981; Jørgensen *et al.*, 1982; Scharrer, 1982; Garehime, Pecaro and Green, 1983; Zech and Strother, 1983; Griffen, Hoots and Carter, 1987; Shurafa and MacIntosh, 1987). Zech and Strother (1983) and Shurafa and MacIntosh (1987) recommended sequential use of PCC and systemically administered antifibrinolytic drugs due to the risk of development of thromboembolic complications by simultaneous administration of PCC and systemically administered antifibrinolytics. As an alternative to sequential use of the two substances, Garehime, Pecaro and Green

(1983) recommended that the patients should be carefully monitored during treatment, under which circumstances simultaneous use might be considered. However, other treatment modalities, including a combination of non-activated PCC and systemic antifibrinolytic treatment, have also been recommended (Cudzinowski, 1979; Shurafa and MacIntosh, 1987), or use of factor VIII concentrate combined with systemic antifibrinolytic treatment (Redding and Stiegler, 1983). In a patient with low-titer inhibitor undergoing extensive periodontal surgery and dental extractions, Sindet-Pedersen *et al.*, (1988) utilized infusion of factor VIII concentrate to neutralize the factor VIII activity combined with local and systemic antifibrinolytic treatment with tranexamic acid. Recently, reports on the management of these patients utilizing factor VIIA or recombinant factor VIIA replacement therapy combined with tranexamic acid have emerged in the literature (Hedner and Kisel, 1983; Ingerslev *et al.*, 1991, 1993). These reports indicate that recombinant Factor VIIA may constitute a viable alternative to activated PCC.

Regarding maxillofacial trauma, only few anecdotal reports about hemophilic patients with inhibitors are available in the literature (Wepner, Bukal and Beck-Mannagetta, 1979; Blatt *et al.*, 1984; Sindet-Pedersen, Stenbjerg and Ingerslev, 1987). The report by Sindet-Pedersen, Stenbjerg and Ingerslev describes management of a patient with inhibitors to factor VIII with bilateral fractures of the mandible; this was successfully treated by a combination of activated PCC, systemic and local antifibrinolytic treatment, antibiotic treatment, and conservative treatment of the fractures employing dental archbars.

Summarizing the above-mentioned data, activated PCC or recombinant factor VIIA seems to be the treatment of choice when hemophilia patients with inhibitors are to be treated for bleeding in the oral cavity. However, the risk of development of complicating disseminated intravascular coagulation with simultaneous administration of activated PCC and systemically administered antifibrinolytics should be emphasized. As an alternative, local administration only of an antifibrinolytic might be considered (Sindet-Pedersen, Stenbjerg and Ingerslev, 1987).

Dental disease

Disease in the oral cavity is dominated by two conditions caused by oral bacteria – dental caries and gingivitis/periodontitis.

DENTAL CARIES

Dental caries develops as a result of bacteria accumulating on dental surfaces which are not sufficiently cleaned at regular intervals. If these bacteria are allowed to accumulate, the metabolic products include organic acids which dissolve the enamel or dentine of the teeth. The end-result may be that the lesion continues into the pulp of the tooth, resulting in the development of pulpitis. Pulpitis usually causes necrosis of the dental pulp and this necrotic pulp will always be infected by the bacteria, generating the lesion. The end-stage of dental caries is the development of an infectious process, destroying the bone around the apex of the tooth, and eventually abscess formation.

GINGIVITIS/PERIODONTITIS

Gingivitis develops as result of bacteria accumulating along the gingival margin. If this bacterial plaque is not removed at regular intervals, an inflammation develops in the soft tissues surrounding the teeth. When this process has persisted for longer periods of time the infection may result in destruction of the tooth supporting tissues – periodontal ligament and alveolar bone. The end-stage is total periodontitis, where all tooth supporting tissues are destroyed, in which case the tooth is spontaneously exfoliated. However, during the progression of this bacteria-induced disease abscesses may also form in the periodontal tissues.

OTHER PATHOLOGIC CONDITIONS IN THE ORAL CAVITY

A rather frequently occurring problem in younger patients is the presence of retained teeth or semiretained teeth (wisdom teeth). Such not fully erupted teeth, which have erupted to a degree where there is communication to the oral cavity, will be associated with an infection in the pericoronary space (pericoronitis); particularly in the lower jaw around wisdom teeth this problem can, in the most severe cases, develop into a serious infection problem.

Dental procedures in the hemophilic patient

Although several papers have been published in the past on the subject of dental management of the hemophilic patient (e.g. Snyder and Penner, 1970; Ramström and Blombäck, 1971; Lewis, 1973; Agrestini *et al.*, 1981; Geffner and Porteous, 1981; Saunders, 1982; Sonis and Musselman, 1982; Katz and Terezhalmy, 1988; McKown and Shapiro, 1991), there are only few data supporting the recommended regimens for dental treatment of hemophilic patients. When considering dental or oral surgical procedures in the hemophilic patient, it is always advisable to apply a team approach, collaborating closely on the treatment plan with the hematologist in charge

of the patient. It should also be remembered that the treatment plan always has to be based on an individual assessment of the patient, because there may be special considerations which may make it necessary to refrain from adhering to the recommended guidelines in the following part of the text. Finally, we advise the application of a procedure-oriented approach based on the anticipated type of bleeding, because the approach to superficial bleeding in the gingiva should certainly be different from a procedure which involves risk of bleeding or hematoma formation into loosely structured soft tissues, such as the floor of the mouth.

In the following text different types of dental procedures are discussed with a problem-oriented approach, focusing on the hemophilic patient. The principles described summarize the guidelines applied to management of such patients in our department for the last 15 years.

ANESTHESIA FOR DENTAL PROCEDURES

Usually, most dental procedures can be undertaken with local anesthesia. Three different types of local anesthesia are employed in dentistry: regional, infiltration and periodontal ligament anesthesia.

Regional anesthesia

Regional anesthesia is employed when a segment of the jaw needs to be anesthetized, for instance for removal of wisdom teeth in the lower jaw where the mandibular nerve (third trigeminal nerve) is anesthetized medially to the ramus of the mandible. It is common for regional nerve blocks to be performed by injecting the local anesthetic deep in the tissues; in the past, the use of regional anesthesia in hemophilic patients has been controversial. For several years we have employed the practice that patients with more than 10% spontaneous factor VIII/IX activity can be anesthetized with regional nerve blocks, and we have not observed any complications with this procedure over the past 15 years. However, in patients with less than this spontaneous factor activity, replacement therapy or DDAVP, raising the factor activity to approximately 10% of normal, have to be employed before the use of regional anesthesia.

Infiltration anesthesia

This type of anesthesia is performed by injecting local anesthetic into the tissues surrounding the teeth and may in most cases be sufficient for the one-rooted teeth and premolars in the anterior parts of the jaws for any dental procedure, including endodontic treatment and simple dental extraction. Due to the fact that the injection is performed superficially in the tissues and any encountered bleeding or hematoma formation may easily be detected shortly after such infiltration analgesia, we do not demand any replacement therapy in hemophilic patients receiving infiltration analgesia; in case bleeding develops, it is easily detected and can be treated with compression or, if needed – which has not been the case – replacement therapy may be instituted.

Periodontal ligament anesthesia

This type of anesthesia is performed by injecting local anesthetic directly into the periodontal ligament, and this may be sufficient for most dental procedures and even extractions in the one-rooted teeth anteriorly in the jaws. In multirooted teeth and in molars, this may not be sufficient for dental extraction, but most endodontic procedures can be accomplished by injecting local anesthetic along the periodontal ligament of the different roots; there is no need for replacement therapy when this procedure is employed because only superficial bleeding develops from the gingival crevice with this type of anesthesia; bleeding can be controlled by compression and/or local antifibrinolytic therapy with tranexamic acid.

Several local anesthetics are available for use in dentistry. However, it should be considered whether surgical procedures should be undertaken using drugs containing a vasoconstrictor because a secondary hyperemia develops some time after administration of the local anesthetic and this may not be an advantage from a hemostatic point of view. We therefore consider it an advantage to avoid vasoconstrictors for oral surgery in such patients.

General anesthesia

There is rarely a demand for general anesthesia in connection with dental procedures; however, in cases with severely impacted third molars or other types of dental pathology involving complex surgical procedures, it may be relevant to institute general anesthesia. In these cases, we usually employ oral intubation and patients will only be treated in general anesthesia when they have a spontaneous level of factor VIII/IX above 10% or have been replaced to this level prior to intubation. We recommend the avoidance of any nasal intubation in patients with hemophilia to prevent development of bleeding from the nasal cavity.

CONSERVATIVE DENTISTRY, ENDODONTICS AND PROSTHODONTIC TREATMENT

Conservative dentistry includes treatment of dental caries with fillings. **Endodontic treatment** includes treatment of the dental pulp; this is most frequently required when dental caries result in necrosis of the pulp. Endodontic treatment may, however, also be necessary after dental trauma where root canal treatment and filling can be required.

Usually, most of the necessary procedures can be undertaken using periodontal ligament or infiltration analgesia, which in itself does not demand any replacement therapy. Endodontic procedures involve removal of the dental pulp. However, bleeding that may be induced by these procedures is so minimal that it does not require replacement therapy. The treatment of dental caries in itself involves bleeding problems only when the cavities are extended to the gingiva, where instrumentation may induce gingival bleeding. Usually, however, this bleeding is of such a character that it can be sufficiently controlled utilizing only antifibrinolytic mouthwash, possibly combined with compression.

Summarizing the procedures undertaken in conservative dentistry and endodontics, these do **not** require replacement therapy; however, cases where it is difficult to achieve sufficient anesthesia by means of periodontal ligament or infiltration anesthesia may demand regional anesthesia, which does necessitates replacement therapy.

Prosthodontic treatment includes treatment with crowns, bridges and removable dentures. The need for adjunctive treatment in these cases depends on the need for anesthesia and whether extending preparations in the teeth below the gingiva are required.

Usually, the preparation of teeth may be undertaken with infiltration or periodontal ligament anesthesia, in which case no replacement therapy is necessary. In cases where preparation of teeth and impression procedures are extended below the gingival margin, the same guidelines for management of bleeding as described under conservative dentistry and endodontic treatment should be followed – use of compression perhaps combined with inhibitor of fibrinolysis, particularly for local application.

PERIODONTOLOGY

Periodontology is the discipline which takes care of diseases in the periodontal tissues, i.e. gingivitis and periodontitis. Only a few reports have been published on hemophilic patients with periodontal problems (Webster, Roberts and Penick, 1968; Eastman, Nowakowski and Triplett, 1983; Michaelides, 1983; Sindet-Pedersen, Stenbjerg and Ingerslev, 1988; Sindet-Pedersen et al., 1988). The procedures employed in this discipline include oral hygiene measures, polishing, removal of calculus, also below the gingival margin, and in severe cases, periodontal surgery.

Oral hygiene measures and polishing of teeth do not necessitate any therapy; in case bleeding develops it will be superficial from the gingiva and should be treated by means of compression and, if necessary, local antifibrinolytic therapy alone. In cases where subgingival removal of calculus is indicated, it is frequently necessary to employ local anesthesia, which should be done in the form of periodontal ligament or infiltration local anesthesia. In such cases most incidences of bleeding can be controlled without any replacement therapy, the bleeding is superficial and there will not be any development of hematomas deep in the tissues; compression and local antifibrinolytic treatment will also be sufficient under these circumstances.

In cases where periodontal surgery is indicated, it is usually relevant to employ regional anesthesia, and since mucoperiosteum is elevated during the procedures patients should not be treated if they have a Factor VIII/IX level less than 10% at the time of surgery. Meticulous hemostasis should be undertaken during the procedure and periodontal packs should be used after the procedure in order to minimize hematoma formation and bleeding. In such cases, systemic and local antifibrinolytic treatment should also be administered for a period of approximately 1 week following the procedure.

It has recently been established that periodontitis has a more rapid progression among patients with human immunodeficiency virus (HIV) infection than non-immunologically compromised patients; for this reason this problem necessitates particular attention in hemophilic patients with known HIV infection.

ORTHODONTIC TREATMENT

Orthodontic treatment involves tooth movements in cases of malocclusion or malpositioned teeth (Grossman, 1975; Williams, 1992). Treatment requires the use of brackets which can be bonded directly to the enamel of the teeth and orthodontic bands which frequently are in the vicinity of the marginal gingiva. All patients undergoing orthodontic treatment should commit themselves to meticulous oral hygiene due to the fact that the orthodontic equipment is plaque-retaining, so caries may develop in relationship to the orthodontic equipment or gingivitis may develop as a result of plaque accumulation on the orthodontic equipment. Apart from this special measure, utilization of orthodontic brackets bonded directly to the enamel does not necessitate any special measures. In cases where orthodontic bands are employed, gingival bleeding may develop during their insertion and removal; this may be treated by means of compression and local antifibrinolytic therapy alone. Finally, it should be emphasized that the orthodontist treating hemophilic patients should be very careful when employing orthodontic equipment so that no sharp parts of the equipment induce mucosal bleeding from the soft tissues in the mouth.

ORAL SURGICAL PROCEDURES

Oral surgery includes a wide range of procedures performed in the oral cavity (dentoalveolar surgery), ranging from simple dental extractions to removal of complicated retained teeth and treatment of dental and facial trauma.

Dental extractions

Usually, an uncomplicated dental extraction can be undertaken in one-rooted teeth (i.e. incisors, canines, and premolars) using infiltration or periodontal ligament anesthesia. In these cases, it is advisable to pack the dental alveolus with some kind of resorbable local hemostatic (i.e. collagen) which exerts compression on bleeding vessels within the dental alveolus; also, a suture from the buccal to the lingual gingiva is advisable as this both retains the hemostatic in the dental socket and exerts compression on the gingival margin, thus improving hemostasis. A combination of oral and local antifibrinolytic treatment is usually employed in these cases to improve hemostasis. In the case where multiple teeth have to be removed in the same session, we recommend the mobilization of a mucoperiosteal flap, packing the alveoli with some kind of resorbable hemostatic material and approximating the flaps over the area to a tight soft-tissue closure by sutures.

Retained teeth

Removal of retained teeth usually necessitates the employment of regional anesthesia as well as local infiltration. We prefer the factor activity of the patient to be within the range of approximately 10% at the time of surgery, no matter how it has been achieved, by means of replacement therapy or DDAVP. The most frequently occurring retained tooth, also in hemophilic patients, is the third molar. Even though a conservative approach may be relevant in many cases, several patients develop infection in the pericoronary space around third molars, which are not fully erupted for which reason these teeth have to be removed. It is a well-known fact that third molars may be rather complicated to remove surgically, particularly in the elderly patient. For this reason, we employ the policy that patients are reviewed when they are around the age of 18, when root formation around the third molars is not yet completed, and at this point it is determined whether there is any possibility of the third molar erupting into the oral cavity with a healthy soft-tissue condition around it (i.e. no pericoronitis); if this is not the case, the tooth is usually removed at this age since it is less technically complicated to remove the third molars before the root has been fully formed than afterwards. We do not recommend the use of the lingual split technique in such cases; instead, we do an incision from the anterior edge of the ramus of the mandible along the buccal surface of the third molar. We reflect the soft tissues minimally on the lingual aspect of the mandible due to the risk of development of hematomas in the posterior parts of the floor of the mouth; this may be potentially life-threatening. Of course, careful hemostasis is achieved during surgery and the alveolus is packed with a resorbable hemostatic before the tissues are sutured with a tight closure over the hemostatic. This same procedure applies in principle to any anatomic region in the oral cavity where retained teeth have to be removed; however, it is always advisable to mobilize tissues and expose teeth from a visible area without too large an amount of loosely structured soft tissues, such as in the floor of the mouth, due to the fact that hematomas are detected much easier and earlier in such an area than in loosely structured tissues.

Other oral surgery procedures

These include procedures such as soft-tissue biopsies, endodontic surgery (apicectomies) in teeth with peri-apical infections and removal of minor pathology. All these procedures should in principle be treated in accordance with the principles described under the section on removal of retained teeth above as they commonly involve either regional anesthesia or surgical incisions in loosely structured soft tissues.

DENTOFACIAL TRAUMA

In patients with dental trauma without any soft-tissue involvement the principles described for conservative dentistry and endodontic treatment should be employed. In such cases, it is the type of anesthesia necessary for treatment that usually determines on which regimen the patient has to be treated.

In patients with dental trauma also involving soft tissues or significant gingival bleeding, replacement therapy to approximately 10% should be employed at the time of trauma in patients having less than 10% factor VIII/IX activity to stop the bleeding and make it possible to achieve hemostasis, in conjunction with suturing of the lesions of the soft tissues. Repositioning and fixation of loose teeth is done in accordance with the principles usually employed for such problems.

In patients with more substantial lesions in the facial skeleton, such as a fracture of the jaw, limited experience has been described in the literature. It is, however, important to make a comprehensive treatment plan for the hemophilic patient together with the hematologist. If a conservative approach, i.e. only use of dental arch bars, can be used, this should be done. However, in cases with severe dislocation of mandibular fractures and comminuted cases it is relevant to consider open reduction and osteosynthesis by means of miniplates. This should, of course, be undertaken under a relevant replacement therapy regimen and, again, sufficient hemostasis has to

be obtained during the procedure, particularly to prevent bleeding deep into the soft tissues in the floor of the mouth. Patients with fractures of the jaws usually have to be given general anesthesia. However, it is not possible to achieve a proper occlusion with the patient being orally intubated. On the other hand, the extent of the surgical procedure may modify the guidelines for replacement therapy and this has to be assessed on an individual basis.

ADJUVANT MEDICAL TREATMENT FOR HEMOPHILIC PATIENTS UNDERGOING ORAL SURGERY.

Antifibrinolytic treatment

In patients with hemophilia who are to undergo oral surgery, we advise in all cases the use of a combination of systemic and local antifibrinolytic treatment. Our treatment regimen consists of 25 mg tranexamic acid per kg body weight orally 4 times a day for some days after the procedure, combined with tranexamic mouthwash 10 ml 5% solution 4 times a day for 7 days following surgery.

Adjunctive antibiotic therapy

The adjunctive administration of antibiotic therapy to hemophilic patients undergoing oral surgery has been recommended in several studies. Unfortunately, no controlled studies have been conducted to evaluate the influence of antibiotics on the incidence of bleeding. However, a decrease in postoperative bleeding from 39 to 20% under a treatment regimen consisting of replacement therapy and EACA has been observed as a result of adding antibiotics to the treatment regimen (Walsh *et al.*, 1971). That antibiotics have been recommended to be used routinely in hemophilic patients undergoing oral surgery (Ramström and Blombäck, 1975; Ramström, 1984; Ramström *et al.*, 1989) has been based on the argument that infection induces inflammation which in the local environment may increase the fibrinolytic response and thereby the risk of bleeding. On the other hand, it has also been observed that local hemostatics applied into surgical wounds without using simultaneous antibiotic therapy could be rejected due to infection and result in rebleeding (Ramström and Blombäck, 1975).

No acetylsalicylic acid or non-steroidal anti-inflammatory drugs are used as analgesics in hemophilic patients. Instead, acetaminophen eventually combined with narcotic drugs, is used for pain control. All patients who undergo oral surgical procedures also use chlorhexidine mouthwash twice daily for a week following surgery in order to reduce the microflora in the oral cavity.

Sedation

Frequently in the past, patients with hemophilia have experienced bleeding problems in conjunction with procedures in the oral cavity, for which reason they may fear the procedure. In such cases, we administrate anxiolytic drugs, preferably benzodiazepines, either orally or intravenously to reduce the patient's fear and anxiety.

ORAL PATHOLOGY

Hemophilic patients may also demonstrate oral pathologic conditions such as oral *Candida* infection or other disorders of the oral mucosa. It is relevant to remember that recurrent oral *Candida* infections may be a sign of a compromised immunologic status and such recurrent clinical problems should lead to an offer to the patient of further examination of the immune system after consultation with the hematologist in charge of the patient. Also, hairy leukoplakia and Kaposi's sarcoma have within recent years been described in the oral cavity in HIV-infected individuals. For these reasons, a careful examination of the oral cavity, including the oral mucosa, should be a natural part of any dental examination of a patient with hemophilia.

THE PEDIATRIC DENTAL PATIENT AND PREVENTION OF DENTAL DISEASE

The dental procedures, which have to be undertaken in a child with hemophilia, have been described previously in this text; the guidelines described for management of the problem should, in principle, be the same in the pediatric patient, with the exception that there may be a more frequent need for general anesthesia. It should be emphasized that it is very important to organize a regular recall schedule so that as early as possible they, together with their parents, are instructed in relevant oral hygiene measures in order to prevent the development of disease (Steinle and Kisker, 1970; Nakai, Peterson and Law, 1974; Hobson, 1981; Ublansky, 1992).

Exactly the same measures for oral hygiene should be employed in a hemophilic child as in a non-hemophilic child, with the special remark that oral hygiene is even more important in the hemophilic child because simple gingivitis may result in repeated gingival bleeding problems with subsequent necessary therapy. In the general population, it has been possible to achieve a very low occurrence of dental disease by introducing a combination of oral hygiene measures, fluoridized toothpaste or other fluoridized agents, combined with dietary advice. This is also possible to achieve among hemophilic patients, for which reason a regular recall program with relevant instruction in oral hygiene procedures of the child as well as the parent, dietary instruction and use of appropriate fluoridized agents, depending on the fluoride content in drinking water, should be an integrated part of managing the hemophilic patient. In this way, the need for later procedures necessitating extensive measures, including replacement therapy and hospitalization, may be avoided.

Acknowledgement

My warmest thanks to my secretary, Ms Lisbeth Nielsen, for her assistance in the preparation of the manuscript.

References

Agrestini, F., Mariani, G., Capozzi, L. *et al.* (1981) A comprehensive programme for dental care in haemophilia. *Haemostasis*, **10** (suppl. 1), 282–284.

Albrechtsen, O.K. and Thaysen, J.H. (1955) Fibrinolytic activity in human saliva. *Acta Physiol Scand*, **35**, 138–145.

Astrup, T and Brakman, P. (1975) Tissue repair and vascular disease in haemophilia, in *Handbook of Hemophilia* (eds K.M. Brinkhous and H.C. Hemker), Excerpta Medica, Amsterdam, pp. 285–299.

Atterbury, R.A. (1979) Past and present practices of hemostasis in dentistry and oral surgery. *Bull Hist Dent*, **27**, 15–21.

Baudo, F., de Cataldo, F., Gatti, R. *et al.* Local hemostasis after tooth extraction in patients with abnormal hemostatic function. Use of human fibrinogen concentrate. *Haemostasis*, **15**, 402–404.

Baudo, F., de Cataldo, F., Landonio, G. and Muti, G. (1988) Management of oral bleeding in haemophilic patients. *Lancet*, **2**, 1082.

Berry, E.W. and Berry, P.R. (1993) DDAVP – clinical use and therapeutic limitations in patients with congenital bleeding disorders: the Auckland experience, in *Desmopressin in Bleeding Disorder* (eds G. Mariani, P.M. Manucci and M. Cattaneo), NATO ASI Series, Series A: Life Sciences, vol. 242, Plenum Press, New York, pp. 249–260.

Berry, P.R., Coster, A.B. and Berry, E.W. (1977) Local use of epsilon-aminocaproic acid in dental therapy. *Thromb Haemost* **38** (suppl. 1), 373.

Biggs, R., Mattews, J.M., Rush, B.M. *et al.* (1965) Further experience in use of human antihaemophilic globulin (H.A.H.G.) for the control of bleeding after dental extraction in haemophilic patients. *Lancet*, **1**, 970–974.

Birkedal-Hansen, H. and Taylor, R.E. (1983) Production of three plasminogen activators and inhibitor in keratinocyte cultures. *Biochim Biophys Acta*, **756**, 308–318.

Birn, H. and Fejerskov, O. (1971) Fibrinolytic activity of human oral epithelial cells. A preliminary report. *Scand J Dent Res*, **79**, 381–386.

Björlin, G. and Nilsson, I.M. (1963) Oral surgery in patients with coagulopathies. *Acta Odontol Scand*, **21**, 99–139.

Björlin, G. and Nilsson, I.M. (1965) Oral surgery in patients with coagulopathies. II. *Odontol Rev*, **16**, 216–237.

Björlin, G. and Nilsson I.M. (1968) Fibrinolytic activity in alveoli after tooth extraction. *Odontol Revy*, **19**, 197–204.

Blatt, P.M, White, G.C., McMillan, C.W. and, Webster, W.P. (1984) Failure of activated prothrombin complex concentrates in a hemophiliac with an anti-factor VIII antibody. *J Am Med Assoc*, **251**, 67.

Blombäck, M. and Ramström, G. (1971) Blödarsjuka med hensyn speciellt till odontologiska problem. *Tandläkartidningen*, **12**, 449–455.

Borea, G., Montebugnoli, L., Capuzzi, P. and Magellis, C. (1993) Tranexamic acid as a mouthwash in anticoagulant-treated patients undergoing oral surgery. *Oral Surg Oral Med Oral Pathol*, **75**, 29–31.

Cooksey, M.W., Perry, C.B. and Raper, A.B. (1966) Epsilon-aminocaproic acid therapy for dental extractions in haemophiliacs. *Br Med J*, **2**, 1633–1634.

Cudzinowski, L. (1979) Circulating antibodies in factor VIII deficiency hemophilia: report of a case. *J Dent Child*, **46**, 54–56.

De la Fuente, B., Kasper, C.K., Rickles, F.R. and Hoyer, L.W. (1985) Response of patients with mild and moderated hemophilia and von Willebrand's disease to treatment with desmopressin. *Ann Intern Med*, 6–14.

Eastman, J.R., Nowakowski, A.R. and Triplett, E.A. (1983) DDAVP: review of indications for its use in the treatment of factor VIII deficiency and report of a case. *Oral Surg*, **56**, 246–251.

Evans, B.E. (1977) Local hemostatic agents. *NY J Dent*, **47**, 109–114.

Findlay, I.A. and Nicholl, B. (1960) Tooth extraction in patients with hemophilia. *Oral Surg Oral Med Oral Pathol*, **13**, 116–1180.

Forbes, C.D., Barr, R.D., Reid, G. *et al.* (1972) Tranexamic acid in control of haemorrhage after dental extraction in haemophilia and Christmas disease. *Br Med J*, **2**, 311–313.

Garehime, W.J., Peacaro, B.C. and Green, D. (1983) Use of activated prothrombin complex concentrate in a severely hemophilic patient with factor VIII inhibitor. *J Oral Maxillofac Surg*, **41**, 262–264.

Geffner, L. and Porteous, J.R. (1981) Haemorrhage and pain control in conservative dentistry for haemophiliacs. *Br Dent J*, **151**, 256–258.

Gersel-Pedersen, N. (1982) Fibrinolytisk aktivitet i saliva og blod i relation til oral kirurgi og alveolitis sicca dolorosa. Thesis Odontologisk Boghandels Forlag, Copenhagen, pp. 1–198.

Ghirardini, A., Christolini, A., Tirindelli, M.C. *et al.* (1988) Clinical evaluation of subcutaneously administered DDAVP. *Thromb Res*, **49**, 363–372.

Grasser, H. and Ackerman, K. (1977) Anwendungsmöglichkeiten von Laserstrahlen in der zahnärztlichen Chirugie. *Dtsch Zahnarztl Z*, **32**, 512–515.

Griffen, A.L., Hoots, W.K. and Carter, A.B. (1987) Activated prothrombin complex concentrates in the management of the hemophilic patient with factor VIII inhibitor: case report. *Pediatr Dent*, **9**, 321–324.

Grossman, R.C. (1975) Orthodontics and dentistry for the hemophilic patient. *Am J Orthodont*, **68**, 391–403.

Hanna, W.T., Madigan, R.R., Miles, M.A. and Lange, R.D. (1981) Activated factor IX complex in treatment of surgical cases of hemophilia A with inhibitors. *Thromb Haemost*, **46**, 638–641.

Hausamen, J.E., Bruster, H.T., Riech, P. *et al.* (1970) Zahnextraktionen unter Substitutionsbehandlung bei Hämophilie. *Dtsch Zahnartzl Z*, **17**, 317–320.

Hobson, P. (1981) Dental care of children with haemophilia and related conditions. *Br Dent J*, **151**, 249–253.

Ingerslev, J., Feldstedt, M. and Sindet-Pederson, S. (1991) Control of haemostasis with recominant factor VIIa in patient with inhibitor to factor VIII. *Lancet*, **338**, 831–832.

Ingerslev, J., Sneppon, O., Knudsen, L. and Sindet-Pedersen, S. (1993) Efficacy of recombinant factor VIIa (rVIIa) in surgical procedures in haemophilia A patients with inhibitors and congenital factor VII defiency. 24. Hämophilie-symposion, Hamburg 1993.

Johansen, J. Dentoalveolær kirurgi hos hemofilikere. *Nor Tannlaegeforen Tid*, **79**, 535–545.

Jørgensen, J., Stenbjerg, S., Skottun, T. and Tauris, P. (1982) Total dental extraction in a patient with factor VII inhibitor, in *Activated Prothrombin Comple Concentrates. Managing Hemophilia with Factor VIII Inhibitor* (eds G. Mariani, M.A. Russo and F. Mandelli), Praeger, New York, pp. 176–179.

Kaneda, T., Shikimori, M., Watanabe, I. *et al.* (1981) The importance of local hemostatic procedures in dental extractions and oral mucosal bleeding of hemophiliac patients. *Int J Oral Surg*, **10**, 266 –271.

Katz, J.O. and Terezhalmy, G.T. (1988) Dental management of the patient with hemophilia. *Oral Surg Oral Med Oral Pathol*, **66**, 139–144.

Kinnby, B., Lecander, I. and Martinsson, G. (1991) Tissue plasminogen activator and placental plasminogen activator inhibitor in human gingival fluid. *Fibrinolysis*, **5**, 239–242.

Kjaeldgaard, A. and Kjaeldgaard, M. (1986) Immunological characterization of plasminogen activators in human mixed saliva. *Acta Physiol Scand*, **126**, 443–447.

Kjaeldgaard, M. and Kjaeldgaard, A. (1987) Immunological characterization of plasminogen activators in human parotid saliva. *Arch Oral Biol* **32**, 855–857.

Kjaeldgaard, A., Kjaeldgaard, M. and Gaffney, P. (1989) Presence of a fast-acting specific inhibitor of plasminogen in human parotid saliva. *Acta Physiol Scand*, **137**, 379–383.

Kjaeldgaard, M., Lagerlöf, F. and Kjaeldgaard, A. (1989) Effect of flow rate on tissue plasminogen activator activity in human parotid saliva. *Arch Oral Biol*, **34**, 621–623.

Lewis, B. (1973) Dental care in the hemophiliac. *JADA*, **87**, 1411–1415.

Lowe, G.D.O. and Small, M. (1988) Stimulation of endogenous fibrinolysis, in *Tissue-type Plasminogen Activator (t-PA): Physiological and Clinical Aspects*, vol. II (ed. C. Kluft), CRC Press, Boca Raton, 129–169.

Luke, K.H. (1992) Comprehensive care for children with bleeding disorders – a physician's perspective. **58**, 115–118.

McIntyre, H., Nour-Eldin, F., Israel, M.C.G. and Wilkinson, J.F. (1959) Dental extractions in patients with haemophilia and Christmas disease. *Lancet*, **2**, 642–646.

McKown, C.G. and Shapiro, A.D. (1991) Oral management of patients with bleeding disorders. Part 2: Dental considerations. *JIDA*, **70**, 16–21.

Mannucci, P.M. (1986) Desmopressin (DDAVP) for treatment of disorders of hemostasis. *Prog Hemost Thromb*, **8**, 19–45.

Mannucci, P.M., Ruggeri, Z.M., Pareti, F.I. and Capitanio, A. (1977) 1-Deamino-8-D-arginine-vasopressin: a new pharmacological approach to the management of haemophilia and von Willebrand's disease. *Lancet*, **1**, 869–872.

Mannucci, P.M., Fedrici, A., Vigano, S. and Cattaneo, M. (1979) Multiple dental extractions with a new prothrombin complex concentrate in two patients with factor VIII inhibitors. *Thromb Res*, **15**, 359–364.

Marder, V.J. and Shulman, N.R. (1966) Major surgery in classic hemophilia using fraction I. Experience in twelve operations and review of the literature. *Am J Med*, **41**, 56–75.

Mariani, G., Ciavarella, N., Mazzucconi, M.G. *et al.* (1984) Evaluation of the effectiveness of DDAVP in surgery and in bleeding episodes in haemophilia and von Willebrand's disease. A study of 43 patients. *Clin Lab Haematol*, **6**, 229–238.

Maycock, W.'dA., Evans, S., Vallet, L. *et al.* (1963) Further experience with a concentrate containing human antihaemophilic factor. *Br J Haematol*, **9**, 215–235.

Michaelides, L. (1983) Die ambulante Behandlung von Hämophilie-Patienten mit Parodontalerkran-kungen. *Int J Parodontol Restaur Zahnheilkunde*, **5**, 65–73.

Moody, G.H. (1982) The source of plasminogen activator in human saliva. *Arch Oral Biol*, **27**, 33–37.

Nakai, T.R., Peterson J.C. Jr., and Law, D.B. (1974) Current concepts in the management of the hemophilic pedodontic patient. *J Dent Child*, **31**–36.

Nakajima, T., Tomizawa, M., Hasegawa, S. *et al.* (1978) Topical application of antihemophilic factor after dental extractions in hemophilic patients. *J Oral Surg*, **36**, 873–877.

Niessner, H. and Korninger, C. (1983) 1-Deamino-8-D-arginine-vasopressin – an alternative in the management of mild haemophilia A and von Willebrand's disease. *Wien Klin Wochenschr*, **95**, 753–757.

Ogston, D. (1984) *Antifibrinolytic Drugs. Chemistry, Pharmacology and Clinical Usage*, John Wiley, Chichester.

Orr, J.A. and Douglas, A.S. (1957) Dental extraction in haemophilia and Christmas Disease. *Br Med J*, **1**, 1035–1039.

Pizzoni, D., Coitellaro, M. and Mannucci, P.M. (1973) Replacement therapy and local measures for dental extractions in haemophiliacs: a comparison of various schemes of treatment. *Excerpta Med*, **252**, 242–244.

Preston, F.E., Dinsdale, R.C.W., Sutcliffe, D.J. *et al.* (1977) Factor VIII inhibitor by-passing activity (Feiba) in the management of patients with factor VIII inhibitors. *Thromb Res*, **11**, 643–651.

Rakocz, M., Mazar, A., Varon, D. *et al.* (1993) Dental extractions in patients with bleeding disorders. *Oral Surg Oral Med Oral Pathol*, **75**, 280–282.

Ramström, G. (1975) Fibrinolytic activity in the saliva of patients with coagulation disorders. *Swed Dent J*, **68**, 49–54.

Ramström, G. (1984) Contamination of oral wounds with saliva and bacteria. *Scand J Haematol*, **33** (suppl. 40), 423–427.

Ramström, G. and Blombäck, M. (1975) Tooth extractions in hemophiliacs. *Int J Oral Surg*, **4**, 1–17.

Ramström, G., Blombäck, M., Egberg, N. *et al.* (1989) Oral surger in patients with hereditary bleeding disorders. A survey of treatment in the Stockholm area. (1974–1985) *Int J Oral Maxillofac Surg*, **18**, 320–322.

Ramström, G., Sindet-Pedersen, S., Hall, G. *et al.* (1993) Prevention of post-surgical bleeding in oral surgery using tranexamic acid without dose modification of oral anticoagulants. *J Oral Maxillofac Surg*, **51**, 1211–1216.

Redding, S.W. and Stiegler, K.E. (1983) Dental management of the classic hemophiliac with inhibitors. *Oral Surg Oral Med Oral Pathol*, **56**, 145–148.

Reid, W.O., Lucas, O.N., Francisco, J. *et al.* (1964). The use of epsilonaminocproic acid in the management of dental extractions in the hemophiliac. *Am J Med Sci*, **248**, 184–188.

Rizza, C.R. (1980) Inhibitors of fibrinolysis in the treatment of haemophilia in (ed. J.F. Davidson) Fibrinolysis and its inhibition. *J Clin Pathol*, **33** (suppl. 14), 50–54.

Roberts, H.R., and Cromartie, R. (1984) Overview of inhibitors to factor VIII and IX, in *Factor VIII Inhibitors* (ed. L.W Hoyer), Alan R. Liss, New York, pp. 1–18.

Rodeghiero, F., Castaman, G., Giustolisi, R. and Mariani, G. (1993) Multicentre evaluation of a new concentrated desmopressin preparation (Emosint) administered intravenously or subcutaneously: analysis of biological responses and side-effects in 49 patients with hemophilia A and von Willebrand's Disease, in *Desmopressin in Bleeding Disorders* (eds G. Mariani, P.M. Mannucci, Cattaneo), NATO ASI Series, Series A: Life Sciences, Life Sciences, vol. 242, Plenum Press, New York, pp. 261–266.

Saulnier, J., Marey, A., Horellou, M.H. *et al.* (1994) Evaluation of desmopressin for dental extraction in patients with hemostatic disorders. *Oral Surg Oral Med Oral Pathol*, **77**, 6–12.

Saunders, S. (1982) A management perspective in the treatment of hemophilia. *Dent Hygiene*, **56**, 32–39.

Scharrer, I. (1982) Multiple dental extractions with Feiba in a patient with factor VIII inhibitor, in *Activated Prothrombin Complex Concentrates. Managing Hemophilia with Factor VIII Inhibitor* (eds G. Mariani, M.A. Russo, F. Mandelli), Praeger, New York, pp. 180–181.

Schmid, J. and Chambers, D.A. (1989) Molecular characterization of plasmino-gen activator in human supragingival plaque. *Arch Oral Biol*, **34**, 17–21.

Schulte, W. and Vorbauer, J. (1965) Fibrinolytische Effeke beim Kontakt von Speichel und Blut. *Dtsch Zahn Mund Kieferheilkd Zentrabl Gesamte*, **44**, 23–36.

Shurafa, M. and MacIntosh, R.B. (1987) Management of dental extractions in two hemophilia A patients with factor VIII inhibitor. *J Oral Maxillofac Surg*. **45**, 698–701

Sindet-Pedersen, S. (1987) Distribution of tranexamic acid to plasma and saliva after oral administration and mouth rinsing: a pharmacokinetic study. *J Clin Pharmacol*, **27**, 1005–1008.

Sindet-Pedersen, S. (1991) Haemostasis in oral surgery – the possible pathogenetic implications of oral fibrinolysis on bleeding. Experimental and clinical studies of the haemostatic balance in the oral cavity with particular reference to patients with acquire and congenital defects of the coagulation system.

Sindet-Pedersen, S., Gram, J. and Jespersen, J. (1987) Characterization of plasminogen activators in unstimulated and stimulated human whole saliva. *J Dent Res*, **66**, 1199–1203.

Sindet-Pedersen, S., Ingerslev, J., Ramström, G. and Blombäck, M. (1988a) Management of oral bleeding in haemophilic patients. *Lancet*, **2**, 566.

Sindet-Pedersen, S., Ingerslev, J., Ramström, G. and Blombäck, M. (1989a) Management of oral bleeding in haemophilic patients. *Lancet*, **1**, 325.

Sindet-Pedersen, S., Ramström, G., Bernvil, S. and Blombäck, M. (1989b) Hemostatic effect of tranexamic acid mouthwash in anticoagulant-treated patients undergoing oral surgery. *N Engl J Med*, **320**, 840–843.

Sindet-Pedersen, S., Gram, J. and Jespersen, J. (1990) The possible role of oral epithelial cells in tissue-type plasminogen activator (t-PA) related fibrinolysis in human saliva. *J Dent Res.* **69**, 1283–1286.

Sindet-Pedersen, S. and Stenbjerg, S. and Ingerslev, J., (1987) Treatment of bilateral fracture of the mandible in a hemophilic patient with inhibitor to factor VIII. *J Oral Maxillofac Surg*, **45**, 537–540.

Sindet-Pedersen, S., Stenjerg, S. and Ingerslev, J. (1988) Control of gingival hemorrhage in hemophilic patients by inhibition of fibrinolysis with tranexamic acid. *J Periodont Res*, **23**, 72–4.

Sindet-Pedersen, S., Stenbjerg, S., Ingerslev, J. and Karring, T. (1988) Surgical treatment of severe periodontitis in a hemophilic patient with inhibitors to factor VIII. Report of a case. *J Clin Periodontol*, **15**, 636–638.

Sixma, J.J. and Van den Berg, A. (1984) The haemostatic plug in haemophilia A: a morphological study of haemostatic plug formation in bleeding time skin wounds of patients with severe haemophilia A *Br J Haematol*, **58**, 741–753.

Snyder, D.T. and Penner, J.A. (1970) Preventive and restorative dental care for the hemophiliac. *J Mich Dent Assoc* **52**, 6–8.

Sonis, L. and Musselman, R.J. (1982) Oral bleeding in classic hemophilia. *Oral Surg Oral Med Oral Pathol*, **53**, 363–366.

Southam, J.C. (1981) Autographic study of fibrinolytic activity of rat oral epithelium. *Arch Oral Biol*, **26**, 831–835.

Stajcic, Z. (1985) The combined local/systemic use of antifibrinolytics in hemophiliacs undergoing dental extractions. *Int J Oral Surg*, **14**, 339–345.

Steinberg, S., Levin, J. and Bell, W.R. (1984) Evidence that less replacement therapy is required for dental extractions in hemophiliacs. *Am J Hematol*, **16**, 1–13.

Steinle, C.J. and Kisker, C.T. (1970) Pediatric dentistry for the child with hemophilia. *N Engl J Med*, **283**, 1325–1326.

Suzuki, H., Takeuchi, M., Sumi, Y. *et al.* (1983) Local haemostasis for oral bleeding in patients with coagulopathy. *Lancet*, **2**, 1362–1363.

Tavenner, R.W.H. (1968) Epsilon-aminocaproic acid in the treatment of haemophilia and Christmas disease with special reference to the extraction of teeth. *Br Dent J*, **124**, 19–22.

Taylor, R.G., Doku, H.C. and Romero, J. (1964) Direct determination of fibrinolytic activity of human saliva. *J Dent Res*, **43**, 86–91.

Törteli, A. (1967) Untersuchungen über die fibrinolytische Wirkung des Speichels. *Dtsch Stomatol*, **17**, 96–107.

Ublansky, J.H. (1992) Comprehensive dental care for children with bleeding disorders – a dentist's perspective. **58**, 111–114.

Vinckier, F. and Vermylen, J. (1985) Dental extractions in hemophilia: reflections on 10 years experience. *Oral Surg Oral Med Oral Pathol*, **59**, 6–9.

Wahl, G. and Budde, U. (1982) Oralchirurgische Eingriffe beim von Willebrand-Jürgens Syndrom. *Dtsch Zahnartzl Z*, **37**, 33–38.

Walsh, P.N., Rizza, C.R., Matthews, J.M. *et al.* (1971) Epsilon-aminocaproic acid therapy for dental extractions in haemophilia and Chrismas disease: a double blind controlled trial. *Br J Haematol*, **20**, 463–475.

Walsh, P.N., Rizza, C.R., Evans, B.E. and Aledort, L.M. (1975) The therapeutic role of epsilon-aminocaproic acid (EACA) for dental extractions in hemophiliacs. *Ann NY Acad Sci*, **240**, 267–276.

Warrier, A.I. and Lusher, J.M. (1983) DDAVP: a useful alternative to blood components in moderate hemophilia A and von Willebrand disease. *J Pediatr*, **102**, 228–233.

Webster, P. and Roberts, H.R. (1970) Dental treatment of patients with hemorrhagic disorders, in *The Hemophiliac and His World*, Karger, Basel, pp. 139–148.

Webster, P., Roberts, H.R. and Penick, G. (1968) Dental care of patients with hereditary disorders of blood coagulation. *Mod Treat*, 93–110.

Wefers, H., Körbner, I., Arends, P. and Sutor, A.H. (1981) Zahnärztlich-chirurgische Eingriffe bei Hämophilie, v. Willebrand-Jürgens-Syndrom und Thrombozytenfunktionsstörung unter Verwendung von Fibrinkleber und DDAVP. *Dtsch Z Mund Kiefer Gesichtschir*, **5**, 311–317.

Wepner, F., Bukal, J. and Beck-Mannagetta, J. (1979) Über die Anwendung des Fibrinklede systems im dentoalveolären Bereich bei hämorrhagischen Diathesen. *Dtsch Z Mund Kiefer Gesichtschir*, **3**, 46S–49S.

Wepner, F., Fries, R. and Platz, H. (1982) The use of the fibrin adhesion system for local hemostasis in oral surgery. *J Oral Maxillofac Surg*, **40**, 555–558.

Williams, B.J. (1992) Modified orthodontic treatment goals in a patient with multiple complicating factors. *Special Care Dentistry*, **12**, 251–254.

Williamson, R. and Eggleston, D.J. (1988) DDAVP and EACA used for minor oral surgery in von Willebrand disease. *Aust Dent J*, **33**, 32–36.

Wishart, C., Smith, C.A., Honey, G.E. and Taylor, K.B. (1957) Dental extraction in haemophilia. *Lancet*, **2**, 363–366.

Wörner, H. (1972) Operative Eingriffe am Kiefer bei Kranken mit Hämophilie. *Dtsch Med Wochenschr*, **97**, 1182–1187.

Wutka, P. (1978) Erfahrungen mit dem Fibrinklebesystem bei der Versorgung von Extraktionswunden Hämophiler Patienten. *Osterr Z Stomatol*, **75**, 450–452.

Wünschmann-Henderson, B. and Astrup, T. (1972) Relation of fibrinolytic activity in human oral epithelial cells to cellular maturation: the influence of smoking. *J Pathol*, **108**, 293–301.

10 MUSCULOSKELETAL BLEEDING IN HEMOPHILIA

R. Madhok

Recurrent musculoskeletal bleeding is the most frequent manifestation of severe hemophilia. Most patients with a moderately severe deficiency will have had a muscle or joint bleed and virtually all those with a severe deficiency have repeated spontaneous hemarthrosis and muscle hematoma. The resulting arthritis, combined with muscle contractures, is the main cause of disease-related morbidity and need for clotting factor concentrate transfusion (Arnold and Hilgartner 1977; Plate 1). No other site of hemophilic bleeding matches the suffering from pain and disability as well as the financial cost in management.

With the availability of clotting factor concentrates, there have been substantial changes both in the natural history and management of hemophilic arthritis. First, with home therapy, prompt treatment with clotting factor concentrates appears to have delayed rather than avoided the onset of degenerative arthritis (Guenthner *et al.*, 1980). With prophylactic treatment there is accumulating evidence that the chronic arthritis is avoidable (Nilsson *et al.*, 1992, Aledort *et al.*, 1995). Second, in patients with established arthritis, treatment strategies used in other types of arthritis can be adapted to manage end-stage chronic hemophilic arthritis. Third, the treatment of chronic hemophilic synovitis remains uncertain.

In this chapter the clinical features, pathogenesis and management of musculoskeletal bleeding in hemophilia are reviewed.

History of hemophilic arthritis

The association between joint disease and hemophilia was recognized as a feature of the disease in several of the early descriptions, including that by Otto in 1803. The credit of attributing intra-articular bleeding as the cause of joint swelling in hemophilia was first postulated by Dubois in 1838. However, this was not the prevailing view. Lane (1840), for example, who was the first to use blood to treat bleeding in hemophilia, regarded gout as a cause and Grandidier in 1855 also considered gout and rheumatism as an explanation.

Proof that blood may be causative was provided by Assman in 1869; he aspirated blood from a swollen joint. In the same year Reinert (1869) described blood discharging from a hemophiliac's shoulder that was also infected. Poncet (1871) confirmed the association in a pathologic study of a boy who died of bleeding subsequent to an arthrotomy for knee swelling.

Legg (1872) gave the earliest and most erudite description of the joint disease in hemophilia when he described five hemophiliacs under his care and reviewed the published literature. He not only described the joints most commonly affected but also the three stages of the joint involvement and considered arthritis as a diagnostic feature of hemophilia. This work finally dismissed the view that gout was a cause of the arthritis. A conservative non-surgical approach to managing the arthritis was advocated by Legg (1872). Finlayson (1882) from the Western Infirmary in Glasgow described arthritis in three generations of a family with hemophilia in 1882.

Konig (1892), after operating on two patients, wrote an authoritative description of the pathologic changes in affected joints. Interestingly, his preoperative diagnosis was tuberculosis. He, like Legg, proposed three distinct stages in the evolution of the joint disease, advised conservative measures in the treatment and strongly cautioned against surgery and the use of leeches.

Several other authors also contributed: Shaw (1897) in the UK described a single patient with chronic hemophilic arthritis of the elbows and knees. He also aspirated blood from his patient's joint as well as providing the earliest description of the radiological features. Ryerson

Hemophilia. Edited by C.D. Forbes, L. Aledort and R. Madhok. Published in 1997 by Chapman & Hall, London. ISBN 0 412 63820 7

(1906) was the first to describe the findings in the North American literature.

Jordan's (1958) pioneering work in the rehabilitation of hemophiliacs with chronic arthritis by adopting approaches such as the Quengel brace (which was at that time of value in those who had survived the ravages of acute poliomyelitis infection) established the basis for further work in managing chronic hemophilic arthritis.

Why do hemophiliacs bleed into joints?

Any explanation for the frequent occurrence of bleeding into joints must reconcile not only why joint bleeds are so frequent compared to other sites, but also the predisposition of the knees, ankles and elbows to bleeding relative to other joints.

No single factor provides a satisfactory explanation. Anatomical, biochemical as well as mechanical factors all probably contribute to the initial bleed as well as to the persistence of the arthritis.

The presentation of joint bleeding at the time the child starts to weight-bear, the more frequent occurrence of bleeds into the lower than the upper limbs and the presence of more severe arthritis on the dominant side strongly suggest that mechanical factors are important. The more frequent occurrence of bleeds into hinge rather than the ball-and-socket joints further suggests that mechanical factors are important.

Bleeding probably arises from the subsynovial plexus of capillaries that form numerous loops at the juxta-cavitary surface of the joint (Davies and Edwards, 1948). These capillaries differ from the deeper subsynovial capillaries in that they are fenestrated to allow rapid exchange of solutes and water (Levick and Sinaje, 1987), a feature that may also predispose to bleeding. There is no obvious difference in the ultrastructure of synovium between those joints predisposed to bleeding. However, the overall arrangement of synovium in the knee, ankle and elbow into a pleated membrane with recesses and pouches (rather than a sleeve-like covering, as in the hip and shoulder) may make the synovium of these joints more vulnerable to mechanical entrapment and injury.

The absence of thromboplastic activity in synovium (Harrold, 1961) combined with the deficiency in the extrinsic pathway coagulation, may also contribute to joint bleeding.

Although normal synovium has some fibrinolytic activity, Pandolfi *et al.* (1972) reported that synovium obtained from hemophiliacs undergoing synovectomy has an increased fibrinolytic potential. This may perpetuate bleeding in a joint in which recurrent hemarthosis has previously occurred.

What remains unexplained is why some hemophiliacs, despite a similar deficiency in circulating factor levels, have less frequent hemarthrosis (Rainsford and Hall, 1975). There is no difference between hemophiliacs in joint laxity (Patrick *et al.*, 1982) but, in one study (Bern *et al.*, 1979), height irrespective of age was directly related to the frequency of hemarthrosis. Psychological adjustment may be important but no formal studies have been undertaken.

Clinical features of hemophilic arthritis

There are three sequential stages in the progression of hemophilic arthritis: acute hemarthrosis, chronic synovitis and degenerative change.

ACUTE HEMARTHROSIS

The severity of circulating factor deficiency correlates directly with the frequency of joint bleeding. Although bleeding can occur into any diarthrodial joint, the knees, elbows and ankles of the dominant side are the most frequent sites. The diagnosis of an acute hemarthrosis in a known hemophiliac is not difficult. Most patients are aware of a bleed before any clinical signs are present and prior to the characteristic acute pain. The premonitory symptoms vary between patients. With bleeding into the joint cavity, the joint is swollen, held in flexion and its use limited.

Difficulties in diagnosis may arise in distinguishing a hip hemarthrosis from an iliopsoas or gluteal hematoma and in those with chronic arthritis. The patient with chronic arthritis is often not able to distinguish an acute exacerbation of arthritic pain from a hemarthrosis and clinical examination is of limited value as the fibrosed joint capsule will contain bleeding and swelling may be absent.

In the absence of trauma, no further investigations are necessary to confirm the diagnosis. An X-ray to exclude a fracture may be necessary if significant trauma is suspected. To detect soft tissue injuries such as ligamentous or meniscial damage, the resolution offered by magnetic resonance imaging may be more helpful. In human immunodeficiency virus type 1 (HIV-l)-positive patients, a septic arthritis needs to be considered and, if suspected, arthrocentesis is indicated.

CHRONIC SYNOVITIS

The onset of this stage can be difficult to date. In a few patients the synovitic stage may arise after a large hemarthrosis or one inadequately treated. As with acute hemarthrosis, the most frequently affected joints are the knees, ankles and elbows. The involved joint is often the target of previous bleeds.

The clinical features arise due to a cycle of bleeding leading to synovitis that predisposes to further bleeds. Presentation is with a persistently swollen joint that is

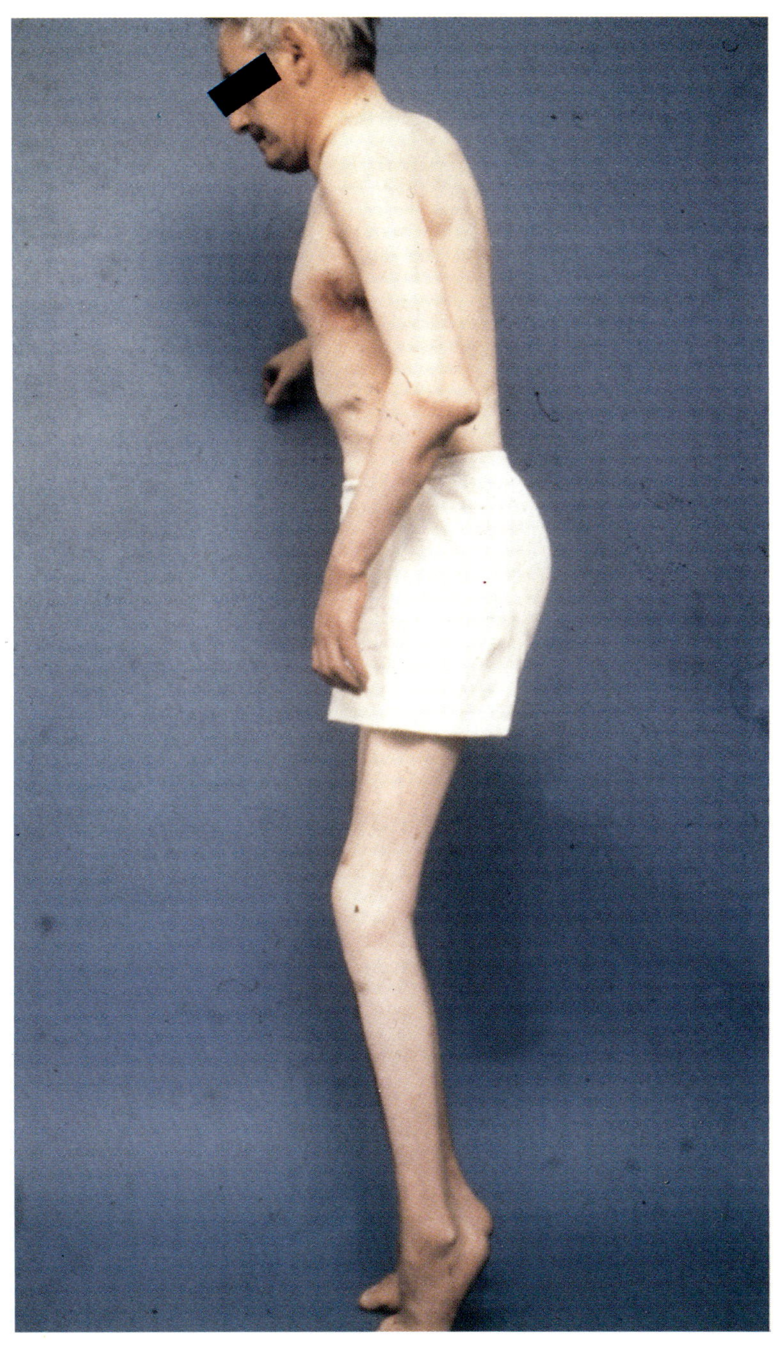

Plate 1 Patient with severe hemophilic arthritis and muscle contractures leading to equinus deformities.

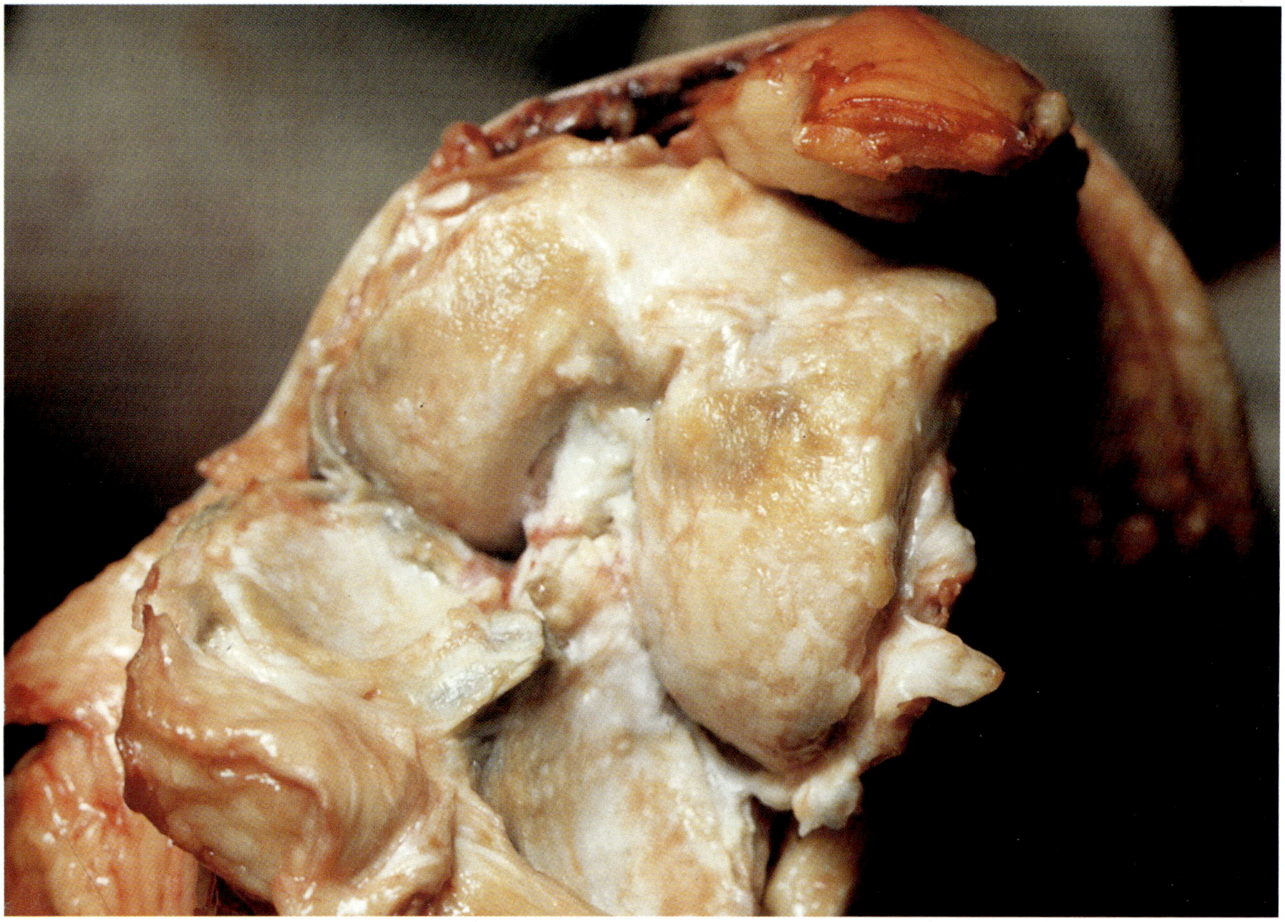

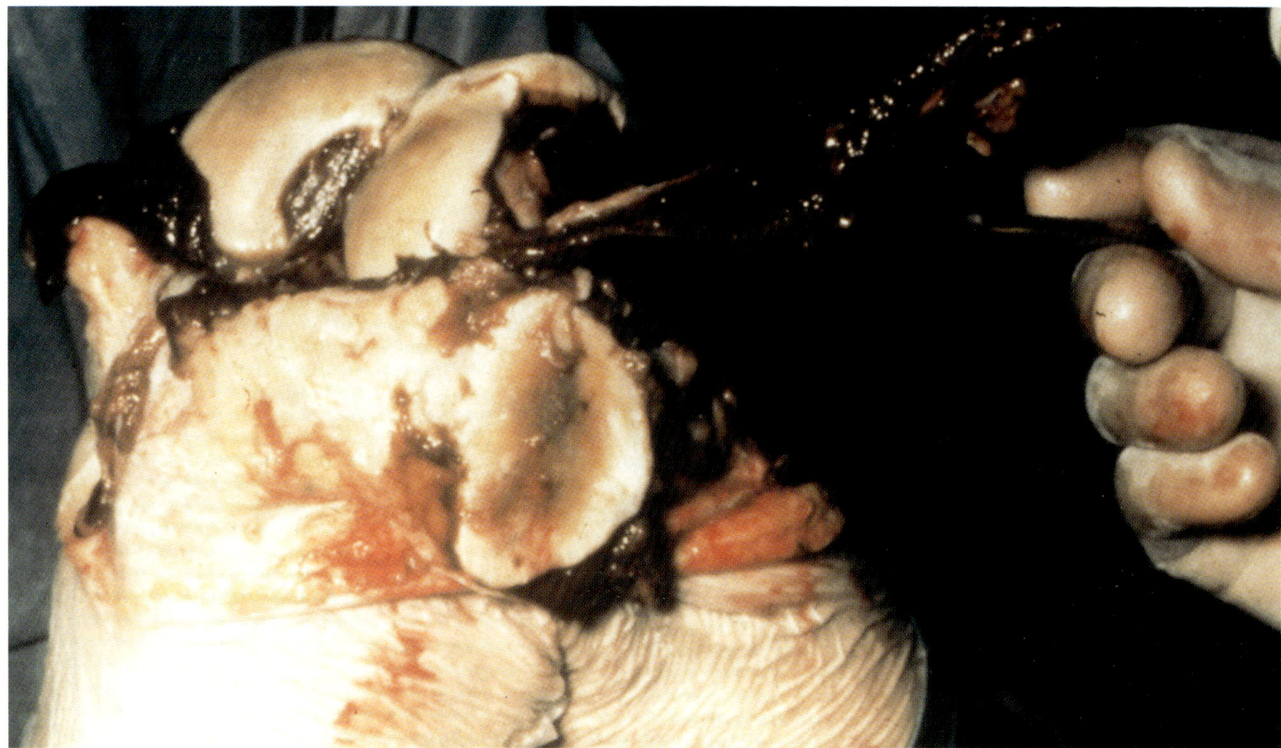

Plate 2   Pitting and gross erosion of cartilage, exposing underlying chondral bone seen at arthroplasty of the knee joint.

Plate 3   Synovial proliferation and staining of the synovium and cartilage by hemosiderin seen in a knee joint during surgery.

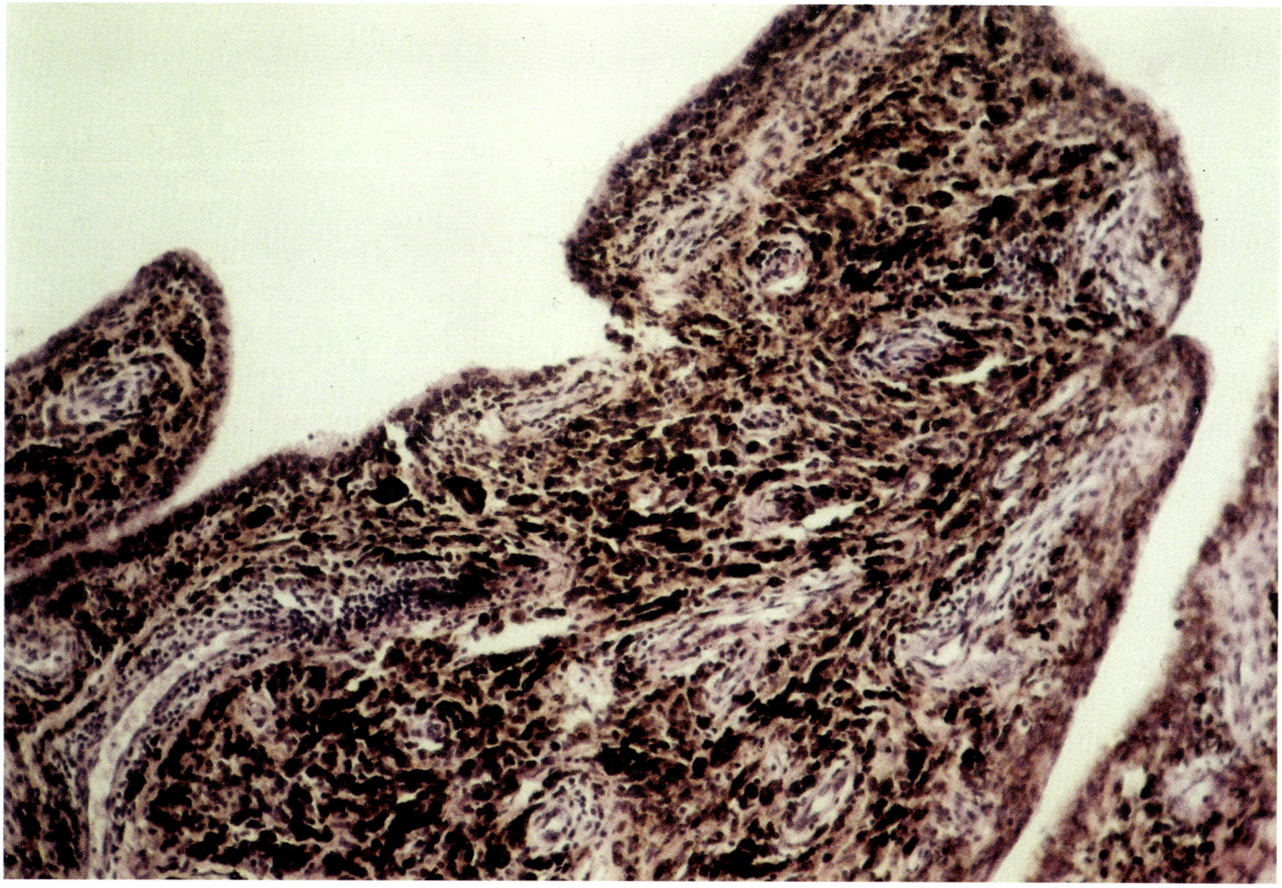

Plate 4   Microscopic view of the villous proliferation of synovium. There is marked synovicite hypertrophy and increased vascularity of the synovium. (Hematoxylin and eosin staining.)

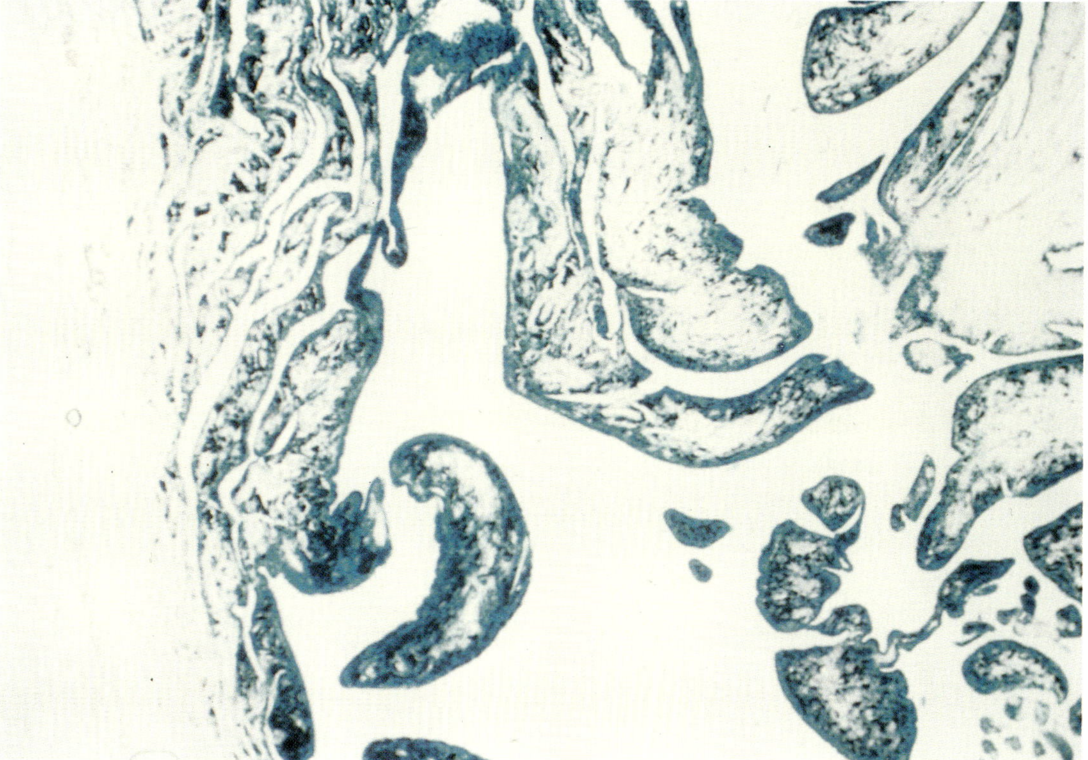

Plate 5   Microscopic view of the synovium showing the synovial and subsynovial iron deposition. (Prussian blue stain.)

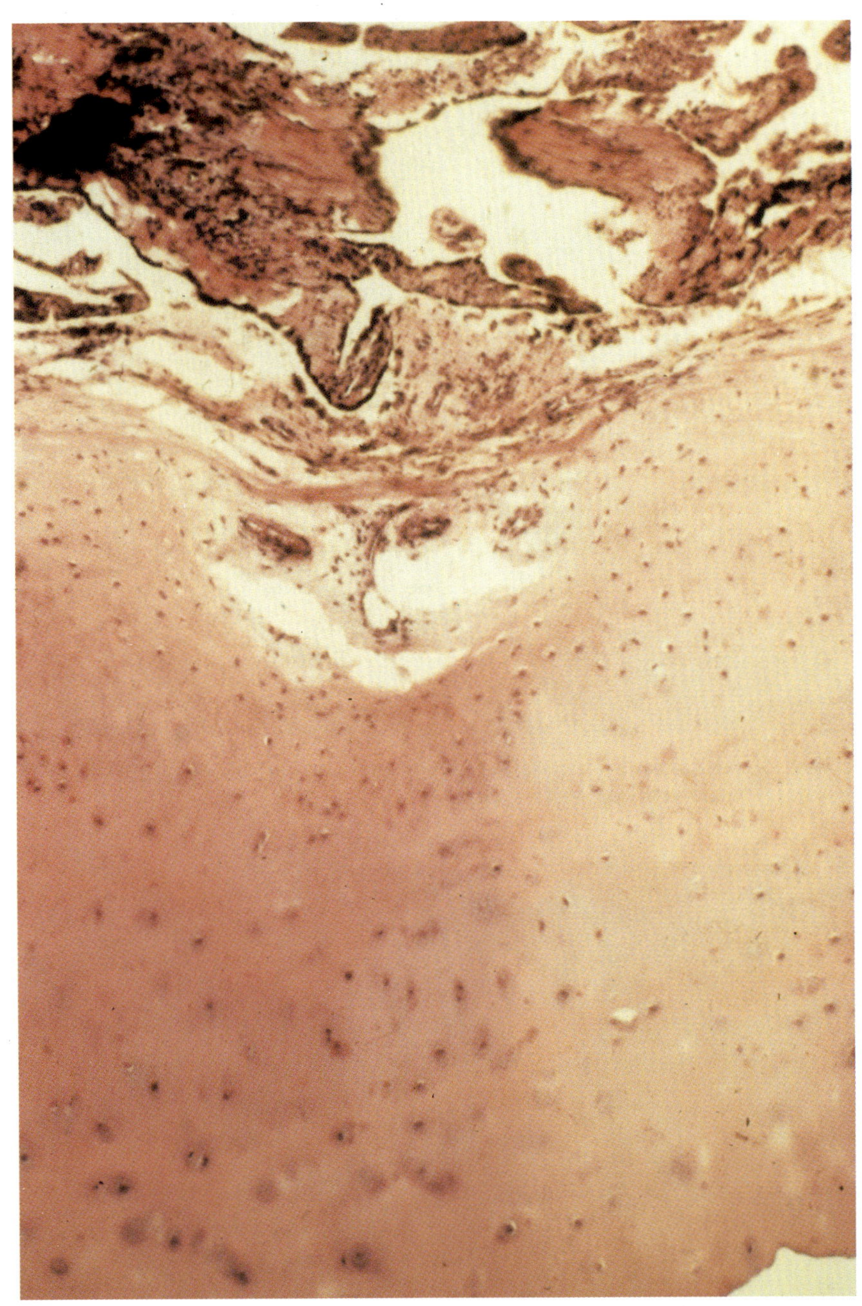

Plate 6 Microscopic view of the cartilage showing chondrocyte irregularity and erosion of the surface by overlying pannus formation. (Hematoxylin and eosin staining.)

painless or only intermittently painful. The pain is usually less severe than that of an acute hemarthrosis. Swelling is due to synovitis as well as an effusion. Wasting of the periarticular muscles may be present, with no significant limitation in the range of movement. The history and clinical findings establish the diagnosis. X-rays are useful in defining the extent of cartilage erosion and bone damage rather than in making the diagnosis.

The synovitic stage often persists for months to years and the size of the effusion may fluctuate depending on the amount of intra-articular bleeding. Fibrotic tissue eventually supervenes in the areas of synovial hyperplasia.

DEGENERATIVE ARTHRITIS

An arbitrary definition of degenerative arthritis is the persistence of chronic synovitis for more than 6 months (Arnold and Hilgartner, 1977). The late clinical features are those of an end-stage joint due to synovitis from any cause (Plate 2). The deformities in hemophilia are, however, more severe because the destructive process has its onset before the epiphyses have fused and because of the presence of muscle contractures due to previous muscle hematomas and disuse atrophy.

The earliest radiological sign of degenerative arthritis is loss of joint space. As cartilage loss progresses, secondary osteoarthritic changes supervene. This is radiologically manifest as subchondral sclerosis and cyst formation as well as the presence of osteophytes at the joint margin.

In developed countries there are two overlapping groups of hemophilic patients with chronic or degenerative arthritis. In the first group are patients who were teenagers or young adults when cryoprecipitate or clotting concentrates became available and therefore already had established arthritis in several joints. The second group consists of patients, now in their late 20s and 30s, in whom bleeding episodes were treated on a demand basis and who are now showing evidence of chronic arthritis in one or two joints.

Pathology of hemophilic arthritis

Several of the early descriptions of arthritis in hemophilia included the morphologic changes. A better understanding of the pathogenesis has only recently been acquired. It has its foundations in the descriptive pathology of joint disease in dogs with hemophilia (Swanton, 1959). The early changes were described in studies on synovium obtained from individuals with traumatic hemarthrosis but without hemophilia (Roy and Ghadially, 1966). Detailed descriptive and functional studies on synovium from hemophiliacs obtained at surgery have characterized some of the mediators of cartilage damage (Mainardi *et al.*, 1978; Stein and Duthie 1981; McLardy-Smith *et al.*, 1984). Experimental animal work in which autologous

blood is repeatedly injected into the joint has provided an insight into the mechanism of cartilage damage (Madhok *et al.*, 1988). To appreciate fully the extent and the nature of change in hemophilic synovium requires first a brief description of normal synovium.

NORMAL SYNOVIUM

Normal adult synovium is a relatively acellular tissue with two distinct layers. The intima or synovial lining is usually only one to three cell layers thick. It does not function as a true boundary of the joint cavity as the cells are only loosely attached to each other and lack a basement membrane. Two distinct types of synovicytes are present. Type A cells are macrophage-like and probably of bone marrow origin, whereas type B cells have a fibroblast cell-like morphology and are of presumed mesenchymal origin. They possess a prominent secretory machinery and synthesize primarily glycosaminoglycans like hyaluronic acid that provides the lubricant properties to synovial fluid.

The subintimal layer is acellular and contains fat cells, fibroblasts which are morphologically different from the type B synovicites and scattered blood vessels. The matrix proteins include fibronectin, collagen and proteoglycans.

ACUTE HEMARTHROSIS

The earliest pathologic finding of an intra-articular bleed is the presence of small hemorrhages usually within synovial villi (Swanton, 1959). These apparently never coalesce into hematoma but rupture into the joint cavity (Swanton, 1959). An acute inflammatory infiltrate may surround larger intrasynovial hemorrhages (Swanton, 1959). After the first 3–4 days, intra-articular blood provokes a mild perivascular inflammatory response (Roy and Ghadially, 1967). The initial inflammatory exudate consists primarily of neutrophils, after which mononuclear cells predominate (Roy and Ghadially, 1967). Radionucleotide studies in hemophiliacs with hemarthrosis indicate that the inflammatory response is often slow to resolve (Forbes *et al.*, 1972). In parallel with the inflammatory response, there is hyperplasia and hypertrophy of type B synovicytes manifest as villous projections into the joint space (Roy and Ghadially, 1967).

Type A cells phagocytose erythrocytes sequestered within the joint cavity, while others pass between the synovial cells into the subintimal layer. The phagocytosed red cells are broken down into whorled membranous bodies and siderosomes, which are single-layer lysomes and contain iron in the form of hemosiderin. These are late changes and become more marked weeks after the hemarthrosis (Roy and Ghadially, 1967).

Macroscopically, the cartilage surface may appear normal but on electron microscopy iron also accumulates within the more superficial chondrocytes. These cells also show evidence of intracellular degeneration (Hough, Banfield and Sokoloff, 1976). The mechanism by which iron enters chondrocytes is not known.

CHRONIC SYNOVITIS

With repeated bleeds the synovial changes described during an acute hemarthrosis become more intense and the process at some point becomes self-perpetuating, with bleeding provoking a synovial reaction that results in further small intrasynovial hemorrhages as well as bleeding into the joint that results in a further synovial reaction.

Macroscopically, the synovial membrane thickens, and is nodular with friable synovial fronds projecting into the joint cavity discolored due to hemosiderin deposition (Plate 3). Over the central areas of cartilage there is deposition of brown pigment suggestive of iron. The microscopic changes include synovicyte hyperplasia (Plate 4), hemosiderosis (Plate 5), a marked angiomatous reaction and subintimal fibrosis.

The increase in cell numbers is due to marked type B synovicyte hyperplasia that is manifest as villous projections. At the cartilage–synovium junction the hyperplastic synovium is adherent to the joint margin and is described as pannus. The hemosiderosis is both intra- and extracellular and is present in both the intimal and subsynovial layers. The intracellular iron is contained within siderosomes that have the same morphology as those present during acute hemarthrosis but are occasionally larger (Stein and Duthie 1981). The macrophages containing iron have few organelles and those present are abnormal.

In the subsynovial layer there is a marked angiomatous reaction predisposing to further intrasynovial and intra-articular bleeding. Other changes include fibrosis that is proportional to the number of intra-articular bleeds (Roy and Ghadially, 1967). A perivascular inflammatory reaction is also present which, in experimental animal studies, consists of primarily mononuclear cells (Madhok *et al.*, 1988). In both experimental models (Madhok *et al.*, 1988) and hemophilic synovium (Andes *et al.*, 1984) immunofluoresence studies do not show immunoglobulin or complement deposits, which suggests that the changes are not antibody-mediated, as had been suggested (Arnold and Hilgartner, 1977)

DEGENERATIVE ARTHRITIS

In hemophilic arthritis, three overlapping mechanisms of cartilage damage appear to occur: superficial pannus, central degradation and deep marginal erosion (Madhok *et al.*, 1988). Pannus is the soft tissue that replaces the surface of cartilage encroaching it from the periphery (Plate 6). It is adherent to the cartilage surface and locally invasive. Histologically, the tissue consists of mesenchymal type cells, the precise origin of which is not clear.

In the central areas of the joint, the cartilage loss is multifactorial, probably initiated by sequestered neutrophils at the time of hemarthrosis. As synovium proliferates in response to repeated bleeds, the release of chondrolytic enzymes will also contribute. The intracellular accumulation of iron in chondrocytes (in the form of siderosomes and free ferritin granules in the cytoplasm) is also likely to play an important part.

Deep cartilage erosion with bone erosion occurs by several mechanisms. Soft tissue from the cartilage–synovium junction may undermine cartilage directly and may also occur at sites distant from the synovium by invasion through the subchondral plate.

Synovitis results in bone loss in two ways. The initial bone loss is periarticular which, in part, results from disuse and to the release of local bone-resorbing mediators released by inflamed synovium. With the persistence of synovitis, focal cortical bone erosions occur in the areas where synovium is contiguous with periostium. The synovitis eventually extends into spongy bone undermining the articular catilage surface. Bone replacement also occurs by the formation of cystic cavities below subchondral bone that communicate with the joint surface through a cartilage defect.

Several aspects of the pathogenesis of hemophilic arthritis however still remain unclear. First, the response of synovium to intra-articular blood is poorly understood; in particular, the blood components that initiate and perpetuate the synovitis are not known. Second, the mediators that result in cartilage breakdown need to be further defined. Third, the mechanisms by which chondrocytes take up iron is not yet explained.

Management of hemophilic arthritis

The main aims of treating hemophilic arthritis include symptom relief, prevention of the progression of the joint damage, and maintenance of function. These goals can be achieved by early treatment of hemarthrosis and by limiting the effects of chronic synovitis. In the patient with degenerative arthritis function can be improved by surgical and physical methods with adequate hemostatic cover.

ACUTE HEMARTHROSIS

Management of an acute hemarthrosis requires transfusion with clotting factor concentrates and provision of adequate analgesia. Replacement therapy should aim to achieve plasma levels of between 30 and 40% of normal for factor VIIIc-deficient patients (25–40 u/kg). For factor IX-deficient patients (20–30 u/kg), target levels of

20–30% of normal will cover most hemarthrosis. Shoulder and hip bleeds often require higher levels for more prolonged periods. Home therapy will allow earlier treatment of bleeds.

If there is a large tense hemarthrosis or if joint sepsis is suspected arthrocentesis may be necessary but does not slow the progression of hemophilic arthritis (Ingram, Matthews and Bennett, 1972). The procedure should only be performed by someone experienced in performing joint aspirates using an aseptic technique and only after adequate clotting factor concentrate replacement.

Systemic corticosteroid treatment has been evaluated in dampening the intra-articular inflammatory response after an acute hemarthrosis. The benefits are short lived but because of frequent side-effects their use is limited and not advocated (Kinker and Burke, 1970).

Pain is the main factor determining the rate at which activity is resumed. Mobilization should be encouraged once bleeding has stopped and the acute pain has subsided. Temporary immobilization with a splint is only appropriate if there is a significant flexion deformity to provide symptom relief. If a flexion contracture persists then its conservative correction may be necessary. In the knee, serial plaster-of-Paris splints, jet splinting or a Quengel cast are useful methods. Choice should be influenced by familiarity with the method and applied only after adequate clotting factor replacement. Ankle equinus contractures of recent onset can be corrected by serial splinting but if of longer duration surgery to the Achilles tendon may be appropriate.

CHRONIC SYNOVITIS

Chronic synovitis is due to a cycle of bleeding producing synovicyte hypertrophy that leads to further bleeding. Once established, the mainstay of treatment is to prevent further bleeding as well as consideration of measures to suppress synovicite proliferation.

Prophylactic clotting factor concentrate replacement may prevent further joint bleeding. To reduce the demand for clotting factor concentrate as well as to prevent further articular damage, surgical and radiochemical synovectomy have been tried. Storti *et al.* (1969) were the first group to use open synovectomy. Subsequently, several groups reported their short-term results (Pietrogrande, Dioguardi and Mannucci, 1972; Kay *et al.*, 1981; Mastuda and Duthie, 1984; Post *et al.*, 1986; Montage *et al.*, 1986). Comparisons of outcome are difficult to make because of the differences in patient selection. Most report a reduction in the use of clotting factor concentrates. One consequence is loss in the range of movement. Only one group (Traldi *et al.*, 1986) has reported their 20-year results in 89 patients and 266 joints (164 knees, 64 elbows, 55 ankles, 6 shoulders and 1 hip). The results show an improvement in the range of joint movement and in radiologic outcome as well as reduction in the number of hemarthrosis. The outcome was better in those patients operated on with no radiological damage. Disappointingly, these results are difficult to interpret fully because of the paucity of information in the report.

Arthroscopic synovectomy is a less traumatic procedure but there is a high incidence of postoperative hemorrhage. In the largest series of 20 knee synovectomies reported by Wiedel *et al.* (1986) from three centers, there was no significant loss in the range of joint movement in 12 patients, in five there was an improvement but in three patients significant postoperative complications arose with a loss in the range of movement that was significant enough to affect function.

The value of synovectomy in hemophilic arthritis is not resolved. Arguments against undertaking synovectomy include its questionable long-term value and a loss in the range of movement in some. These patients are difficult to identify prior to surgery and also in our experience there is patient reluctance to undergo the procedure. Other factors that probably have influenced the use of this procedure include the expanding role of reconstructive surgery and the availability of increasing amounts of clotting factor concentrates.

An alternative to surgical synovectomy used successfully by some centers is radiation synovectomy. The principle of this procedure is to place a β-emitting radiopharmaceutical into the joint to suppress the synovial response. A good to moderate response as assessed by the physician in charge is reported in most series (Deutsch, Brodeck and Deutsch, 1993). The limitations of this procedure include an unacceptable radiation exposure to the liver, spleen and draining inguinal lymph nodes. Despite this exposure, as yet no long-term consequences have been reported.

DEGENERATIVE ARTHRITIS

Management goals in the patient with degenerative arthritis include providing relief of symptoms and improving functional ability. These are best achieved by a team approach involving the input of several medical and paramedical groups. Our team, for example, in addition to the hemophilia consultant consists of a hemophilia nurse specialist, a dedicated physiotherapist, social worker, hematologist, rheumatologist and orthopedic surgeon. In our patient cohort two overlapping groups of patients with degenerative arthritis can be defined.

The typical patient with severe chronic arthritis in several joints is often between 40 and 60 years old, has a history of frequent muscle and joint bleeds and complains of chronic pain in several joints as well as stiffness and reduced functional ability. Adequate analgesia in this group can be difficult to provide and previous drug habituation (which complicates the assessment) may be important. Non-steroidal anti-inflammatory drugs may be a useful adjunct in those in whom stiffness is an additional symptom; several have been evaluated and are of value as well as safe in the short term. Most safety information is available for ibuprofen, which has the additional advantage of being the least likely to cause gastrointestinal damage; it has a flexible dosage regime as well as a short half-life (Steven *et al.*, 1985).

In those with severe pain in one joint, particularly if it disturbs sleep, orthopedic surgery may be of value. Such patients often have already adapted to their disability and rehabilitation with particular attention to altering their environment and provision of aids to maintain their independence are acceptable goals.

Reconstructive surgery including joint arthroplasties has been undertaken in hemophiliacs (Duthie and Dodd, 1994). Surgery should only be performed in a center with the facilities and experience in the postoperative care of hemophiliacs and by a surgeon with an interest in and an understanding of the difficulties faced by hemophiliacs. The long-term results of knee and hip arthroplasties are encouraging and comparable to those obtained in younger patients with other types of arthritis (Duthie and Dodd, 1994). The procedure of choice in hemophilic arthritis of the elbow is resection of the radial head with a limited synovectomy (Duthie and Dodd, 1994). For ankle arthritis, if non-surgical methods should fail, then fusion of the tibio-talar, including the subtalar joints if necessary, is the preferred option (Duthie and Dodd 1994).

The more challenging patient is the younger patient with pain and limited function in one joint that has been the focus of previous bleeds treated on a demand basis. Complicating the articular problems is the presence of chronic liver disease due to hepatitis C and immuno-deficiency due to HIV-1 infection. Experience in managing such patients is limited both in the outcome of the underlying infections and in the increased risk of postoperative and prosthesis infection.

Septic arthritis

Septic arthritis, although rare in hemophiliacs prior to the HIV-1 epidemic, was described (Houghton, 1977). The estimated incidence in one cohort was 0.05% (Goldsmith *et al.*, 1983). Its occurrence was attributed to the need for frequent venesection, poor venesection technique and the presence of more superficial sites of sepsis.

Coincident with HIV-1 infection in hemophiliacs septic arthritis is more frequently recognized (Bleasel, York and Richard, 1990; Gregg-Smith *et al.*, 1993). Infection in both prosthetic and non-prosthetic joints is described. The most frequently isolated organisms have been Gram-positive cocci, both *Staphylococcus aureus* and strepto-

cocci, although Gram-negative infections as well as more unusual organisms have been causative.

Differentiating septic arthritis from a hemarthrosis may be initially difficult and should be considered if there are concomitant constitutional symptoms to suggest infection. Pyrexia and failure of the acute symptoms to settle soon after treatment with clotting factor concentrate should further raise suspicion. X-rays in the early stages are not helpful except to rule out a fracture. The presence of a marked acute-phase response, such as a raised erythrocyte sedimentation rate, plasma viscosity or C-reactive protein level may help but is not diagnostic. Neutrophilia is not present in all cases but if it occurs in the presence of joint pain should lead to consideration of the diagnosis. If sepsis is suspected then aspiration of the joint for Gram stain and culture of the joint fluid is mandatory. In most but not all reported cases the causative organism can be isolated from venous blood cultures.

Specific initial management should consist of broad-spectrum antibiotics covering Gram-positive and negative organisms once the joint has been aspirated. Almost all tested antibiotics achieve satisfactory antimicrobial levels within an inflamed joint. Intra-articular administration of antibiotics is unnecessary and may cause a chemical synovitis.

Drainage of purulent joint effusions is an important component of the successful management of a septic arthritis. Initially closed needle aspiration may be necessary daily, when joint effusions accumulate except in the hip. Surgical intervention is advised only if serial synovial fluid culture is positive on culture.

During the acute phase the joint should be partially immobilized in a functional position, for example the knee should be kept extended by using an external splint. Mobilization should begin immediately the systemic symptoms have resolved and once there is objective evidence of the infection improving initially; muscle-strengthening exercises should be used, progressing from passive movement to active muscle resistance exercises.

The effect of clotting factor concentrates on the progression of hemophilic arthritis

Early studies in small cohorts of patients indicated that hemophilic arthritis was a progressive disorder despite early and adequate treatment of joint bleeds. Other work however indicated that early treatment resulted in a more favorable outcome. To resolve this issue a worldwide observational study using clinical and radiologic scores as the primary outcomes over 5 years was undertaken (Aledort *et al.*, 1995). Of 673 patients entered into the study, full clinical data were available on 477; 378 had initial and final X-rays and 300 had both clinical and radiological data. Mean patient age was 13.5 years, mean total hemorrhages per year were 23, the mean number of weeks on prophylaxis per year was 11 and mean annual dose of clotting factor concentrate was 1278 units.

The main conclusions of this study are:

1. The average number of hemarthroses per patient per year is 15 – that is, less than in previous surveys.
2. On physical examination in 55% of patients the joint disease is progressive, in 21% it remains the same and improves in the remainder. Clinical progression is independent of age, although with increasing age there is more clinical damage that is related to the number of joint bleeds but not to total number of bleeds. Radiologically, progression occurred in 76%, 18% remained the same and 6% improved. Radiologic progression occurs with increasing age and is related to total number of bleeds as well as number of joint bleeds.
3. Increasing clotting factor concentrate use results in a reduced need for hospitalization and days lost from work.
4. Full prophylaxis, that is, patients who received more than 45 weeks of prophylaxis per year, had less time off work, had a reduced need for hospitalization, as well as a favorable effect on the rate of progression of joint disease, both clinically and radiologically. Benefit was observed, even in those with pre-existing joint disease.
5. Intermediate prophylaxis is not better than no prophylaxis in influencing the clinical or radiographic progression of joint disease.
6. In those not receiving prophylaxis the optimal dose for treating a joint bleeds is 25–40 u/kg per bleed.
7. In a minority of patients with severe hemophilia there was no evidence of joint disease either clinically or radiologically at study onset. Half of these patients maintained joint integrity. Patients who progressed did not differ in age or total number of bleeds but had more joint bleeds and significantly fewer received prophylaxis.

Muscle bleeding in hemophilia

Muscle bleeding is the second most frequent cause of spontaneous bleeding in severe hemophilia. In addition to the morbidity their importance lies in the recognition that at some sites complications may arise. These may be potentially irreversible and further contribute to the musculoskeletal disability. Unlike intra-articular bleeding, which in the individual hemophiliac, often occurs repeatedly into a target joint, muscle bleeds occur at random.

FREQUENCY AND SITES OF MUSCLE BLEED

Prior to the more widespread availability of clotting factor concentrates, Favre Gilly (1964) observed that three-quarters of severe hemophiliacs had a significant hematoma and the frequency in any one individual was about two per year.

Muscle bleeds are more frequent in the lower limb, particularly in the ilacus and gluteal regions. In a two-year survey of 48 Spanish severe hemophiliacs admitted to hospital with a intramuscular bleed in whom the site of bleeding was accurately defined by muscle ultrasound, 27 occurred in the iliopsoas muscles, four in the gluteal, seven in the quadricep, seven in gastronemius, two in the forearm muscles and one in pectoralis major (Galindo *et al.*, 1985). The pattern was similar in a cohort followed by Duthie (1994) attending the Oxford hemophilia center.

PATHOLOGY

No detailed studies of the pathologic changes that follow bleeding into muscle in hemophiliacs are available. Duthie (1994) has however described both the early and late changes. Within a few hours of an intramuscular hematoma there is an acute inflammatory response which over time evolves to a fibrotic reaction. Although at the periphery of the bleed myocyte regeneration is present after a large hematoma, no significant regeneration occurs.

Using ultrasound, two types of intramuscular hematomas can be delineated – in the more frequent, blood spreads through the fascial planes and the borders are therefore more difficult to define. After large bleeds there may be a better defined mass consisting of a central cystic mass of unresorbed blood with a surrounding capsule of fibrous tissue.

CLINICAL FEATURES

The diagnosis of intramuscular hematoma in a hemophiliac is not difficult and, as with hemarthrosis, patients are often aware of bleeding before there are any signs. Pain is a later symptom than in hemarthrosis and its onset as well as severity is determined by the site of bleeding. In bleeding confined to a small muscle compartment, more acute and severe pain occurs for the same volume of blood compared to a more accommodating area. On examination, palpation will define the muscle mass, in the surrounding muscle groups, reflex spasm may also be present. Other important physical signs to determine include establishing that there is no associated vascular or neurologic compromise.

COMPLICATIONS

Both vascular and neurologic complications can occur due to muscle bleeding. Duthie (1994) from the Oxford hemophilia center has provided the most comprehensive long-term follow-up of muscle bleeding and its complications.

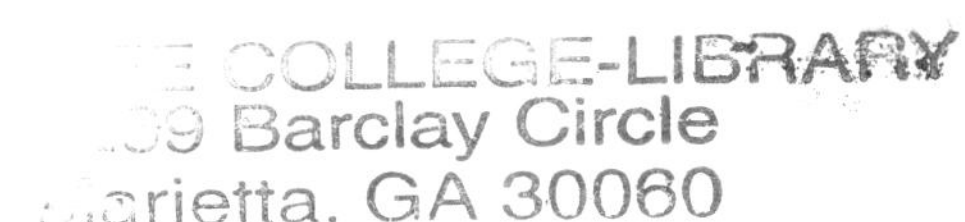

The study documents the outcome and complications of 70 intramuscular hematomas over 3 years in patients requiring inpatient care.

Neurological complications occurred in a third of patients. Of these, 51% were accounted for by femoral nerve palsies, 16% involved the median nerve and 12% the ulnar nerve. In 49% there was full functional recovery, in 21% there was a residual sensory loss and in 16% both a motor and sensory deficit persisted.

With large intramuscular hematomas of the forearm and calf, contractures are more likely to occur than in more proximal bleeds. In the Oxford series muscle contracture as well as neurologic involvement was present in approximately 50%. Bleeds into the more proximal muscle groups were less likely to result in contracture formation. In this cohort no patient developed vascular compromise.

MANAGEMENT

The management of intramuscular bleeding requires adequate replacement therapy with clotting factor concentrate as well as graded rehabilitation. During the acute phase the affected limb should be rested in a functional position and if necessary splinted. Mobilization should begin only when the hematoma has resolved rather than when the pain has subsided to prevent recurrence. If a peripheral nerve palsy is present mobilization should be delayed until there are clear clinical signs of neurologic recovery. Serial splinting may be necessary if a contracture is present.

References

Andes, W.E., Walker, P.D., Edmunds, J.O. and Wulff, K.M. (1984) Haemophilic arthropathy – an immunologic study of synovium. *Scand J Haematol* 33 (suppl. 40), 221–224.

Bern, J.L., Painter, M.J., Aronstam, A. *et al.* (1979) The frequency of bleeding and height in adolescent haemophiliacs. *Thrombos Haemost* 41, 286–290.

Bleasel, J.F., York, J.R. and Richard, K.A. (1990) Septic arthritis in human immunodeficiency virus infected haemophiliacs. *Br J Rheumatol*, 29, 494.

Davies, D.V. and Edwards, D.A.W. (1948) The blood supply of the synovial membrane. *Ann R Coll Surg Engl* 2, 142–186.

Deutsch, E., Brodeck, J.W. and Deutsch, K.F. (1993) Radiation synovectomy revisited. *Eur J Nucl Med* 20, 1113–1127.

Duthie, R.B. (1994) Muscle bleeds and consequences, in *The Management of Musculoskeletal Problems in Haemophiliacs*, 2nd edn (eds R.B. Duthie, C.R. Rizza, P.L.F. Giangrande and C.A.F. Dodd), Oxford Medical Publications, Oxford, pp. 104–116.

Duthie, R.B. and Dodd, A.F. (1994) Reconstructive surgery and joint replacement, in *The Management of Musculoskeletal Problems in the Haemophiliacs*, 2nd edn (eds R.B. Duthie, C.R. Rizza, P.L.F. Giangrande and C.A.F. Dodd), Oxford University Press, Oxford, pp. 189–217.

Favre-Gilly, J. (1964) Experience de cinq ans du Centre Emily Remigy de Montain (Jura) pour jeunes garcons hemophiles. *Hemostase*, 4, 231–257.

Forbes, C.D., Greig, W.R., Prentice, C.R.M. and McNicol, G.P. (1972) Radio-isotope knee scans in haemophilia A and Christmas disease. *J Bone Joint Surg (Br)*, 54B, 468–475.

Galindo, E., Merchon, C.R., Gage, J. and Orban, A. (1985) Ultrasonics in the diagnosis and assessment of the effect of treatment of intramuscular haematomas in haemophiliacs, in *Orthopedic Problems in Haemophilic* (eds S. Dohring and K.P. Schultz), W. Zuckschwerdt, Munich, pp. 56–60.

Goldsmith, J.C., Silberstein, P.T., Fromin, R.E. and Walker, D.Y. (1983) Haemophilic arthropathy complicated by polyarticular septic arthritis. *Acta Haematol (Basel)*, 71, 121–123.

Gregg-Smith, S., Giangrande, P.L.F., Paltnon, R. *et al.* (1993) Septic arthritis in haemophilia. *J Bone Joint Surg* 75B, 368–370.

Guenthner, E.E., Hilgartner, M.W., Miller, C.H. and Vienne, G. (1980) Haemophilic arthropathy: effects of home care on treatment patterns and joint disease. *J Pediatr* 97, 378–382.

Harrold, D.J. (1961) The defect of blood coagulation in joints. *J Clin Pathol*, 14, 305–308.

Hough, A.J., Banfield, W.G. and Sokoloff, L. (1976) Cartilage in haemophilic arthropathy. Ultrastructural and micronalalytical studies. *Arc Pathol Lab Med*, 100, 91–96.

Houghton, G.R. (1977) Septic arthritis of the hip in a haemophilic. Report of a case. *Clin Orthop*, 129, 223–224.

Ingram, G.I.C., Matthews, J.A. and Bennett, A.E. (1972) Controlled trial of joint aspiration in acute haemophilic arthritis. *Br J Haematol*, 23, 649–654.

Kinker, C.T. and Burke, C. (1970) Double blind studies of the use of steroids in the treatment of acute haemarthrosis in patients with haemophilia. *N Engl J Med*, 282, 639–642.

Levick, J.R. and Sinaje, L.M. (1987) An assessment of the permeability of fenestra. *Microvasc Res*, 33, 233–286.

Patrick, J.N., Bern, J.L., Aronstam, A. and Darby, S.C. (1982) An examination of joint laxity in haemophilia. *Injury*, 13, 337–342

Pietrogrande, V., Dioguardi, N.and Mannucci, P.M. (1972) Short term evaluation of synovectomy in haemophilia. *Br Med J*, 378–381.

Post, M. *et al.* (1986) Synovectomy in haemophilic arthropathy; a retrospective review of 17 cases. *Clin Orthop*, 202, 139–146.

Rainsford, S.G. and Hall, A. (1975) Clinical observations and their relationship to laboratory findings in haemophiliacs. *Thromb Diathesis Haemorrh*, 34, 734–740.

Roy, S. and Ghadially, F.N. (1967) Ultrastructure of synovial membrane in human hemarthrosis. *J Bone Joint Surg*, 49A, 1636–1646.

Roy, S. and Ghadially, F.N. (1969) Synovial membrane in experimentally provided chronic haemarthrosis. *Ann Rheum Dis*, 28, 402–413.

Stein, H. and Duthie, R.B. (1981) The pathogenesis of chronic haemophilic arthropathy. *J Bone Joint Surg (Br)*, 63B, 601–609.

Steven, M.M., Small, M., Pinkerton, L. *et al.* (1985) Non steroidal anti-inflammatory drugs in haemophilic arthritis – a clinical and laboratory study. *Haemostasis*, 15, 204–209.

Storti, E., Traldi, A., Tossatti, E. *et al.* (1969) Synovectomy, a new approach to haemophilic arthropathy. *Acta Haematol (Basel)*, 41, 193–205.

Swanton, M.C. (1959) Haemophilic arthropathy in dogs. *Lab Invest*, 8, 1269–1277.

Traldi, A., Melanotte, P.L. Africa, A. *et al.* (1986) Twenty years experience with synovectomy for haemophilic arthropathy, in *Symposium on Orthopaedic Problems in Haemophilia* (eds S. Dohring and K.P. Schultz), W. Zuckschwerdt, Munich, pp. 180–183.

Wiedel, J.D., Gilbert, M.S., Berson, B.L. and Hofmann, A. (1986) Arthroscopy of the knee in haemophilia, in *Symposium on Orthopaedic Problems in Haemophilia* (eds S. Dohring and K.P. Schultz), W. Zuckschwerdt, Munich, pp. 121–127.

11 PSEUDOTUMORS (HEMOPHILIC BLOOD CYSTS)

M.S. Gilbert

A three-page report appeared in the *Lancet* on 10 May 1856 describing 'Extravasation of blood into the calf of the leg; haemorrhagic diathesis; opening of a cavity filled with coagula expanding from the popliteal space above the knee down to the heel.' In this detailed report, Mr Erichsen (1856) described in detail the natural history, pathology and pitfalls of treatment of the hemophilic pseudotumor. It is required reading for anyone interested in this unique musculoskeletal manifestation of hemophilia.

Over 60 years later, Starker (1918), in his classic article, described the lesion and designated it a 'hemophilic subperiosteal hematoma.' Fernandez de Valderrama and Matthews (1965) characterized it as 'a progressive cystic swelling involving muscle, produced by recurrent hemorrhage and accompanied by radiographic evidence of bone involvement.' Gunning (1966), just prior to modern replacement therapy, estimated its incidence at about 1% of severe hemophiliacs. If left untreated, these lesions will destroy soft tissue, replace muscle, cause pressure neuropathy and erode through bone. In its end-stage it can erode through blood vessels and skin, causing death by exsanguination or infection. Therefore, early recognition and treatment are required to prevent a threat to life and limb.

Definition

The terms hemophilic cyst and hemophilic pseudotumor have been used interchangeably in the literature to describe this lesion. The term pseudotumor was first used when these lesions were poorly understood and clinically confused with true tumors. Modern diagnostic imaging has eliminated this diagnostic confusion, and destructive hemophilic cyst would be a more appropriate appellation. Fernandez de Valderrama and Matthews (1965) classified these cysts into three categories:

1. The simple cyst which occurs within the fascial envelope of a muscle or muscles and which is confined by the tendinous attachments.
2. The cyst which develops in a muscle with wide fibrous periosteal attachments and which may progress to give rise to cortical thinning because it interferes with the periosteal blood supply.
3. The pseudotumor which starts as a subperiosteal hemorrhage with stripping of the periosteum from the cortex until this is limited by aponeurotic or tendinous attachments and which then raises or destroys the muscles.

They infer that these are different entities, but it is the author's feeling that they represent different stages of the same entity. The variation is due to the site and extent of the original hematoma. Duthie *et al.* (1972) stated that 'since a haemophilic pseudotumour is clearly not a single pathologic entity, but the response of bone to a haemorrhagic process, the radiologic features will vary depending on the site and extent of the lesion.' I am in agreement with Duthie *et al.* and apply the same reasoning to the changes seen in the soft tissues. The initial lesion is a hematoma which encapsulates before resorption is complete. Once encapsulated, expansion rather than resorption occurs and destruction of muscle and bone begins. It is the encapsulation and locally expansive and destructive nature of these lesions that differentiate them from other lesions and that make them unique to hemophilia.

Natural history and clinical considerations

The spectacular nature of these lesions led to many of them being recorded in the literature before the availability of factor replacement. The natural history is well documented. The vast majority develop in the area

Hemophilia. Edited by C.D. Forbes, L. Aledort and R. Madhok. Published in 1997 by Chapman & Hall, London. ISBN 0 412 63820 7

Table 11.1 Site of hemophilic blood cysts

Site	Steel, Duthie and O'Connor (1969)	Gilbert (1985)	Dohring and Hofmann (1986)	Literature
Pelvis	12	8	3	34
Femur	20	6	6	43
Tibia	3	3	4	10
Calcaneus–talus	4	1	7	12
Foot	1	·		
Scapula			1	2
Humerus		2	2	
Ulna–radius		1	1	
Hand	2			6
Spine		1	1	
Unspecified	4			
Total	47	19	25	100

of the pelvis and thigh. Steel, Duthie and O'Connor (1969) documented this in 32 of 47 lesions, Gilbert (1985) in 14 of 19 lesions, and Dohring and Hofmann (1986) in nine of 25 lesions. The last authors also researched the world literature and the above data are tabulated in Table 11.1.

The superficial aspect of the mass is usually firm, non-tender and adherent to the deep structures. The lack of symptoms accounts for the fact that many remain undiagnosed for years. There was an average delay of 8 years before diagnosis (Gilbert, 1975). A history of trauma was recorded in 62% of cysts of the thigh, but in only 6% of cysts of the pelvis (Gilbert, 1975). However, massive hematomas of the iliopsoas are frequently seen without a previous history of trauma.

The mass, if untreated, enlarges at a variable rate. It may remain static for years, only to enlarge rapidly. The mass will remain asymptomatic until local complications occur. These include nerve compression, pathologic fracture and possible infection. Vascular compromise is rare as the slow development usually distorts rather than compresses adjacent vessels. Compression neuropathy, however, is not uncommon, especially at the pelvis where the femoral nerve is compressed against the inguinal ligament. Sciatic nerve involvement has also been documented.

Pathologic fracture, especially of the femur, has been reported and occurred in one of the author's patients. The spontaneous onset of pain, without evidence of fracture or nerve involvement, may portend the onset of spontaneous infection (Ferenz and Tozzi, 1989). Four untreated cases spontaneously ulcerated through skin and were followed within 1 year by infection, septicemia and death (Gilbert, 1975). Another case eroded in the sigmoid colon with rapid exsanguination. Erosion into the bladder has also been reported (Mauro *et al.*, 1984).

In contrast to these reports is a paper by Stavem *et al.* (1974) subtitled 'Recovery after rupture of cyst wall without necrosis or perforation of the skin.' They demonstrate complete resolution of a proximal tibial pseudotumor with significant bone involvement prior to rupture. The author has observed several cysts which have remained stable for many years, but has not seen one that has resolved spontaneously.

Although not documented, the incidence of cyst formation appears to be decreasing with adequate replacement therapy. Dohring and Hofmann (1986) and Duthie (1994) report that no new pseudotumors have developed in their well-treated population. The author has a similar experience at his center. The only pseudotumors seen recently are in patients with high-level and high-responding inhibitors.

It should be noted that at the present time there are no prognostic signs to predict the clinical course of an established blood cyst. Close clinical follow-up and imaging may be elected, but, if possible, surgical intervention should be considered.

Pathology

The basic pathology of these lesions is an encapsulated hematoma. A fibrous wall surrounds a collection of blood, bloody fluid or coagulum. Small lesions are fluid-filled with thin, fibrous walls that are easily separated from surrounding tissues. More established lesions have thick fibrous walls and are filled with gritty, dark red or brown coagulum (Fig. 11.1). When adjacent to bone, the capsule can cause local erosion and necrosis (Fig. 11.2). It may elevate the adjacent periosteum and stimulate new bone formation. Spicules of bone and areas of clarification can be seen within the fibrous wall. Loculation and daughter cysts are common. The latter, if unrecognized, may be the cause of recurrence following surgery.

Microscopic evaluation confirms a thick fibrous wall. Fernandez de Valderama and Matthews (1965) describe a hemosiderin-filled inner layer, a dense fibrous middle layer and a more vascular outer layer. Duthie (1994) describes inflammatory cells, especially histiocytes containing hemosiderin. The cyst content consists of blood in various stages of degeneration and lysis (Fig. 11.3). Gritty areas contain calcific debris. Steel, Duthie and O'Connor (1969) and the author injected Micropaque into the vessels of amputation specimens. No specific feeding vessels were observed. A large number of small vascular blow-outs were observed, but the significance is unclear.

Diagnostic imaging

CONVENTIONAL RADIOGRAPHY

In the early stages, when confined to the soft tissues, the predominant feature is a soft-tissue mass with obliteration

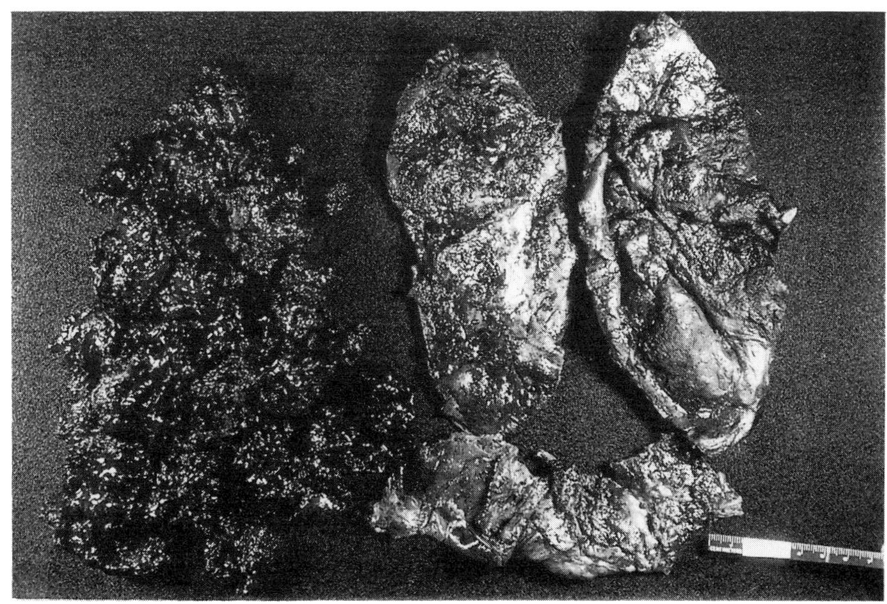

Fig. 11.1 Encapsulated blood cyst with thick fibrous wall and gritty coagulum.

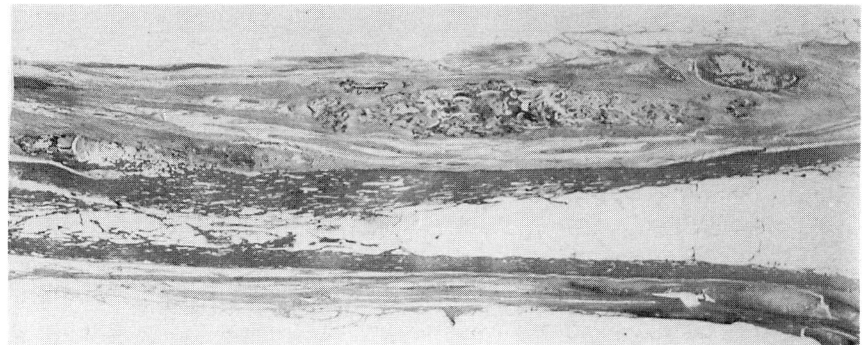

Fig. 11.2 Fibrous wall adjacent to bone causing early erosion.

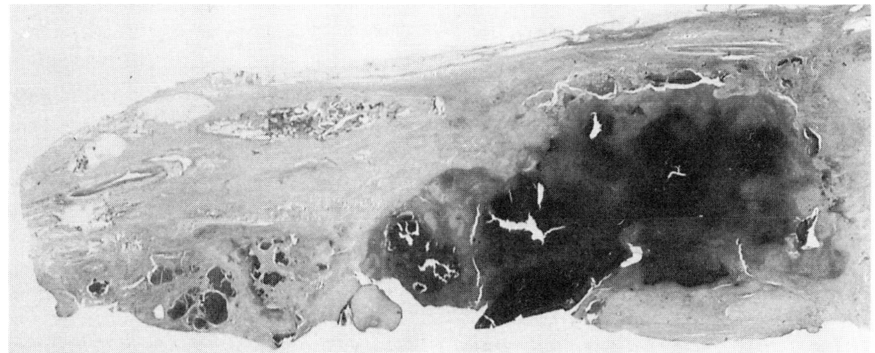

Fig. 11.3 Contents of blood cyst. Coagulum with areas of calcification.

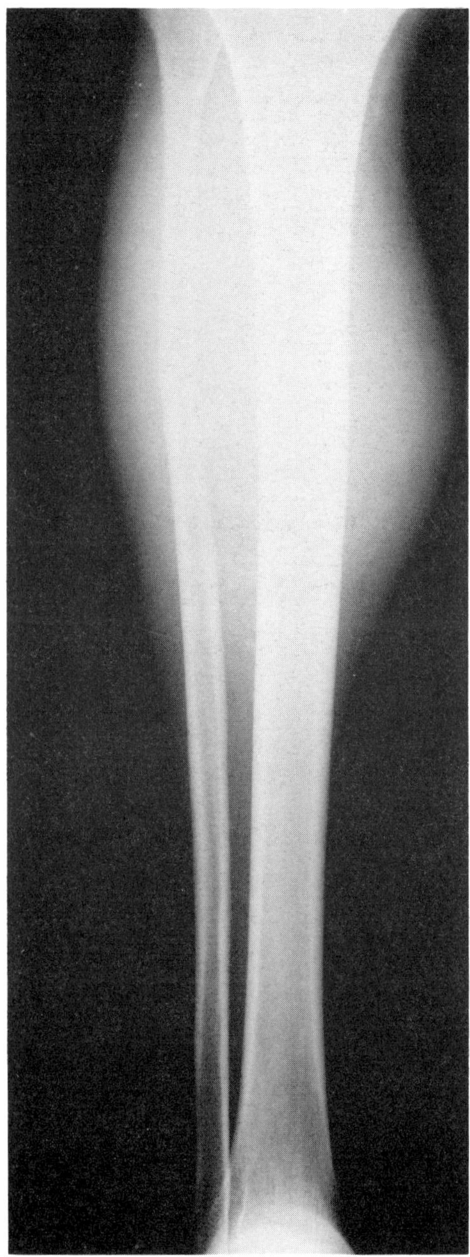

Fig. 11.4 Tribial blood cyst.

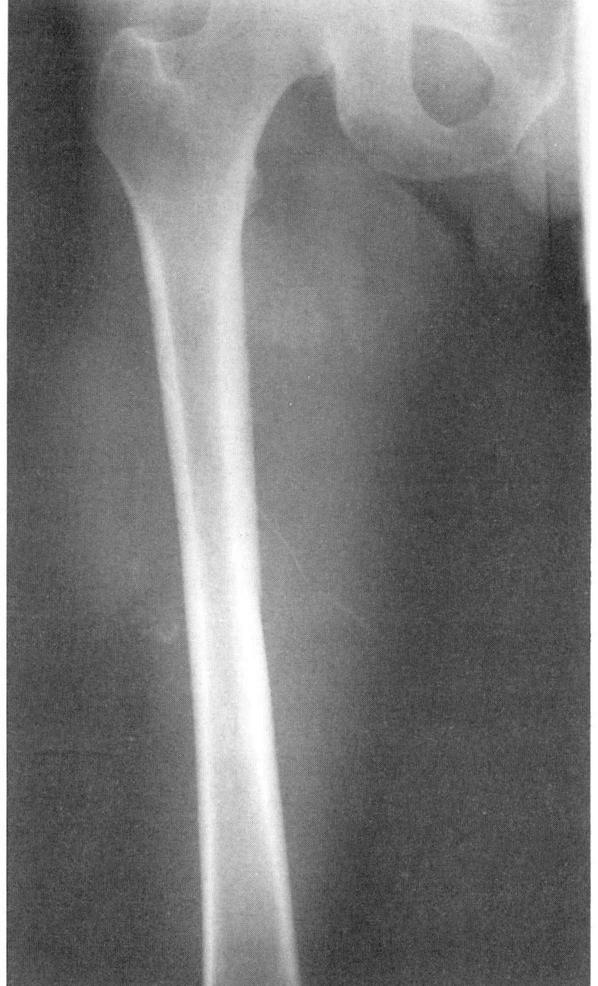

Fig. 11.5 Femoral blood cyst. Note early erosion of lateral cortex.

of normal muscle and fascial planes. Typical examples of a tibial and femoral blood cyst are seen in Figures 11.4 and 11.5, respectively. On close inspection, however, there are early erosive changes of cortical bone and, in Figure 11.5, one can appreciate the multilocular nature of the lesion with calcifications noted lateral to the femur. With progression, destruction of cortical bone and periosteal new bone in the areas of periosteal elevation are seen (Fig. 11.6). Spicules of bone or calcification may be noted within the soft-tissue mass. Similar destruction of a proximal tibia lesion is shown in Figure 11.7. Arteriography will show displacement of the major vessels, but they do not seem to be involved directly with the lesion.

As noted previously on Micropaque injection studies, no feeding vessels have been identified in any of our studies, nor in those reported by Thomas and Walters (1977).

The early diagnosis of a pelvic pseudotumor is almost impossible to make on plain-film radiography. The soft-tissue mass is difficult to evaluate, but the psoas muscle margin may not be identified. In the past, intravenous urography was used to identify the extent of the retroperitoneal mass. With progression, destruction of the ilium is seen. A circular, punched-out lesion in the iliac wing usually corresponds with a dumbbell-shaped lesion which clinically protrudes in the flank area. Progressive destruction of the iliac wing and acetabulum are seen as the lesion advances.

The radiographic imaging of cysts of the small bones of the hand and foot shows a different picture. Rarely is a soft-tissue mass demonstrated. The lesion appears to expand from within the bone, suggestive of an aneurysmal-type lesion. The trabecular pattern is des-

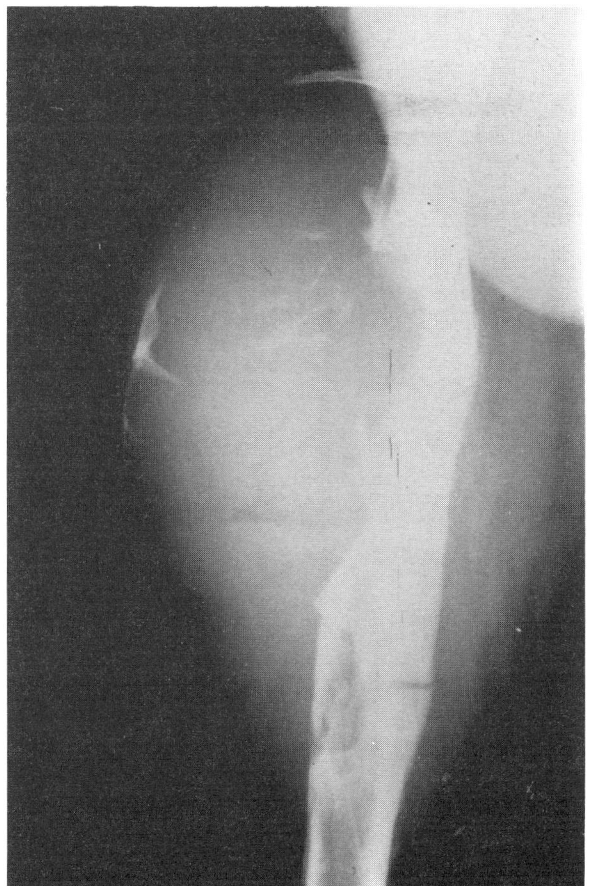

Fig. 11.6 Femoral pseudotumor. Note cortical destruction and spicules of bone in the soft-tissue mass.

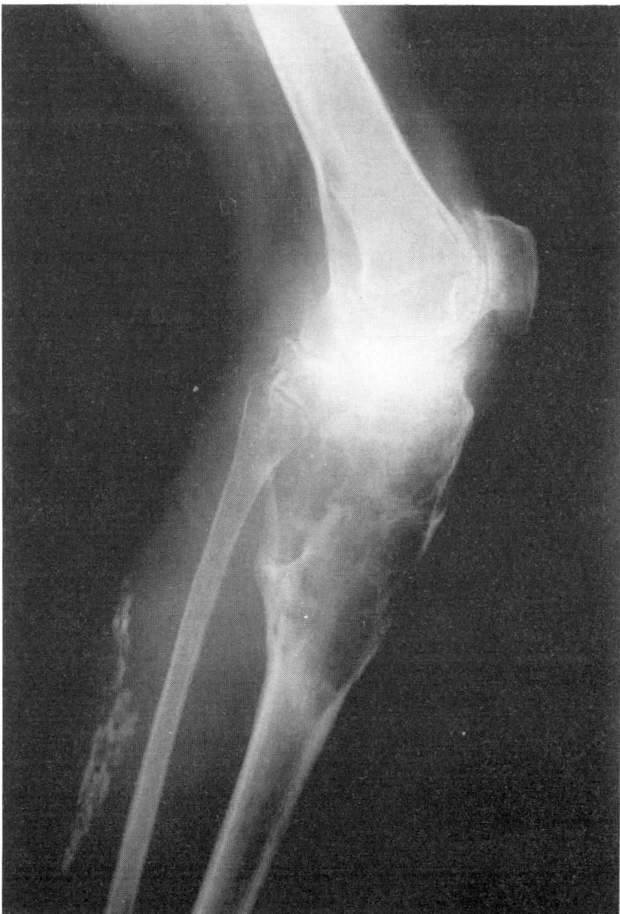

Fig. 11.7 Proximal tibial pseudotumor.

troyed. The picture may be suggestive of infection or a malignancy. Examples are shown in Figures 11.8 and 11.9.

COMPUTED TOMOGRAPHY

Computed tomography is extremely useful in the evaluation of the hemophilic blood cyst (Guilford *et al.*, 1980; Pettersson and Ahlberg, 1982). The typical finding is a soft-tissue mass with a discrete fibrous capsule. This capsule differentiates the true cyst from a resolving hematoma. A typical pelvic pseudotumor is seen in Figure 11.10. The degree of bone destruction is easy to assess and helps define the need for bone grafting in surgery of the long bones. Distortion of neurovascular structures can be traced. Of great importance in the evaluation of blood cysts by computer tomography is the demonstration of loculation and daughter cysts.

MAGNETIC RESONANCE IMAGING

Magnetic resonance imaging is quickly replacing all other diagnostic imaging techniques in the diagnosis and surgi-

cal planning of these cysts. Wilson and Prince (1988) describe a hypointensive rim which corresponds with the fibrous capsule. The different combinations of signal intensities within the cyst reflect the presence of fluid, recurrent bleeding and clot organization which has been shown pathologically. The clear demonstration of the lesion, the detection of multiple cysts and their relationship to bone, blood vessels and nerve prove invaluable in preoperative planning for surgical resection (Hermann, Yeh and Gilbert, 1986).

Different clinical patterns in the adult and the child

Ahlberg (1975) and Gilbert (1975) independently showed that the clinical pattern of hemophilic cysts is different in the adult and the child. The clinical and radiologic picture differs, as does the response to treatment. This differentiation will be outlined, but it must be noted that the distinctions are not always sharp and that exceptions exist. Therefore, each blood cyst must be independently evaluated and the plan of treatment must be based on the unique characteristics of each lesion.

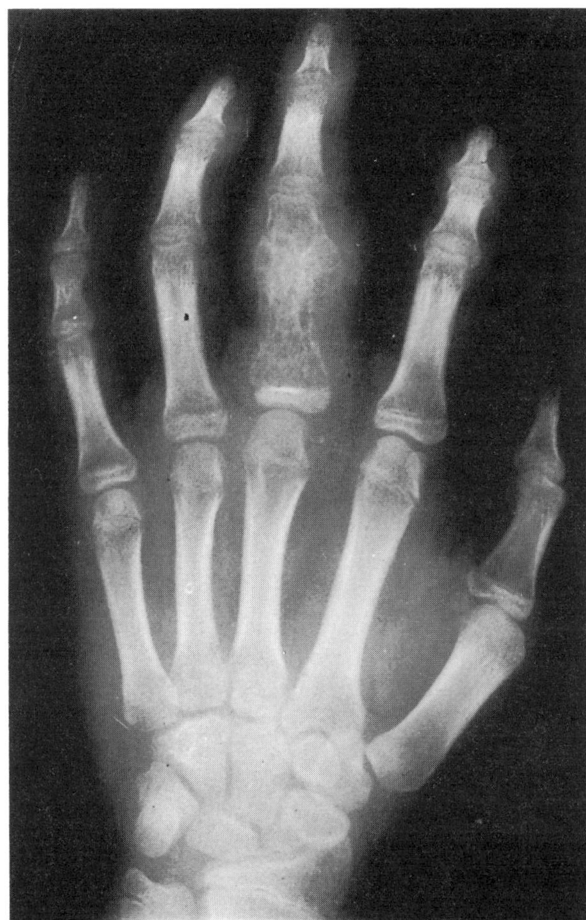

Fig. 11.8 Blood cyst of the phalanx. Immature skeleton.

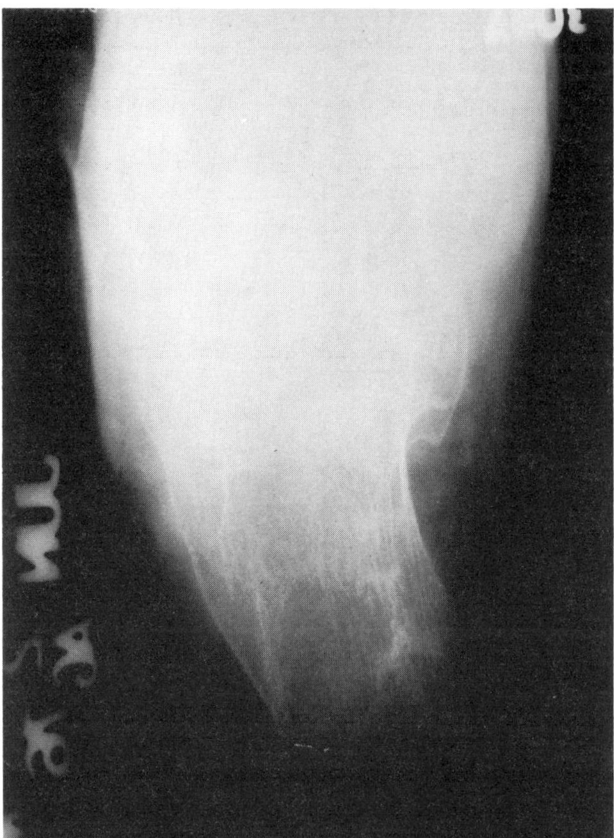

Fig. 11.9 Calcaneal blood cyst.

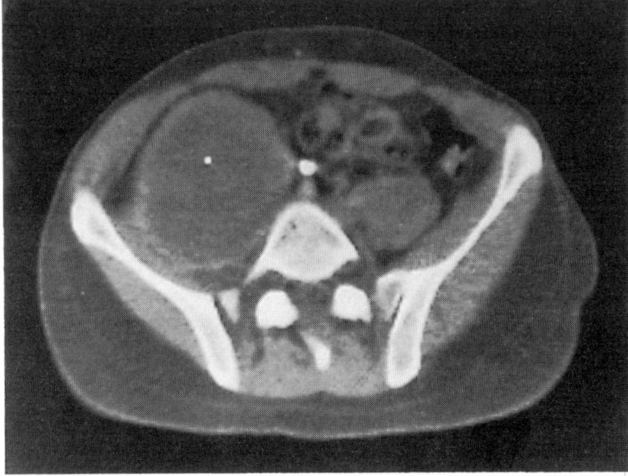

Fig. 11.10 Computed tomography of pelvic blood cyst.

The differentiation of the pseudotumor in the adult and child is a clinical rather than a pathologic differentiation. This is summarized in Table 11.2. However, the differentiation is important in that the treatment plan differs. Most pseudotumors in the adult occur in the proximal skeleton and long bones, especially in the lower extremity in proximity to the pelvis, femur and tibia. Many pseudotumors in the immature skeleton occur in proximity or distal to the wrist and ankle, usually in the small bones of the hand and foot. In the adult, the lesion is usually preceded by a documented, intramuscular hematoma, frequently noted after trauma. In the child, a history of trauma is not common. The X-ray of the child is suggestive of intraosseous hemorrhage with rapid expansion and destruction of bone. In contrast, in the adult, there is a large extraosseous soft-tissue mass which seems to be causing bone destruction by extrinsic pressure. Clinically, the lesions in the child develop rapidly, usually in less than 1 year, while in the adult the development is slow, frequently upward of 10 years.

Another unusual feature is the fact that multiple pseudotumors are common in the child, while in the adult single lesions are common except in the few reported cases of bilateral pelvic cysts. Lastly, the response to treatment is different in that lesions in the child often respond to non-surgical intervention, while the established pseudotumor in the adult requires surgical intervention. This will be discussed in detail in the next section.

Table 11.2 Comparison of hemophilic blood cysts in the adult and child

	Adult	*Child*
Site	Long bones and pelvis	Small bones of hand and foot
Clinical picture	Slow development	Rapid development
	Single bone involvement	Frequent multibone involvement
X-ray picture	Suggests extraosseous hemorrhage	Suggests intraosseous hemorrhage
Response to non-surgical treatment	Poor	Frequently successful

Treatment

Prior to the availability of concentrated products of factor VIII and IX, the surgical treatment of these lesions was accompanied by a high morbidity and mortality. Early attempts at aspiration, evacuation and biopsy were followed by the development of draining sinuses, infection and generalized sepsis. Amputation was required for most advanced lesions. These complications led to various attempts at non-surgical care. Factor replacement and immobilization were reported to be successful by several authors (MacMahon and Blackburn, 1960; Caen, *et al.*, 1964; Favre-Gilly, *et al.*, 1965). Of interest is the fact that most of the cysts that responded to this form of therapy were of the distal skeleton in young patients. There are very few reports documenting successful conservative treatment of advanced cysts of the proximal skeleton in the mature patient. If this course of treatment is undertaken, close follow-up must be maintained to insure that the cyst does not enlarge and threaten pathologic fracture or endanger vital structures.

Radiation therapy has also been successfully reported in distal cysts (Yung Fu Chen, 1965). Brant and Jordan (1972) reported initial success with radiation therapy for established femoral pseudotumors, but several of these patients were followed by this author and the initial shrinkage (probably secondary to radiation fibrosis) was followed by recurrent enlargement and pathologic fracture in one patient. Therefore, this modality of treatment should be reserved for those patients in whom surgery is not feasible.

Surgical excision of the mass is the treatment of choice in most patients. The surgery is a significant undertaking, but relatively safe when performed with proper planning at a major hemophilia center. The surgical approach to these lesions must be individualized.

In the extremity, an attempt should be made to go from normal tissue proximally and not to come down directly upon the lesion. Proximal to the lesion, the blood vessels and nerves should be traced. Frequently, they run around the periphery of the lesion, but loculation may envelop important structures directly in the cyst wall. Therefore, important arteries, nerves and veins must be traced completely before removal of the lesion is undertaken. When these structures are adequately retracted, the mass itself is surgically dissected. Frequently it lies within large muscle masses and there are multiple layers of thin muscle fibers which form a false capsule. The dissection should be carried circumferentially as far as possible. At times this becomes difficult because of the size of the cyst and the fibrous wall can be opened and the cyst contents evacuated. Large parts of the wall can then be removed, allowing easier access to the areas of the pseudotumor adjacent to bone. The bone itself is moth-eaten in appearance and eroded. The wall should be curetted off the bone. If the integrity of the bone is threatened, internal fixation with intramedullary rods should be considered. Bone grafting may be required. However, it has been the author's experience that the raw, bleeding bone heals very well and in several cases in which grafting was planned as a secondary procedure, the lesions healed successfully with immobilization.

The approach to large pseudotumors of the pelvis is carried out with the help of a general surgeon. Before starting the procedure, a ureteral catheter is placed so that it can be palpated easily during the dissection. The patient is then placed with several sandbags under the pelvis and the lower limb is draped free. A flank incision is made extending to the center of the inguinal ligament and then the incision is carried distally. After the muscles are split, the pseudotumor is noted in the retroperitoneum. The femoral nerve may lie anteriorly, medially or directly within the pseudotumor. Therefore, it is dissected free distally and the dissection carried proximally as far as possible. The pseudotumor is dissected, making sure that the course of the iliac vessels and ureter is known at all times. In many lesions, these structures are adherent to the cyst wall and, in these instances, a cuff of tissue is left rather than endanger important structures. At this point, the pseudotumor is usually decompressed. There may be significant destruction of the ilium.

If a large defect is present, closure of the dead space is difficult. In our earliest surgeries, we packed the lesion and went back several days later to remove the packing under anesthesia. Healing occurred by secondary intent. In one lesion, the surgeon mobilized the omentum and obliterated the dead space with the omentum. This allowed primary closure of the wound and this approach is recommended.

Recently, two alternatives to radical surgery have been presented. Fernandez-Palazzi and Rivas (1985) have advocated the aspiration of small cysts and the injection of fibrin-glue to obliterate the cavity. This approach is especially attractive in patients for whom major surgery would be very risky, for example those with high-responding inhibitors and those with advanced human immunodeficiency virus (HIV) disease. Caviglia *et al.* (1994) presented a paper which questioned the necessity to resect the fibrous wall of established blood cysts. He suggested that a laparoscope be introduced into the cavity to evacuate the contents and he then introduced bone graft and fibrin-glue to obliterate the dead space. Short-term follow-up demonstrated healing of several smaller cysts. He did caution that longer follow-up is required but, if successful, this approach could reduce the need for extensive surgery.

Conclusion

The hemophilic blood cyst represents a spectrum of pathology from a simple, encapsulated, intramuscular hematoma to the larger loculated lesion, which destroys muscle and destroys fascial planes to the true pseudotumor which erodes bone and elevates periosteum. Early diagnosis and treatment are required to prevent a threat to the integrity of the skeleton. Conservative treatment may be undertaken but, if there is evidence of enlargement despite conservative care, surgical excision should be undertaken. As with all musculoskeletal complications of hemophilia, the incidence of these lesions is decreasing with early adequate treatment and, hopefully, will be eliminated in the near future.

References

Ahlberg, A.K. (1975) On the natural history of hemophilic pseudotumor. *Journal of Bone and Joint Surgery*, **57A**, 1133–1136.

Brant, E.E. and Jordan, M.H. (1972) Radiologic aspects of hemophilic pseudotumors in bone. *American Journal of Roentgenology*, **114**, 525.

Caen, J., LeClerc, J.C., Patrux, C. *et al.* (1964) Pseudo-tumeurs hémophiliques (à propos de 3 cas). Seance du 22 Juin 1964 Societe Francaise d'Hemotologie.

Caviglia, M. *et al.* (1994) Hemophilic pseudotumur. Is it necessary to resect the pseudocapsule? (Abstract). *XXI Congress of the World Federation of Hemophilia*, Mexico City.

Duthie, R.B. (1994) Haemophiliac cyst formation in the management of musculoskeletal problems in the haemophilias (eds R.B. Duthie, C.R. Rizza, P.L.F. Giangrande and C.A.F. Dodd), Oxford University Press, Oxford, pp. 139–158.

Duthie, R.B., Matthews, J.M., Rizza, C.R. and Steel, W.M., (1972) *The Management of Musculoskeletal Problems in the Hemophilias*, Blackwell, Oxford.

Erichsen (1856) Extravasation of blood into the calf of the leg. *Lancet*, May 10, 511–513.

Favre-Gilly, J., Chatain, R., Trillat, A. and Saint-Paul, E. (1965) Pseudo-tumeur du calcaneume chez un hemophilie. *Hemostase*, 5, 95.

Ferenz, C.C. and Tozzi, J.M. (1989) Sepsis due to an infected pseudocyst of hemophilia. *Clinical Orthopedics and Related Research*, 244, 254–257.

Fernandez de Valderrama, J.A. and Matthews, J.M. (1965) The haemophilic pseudo-tumor or haemophilic subperiosteal haematoma. *Journal of Bone and Joint Surgery*, **47B**, 256.

Fernandez-Palazzi, F. and Rivas, S. (1985) The use of 'fibrin-seal' in surgery of coagulation diseases with special reference to cysts and pseudotumors, in *Orthopedic Problems in Hemophilia, Symposium* (eds S. Dohring and K.P. Schulitz), W. Zuckschwerdt, Munich, pp. 170–179.

Gilbert, M.S. (1975) Hemophilic pseudotumor, in *Handbook of Hemophilia* (eds K.M. Brinkhoust and H.C. Hemker), Excerpta Medica, Amsterdam, pp. 435–446.

Guilford, W.B., Mintz, P.D., Blatt, P.M. and Staab, E.V. (1980) *American Journal of Roentgenology*, **135**, 167–169.

Gunning, A.J. (1966) The surgery of haemophilic cysts, in *Treatment of Haemophilia and Other Coagulation Disorders* (eds R. Biggs and R.G. MacFarlane), Blackwell, Oxford.

Hermann, G., Yeh, M.C. and Gilbert, M.S. (1986) Computed tomography and ultrasonography of the hemophilic pseudotumor and their use in surgical planning.

MacMahon, J.S. and Blackburn, C.R.B. (1960) Hemophilic pseudotumor: a report of a case treated conservatively. *Australian and New Zealand Journal of Surgery*, **29**, 137.

Mauro, Y.A., Vincent, L.M., Mandell, V.S. and Guilford, W.B. (1984) Gas within hemophilic pseudotumors: CT demonstration. *Journal of Computer Assisted Tomography*, **8**, 473–475.

Pettersson, M. and Ahlberg, A. (1982) Computed tomography in hemophilic pseudotumor. *Acta Radiologica Diagnosis*, **23**, 453–457.

Starker, L. (1918) Knochenusur durch ein hamophiles subperiosteles hamatom. *Mitteilungen aus den Grenzegebieten der Medizin und Chirurgie*, **31**, 381–415.

Stavem, P., Eaeberg, O., Kolmannskog, F. and Nokleby, K. (1974) Pseudotumor of bone in a haemophiliac with circulation antibodies to factor VIII. *Scandinavian Journal of Haematology*, **12**, 161–164.

Steel, W.M., Duthie, R.B. and O'Connor, B.T. (1969) Haemophilic cysts. *Journal of Bone and Joint Surgery*, **51B**, 614.

Thomas, M.L. and Walters, H.L. (1977) The angiographic findings in a hemophilic pseudotumor of bone. *Australasian Radiology*, **21**, 346–349.

Wilson, D.A. and Prince, J.R. (1988) MR imaging of hemophilic pseudotumors. *American Journal of Roentgenology*, **150**, 349–350.

Yung Fu Chen (1965) Bilateral hemophilic pseudotumors of the calcaneus and cuboid treated by irradiation: case report. *Journal of Bone and Joint Surgery*, **47A**, 517.

Further reading

Abell, J.M. and Bailey, R.W. (1960) Hemophilic pseudotumor: two cases occurring in siblings. *Archives of Surgery*, **81**, 569.

Auger, M.J., Critchley, M. and McVerry, B.A. (1986) Unusual presentation of a large infected hemophiliac pseudotumor in an autologus indium-III WCB scan. *Clinical Nuclear Medicine*, **11**, 568–569.

Bailey, R. W., Penner, J.A. and Rorte, G.J. (1960) Successful excision of pseudotumor of hemophilia. *Surgical Forum*, **16**, 464–466.

Bailey, R.W., Penner, J.A. and Korte, G.J., (1967) New vistas in the surgery of hemophilia. *Journal of Bone and Joint Surgery*, **49A**, 1009.

Bard, M., Patrux, C., Bourdon, R. *et al.* (1965) Lesions extra-articulaires de type pseudo-tumoral chez l'hemophilie. *Hemostase*, 5, 89.

Bennett, G.A. (1966) Huge mass in great toe with destruction of phalanx in patient with hemophilia, in *Bone and Joint Clinicopathological Conferences of the Massachusetts General Hospital* (eds B. Castleman and J.M. McNeill), Little-Brown, Boston.

Birk, W. (1960) Ossaerer Pseudotumor bei Hemophilie. *Wienishe Klinishe Wochenschrift*, **47**, 72.

Brummelkamp, W.H. (1958) Pseudo-tumeur en cas d'hemophilie. *Arch Chir neerl*, **10**, 263.

Croizat (1965) Discusion sur les pseudo-tumeurs osseuses des hemophilas. *Hemostase*, 5, 99.

Echternacht, A. (1943) Pseudotumor of bone in hemophilia. *Radiology*, **41**, 565.

Egeberg, O., Borchgrevink, C.F. and Hjort, P.F. (1960) Use of animal antihaemophilic globulin in surgery: exarticulation in the hip in a haemophiliac. *Acta Medica Scandinavica*, **167**, 415.

Eibl, M., Fischer, M. and Kuhbock (1965) Pseudotumor des Darmbeins bei Hämophile A. *Deutsche Medizinische Wochenschrift*, **90**, 1965.

Eichler, J. (1966) Tumorahnliche Veranderungen bei *Haemophilie. Fortschritte Rontgenstr*, **104**, 1.

Fessey, B.M. and Meynell, M.J. (1967) Successful amputation through the hip for pseudotumour in severe haemophilia. *British Journal of Surgery*, **54**, 559.

Firor, W.M. and Woodhall, B. (1936) Hemophilic pseudotumor: Diagnosis, pathology and surgical treatment of hemophilic lesions in the smaller bones and joints. *Bulletin of the Johns Hopkins Hospital*, **59**, 237.

Fleming, J.L. (1962) Pseudotumor of hemophilia. *Guthrie Clinic Bulletin (Sayre)*, **31**, 90.

Forfota, E. (1931) Uber die Gelenk und Knochenveranderungen bei Blutern. *Rontgen-u. Lab-Prax* **3**, 399.

Fraenkel, G.J., Taylor, K.B. and Richards, W.C.D. (1959) Haemophilic blood cysts. *British Journal of Surgery*, **46**, 383.

Friedlander, H.L. and Bump, R.G. (1968) Chronic expanding hemotoma of the calf: a case history. *Journal of Bone and Joint Surgery*, **50A**, 1237.

Ghormley, R.K. and Clegg, R.S. (1948) Bone and joint changes in hemophilia: with report of cases of so-called hemophilic pseudotumor. *Journal of Bone and Joint Disease*, **30A**, 589.

Gugler, E. (1961) Zur therapeutischen Ansendung der Fraktion I nach Cohn. *Bibl haemat (Basel)*, **12**, 270.

Hall, M.R.P. (1961) Haemophilia complicated by an acquired circulating anticoagulant: a report of three cases. *British Journal of Haematology*, **7**, 340.

Hall, M.R.P. and Webster, C.V. (1962) The surgical treatment of haemophilic blood cysts. *Journal of Bone and Joint Surgery*, **44B**, 781.

Harrison, J.F. (1964) Haemophilic pseudotumor after fractured femur. *British Medical Journal*, **1**, 544.

Hermann, G., Yeh, M.C. and Gilbert, M.S. (1986) Computed tomography and ultrasonography of the hemophilic pseudotumor and their use in surgical planning. *Skeletal Radiology*, **15**, 123–128.

Horwitz, H., Simon, N. and Bassen, F.A. (1959) Hemophilic pseudotumor of the pelvis. *British Journal of Radiology*, **32**, 51.

Jones, D.M. (1965) Haemophilic blood cyst: report of a case. *Journal of Bone and Joint Surgery*, **47B**, 266.

Kerr, C.B. (1963) *Management of Hemophilia*, N.S.W. Australian Medical, Glebe.

Koepke, J.A. and Brower, T.W. (1965) Chondrosarcoma mimicking pseudotumor of hemophilia. *Archives of Pathology*, **80**, 655.

Larsen, R. (1938) Intramedullary pressure with particular reference to massive diaphysiol bone necrosis. *Annals of Surgery*, **108**, 127.

LeQuesne, L.P., Parker-Williams, E.J., Stewart, J.W. and Worth, R.L. (1967) Successful exclusion of massive, intra abdominal haemophilic pseudo-tumour, with primary wound healing. *Lancet*, **2**, 482.

Lewis, J.H., Cottington, G.M. and Brower, T.D. (1965) The use of plasma fraction 1 to maintain hemostasis following amputation for hemorrhage cyst of the thigh in a severe hemophiliac. *Journal of Bone and Joint Surgery*, **47A**, 333.

MacFarlane, R.G., Mallam, P.C., Witts, L.V. *et al*. (1957) Surgery in haemophilia. The use of animal anti-haemophilic globulin and human plasma in 13 cases. *Lancet*, **2**, 251.

Marder, V.J. and Shulman, N.R. (1966) Major surgery in classic hemophilia using fraction 1. Experience in 12 operations and review of the literature. *American Journal of Medicine*, **41**, 56.

Moseley, J.E. (1963) *Bone Changes in Hemotologic Disorders*, Grune & Stratton, New York.

Nelson, M.G. and Mitchell, E.S. (1962) Pseudo-tumour of bone hemophilia. *Acta Haemat (Basel)*, **28**, 137.

O'Brien, M.M. and Ewing, M.R., (1973) Haemophilia: the natural history of a destructive haematoma over a period of 50 years. *Australian and New Zealand Journal of Surgery*, **43**, 46–48.

Petersen, J., (1947) A case of osseous changes in a patient with hemophilia. *Acta Radioiogica (Stockholm)*, **28**, 323.

Reinecke, and Wohlwill, (1929) Uber Hamophilie Gelenkerkrankung. *Langenbecks Arch klin Chir*, **154**, 425.

Revol, L. (1965) Vaste lacune asseuse pseudo-tumorale de l'aile iliaque par hemotome ancien et recidivant chez un hemophile "B". *Hemostase*, **5**, 87.

Schwartz, E. (1960) Hemophilic pseudotumor of the ilium. *Radiology*, **75**, 795.

Silber, R. and Christensen, W.R. (1959) Pseudotumor of hemophilia in a patient with PTC deficiency. *Blood*, **14**, 584.

Thomas, H.B. (1936) Some orthopedic findings in 98 cases of hemophilia. *Journal of Bone and Joint Surgery*, **18**, 140.

Walker, H.J.S. and Womack, N.A. (1948) Pseudotumor of bone in hereditary pseudohemophilia. *Archives of Surgery*, **56**, 329.

Wesolowski, S.A., Lichtman, H.C. and Sawyer, P.N. (1964) Major surgery on the severe hemophiliac. Lessons in management. *Annals of the New York Academy of Science*, **115**, 505.

Wessler, S. and Avioli, L.V. (eds) (1968) Changes in surgical management of hemophiliacs. *Journal of the American Medical Association*, **206**, 2292.

Wolff, J.P. and Smiley, R.H. (1966) Spontaneous hemotomata of the calf. *Journal of the Oklahoma Medical Association*, **59**, 619.

Witts, L.J. and Allison, P.R. (1960) Haemophilia with cystic haematoma (2 cases). *Proceedings of the Royal Society of Medicine*, **53**, 976.

Yung Fu Chen (1972) Roentgen irradiation for chronic hemorrhage for an ulcer in a hemophiliac. *Journal of Bone and Joint Surgery*, **54A**, 1783.

van Creveld, S. and Kingma, M.J. (1961) Subperiosteal hemorrhage in haemophilia A and B. *Acta Paediatrica (Uppsala)*, **50**, 291–296.

12 HEMOPHILIA AND SPORT

P.M. Jones and B.M. Buzzard

Amongst those with little or no experience of hemophilia care, there is a school of thought that people with the disorder should not undertake strenuous physical activity. In the 1970s this attitude was encompassed in the suggestion that hemophiliacs should live within the bounds of their disorder. By doing so, the argument went, they would do less damage to themselves, require less therapeutic clotting factor and be less expensive to treat.

The argument was flawed in two fundamental ways. First, it was already common experience that people with hemophilia who were confined to bed or immobilized for long periods of time bled more often and needed more treatment than their active but equally affected peers. Second, even in those days of paternalistic medicine, it was trite to suggest that young and active people who happened to have hemophilia should adopt a role of invalidity. That this is what had happened to many of the previous generations of affected men who, without resource to treatment, had been thought to be protected from harm by their relatives and family doctors, was reflected in a poor quality of adult life characterized by dependence on others (Jones, 1980).

The integrity of major synovial joints depends on the health of their anatomy and physiology. Joints are stabilized by their capsules and ligaments and by muscle action exerted through the tendons. Weak muscles result in instability, less protection by muscle bulk and in an increased likelihood of significant accidental trauma. Resilience is lost, along with strength and easy adaptability. Changes resulting from intra-articular bleeding add to the instability; rest and immobility add to muscle weakness. The result is a vicious circle of repeated hemarthroses, each of which adds to the increasing development of chronic hemophilic arthropathy. The longer bleeds take to stop, the more a joint is targeted by repeated bleeding, the more replacement therapy is needed and the greater the likelihood of expensive reconstructive surgery in the future. Coincidentally, in the meantime, the more pain and disability experienced by the patient, and the greater the loss of time at school or work

Review of literature

Although it is nowadays generally agreed that sport should be encouraged in the hemophilic population, the literature is confusing when it comes to recommended physical activity. Before the advent of widely available replacement therapy, Austin, Rolland and Clausen (1961) encouraged swimming as the 'only safe, active sport' for patients with hemophilia. However, by 1974 Boone was stressing that the needs of hemophilic patients undergoing rehabilitation after replacement therapy were the same as those of any patient. She recommended swimming, cycling, tennis, gardening and hiking as good recreational activities. Dietrich (1975) stressed the importance of good musculoskeletal function and encouraged boys with hemophilia to participate in physical education. However, she cautioned against contact sports, citing soccer, wrestling and basketball.

Weigel and Carlson (1975) also considered the question of whether physical activity should be encouraged for the person with hemophilia. Their article was based on the premise that, as hemophilia was a handicapping condition, certain human rights must be recognized, including the 'right to grow up in a world which does not set [him] apart.' They emphasized the life-threatening nature of hemophilic bleeding and the psychologic impact of 'fear of immobility and untimely death' which led to parental imposition of strict rules of behavior. The key problem for parents of hemophiliacs is in drawing a fine line between necessary caution and harmful over-protection.' They stressed the importance of the father

Hemophilia. Edited by C.D. Forbes, L. Aledort and R. Madhok. Published in 1997 by Chapman & Hall, London. ISBN 0 412 63820 7

in the child's development, and of the need to encourage 'healthful activity and reasonably aggressive pursuits. After all, striated muscle is an outlet for emotions and nerve responses.' They emphasized early physiotherapy after bleeding, disuse atrophy and its effects on musculoskeletal function, and the vicious circle of knee bleeding and weakness of the quadriceps group of muscles.

With regard to sports, the authors considered skiing, horseback riding, tumbling and apparatus and soccer dangerous, but recommended archery, fencing, air rifle, badminton, billiards, bowling, golf, social dancing, softball, swimming, table tennis, 'stationary' bicycle riding, walking, hiking, fishing, music and movement, canoeing, sailing, tennis and volleyball. They considered basketball and track and field athletics as 'objectionable.' Swimming and tennis were their major recommendations because these developed coordination as well as muscle strength.

Although, in the light of hemophilia treatment today, Weigel and Carlson's paper placed too much emphasis on the risks of bleeding, this was one of the first comprehensive assessments of exercise and hemophilia. The authors considered the advantages of team sports and of prevention of handicap by developing social awareness and encouraging affected children to become productive members of society. They explained the comprehensive approach to each boy as an individual and the roles of orthopedic surgeon, physical training specialist and the physiotherapist in planning exercise and sports programs.

In 1976 Cole and Jones reviewed the role of the physiotherapist in hemophilia comprehensive care. The stressed the need for the early treatment of bleeds and how the physiotherapist might help the patient maintain or restore normal muscle and joint status. The emphasis in this paper was on encouraging even the most severely affected patients to keep active.

Weissman (1977), describing the work of an American hemophilia center, listed jogging, bicycling, tennis, golf, dancing, croquet, ping-pong, fishing and shuffle board in addition to swimming, which was 'encouraged for all' as suitable activities. Sports not encouraged were soccer, wrestling, jumping rope, basket and volleyball, roller skating, horseback riding and trampoline. However, Lazerson (1975) allowed modified forms of basketball, soccer and baseball, and Seeler, Ashenhurst and Miller (1975) used trampoline as part of their camp program. As Weissman pointed out, these differences in approach were often dictated by the provision of supervision or home therapy programmes. The key to all exercises used in rehabilitation of a hemophilic joint or muscle was slow, gradual progression, with modest incremental increases in resistance.

Weissman reviewed the role of rehabilitation medicine and hemophilia, citing Ahlberg's (1965) finding that in Sweden most musculoskeletal disability had occurred by the age of 15 years. The emphasis in Weissman's paper was on an exercise program designed to respond to bleeds rather than on prevention. He mentioned the roles of hydrotherapy and of the proprioceptive neuromuscular facilitation exercises described by Boone (1966).

Koch, Cohen and Luban (1982) reviewed methods of rehabilitation following knee hemarthroses. They concluded that intensive physiotherapy and exercise, rather than conservative management with immobilization, resulted in increased joint range and strength and fewer bleeds. Exercises recommended included gym work with cycle, treadmill and multigym, swimming, jogging and soccer. The question of the continued motivation needed to persist with an exercise program was addressed by Greene and Strickler (1983) and Varni and Wallender (1984). In Greene and Strickler's study, only a third of 32 patients with hemophilia continued to perform a simple daily exercise regimen 100 days into a treatment plan intended to last 6 months. Varni and Wallender emphasized the role of immediately beneficial results in reinforcing the need for adherence to regular exercise. Once the immediate alleviation of physical symptoms of a bleed occurred there was little positive playback to encourage the continuation of the regimen.

Greene and Strickler (1983) reviewed evidence of the shock-absorbing function of normal lower limb musculature in protecting the knee. They argued that muscle weakness secondary to repeated hemarthroses reduced this protection, making the joint more susceptible to heel strike and other weight-bearing forces. In order to counter this weakness they described a modified isokinetic strengthening, home-based program for the knee flexors and extensors. In a study involving 32 people with hemophilia, they showed that the technique resulted in significant strengthening without additional bleeding. This effect was not confined to patients with minimal arthropathy.

Koch and colleagues (1984) studied the physical fitness of 11 boys with hemophilia aged between 8 and 15 years. They compared results of bicycle ergometry with those of non-hemophilic children. The affected boys performed poorly: the authors concluded that their lack of physical conditioning was due to both the overprotective attitudes of parents and doctors, and to their sedentary lifestyle. The boys with hemophilia had a higher proportion of body fat than the normal boys and had been discouraged from active sport, especially team sport.

Stokes and Young (1984) reviewed the evidence for the reflex inhibition of quadriceps activation by injury to the knee. Their conclusions are fundamental to the management of musculoskeletal problems in hemophilia in which muscle weakness and wasting contribute to joint instability, repeated bleeding and the early development of arthropathy. The basic premise was that immobilization of a joint exacerbated wasting and weakness.

Conversely, early mobilization and exercise helped overcome reflex inhibition and aided recovery (Fig. 12.1).

Muscle inhibition following experimental distension of the knee with sterile saline had previously been demonstrated by de Andrade (1965). As a consequence, the stability of the joint was directly affected by loss of quadriceps power. In addition, when the knee was injured there was thought to be an immediate inhibition of vastus medialis; a protective reflex placed the joint into a slightly flexed position of comfort. Whilst the importance of this mechanism has been questioned, such a reflex would help explain the typical hemophilic stance following a series of knee hemarthroses.

Greenan-Fowler, Powell and Varni (1987) investigated the compliance of 10 children with hemophilia prescribed therapeutic exercise for 1 year. In the first week only half the children did what they had been told. Behavior therapy was used to encourage them and there was 94% adherence to the program during the treatment phase and an initial 84% during the follow-up phase. Thereafter compliance fell as explicit reinforcement decreased.

Most of the exercises prescribed in this program were meant to be carried out at home. Instruction was given both in class and individually. Cycling and swimming were encouraged in addition to three-times-a-week musculoskeletal work-outs. Prizes were offered to children shown to be following their programs. After a week's baseline phase, a 12-week treatment phase began. During this each child was seen regularly and was given praise and encouragement. Parents were involved in helping with this encouragement at home and in the regular

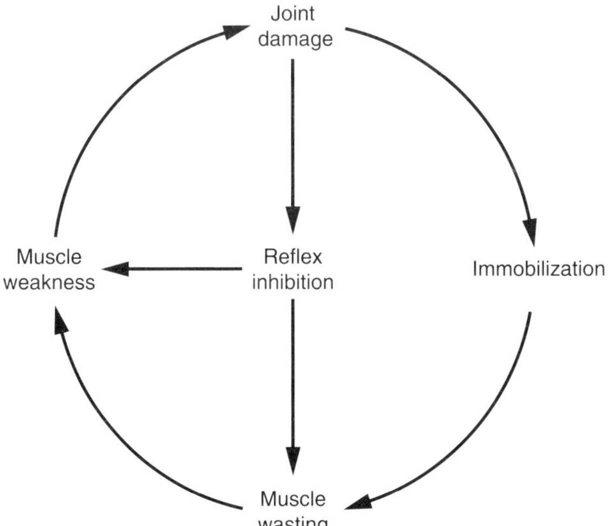

Fig. 12.1 Vicious circles of arthrogenous muscle weakness. Redrawn from Stokes, M. and Young, A. (1984). The contribution of reflex inhibition to arthrogenous muscle weakness. *Clinical Science*, **67**, 714, with permission.

assessment of their children. These weekly sessions included exercise instruction, refreshment and group activity. During the 9-month follow-up phase requirement for attendance was gradually reduced. Towards the end of the study assessment was performed by written response.

The results of this study are of considerable importance. Children will not follow routine exercise regimens unless they receive a high level of encouragement. Even then, as this diminishes, compliance falls away. Whilst the authors discussed how barriers to compliance might be removed, it is clear that only the regular involvement of a friendly adult, or peer pressure, or the fun of a sport and competitive achievement can persuade a child (or indeed an adult) to exercise regularly.

Buzzard and Jones (1988) referred to the importance of regular musculoskeletal assessment with measurement of joint range and muscle strength in people with hemophilia. Evidence of deterioration, muscle wasting or abnormal gait should result in a review of treatment and activity and specialist referral. Early treatment of bleeds was again emphasized, together with the prevention of bleeding by the strengthening and maintenance of good musculature. The authors emphasized the dual needs of enhancing good health and reducing bleeds, and showed how a physical fitness approach to hemophilia management simply reflected the changes in lifestyle and leisure time of the general population. Here the emphasis was on the enjoyment of activity and sport, rather than on regular exercises which people found boring and repetitive. The need for individual assessment and encouragement was crucial, adaptations being suggested by associations between particular activities and bleeding. The value of warm-up and stretching exercises was noted. Whilst advocating the freedom of exercises provided by an enjoyable sport, the authors also noted the need for specific muscle-building exercises before, for instance, joint replacement surgery and following operation.

McLain and Heedrich (1990) reported on the case of a hemophilic teenager inappropriately advised to discontinue his favourite sport, soccer. They urged that decisions like that reached in this case, which was made without the personal involvement of the youngster or his parents (who wanted him to continue to play), could only be reached after the most careful review of all pertinent factors. These should include the type and severity of the hemophilia, the age, experience and emotional maturity and judgment of the affected person, his clinical history and musculoskeletal health, and the perceived risks of performing a particular sport. They emphasized that it is always better to emphasize the sports that can be enjoyed rather than those that should be avoided. Among the sports recommended were track and field athletics, archery, running, tennis and swimming. The not-recommended list included soccer and water polo, as well as rugby and wrestling; surprisingly, boxing was not mentioned. Limited-contact/impact sports not recommended were baseball, basketball, cycling, diving, gymnastics and downhill skiing.

Jones (1995) has reviewed the value of sport for people with hemophilia. Using data collected from a sports survey conducted for the World Federation of Hemophilia (WFH) he emphasized the values of regular physical exercise in terms of well-being and fulfilment. Of 69 sports surveyed in the WFH questionnaire, which was answered by doctors actively working with hemophilia, 10 were recommended by more than 94% of respondents. Similarly, most doctors thought some sports hazardous (Tables 12.1 and 12.2). The tables give general guidance; there are always individual exceptions. For instance, whilst most youngsters will have a go on a skateboard, a few will choose a sport like karate in which to excel. In either case only experience will suggest whether or not there is a detrimental (or beneficial) effect on the underlying bleeding disorder.

Table 12.1 The top 10 sports recommended by doctors. All of those replying put swimming at the top of this list; 94% recommended cycling

Sport	%
Swimming	100
Table tennis	100
Walking	100
Fishing	99
Dance	98
Badminton	98
Sailing	98
Golf	96
Bowls	95
Cycling	94

Table 12.2 The least favored sports. All the doctors were opposed to boxing and 90% thought skateboarding dangerous for someone with severe hemophilia

Sport	%
Boxing	100
Rugby football	99
American football	99
Karate	94
Wrestling	93
Motorcycling	91
Judo	91
Hang-gliding	90
Hockey	90
Skateboarding	90

Prevention of injury

No sport is without risk but this can be reduced by following simple guidelines. Participants should:

1. Know the rules of the sport and abide by them.
2. Learn the skills required by taking regular tuition from experts.
3. Wear clothing, footwear and protection appropriate to the sport.
4. Not play on if injured.

These four basic rules have been explained more fully by Grisogono (1991), who recorded 189 sports injuries to children or adolescents in her physiotherapy practice over a 6-year period. The knee was the site of injury in a third (63) of cases, followed by hip and groin (13), ankle (11), shoulder (9) and elbow (4). Grisogono looked at why children were injured, and listed 15 contributory features, which have been amended below:

1. Children should do sports appropriate to their size and physical characteristics.
2. The type and amount of sport should be in keeping with the child's development.
3. The equipment should fit the child; adult-sized apparatus puts inappropriate loading and stress on the developing body.
4. Fitness training for sport must be tailored to a child's age and understanding, and be applicable to the sport he or she enjoys.
5. Children participating in team sports should be matched for size and development. This can be forgotten in sports requiring a large amount of protective clothing, which can give a false air of confidence to a small boy facing a more mature opponent.
6. Too much sport may be as harmful as too little; overtraining is especially dangerous in activities involving a limited range of repetitive movement.
7. Appropriate protective clothing is essential.
8. Footwear should be of good quality and fit, and appropriate to the sport. Everyone with hemophilia should wear shock-absorbing material in their shoes, in addition to built-in protection devices like air-cavities. Sorbothane soles and/or heels reduce heel strike significantly, and help protect knees as well as ankles from repeated stress. The combination of well-designed footwear, a shock-absorbing layer and sports socks with thickened soles provides both comfort and protection.
9. Skills need learning; inadequate training predisposes the child to injury.
10. Accidents happen when people are not prepared. New sports need to be learnt gradually; warm-ups and warm-downs are integral parts of any sport.
11. Sports should be adequately supervised.

12. Sport requires discipline, to protect both the individual and others.
13. The environment should be safe, with surfaces and surroundings suitable for the sport.
14. Children should be taught never to try and 'play through' an injury.
15. Sport becomes dangerous when the participant is over-tired and lacks concentration and co-ordination.

If an activity regularly provokes bleeding, a cause should be sought. Changes in footwear or technique, or a period of rest and retraining may be effective. Only if the problem persists should a change to another sport be considered.

Prophylaxis with clotting factor is not a prerequisite for sport. Many people with severe hemophilia maintain high levels of activity without any replacement therapy, only treating themselves in the event of injury. The use of desmopressin (DDAVP) in order to boost factor VIIII C levels before activity is contraindicated. Levels will rise anyway with exercise in mildly affected people, and the antidiuretic effect of the drug could complicate the maintenance of fluid balance, especially in children and if the sport is vigorous, or performed at high ambient temperatures.

Local hemostatic therapy

Minor open trauma in hemophilia, including small cuts and abrasions, can usually be treated in exactly the same way as in the non-hemophilic patient without recourse to systemic therapy. However, local hemostatics are rarely effective except perhaps in the nose. Epistaxis can sometimes be controlled with antifibrinolytic (cyklokapron) drops.

Local hemostatics include epinephrine, topical thrombin, fibrin-glue and pastes made up from factor VIII or IX concentrates. They have a use in the control of hemorrhage in patients with inhibitors in whom systemic therapy may be ineffective. However, when applied to open wounds, they are washed away by escaping blood. Pressure bandaging over a non-adhesive dressing may increase their effectiveness.

Larger wounds may be closed in a variety of ways, including sutures, clips, sterile adhesive strips and cyanoacrylic glue. However, in hemophilia, later wound disruption may occur as a result of secondary hemorrhage if clotting factor replacement is not also used. One injection, supported by 3 days of oral antifibrinolytic therapy, is recommended. Systemic antifibrinolytics should be used with caution in immobile patients with factor IX deficiency treated with a prothrombin complex concentrate (PCC).

Supervision of people with hemophilia and assessment of trauma

The first aid and assessment of someone injured during sport are exactly the same whether or not they have hemophilia. It is important that this is known by teachers and trainers who might otherwise assume that the proper management of a sports injury is of secondary importance to the underlying bleeding disorder. When writing to the staff of schools or sports facilities this fact should be stressed (Jones, 1995).

The person supervising a sport should know how to contact the relevant hemophilia center staff so that help can be obtained in the event of serious injury, especially if this involves the head. In practice this information is conveniently provided by making the supervisor aware of the affected person's identity card. In the UK this card, which contains details of diagnosis and suggested therapy, is given to each patient at diagnosis of a hereditary hemorrhagic disorder.

Affected people involved in outdoor activities like sailing, climbing or skiing should always carry identification and details of their disorder with them. Whilst first aid is conveniently carried out at the sports facility and in the casualty room of the local doctor's practice or hospital, hemophilia therapy means the early involvement of the nearest center. Lines of communication should be clear, and anyone participating in sport should know where to go first if injury occurs. Most large comprehensive care centers are used to coping with casualties at first hand, treating both the injury and the hemophilia. If a casualty department usually provides the initial site for management, staff should know that replacement therapy must be given on presentation in order to prevent untoward bleeding. It is imperative that no one waits for the appearance of physical signs before starting appropriate hemophilia treatment. Radiology and other investigation should be performed as required in assessment of the injury and not because of the hemophilia.

Decisions on whether to admit someone to hospital should be dictated by the nature of the injury, the severity of the hemophilia and the need for repeated or continuous treatment. Guidelines for admission include the development of large-muscle hematoma or hemarthrosis of a major joint, as well as possible internal damage demanding skilled orthopedic assessment and possible surgery. In youngsters the differential diagnosis of a sports injury will include Osgood–Schlatter's disease (knee) and Sever's disease (ankle), both disorders caused by repeated mechanical force on growing bone. Avulsion fracture, slipped epiphyses, Perthes disease and benign hip syndrome may also present following the history of an injury. Iliopsoas bleeds, which may present as possible hip lesions, are common in the hemophilic adolescent. Diagnosis depends on the demonstration of sensory loss in the distribution of the femoral nerve in someone holding his hip in flexion in order to ease the pain. Hip rotation is normal. Iliac fossa tenderness is often acute, and on the right side can mimic appendicitis. Hospital admission in these cases is mandatory because full recovery can only be achieved by intensive physiotherapy following at least 1 week's clotting factor replacement therapy. Sensory loss may take many months to disappear. More important, quadriceps wasting and weakness may be profound, and affect the stability of the knee and the patient's gait for over a year.

Attention should always be paid to the condition of the affected joint prior to an accident. Previous injury or bleeding with subsequent arthropathy may have altered the normal alignment of bones, and there may be mechanical restrictions on joint range and movement. Attempts to force an already damaged joint into a normal range of activity will only increase disability. Fractures in someone with hemophilia heal normally after conventional treatment. Clotting factor cover is, of course, required for manipulation and if there is any associated bleeding. However, once a closed fracture has been immobilized, 3 days' cover is usually adequate. There is no place for concomitant antifibrinolytic therapy.

If pain is not controlled by local measures, the first analgesic of choice is acetaminophen. Whilst aspirin is contraindicated because of its effects on platelet function and gastric mucosa, the non-steroidal anti-inflammatory drugs (NSAIDs) may be useful in the control of pain and inflammation following musculoskeletal injury. If an NSAID is used it should only be taken orally after food or a glass of milk and not repeated if there is gastric discomfort or pain. Previous evidence of peptic ulceration is an absolute contraindication.

Rehabilitation usually starts with a return to activity 24 h postinjury. Isometric exercise of increasing intensity leads to active exercise as the wound heals. The procedure is a balance between protecting the wound and providing the maximum possible movement. It is very important that all unaffected joints and muscles are regularly exercised during recovery. If this is not done in someone with hemophilia, especially if they are bed-bound, bleeds of inactivity start within a week or so, and are difficult to control with replacement therapy alone.

Treatment of common sports injuries

In general, the acute treatment of all sports injuries is the same. The application of ice for 15 min relieves pain and reduces bleeding into injured tissues through vasoconstriction. Compression, usually by crêpe bandaging for the first day postaccident, continues to limit bleeding. Elevation at this time adds to this by lowering venous hydrostatic pressure. To ice, compression and elevation (acronym: ICE) should be added rest (RICE), but only for

a few specific injuries. Most respond better with an early return to activity.

When using an icepack, care must be taken to protect underlying skin from ice burn by wrapping the pack in a wet towel. Similarly, the instructions for use of proprietary chemical cold packs should be followed carefully. There is no contraindication to the direct application of cooling sprays to someone with a bleeding disorder.

Guidelines for the management of commonly encountered conditions are give in Table 12.3. Obviously, hemophilia replacement therapy should be given whenever bleeding supervenes. Some chronic lesions unassociated with bleeding (tennis elbow, tendinitis) should not require hemostatic cover.

When indicated, the earlier specific hemophilia treatment is given after injury the better. This principle applies even if prophylactic therapy preceded activity because the clotting factor present is unlikely to be sufficient to control an acute bleed. In addition, what circulating factor there is will be depleted rapidly in response to the trauma. Speed of replacement therapy is probably more important than dose. The latter is very individual and depends on knowledge of usual response in a particular patient. Rule-of-thumb recommendations are for around 1000 iu of factor VIII or IX for children, and 2000 iu for adults.

In general, factor VIII should be given 8–12 hourly for at least the first 48 h after a major sports injury. Dosage and frequency can then be tailed off, but severe blows and sprains and the appearance of physical signs of intramuscular hemorrhage or hemarthrosis require twice-daily treatment for a week or more. Factor IX dosage may need to be higher than theoretically calculated initially. If the injury is severe the patient's response to an injection should be checked by assay. Factor IX may be required 12-hourly in the first 2 days. Less replacement therapy will be required if a continuous infusion is set up, instead of relying on pulsed treatment. If continuous infusion is used, laboratory monitoring by random assay is necessary to ensure that hemostatic levels are being achieved.

High body weight, whether through muscular development or obesity, and injury or bleeding in a previously damaged site dictate high and more prolonged replacement therapy.

Infection control

Normal hygiene, together with the sensible precaution of refraining from activity whilst overtly bleeding, prevents cross-infection during sport. The three known major pathogens associated with previous blood product therapy, hepatitis B and C and human immunodeficiency virus (HIV), gain access to the body by inoculation of infected material into the recipient's bloodstream. Parenteral transmission thus requires injury to both donor and

Table 12.3   Treatment of common sports injuries

(a) Upper limb

Injury	*Suggested physiotherapy*
Bursitis/tendinitis of shoulder complex (impingement syndrome)	Pain relief (electrotherapy)
	Maintenance exercises
	Deep frictional massage
	Refer to doctor for injection if indicated
Tennis/golfer's elbow	Deep frictional massage
	Pain relief (electrotherapy, ultrasound, pulsed short-wave diathermy)
	Manipulation if appropriate
	Cuff
	Reduction in aggravating activities
Hematoma (forearm)	Elevation
	Pulsed short-wave diathermy
	Active exercises of fingers, wrist, elbow
	Deep frictional massage

(b) Lower limb

Injury	*Suggested physiotherapy*
Hematoma of quadriceps or calf	Bedrest
	Pulsed short-wave diathermy or ice at home
	Elevation progressing to partial weight-bearing with crutches
	Deep frictional massage
	Static muscle contractions
	Gradual muscle stretches
	Must have full range of movement and no pain before returning to sport
Anterior knee pain	McConnell taping and vastus medialis re-education exercise
	Pain relief using ice, pulsed short-wave diathermy
	Patella mobilizations
Torn meniscus	**Post arthroscopy**
	Pulsed short-wave diathermy, ice
	Quadriceps exercises, especially inner range
	Specific muscle retraining if necessary
	Home exercise and advice on returning to sport
Anterior cruciate ligament instability or deficiency	Hamstring exercises
	Balance exercises
	Proprioception exercises

Table 12.3 (Continued)

(b) continued

Injury	*Suggested physiotherapy*
Peronei tendinitis	Deep frictional massage
	Electrotherapy
	Strapping
	Proprioception exercises
Tibialis posterior tendinitis	Deep frictional massage
	Electrotherapy (pain relief)
	Calf stretches
	Proprioception exercises
	Biomechanical assessment
Gastrocnemius tear–'tennis leg'	**First stage**
	Inner-range static contractions
	Pulsed short-wave diathermy
	Deep frictional massage
	After 2 weeks
	Increase deep frictional massage
	Start stretches
	Advice re: warm-up and stretching
Sprained ankle	Rest, ice, compression, elevation (RICE)
	Strapping, ultrasound, deep frictional massage Partial weight-bearing progressing to full weight-bearing
	Active exercises; proprioception and balance retraining

(c) Other

Injury	*Suggested physiotherapy*
Plantar fascitis	Rest
	Heel pads
	Gastrocnemius and soleus stretches
	High-dose ultrasound
	Strapping
Whiplash	Pain relief (usually heat)
	Collar ±
	Mobilization/manipulation
	Cervical spine exercises
	Neck-care advice

Table 12.4 Infection control checklist

Cover wounds with waterproof adhesive dressings

Stop activity if bleeding, and leave the playing area

Only restart activity when bleeding has stopped and the wound has been dressed

Use once-only disposable materials for first aid

Wear gloves for first-aid treatment of bleeding and when clearing up

Hot soapy water and/or disinfectant make contaminated surfaces safe

Dispose of any used materials carefully

Contaminated clothing should be cleaned on the washing-machine hot cycle

Showers are preferable to communal baths

recipient. Even if both are actively bleeding during contact, the chances of transmission are remote. In the words of one national authority, 'wounds tend to bleed outwards, not inwards' (Scottish Sports Council, 1989).

Whilst there have been reports of hepatitis B transmission through sport, notably orienteering, only one case of possible HIV transmission is known. This involved a collision between two soccer players in an amateur match in Italy. Both bled from head wounds. One player was known to be HIV-antibody-positive; the other seroconverted later. Other than the accident no other risk factors were known.

There is therefore no need to ban people with hemophilia from participating in team sport, even if they are infected with hepatitis or HIV. The UK Health Education Authority (1992) cautions HIV-antibody-positive people from taking part in 'robust contact sports' like rugby or boxing, but this is not the province of the person with hemophilia anyway. The Authority concludes 'with the many sporting activities where there is a minimum risk of injury, people with HIV who are fit and well should be freely able to participate if they want to.' In keeping with more general advice, there is no requirement to disclose confidential personal information to trainers, team mates or clubs, and absolutely no requirement for prospective testing by any sports organization. HIV-infected people should, however, be aware of some national restrictions if they aim to compete abroad. Notoriously, the USA requires admission of infection and the issue of a waiver to certain visitors.

In 1989 the World Health Organization issued a consensus supporting the concept of sport for all, even if HIV-infected. The statement emphasized the very low risk of transmission, and gave guidelines on hygiene and testing.

Cross-infection guidelines

These are straightforward (Table 12.4). Wounds that may bleed (recent cuts or grazes) must be covered with waterproof adhesive dressings. Injuries that result in bleeding

must be attended to promptly as should spontaneous nosebleeds. The days of the universal 'magic sponge' are over; individual players should be treated with disposable absorbent materials and fresh water. The person giving first aid should wear disposable gloves. Players should leave the field until bleeding stops and is unlikely to restart. Open wounds that have been bleeding must be covered.

When appropriate, contaminated surfaces should be washed over with hot soapy water and a hypochlorite solution. Gloves should be worn and paper towels should be disposed of carefully. Soiled clothing should be washed using the hot cycle of a washing machine.

It is important to reassure those involved in giving first aid that mouth-to-mouth resuscitation is safe and should never be withheld. Cheap, disposable plastic mouth valves should be kept in the first-aid kit.

Those with hemophilia are just as prone to sports injuries, infections and temptations as anyone else. Trainers and others in authority at clubs or camps should be aware of this and plan accordingly. Everyone should be aware of the sexual and intravenous drug transmission risks of hepatitis B and HIV, and of the precautions needed to prevent this transmission. Otherwise most of the rules of hygiene suggested for HIV should raise the awareness of everyone concerned with sport, and help prevent infection with other, far commoner conditions. The overall diagnosis and management of these have been reviewed by Diop Mar (1988) and Strauss (1988), and by Sharp (1994).

References

Ahlberg, A. (1965) Hemophilia in Sweden VII. Incidence, treatment and other musculo-skeletal manifestations of hemophilia A and B. *Acta Orthop Scandanavica* (suppl. 77).

Austin, E., Rolland, W. and Clausen, D. (1961) Use of physical modalities in the treatment of orthopaedic and neurologic residuals in hemophilia. *Arch. Phys. Med Rehab*, **42**, 393–397.

Boone, D.C. (1966) Physical therapy aspects related to orthopaedic and neurologic residuals of bleeding. *Phys Ther*, **42**, 1272–1281.

Boone, D.C. (1974) Management of musculoskeletal problems of hemophilia. *Phys Ther*, **54**, 122–127.

Buzzard, B.M. and Jones, P.M. (1988) Physiotherapy management of haemophilia: an update. *Physiotherapy*, **74**, 221–226.

Cole, S. and Jones, P. (1976) Physiotherapy in haemophilia. *Physiotherapy*, **62**, 217–221.

de Andrade, J.R. (1965) Joint distension and reflex muscle infiltration in the knee. *J Bone Joint Surg*, **47**, 313–322.

Dietrich, J.L. (1975) Rehabilitation and nonsurgical management of musculoskeletal problems in the hemophilic patient. *Am NY Acad Sci*, **240**, 328–337.

Diop Mar, I. (1988) Infectious diseases in tropical climates, in *The Olympic Book of Sports Medicine*, vol. 1 (eds A. Dirix, H.G. Knultgen and K. Tittel), **4**, 583–588.

Greenan-Fowler, E, Powell, C. and Varni, J.W. (1987) Behavioural treatment of adherence to therapeutic exercise by children with haemophilia. *Arch Phys Med Rehab*, **68**, 846–849.

Greene, W.B. and Strickler, E.M. (1983) A modified isokinetic strengthening program for patients with severe hemophilia. *Dev Med Child Neurol*, **25**, 189–196.

Grisogno, V. (1991) *Children and Sport*, John Murray, London.

Jones, P. (ed.) (1980) *Haemophilia Home Therapy*, Pitman Medical, London.

Jones, P. (1996) *Living with Haemophilia*, 4th edn, Oxford University Press, Oxford.

Koch, B, Cohen, S, and Luban, N.C. (1982) Hemophiliac knee: rehabilitation techniques. *Arch Phys Med Rehab*, **63**, 379–382.

Koch, B, Galioto, F.M., Kelleher, J. and Goldstein, D. (1984) Physical fitness in children with hemophilia. *Arch Phys Med Rehab*, **65**, 324–326.

Lazerson, J. (1975) It's a new ballgame for hemophiliac youngsters. *Phys Sports Med* **3**, 63–65.

McLain, L.G. and Heedrich, F.T. (1990) Hemophilia and sports: guidelines for participation. *Phys Sports Med*, **18**, 73–80.

Scottish Sports Council (1989) *Infections and Sports: A Short Guide to the Dangers and Precautions,* SSC, Edinburgh.

Seeler, R., Ashenhurst J. and Miller, J. (1975) A summer camp for hemophiliacs. *J Pediatr*, **87**, 758–759.

Sharp, J.C.M. (1994) Infections in sport, in *ABC of Sports Medicine. British Medical Journal*, **308**, 1702–1706.

Stokes, M. and Young, A. (1984) The contribution of reflex inhibition to arthrogenous muscle weakness. *Clin Sci*, **67**, 714.

Strauss, R.H. (1988) Infectious diseases in temperate climates, in *The Olympic Book of Sports Medicine*, vol. 1 (eds A. Dirix, H.G. Knultgen and K. Tittel), pp. 589–602.

United Kingdom Health Education Authority (1992) *Sport and HIV: A Kitbag Guide for Managers, Coaches and Players,* HEA, London.

Varni, J.W. and Wallender, J.L. (1984) Adherence to health-related regimens in pediatric chronic disorders. *Clin Psychol Rev*, **4**, 585–596.

Weigel, N. and Carlson, B.R. (1975) Physical activity and the haemophiliac: yes or no? *Am Corr Ther J*, **29**, 197–205.

Weissman, J. (1977) Rehabilitation medicine and the hemophilic patient. *Mount Sinai J Med*, **44**, 359–370.

World Health Organization (1989) *Consensus Statement on AIDS and Sport*, WHO, Geneva.

13 VISCERAL BLEEDING

M.J. Inwood

Historical reviews of hemophilia emphasize the relative frequency of joint hemorrhages and other closed-space hemorrhages but have given little significance to visceral hemorrhages (Ingram, 1976). Similarly, reviews of causes of death in hemophilia state a relatively low incidence of death due to visceral bleeding. Aronson (1988), in reviewing causes of death in hemophilia A patients in the USA from 1968 to 1979 demonstrated that in association with an overall increase in the median age at death compared to historical controls, visceral bleeding accounted for a very small fraction of such deaths. Gastrointestinal bleeding accounted for 4% of deaths as compared to 2.5% in a comparable group of non-hemophiliacs. Genitourinary bleeding deaths in hemophilia was 1% compared to 0.6% in the corresponding non-hemophilia population. Cirrhosis was considered to be a significant cause of death in hemophilia; undoubtedly this could present with gastrointestinal symptoms and signs. In the seven deaths noted in this survey secondary to renal causes, none were ascribed to intrarenal hemorrhage.

A more recent survey of causes of death among people with hemophilia A reported digestive system disease as a cause of death in 5% of individuals (Chorba *et al.*, 1994). The cause of death was as described on the death certificate and it is very likely that a number of these individuals could well have had human immuno-deficiency virus (HIV)/hepatitis C virus (HCV)-related disease with gastrointestinal hemorrhage secondary to hepatic disease. Such data present a number of difficulties in identifying the actual cause of death as primarily due to renal disease and hemorrhage in hemophilia. Nevertheless, the authors clearly proved the close relationship between HIV-1 infection and the increased death rate among the hemophilia population in the years 1968 to 1989. They also noted that this same group of individuals would have had an increased rate of sero-positivity to hepatitis B and C virus which, in turn, could be related to visceral bleeding as a cause of death.

In considering the complications of hemophilia which can cause significant morbidity and mortality, recent reviews tend to de emphasize genitourinary and gastrointestinal bleeding as a common problem in the management of hemophiliac bleeding (Furie, Limentani and Rosenfield, 1994). Hematuria is considered to be a common problem but one which does not require energetic factor therapy. Gastrointestinal bleeding is considered not to be a common problem and usually responds to 50% replacement factor levels.

All the above considerations suggest that visceral bleeding in hemophilia is a relatively uncommon complication and, therefore, generally does not cause a great deal of concern to the attending physician. This chapter will, however, emphasize that if visceral bleeding occurs it is necessary for the attending physician to ensure that a diligent search is made to identify the precise cause when possible in association with appropriate prompt replacement therapy. Hemoptysis is still considered to be a very unusual cause of bleeding in hemophilia but it has probably increased as a concomitant problem since the advent of HIV-associated opportunistic infections of the pulmonary tract. Therefore, this chapter will primarily examine the causes and treatment of genitourinary and gastrointestinal hemorrhage, with mention being made of hemoptysis primarily as a symptom of other underlying disease in the hemophiliac. In general, these three manifestations of hemorrhage occur more commonly in the severely affected factor VIII and factor IX deficiencies. They are rarely, if ever, seen in mildly affected individuals in the absence of concomitant trauma or other disease processes.

Finally, the diagnosis of visceral bleeding in hemophilia has been much improved by the advent and increasing

Hemophilia. Edited by C.D. Forbes, L. Aledort and R. Madhok. Published in 1997 by Chapman & Hall, London. ISBN 0 412 63820 7

sophistication of non-invasive diagnostic procedures, thus, making management of this complication of hemophilia very much easier to treat compared to the decades prior to 1980. Diagnosis before 1970 was principally related to roentgenography, clinical acumen and invasive diagnostic procedures, including laparotomy and other surgical procedures. All of these procedures were not without risk when considering that they were performed under the cover of lower-potency concentrates, or indeed, lack of concentrates. The new era of high-potency concentrates and a wide variety of non-invasive diagnostic procedures have increased survival due to such hemorrhage. Unfortunately, visceral bleeding in hemophilia has been complicated by the emergence of two significant viral infections – HIV and HCV, both of which can provide for significant bleeding problems, particularly in the gastrointestinal and pulmonary tracts.

Gastrointestinal bleeding

The most recent review of patterns of gastrointestinal hemorrhage in hemophilia is by Mittal and workers (1985), reviewing 243 patients with factor VIII and factor IX deficiency registered with the Hemophilia Center of Western Pennsylvania between 1973 and 1982. It is important to note that this review was performed before the onslaught of HIV infection and before the identification of HCV as the main cause of hepatitis in the multitransfused hemophiliac. The causes of gastrointestinal hemorrhage were peptic ulcer in 28.5% of individuals, gastritis in 11%, bowel hematoma in 5% and a number caused by a wide variety of other conditions including reflux esophagitis, bleeding varices, Mallory–Weiss syndrome, diverticulosis, non-specific proctitis, rectal hemorrhoids and rectal fissure. A total of 38% of all episodes had an unknown site of hemorrhage either due to non-detection of the bleeding site or sites or because no work-up had been performed prior to or during treatment. It was also noted that retroperitoneal hemorrhage could present with abdominal pain.

Diagnosis was principally confirmed by gastrointestinal tract endoscopy, conventional radiology, computed tomography (CT) or ultrasonography of the abdomen. Prior to Mittal's review a thorough assessment of gastrointestinal bleeding in hemophilia had been completed by Forbes and coworkers in 1973. They noted that gastrointestinal hemorrhage had been the second commonest cause of spontaneous bleeding in a number of publications prior to 1966 and that it was considered that approximately one-third of deaths in the hemophiliac population resulted from uncontrolled intestinal hemorrhage or its sequelae. In many cases no local source of bleeding could be found. They noted that in many cases operative intervention was necessary, concomitant with massive hemorrhage and performed with either inappropriate or non-availability of concentrates. Fortunately, in a few years prior to their review there had been dramatic changes in the availability of concentrates and, thus, in their opinion, it seemed reasonable to reassess the prognosis of gastrointestinal hemorrhage in patients with hemophilia. Therefore, in a retrospective study of adult patients in the western region of Scotland it was found that 32 patients had experienced 107 episodes of hematemesis or melena. This represented an incidence of 25% of the patients at risk. The commonest cause was peptic ulceration, demonstrated in 53% of these patients by serial barium meal examinations. The diagnostic cause of bleeding on the first occasion remained a problem as in only 9 out of 32 patients was a probable cause shown. Bleeding as the result of ingestion of salicylates or alcohol was uncommon.

When dyspeptic symptoms were used to divide patients into two subgroups it was found that there was a significantly higher number of patients with a severe grade of hemophilia who were eupeptic when they bled, whereas in the dyspeptic group there was a significantly higher number of moderately affected patients. In this series of patients emergency surgical procedures were not common compared to the authors' historical review. All acute bleeding episodes were controlled by plasma or plasma concentrate and elective surgery performed as necessary. Only one patient died of hemorrhage and he was shown to have a potent factor VIII inhibitor. Their comment at that time was that it was apparent that modern treatment with modern plasma concentrates had substantially altered the prognosis of gastrointestinal hemorrhage in patients with coagulation defects. However, in a prophetic statement they further noted that the use of concentrates introduced the hazards of serum hepatitis. We now know that this was further complicated by the advent of HIV infection in the early part of the 1980s. Furthermore, the use of non-steroidal anti-inflammatory agents in the treatment of hemophiliac arthropathy has probably further increased the risk of gastrointestinal hemorrhage (see below).

Gastrointestinal hemorrhage is a well-appreciated complication of oral anticoagulant therapy and it is of interest to note that gastrointestinal bleeding has revealed mild cases of hemophilia (Baele, Milo and Barbier, 1973). Equally, stress, because of its association with peptic ulceration, has also been related to bleeding episodes in hemophilia and in particular gastrointestinal bleeding (Perrin, MacLean and Janco, 1988). Acute abdominal pain presenting clinically as an intramural hematoma (see below) has been suggested as a reason to exclude acquired and hereditary disorders of coagulation (Roy, Tillyer and Colvin, 1988).

Intra-abdominal hemorrhage in patients with hemophilia may mimic many intra-abdominal conditions. Jones and Kitchens in 1984 emphasized the fact that, although intramural hematoma and peptic ulceration were probably the two main causes of gastrointestinal hemorrhage in the hemophiliac or individuals with acquired coagulation disorders, there were many other conditions which, because of the underlying hemophiliac condition, could masquerade as gastrointestinal bleeding, e.g. ruptured aortic aneurysm, tumor or abscess. In addition, Sitaram *et al.* (1990) emphasize that pre-existing gastrointestinal lesions, e.g. jejunal hemangioma, granulomatous bowel disease, appendicitis, Meckel's diverticulum and other gastrointestinal lesions, could be uncovered by the underlying coagulation disorder. Salomon and Tatarski (1965) state that unexplained chronic intestinal hemorrhage must require the ruling out of other coagulation disorders, both of an acquired and congenital type. They presented a case of von Willebrand's disease who originally presented with chronic intestinal hemorrhage of unknown origin.

This chapter recognizes the change in the patterns of gastrointestinal bleeding now that the use of prophylactic concentrate therapy in severely affected hemophiliacs is becoming most common. It emphasizes the reduced occurrence of intramural gastrointestinal hemorrhage, iliopsoas hemorrhage, retroperitoneal hemorrhage, pseudotumor of the abdomen presenting with abdominal findings and peptic ulceration because of therapy changes and improvements. In addition, comments will also be directed to the impact of HIV and HCV infections in gastrointestinal hemorrhage.

INTRAMURAL GASTROINTESTINAL HEMORRHAGE

This is a specific and dramatic clinical presentation also well-appreciated as a complication during oral anticoagulation and has been described as a non-surgical acute abdomen due to intramural bowel hematoma (Salomon and Tatarski, 1985). The patient shows clinical signs of bowel obstruction and presents in extreme pain with either localized or diffuse visible hyperperistalsis and an often palpable mass. This presentation has very often in past years been confused with bowel obstruction due to other causes. Nevertheless, the incidence of this complication in severely affected factor VIII and factor IX deficiencies not on prophylactic therapy is common enough that it is important that any clinician dealing with the hemophiliac must be aware of its presentation and the need to avoid any form of surgical intervention until otherwise proven.

Griffin *et al.*, in a review of this syndrome in 1986, emphasized that in the clinical presentation, cramping abdominal pain, nausea, vomiting, obstipation and abdominal distension were often present. The small intestine is most often involved with the jejunum as the most common site. Stomach and esophagus are rarely involved but are described (Oldenburger and Gundlach,

1977; Elland, Han and Hicks, 1978; Gordon *et al.*, 1981). Sigmoid and other segments of the colon are even more rarely involved (Harrison *et al.*, 1972). Generally speaking, intramural hematoma presenting in the upper gastrointestinal tract will often be associated with hematemesis. Intramural hemorrhage into the lower bowel can often present with bright red rectal bleeding (Pauly, Watson-Williams and Trudeau, 1987). It has been further emphasized by many of the authors who have presented cases with this syndrome that the patient will present with the signs of an acute surgical abdomen in the absence of visible bleeding and that the bleeding will occur subsequently, probably as a result of necrosis of the mucosal layers of the intestine with blood exiting from the hematoma into the lumen of the bowel.

Diagnosis

If gross blood is not present in the stool, appropriate tests for occult blood should be performed in order to assess whether or not there is leakage from the intramural hematoma. As has already been stated the palpable mass may after several days' duration discharge into the bowel through a rupture in the mucosal layer with the sudden appearance of blood. Occasionally hemorrhage can occur through the serosal surface of the intestine with subsequent free blood and clot being found in the peritoneal cavity. Conventional roentgenographic examination for abdominal symptoms from intramural hematoma or for any other cause of abdominal pain should include plain roentgenograms of the abdomen with a small-bowel series or a barium enema examination or both. As intramural bleeding is more often found in the small-bowel than the colon a barium meal with small-bowel follow-through will often demonstrate in the area of the hematoma straightened mucosal folds. These are sharply outlined with narrow troughs in between, resulting in a 'picket fence' or 'stacked coin' appearance (Dodds, Spitzer and Friedland, 1970). The affected bowel is moderately rigid, its wall thickened and peristalsis is frequently absent or diminished. Mesenteric bleeding often contributes to variable degrees of luminal narrowing but complete obstruction is infrequent. Localized masses or contour defects are seldom present in hemophiliac intramural bleeding. Once bleeding is controlled and reabsorption of the intramural hematoma and secondary edema has occurred, the obstruction is relieved and the initial roentgenographic findings resolve.

The advent of ultrasound diagnosis of abdominal pathology has now allowed this technique largely to replace the roentgenographic procedures, in particular the contrast medium procedures. Lee, Brickman and Avecilla in 1977 attributed a diagnosis of intramural hematoma to a typical sonographic pattern consisting of a series of strong echoes in the center of an anechoic mantle. The anechoic mantle is considered to be the thickened bowel wall and the strong cluster of central echoes represents the considerable difference in impedance between the wall and the lumen. While this sign has been reported in connection with tumors and inflammatory disease, including abscess formation, it is such a characteristic finding in intestinal hematoma that it allows for confident conservative management of the hemophiliac presenting with an acute surgical abdomen.

Morimoto and coworkers (1988) have confirmed these findings and also demonstrate the characteristic ultrasound findings in gastric and duodenal hematoma. Their cases showed echogenic masses posterior to the gastric wall. The hematoma was confirmed by CT, which also demonstrated a high-density mass in the same location. Contrast medium was used to reveal the disappearance of the mucosal fold in the posterior wall of the stomach in one of their cases, thus, demonstrating that a series of investigations often has to be employed to confirm the diagnosis. They emphasized that the gastric, duodenal and intestinal walls are thickened and show characteristic hypoechoic changes which allows for simple non-invasive monitoring of often relatively large and complex hemorrhages. However, while easy to detect, these ultrasonographic observations are not entirely specific in the hemophiliac as they can be seen with various neoplasms and inflammatory lesions which could be associated with concomitant HIV or HCV infection. As Morimoto *et al.* (1988) demonstrated, while barium studies may show the point of obstruction and its relationship to the remainder of the intestine if the lesion has not evacuated itself into the bowel, CT and ultrasound reveal the extent of bleeding more clearly. In the case of the upper bowel, tracking of hemorrhage into the retroperitoneal tissues can be quite extensive.

Management

The immediate need is to initiate conservative management for bowel obstruction. Immediate replacement of the deficient clotting factor to at least 0.50 u/ml (50%) or preferably 1.0 u/ml (100%) is necessary. Continuous infusion of factor concentrate will rapidly achieve a steady-state factor level and is the method of choice in controlling both gastrointestinal and genitourinary bleeding, particularly if invasive diagnostic or surgical procedures are to be used. The patient is given appropriate fluid and electrolyte replacement while fluids are withheld by mouth. The patient is started on a 'by mouth' diet once the intramural hemorrhage is under control and signs of obstruction have been completely resolved.

RETROPERITONEAL HEMORRHAGE

Retroperitoneal hemorrhage has been well-appreciated as a significant cause of occult bleeding in the severely affected hemophiliac. Besides being associated with blunt and penetrating trauma, retroperitoneal hemorrhage will often present as an acute surgical abdomen with diffuse periumbilical pain, flexing of the lower extremities with tracking of bleeding into the lower fascial planes (Fig. 13.1). The degree of bleeding can be severe enough

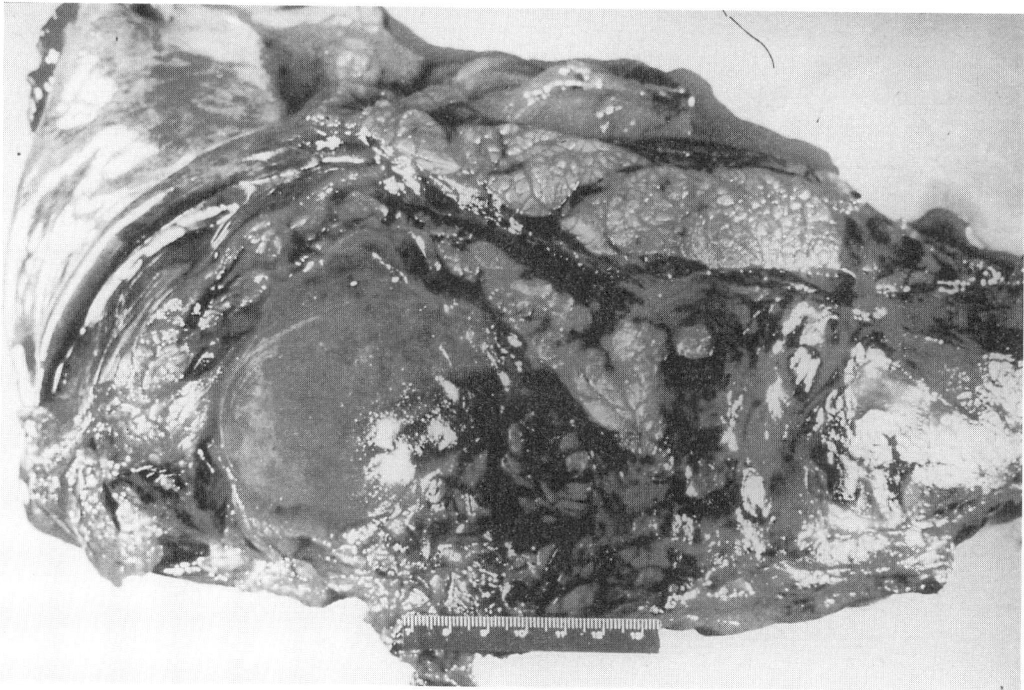

Fig. 13.1 Massive retroperitoneal hemorrhage. An autopsy specimen showing the large infiltrating hematoma in the retroperitoneal tissues of a severely affected factor VIII-deficiency hemophiliac with a factor VIII inhibitor.

to cause significant hypotension and systemic intravascular volume changes requiring energetic and acute resuscitation. The extent of and tracking of the hemorrhage between fascial planes will often require replacement with red cells (Fig. 13.2). It can often masquerade, as in common with the other causes of gastrointestinal bleeding in hemophilia, with a number of other conditions including appendicitis (Aronstam, 1985). If associated with significant intravascular volume changes it must be considered part of the differential diagnosis of a significant intra-abdominal hemorrhagic catastrophe.

Diagnosis

Survival of the patient often depends on rapid and accurate diagnosis (McCort, 1976). Tracking into the retroperitoneal tissues will cause significant changes which can be seen using conventional roentgenographic, ultrasound and CT examination. Conventional radiologic

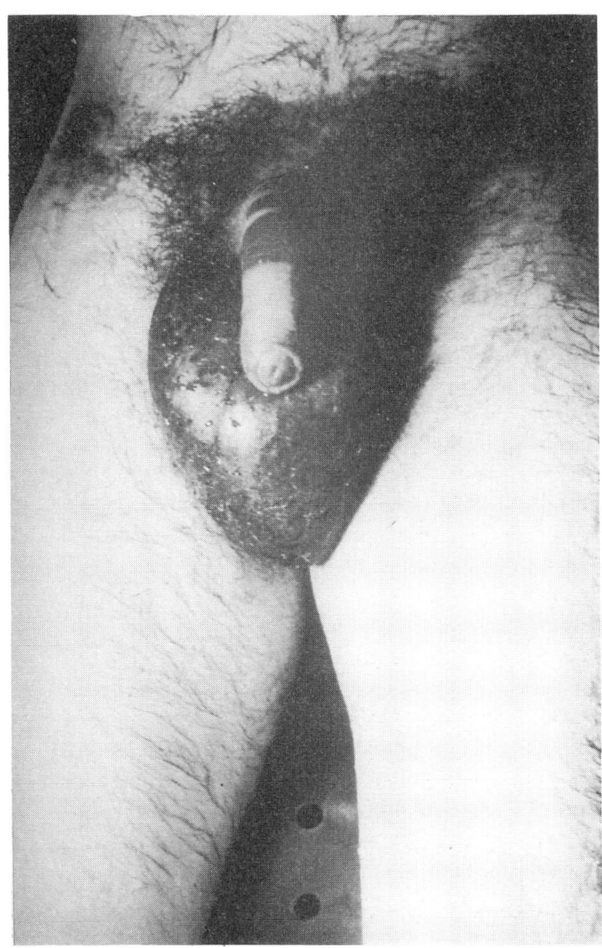

Fig. 13.2 Retroperitoneal hemorrhage with tracking of dependent hemorrhage into the scrotal sac. Note the superficial hemorrhage also in the inguinal crease which emanated from a fatal retroperitoneal hemorrhage in a severely affected factor VIII-deficient hemophiliac with an inhibitor.

examination will include blurring of the outlines of the iliopsoas with or without impairment of renal flow on intravenous pyelogram studies. Ultrasound examination will demonstrate changes in echo patterns in the retroperitoneal tissues independent of bowel outline. CT examination shows characteristic displacement of the retroperitoneal tissues by blood using appropriate cross-section imaging.

Management

The immediate assumption must be to consider intra-abdominal bleeding as the cause of the abdominal findings and immediately to replace the deficient factor to a minimum of 0.50 u/ml (50%) and a maximum of 1.0 u/ml (100%), preferably given by a continuous infusion method. Subsequently, upon confirmation of the diagnosis it is important to monitor the individual's factor VIII or factor IX levels until the clinician is satisfied that there is no evidence of further bleeding and that the abdominal symptoms and signs have fully resolved. This is confirmed by appropriate non-invasive serial imaging. Even small retroperitoneal hemorrhages must be treated energetically in order to prevent compression of the ureters and other retroperitoneal structures (see below). In the individual who presents with evidence of systemic hypotension, energetic resuscitation with appropriate intravenous fluids and red cells along with factor replacement must be commenced.

ILIOPSOAS HEMORRHAGE

This hemorrhage is included here because the clinical presentation of an iliopsoas hemorrhage, even though presenting with characteristically a flexed lower extremity on the side of the hemorrhage along with a femoral nerve lesion, can often present initially with localized right lower quadrant pain. The important consideration is that any person with hemophilia who presents with right lower quadrant pain should always have an alternate clinical diagnosis considered other than appendicitis, with the often surgical indication for immediate appendectomy (McCoy and Kitchens, 1991). In addition, the very large muscle mass inside the abdomen lends itself to rapid loss of blood and this can often cause significant intravascular volume instability, causing further diagnostic confusion (Aronstam, 1985).

Diagnosis

Iliopsoas hematoma provides for a classic ultrasound diagnosis (Figs 13.3 and 13.4). However, urinalysis, roentgenography of the lumbar spine, pelvis and hip and intravenous pyelogram may all be necessary to confirm the diagnosis. If the ultrasound shows a hypoechoic area

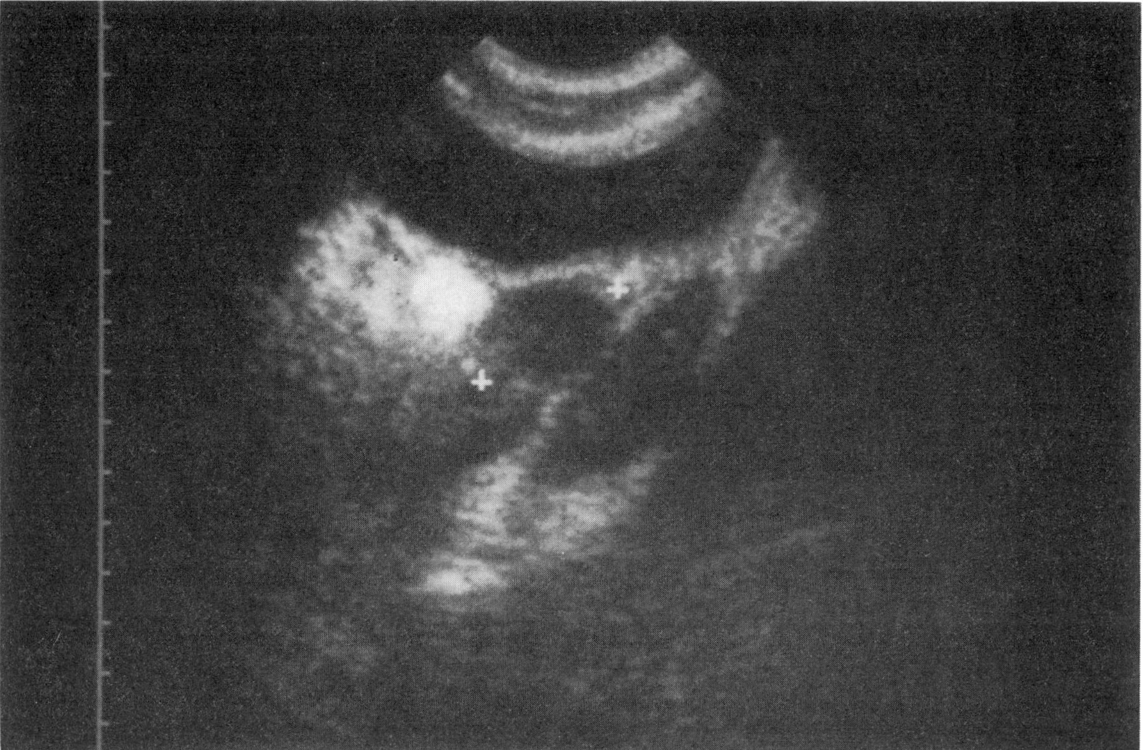

Fig. 13.3 Iliofemoral hemorrhage in a severely affected factor VIII-deficient hemophiliac. This sagittal/oblique ultrasound has the cursors demarcating the hypoechoic hemorrhage with the bladder outlined superior to the cursors.

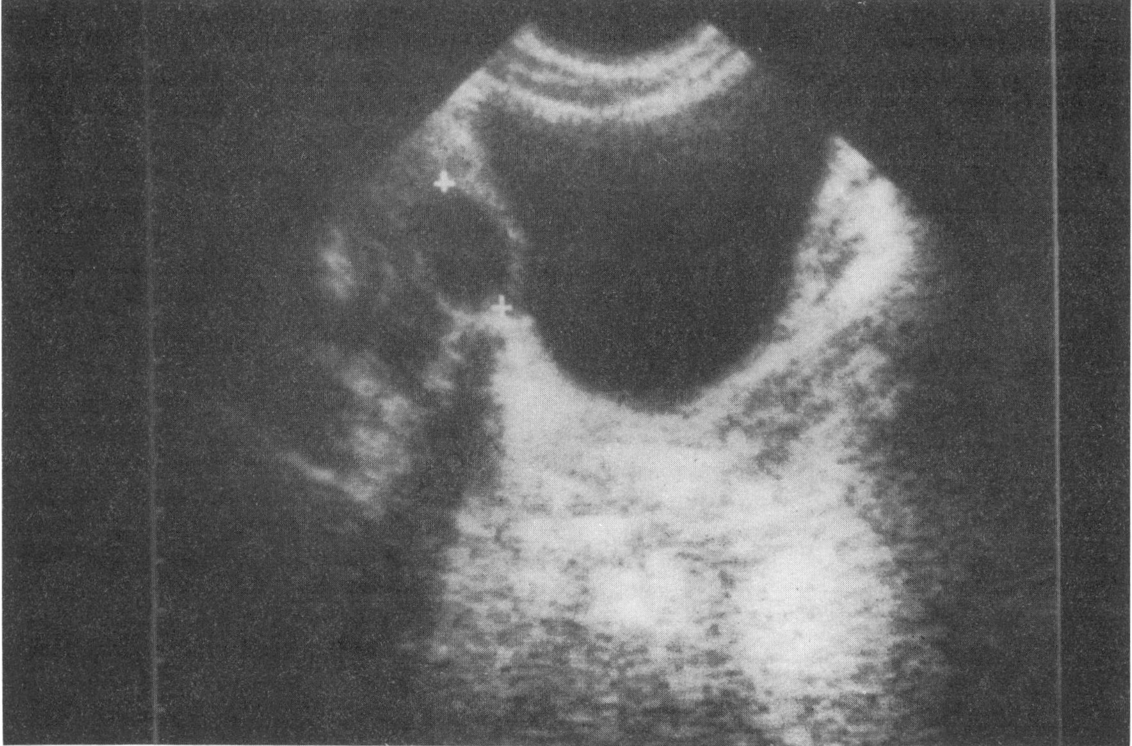

Fig. 13.4 Iliofermal hemorrhage in a severely affected factor VIII-deficient hemophiliac. This transverse image from ultrasound examination shows the cursors outlining a hypoechoic mass situated in the region of the right iliopsoas muscle. The differential diagnosis for this mass would also have to include an abscess and lymphadenopathy as well as hemorrhage.

within the iliopsoas muscle, this generally suffices to prove the diagnosis in association with its clinical presentation. Conventional plain abdominal radiology will often show a blurred psoas shadow with intravenous pyelography demonstrating displacement of the ureter and/or pressure on the bladder wall. CT scanning will again show excellent delineation of the intramuscular hemorrhage. The author has also used magnetic resonance imaging (MRI) to advantage in this situation. Its use has not been documented in the literature to date (Heim *et al.*, 1982).

Management

Veltkamp (1975) made an interesting observation with regard to iliopsoas hemorrhage masquerading as acute appendicitis. He stated that, as always, there is the dilemma in choosing between inflammation and bleeding in the right lower quadrant. His advice was always to await the effect of infusion therapy with benefit apparent within 6–12 h. It was considered that conservative treatment of appendicitis was not unreasonable and noted 'the traditional argument between Dutch doctors at sea, over surgical or conservative treatment of appendicitis had never been settled'. These statements were made prior to the advent of the more specific imaging techniques of ultrasound and CT. Replacement therapy, as previously described, with appropriate concentrates to a minimum level of 50% (0.5 u/ml) is necessary.

PSEUDOTUMOR WITH GASTROINTESTINAL MANIFESTATIONS

Coon and Penner (1981) noted that abdominal hemophilic pseudotumors are rare but frequently present with disabling and life-threatening complications in patients with severe hemophilia. Often these people will document progressive increasing disability from severe abdominal pain, which may or may not be associated with evidence of other nerve compression and/or lower-extremity swelling. Therefore, in any hemophiliac, particularly severely affected, who presents with ill-defined abdominal pain, a full investigation should be undertaken not only to exclude causes of intra-abdominal bleeding which have already been alluded to but also to exclude pseudotumor formation in the pelvic/bony structures.

Diagnosis

Conventional roentgenographic examination should reveal the abnormal bony expansion with subsequent compression on intra-abdominal structures which in turn is considered to be the cause of the abdominal symptoms. CT and MRI will provide for confirmation of diagnosis

(Hampton *et al.*, 1990). The radiologic features of pseudotumors relate directly to the pathologic process. A soft-tissue mass of variable size is usually evident and may be calcified or ossified. With skeletal involvement there is commonly bone erosion or destruction with periosteal elevation and formation of bony struts related to the mass of the pseudotumor (Bonner Guilford *et al.*, 1980). Acute bleeding into the abdomen can also occur which could then present with clinical findings of a peritonitis. In the most advanced cases it is possible that fistula formation and masses may be noted in the abdominal wall.

Management

Management is described in Chapter 11.

PEPTIC ULCERATION

In general, peptic ulceration with gastrointestinal blood loss in the hemophiliac is commonly associated with the use of anti-inflammatory medications. Although studies have been performed to demonstrate the relative safety of specific anti-inflammatory agents, with regard to occult gastrointestinal blood loss it is reasonable to expect that either due to idiosyncratic reactions or to the abuse of such medications this is not an unreasonable consideration in the hemophiliac with arthropathy using such agents (Inwood, Killackey and Startup, 1983). Thould, Keeling and Murrell (1982), investigating gastric microbleeding with Benoxaprofen, found that patients with hemophilia had no significant increase in gastrointestinal blood loss with the use of this medication when compared to the use of a placebo. However, studies have been limited in terms of the various anti-inflammatory medications available and peptic ulcer secondary to non-steroidal anti-inflammatory agents in the hemophiliac has been described (Thould, Keeling and Murrell, 1982). Clinical presentation is as for the non-hemophiliac patient. Certainly dyspepsia and reflux esophagitis in a hemophiliac taking anti-inflammatory medications must be considered of significance and investigated accordingly.

Diagnosis

Gastric endoscopy is the procedure of choice and now replaces, in large part, conventional roentgenographic examination.

Management

In the presence of upper gastrointestinal hemorrhage and prior to gastroscopy, urgent factor replacement to a minimum level of 0.50 u/ml (50%) is necessary. Once ulceration has been demonstrated, conventional treatment using appropriate mucosal-protective agents and continuing factor replacement allow for rapid resolution of the lesion.

HEPATIC DISEASE AS A CAUSE OF GASTROINTESTINAL HEMORRHAGE

Chapter 24 describes the effects of hepatic disease on the hemophiliac. It is of interest to note that abnormalities in the liver, and for that matter, spleen, were well-appreciated many years ago (Meyer *et al.*, 1983). It is now evident that most of these changes and the complications thereof relate to infection with either hepatitis B virus or, more recently and more commonly, HCV infection causing varying degrees of hepatic disease, including cirrhosis. All of the intra-abdominal bleeding syndromes associated with hepatitis and cirrhosis are to be expected and these will include upper gastrointestinal hemorrhages such as esophageal varices with hematemesis as opposed to bright red rectal bleeding as a consequence of enlarged and congested hemorrhoidal veins (Singh *et al.*, 1993). It would therefore seem reasonable, in any hemophiliac presenting with either upper or lower gastrointestinal bleeding, to exclude significant hepatic disease as part of the initial investigations.

HEMOPHILIC GASTROINTESTINAL BLEEDING AND HIV INFECTION

It is now evident that a wide variety of gastrointestinal manifestations are present in HIV infection and, specifically, acquired immunodeficiency syndrome (AIDS; Tanowitz, Simon and Wittner, 1992). Therefore it is not unexpected that the literature is now beginning to correlate gastrointestinal bleeding and HIV disease in hemophiliacs who have been infected with blood products prior to the availability of viral-attenuated concentrates (Garcia-Pagan *et al.*, 1988). Cappell and Seller reported endoscopy findings in 50 consecutive HIV seropositive patients who underwent endoscopy for gastrointestinal bleeding. They concluded from their study that, not only was endoscopy an important and indicated procedure in such patients, but also that such patients have an exceedingly poor prognosis with the mortality from gastrointestinal bleeding in this group being 39% as compared to 8.3% in a non-HIV-infected population. Furthermore, bleeding in the hemophiliac concomitantly infected with HIV disease would correspondingly be more severe. Warrier *et al.* (1994) reviewed 30 HIV-reactive patients with hemophilia or severe von Willebrand's disease for the spectrum of gastrointestinal and hepatic manifestations. Gastrointestinal symptoms occurred in nine patients, six had upper gastrointestinal bleeding, two had lower gastrointestinal bleeding, two had bloody diarrhea and two had chronic pancreatitis with a clinical presentation of an acute abdomen. They noted that the upper gastrointestinal hemorrhages were secondary to esophagitis, gastritis, esophageal varices and nonsteroidal anti-inflammatory medication use. The lower gastrointestinal hemorrhages were secondary to a solitary sigmoid ulcer and colitis in turn related to opportunistic organisms associated with HIV infection. However, they noted that, except for the one case of cytomegalovirus esophagitis and one case of *Cryptosporidium* diarrhea, no other infectious etiology was found to account for the bleeding. It is of interest to note that HCV was present in 78% of the hemophiliac patients surveyed in this study. Their conclusion was that gastrointestinal bleeding and hepatic manifestations were commonly seen in HIV-seroreactive hemophiliacs with CD4 counts of less than 500.0/ml. Their other concern in these patients was the presence of thrombocytopenia and coagulopathy secondary to hepatic disease and concomitant with their pre-existing hereditary coagulation defect.

Genitourinary bleeding

In 1975 Singer reviewed the renal and urologic complications of hemophilia. He made the following prophetic statement;

> The discriminating reader of this chapter will cautiously study the materials presented and interpret them with care. The literature has not presented a complete critical analysis of the hemophiliac and his renal problems. Consequently, many opinions and recommendations for therapy are unfortunately outdated, based on small series or reported with varied biases. The data is presented so that the physician can improve on the care and therapy offered to his patient in order that accurate diagnosis and therapy may be undertaken without causing undue harm to the patient.

An introductory comment made by Lazerson 1 year after Singer's review stated;

> Hematuria is one of the major clinical hemorrhagic manifestations of hemophilia which eventually affects the majority of patients. Although this can often be a distressing problem to the patient, treatment, including plasma concentrate replacement, bed rest, adequate hydration and the use of prednisone, is usually effective. Until recently, except for the patient who developed an obstructive uropathy secondary to clots lodged in the ureters and/or urethra, very little attention was given to the etiology of hematuria.

These two statements have not been improved upon in the intervening 20 years, with no major study devoted to the natural history of renal bleeding in hemophilia since the early 1980s (see below). However, since these two reviews there has been a significant increase in the sophistication of diagnostic and therapeutic methods and materials. Paradoxically, because of these advances, genitourinary bleeding in hemophilia has probably been given further short shrift. Nevertheless, it is important that even with improved care of particularly the young and adolescent hemophiliac, unexplained hematuria or unexpected renal symptoms or signs are thoroughly investigated. For the adult who has been concomitantly HIV- or HCV-infected there are a number of renal considerations which must be included in the routine care of such individuals (see below).

INCIDENCE OF GENITOURINARY BLEEDING

Information concerning incidence, although outdated, has basically been concerned either with cataloging the incidence of hematuria in patient groups or noting the occurrence of abnormalities affecting the urinary tract. Lazerson, in his 1976 review, provided information on 88 patients studied at the Children's Hospital of Los Angeles. The overall incidence of hematuria was 25%. Gross hematuria occurred almost exclusively in children older than 5 years and with less than 1% coagulant factor activity. No evidence of microscopic hematuria preceding the occurrence of gross hematuria was reported in any of the patients studied, although the opposite was usually observed with recurrences of hematuria. In the opinion of that author it was not unusual to observe microscopic hematuria as opposed to macroscopic hematuria in children and, with increasing age (after 10 years), almost twice as many children developed hematuria. In extrapolating these numbers from children to adults Singer noted that a variety of general studies had shown gross and/or microscopic hematuria to be present in up to 70% of adult hemophiliacs. Prentice and coworkers, including an editor of this volume (CDF), demonstrated that, in their series of 35 patients reported in 1971, again 70% showed either gross or microscopic hematuria exclusive of any other renal abnormalities demonstrated. As a general statement, it can now be probably stated that with the advent of prophylactic therapy (described elsewhere in this volume), the incidence of microscopic hematuria has greatly diminished, which in turn probably relates to Lazerson's original observations that hematuria is increased in individuals with less than 1% factor activity. In his 23 patients with greater than 5% activity no hematuria was noted. This would certainly be in keeping with the experience of this writer over the years in noting increasing bouts of hematuria as age increases and universally associated with severely affected individuals in the absence of other pre-existing genitourinary disease or abnormality.

MECHANISM OF BLEEDING

Both Lazerson and Singer emphasize that any individual presenting with hematuria must be assessed using the dif-ferential diagnosis of hematuria. Causes include trauma, infection, various forms of nephritis (which becomes more important in HIV affected individuals; see below, congenital structural defects, medications and other miscellaneous disorders, including sickle-cell disease and renal vein thrombosis. The latter conditions, although admittedly exceedingly rare, can still affect the individual with hemophilia. It is emphasized by a variety of workers that a careful investigation must be made in order to exclude causes other than hemophilia. Forbes *et al.* (1971) provide such an example in describing a case of rupture of the ureter due to a crush injury in a young male with severe hemophilia. They recommend that appropriate investigations must be performed to explain a recent onset of hematuria which cannot be related to solely the hemostatic defect of the individual.

A variety of theories have been advanced to explain spontaneous hematuria in the hemophiliac in the absence of other predisposing genitourinary abnormalities. It is well-appreciated that urokinase has the ability to activate plasminogen and thus the fibrinolytic system. Blood clots which often occur as a natural part of ongoing hemostasis in the severely affected hemophiliac can trigger urokinase activity. This was capitalized on by Gourdeau and Denton in 1970; they proposed that the mechanism of hematuria in hemophilia involved the reaction of the glomeruli capillary tufts to a variety of insults such as trauma, allergy, infection and/or toxins which, because of the decrease in hemostatic ability of the patient, caused the escape of red cells into the urine. Such a concept has not been validated, even though Lazerson noted that steroids appear to be more effective for treatment of hematuria in hemophilia than coagulation factor replacement (see below).

Immune injury to the kidney has also been implicated in causing hematuria in patients with hemophilia. The availability of coagulation factor replacement therapy and the knowledge that until recent times such concentrates were mixtures of a variety of active and partially denatured proteins suggest that a temporal relationship could exist between the increasing use of plasma concentrate and development of hematuria. As stated by Lazerson, coagulation concentrates may represent a large antigenic stimulus leading to antibody production and thus the development of immune complexes. Such a theory is attractive because of the demonstration that multiple transfused hemophiliacs develop antibodies to a variety of proteins.

Lazerson, in his 1976 review, presented a study of 24 patients with severe hemophilia, nine of whom had a history of chronic hematuria. Serum complement levels showed a statistically significant difference between patients with or without a history of gross or microscopic hematuria before and within 45 min of infusion of cryoprecipitate. There was no difference between patients on a prophylactic or as-needed cryoprecipitate infusion program. At the time of the study none of the patients had evidence of renal dysfunction.

LONG-TERM CONSEQUENCES OF GENITOURINARY BLEEDING

It would not be unreasonable to expect that, if severely affected hemophiliacs have hematuria starting from relatively early age, as time progressed they would present with increasingly serious renal abnormalities. The first significant study to test this assumption was that of Prentice and coworkers (including CDF), who initially described the abnormalities presenting in 35 hemophiliacs aged between 13 and 77 years in 1971. A series of clinical tests were performed, including blood urea nitrogen levels, creatinine clearance, quantitative urinary protein plus urinary leukocyte and erythrocyte cell excretion studies. Radiographic studies included renography and intravenous pyelography. The patient had to be hematuria-free for at least 2 weeks prior to testing. Only eight patients of the group had completely normal tests. A total of 38% had abnormal pyelograms, 21% had an abnormal renogram and 26% had a reduced creatinine clearance. Some 20% showed increased evidence of red cell excretion. Severe hemophiliacs with frequent hematuria yielded the most abnormalities, as also seen in Lazerson's series (Lazerson, 1976). However, five of 12 patients had no antecedent history of hematuria but had filling or obstructive defects present. None of the patients had a urinary tract infection.

In view of the great interest at that time in the use of antifibrinolytics in the treatment of hematuria it was noted that those individuals who had been treated with ε-aminocaproic acid (EACA) did not have an increased number of abnormalities. These results were also, in general, confirmed by another group in Birmingham, UK (Dholakia and Howarth, 1979).

Clearly it was of interest to know whether or not the radiographic and/or renal abnormalities were transient and of long-term clinical importance. Therefore, in 1982, Forbes and coworkers (Small *et al.*, 1982) reassessed biochemically and radiologically 27 of the patients from the two centers who had been previously investigated and noted to have abnormal radiographic changes. In addition, they also investigated a new series of 30 hemophiliacs who had been adequately treated by on-demand or self-therapy for at least 5 years prior to the study in order to determine if the incidence of renal abnormalities had decreased as a consequence of more active replacement treatment. This important study was able to demonstrate that, of the 27 original patients, one-third had a renal radiographic abnormality but only two had abnormalities persisting since the 1970s and attributable to renal bleeding. They considered isotope renography a

sensitive indicator of renal abnormality, whereas a history of hematuria was a poor discriminant for patients with abnormal intravenous urograms or impaired creatinine clearance. Their conclusion in this cohort of patients was that hematuria was not associated with progressive loss of renal function and its natural history in hemophilia is probably benign in the absence of other confounding renal problems. It also confirmed that hematuria was still a common complaint occurring in 67% of the follow-up group and 40% of the more intensively treated new patient group.

The results of the follow-up intravenous urography in 10 patients with abnormal findings in the first study showed that these abnormalities were due to a variety of changes, primarily in the pelviureteric junction, the pelvis or calyces of the kidneys. There was one bilateral hydronephrosis which was considered secondary to retroperitoneal fibrosis secondary to a retroperitoneal bleed or bleeds in the past. Of interest is that in the follow-up group the majority of the ureteric abnormalities were found to have reverted to normal, as were two pelviureteric and calyceal abnormalities. Hypertension, despite the high incidence of renal abnormality, occurred with a frequency in this patent group equivalent to that of the general population. Four patients had hypertension and only one had evidence of target organ damage as indicated by left ventricular hypertrophy. In comparing the 27 patients followed since 1969, and the 30 new patients, no significant differences were noted in comparing aspects of their renal function. Hematuria was noted in 67% of the follow-up population versus 40% in the new population. Hypertension, creatinine clearance, abnormal intravenous urograms and congenital anomalies were approximately the same in each cohort. No patient in either group had proteinuria or evidence of infection. The study is reported in detail because it represents the best comparison to date of hemophiliacs on long-term follow-up of hematuria or genitourinary abnormalities. It shows that no significant long-term sequelae were demonstrated and this, in all likelihood, is the opinion of most physicians treating persons with hemophilia today.

In addition, there are scattered reports which demonstrate that genitourinary bleeding, even though associated with abnormal diagnostic tests, can resolve rapidly. Patriquin (1980) reported a case of proven ureteric hemorrhage in a hemophiliac using two sequential intravenous urograms. He was able to demonstrate that hematuria associated with an intramural hemorrhage rapidly resolved with the disappearance of hematuria and the complete resolution of the previous abnormal urographic findings.

Conversely, there is a disturbing report by Gomperts, Malekzadeh and Fine (1981) in which they describe hematuria as a frequent and persisting feature in a hemophiliac from the age of 5 years. Anemia and proteinuria were first detected at 13 years of age. The patient proceeded to hemodialysis at 15 years of age. Subsequently a cadaver donor renal transplant was carried out after 3 months of hemodialysis. The allograph rejected after 3 months and the patient was maintained for another 8 years on hemodialysis. To complete this saga, a second cadaver donor allograft was carried out at 23 years of age. Clearly chronic renal failure can occur in hemophilia but these workers were not able directly to incriminate the chronic hematuria as the initial cause, even though no other etiology was found for the end-stage renal failure.

A final observation on the significance and long-term consequences of genitourinary bleeding in hemophilia was made by Veltkamp (1975), who noted that he had found much more serious kidney damage in hemophilic dogs than had been reported in humans. One hemophilic dog showed on autopsy a completely destroyed kidney which had been replaced by an organized hematoma. This suggests that significant renal disease can probably still occur with subsequent structural abnormality.

Diagnosis

As recommended for gastrointestinal bleeding, it is agreed that all the usual diagnostic procedures which are used to assess renal function and genitourinary tract integrity should be used in the hemophiliac with appropriate factor coverage for any potentially invasive procedure. As it is evident that microscopic hematuria is considered a complication of severely affected persons with hemophilia it is reasonable, as part of their overall comprehensive annual hemophilia assessment, that routine urinary microscopy, including urinary protein, glucose and other screening tests, should be performed at that time along with blood urea and creatinine serum levels. The advantage of having such serial assessments made as part of the annual comprehensive assessment is that if there is a significant change in any of these parameters the patient should be investigated with exactly the same approach as one would use for any non-hemophiliac patient with the same abnormalities.

A major difficulty relates to the indications for investigation of patients who present with repeated episodes of macroscopic hematuria. Mention has already been made of the important work performed by investigators from the UK in assessing the value of performing repeated procedures in the investigation of hematuria in the hemophiliac (Prentice *et al.*, 1971; Forbes and Prentice, 1977; Small *et al.*, 1982). We also have to accept that the majority of changes that have been noted in the urinary tract have been itemized on the basis of radiologic examination. Dholakia and Howarth in 1979 provided information on 28 hemophiliacs who were investigated with a total of 59 radiological examinations of the urinary tract, including 41 intravenous urograms. In 10 patients (36%), abnormalities were demonstrated in the urinary tract, six patients showed changes of hydronephrosis, one a non-functioning kidney and in two patients blood clots were shown in the collecting system. These abnormalities were again more common in clinically severe hemophiliacs while normal urographic appearances were more common in clinically mild cases. The cause of hydronephrosis was considered due to extrinsic compression, whether renal or ureteric or intrinsic from clot retention. In some cases the cause was not evident and it was suggested that in these the hydronephrosis may result from organization of a retroperitoneal hematoma with subsequent periureteric fibrosis. This investigation showed the importance of performing plain radiographs and intravenous urograms. CT scanning now furnishes an elegant display of retroperitoneal hematoma and is particularly valuable in demonstrating its effects on the renal tract. Access to isotope scanning, CT and MRI scanning has provided for increasing definition of the abnormalities in problematic renal symptoms and signs in the hemophiliac.

Nevertheless, Dholakia and Howarth (1979) were able to demonstrate using relatively simple radiologic techniques that obstructive uropathy was the most common abnormality in their series, which would certainly be in agreement with a number of the findings of *Prentice et al.* (1971). They demonstrated the existence of both renal hematoma, be they intrarenal or within the renal pelvis or collecting systems. Conventional radiology also allowed them to demonstrate the importance of ruling out retroperitoneal hematoma as the cause of acute or chronic renal changes. They had no radiologic evidence of renal papillary necrosis or changes secondary to pyelonephritis in their cases. Wright, Matthews and Brock (1971) have also presented a series of patients with hematuria where the abnormalities were again demonstrated by primary radiological examinations (Beck and Evans, 1972). Their results are in agreement with previous studies. Of interest is that several of these investigators noted that cystoscopy and ascending pyelouterography should be avoided because of the danger of further hemorrhages complicating instrumentation. It is now considered reasonable that the hemophiliac who has ongoing clinical bleeding from an unidentified genitourinary lesion should be exposed to such investigations provided that adequate coverage (at least 0.50 u/ml, 50%) when the appropriate factor concentrate is used. On an anecdotal basis it is reasonable to state that this type of procedure can be very helpful, particularly in vesicular bleeding, and it allows for biopsies to be taken as required.

Therefore, the final comment must be that in the diagnosis of the hemophiliac with unexplained genitourinary bleeding the standard of urologic diagnostic practise as used in any given facility must be used.

Management

A reasonable statement would be that no therapy should be initiated until there is a precise diagnosis of the cause of genitourinary bleeding with the hemophiliac. Unfortunately, or fortunately, as is now evident to many workers, appropriate factor VIII replacement is often initiated, e.g. 20–50% plasma level (0.02–0.05 u/ml) as severely affected individuals, certainly in North America and Europe, are often on self-infusion therapy. Equally, if they are facing a diagnostic procedure of any invasive nature, coverage of similar magnitude will also be given. Subsequently, once the diagnosis is made of either a correctable or non-correctable cause of the bleeding, one should then proceed with either the appropriate procedure or conservative management.

Therefore in the majority of hemophiliacs, as already emphasized, no specific cause for the bleeding will be found, even though there may be concomitant renal abnormalities present as a result of previous bleeding. As a result, conservative management of the bleeding is often the choice of the attending physician. In general, this conservative therapy is based upon the three principles of rest, adequate fluid intake to provide for adequate renal output and in most instances concomitant factor replacement to a minimum of a 50% (0.50 u/ml) level. Most cases of hematuria of unexplained origin will settle down very quickly on this regimen and rest alone with adequate fluid intake allowing for a urinary output of at least 100 ml/h during the waking hours may well be sufficient (Singer, 1975). The difficulty arises when the hematuria becomes intractable and no correctable cause can be found. In most cases replacement therapy is continued with the hope that the bleeding will eventually remit. This obviously causes a number of difficulties for the patient, who may be otherwise unaffected by the painless hematuria. Conversely, with replacement therapy patients may well suffer renal colic because of the variety of clots occurring in the genitourinary system. Analgesia and continuous bladder irrigation will require hospitalization and often transfusion with red cells as well as factor concentrate. It is not surprising, therefore, that alternatives have been sought either to reduce the degree of bleeding or to decrease the degree of disability.

In this situation, the use of steroids has been advocated by a number of workers. The basis for this therapy was originally related to the consideration that a variety of insults occurred to the glomerular–capillary tuft, including immune complex injury. Certainly, from an empiric point of view, prednisone in the order of 1–2 mg/kg has been advocated and used by a variety of workers in dealing with intractable hematuria (Gourdeau and Denton, 1970; Lazerson, 1976). Whether or not it has proven benefit has yet to be elucidated. Equally, whether or not it should be used for incidental hematuria or episodic non-complicated hematuria is a matter of opinion. This writer reserves its use in intractable non-correctable hematuria where conventional therapy of rest, increased urinary output and factor replacement has not been of benefit in the absence of a definable bleeding lesion.

The use of antifibrinolytic agents has been a matter of significant discussion. Originally, EACA and, later, tranexamic acid (AMCA) were considered to be useful in the treatment of hemophiliacs (Singer, 1975; Lazerson, 1976). From a pathophysiologic aspect, if there was no specific source of bleeding found which could be corrected, the combination of the decreased clotting ability of the patient coupled with the presence of urokinase in the urine and renal tissues would cause an already disturbed clot to be washed away, thus, preventing adequate hemostasis. However, it was also recognized that a possible risk of antifibrinolytic treatment could be an unusual resistance to clot dissolution and, thus, obstruction would occur in the renal tract. Enthusiasm undoubtedly decreased for EACA as the result of a variety of such complications being reported and these are thoroughly reviewed by Singer (1975). Complications included bilateral renal cortical necrosis, diffuse capillary thrombosis and insoluble fibrin plugs in the collecting systems, resulting in anuria and/or hydronephrosis. Consequently, EACA and AMCA were specifically contraindicated by their respective manufacturers in the treatment of renal bleeding.

Nevertheless – and this is where invasive diagnostic procedures are important and should be used whenever necessary – if a vesicular (bladder) lesion is the source of bleeding, this writer has found it of great benefit to use either direct bladder irrigation with AMCA and/or systemic AMCA therapy in the recommended doses in arresting such bleeding. It must be emphasized that if this is to be used it must be considered a treatment of last resort, with hospitalization and anemia being ongoing problems for the patient. The precautions which must be followed involve an adequate diagnostic work-up including cystoscopy and ascending pyelouterography. If bilateral renal and ureteric bleeding has been completely excluded as the cause of the ongoing hematuria and a specific bleeding site or sites has been identified in the bladder, continuous bladder irrigation must be initiated and continued while on antifibrinolytic therapy. Intravenous fluid administration must be given in order to maintain a renal output of a minimum of 100 ml/h. If all of these caveats are followed it has been found on an anecdotal basis that this procedure has been extremely useful, particularly in patients who have an associated factor inhibitor.

Mention must be made that the use of ancillary techniques to arrest bleeding should be used whenever technically feasible and available. Klamut *et al.* (1979)

reported a case of intractable renal bleeding treated with percutaneous, transcatheter, renal-arterial embolization. The treatment proved to be life-saving and 18-month follow-up revealed no evidence of hypertensive renal disease, infection or recurrent bleeding. This case emphasizes again that the hemophiliac should not be denied conventional or exceptional treatment.

RENAL DISEASE WITH HIV AND HCV INFECTION

It is now recognized that renal disease is often a complication of HIV disease, particularly in those patients who have progressed to AIDS. A wide variety of primary glomerular lesions have been described which result in nephrotic syndrome with or without renal insufficiency. Hematuria may often be a presenting symptom in such a situation. Nephrocalcinosis, acute pyelonephritis due to a wide variety of infections and neoplasms have all been reported (Sreepada Rao, 1995). Therefore, it would be reasonable that in the concomitantly HIV-infected hemophiliac all such diagnoses should be considered.

A number of renal lesions have been described in association with hepatitis virus infection, e.g. hepatitis B virus and HCV (Michel *et al.*, 1992). This again serves to demonstrate that hematuria in such seroreactive individuals must be of increased concern until otherwise proven. It is important to note that many of the surveys of hemophilia populations were performed prior to the advent of HIV and before the characterization of Hepatitis B virus and, more recently, HCV disease. As such, this represents another dimension with which the diagnostician is confronted when considering the cause of hematuria in the hemophiliac.

Hemoptysis

Hemoptysis is not considered to be a feature of hemophilia. When it occurs it is usually the result of bleeding in the proximal respiratory tract, e.g. retropharyngeal, oral lesions or epistaxis. Nevertheless, it has been noted that severe coughing spells, for example·in bronchitis or whooping cough, can lead to an increase in the pressure of blood in the head and neck and may precipitate bleeding from these areas (Jones, 1974). However, anecdotal cases have been noted which probably represent true *de novo* bleeding from the lung parenchyma. Veltkamp (1975) noted that hemoptysis in the hemophiliac was symptomatic of underlying lung disease, e.g. chronic bronchitis or bullous emphysema. He referred to these cases as having a 'locus minoris resistentiae', responsible for the precipitation of hemorrhage.

This would have been an entirely satisfactory explanation as, in the opinion of most practicing hematologists caring for hemophiliacs over extended periods of time,

hemoptysis is not considered to be a common presenting symptom. Unfortunately, with the advent of HIV infection, it is now quite evident that hemoptysis is not an uncommon concomitant symptom in HIV seroreactive hemophiliacs. There are a large number of causes in the HIV-infected individual and *Pneumocystis carinii* is by no means an uncommon cause, even in the non-hemophiliac patient (White and Zaman, 1992). It again emphasizes, as has been the case for gastrointestinal and genitourinary bleeding in the hemophiliac, that HIV disease adds another dimension to causes of bleeding and that hemoptysis in such an individual must be taken as an ominous sign of HIV-induced complications until otherwise proven.

References

Aronson, D.L. (1988) Cause of death in hemophilia A patients in the United States from 1968 to 1979. *American Journal of Hematology*, **27**, 7–12.

Aronstam, A. (1985) *Haemophilic Bleeding*, Baillière Tindall, London, pp. 65–66.

Baele, G., Milo, R. and Barbier, F. (1973) Gastrointestinal bleeding revealing a minor form of haemophilia A in an elderly patient. *Tijdschr-Gastroenterology*, **16**, 372–377.

Beck, P. and Evans, K.T. (1972) Renal abnormalities in patients with haemophilia and Christmas Disease. *Clinical Radiology*, **23**, 349–354.

Bonner Guilford, W., Mintz, P.D., Blatt, P.M. and Staab, E.V. (1980) CT of hemophilic pseudotumors of the pelvis. *American Journal of Radiology*, **135**, 167–169

Cappell, M.S. and Geller, A.J. (1992) The high mortality of gastrointestinal bleeding in HIV-seropositive patients: a multivariate analysis of risk factors and warning signs of mortality in 50 consecutive patients. *American Journal of Gastoenterology*, **87**, 815–824.

Chorba, T.L., Holman, R.C., Strine, T.W. *et al.* (1994) Changes in longevity and causes of death among persons with hemophilia A. *American Journal of Hematology*, **45**, 112–121.

Coon, W.W. and Penner, J.A. (1981) Management of abdominal hemophilic pseudotumor. *Surgery*, **90**, 735–740.

Dholakia, A.M. and Howarth, F.H. (1979). The urinary tract in haemophilia. *Clinical Radiology*, **30**, 533–538.

Dodds, W.J., Spitzer, R.M. and Friedland, G. W. (1970) Gastrointestinal roentgenographic manifestations of hemophilia. *American Journal of Roentgenology Radium Therapy and Nuclear Medicine*, **110**, 413–416.

Eiland, M., Han, S.Y. and Hicks, G.M. (1978) Intramural hemorrhage of the small intestine. *Journal of the American Medical Association*, **239**, 139–142.

Forbes, C.D. and Prentice, C.R.M. (1977) Renal disorders in haemophilia A and B. *Scandinavian Journal of Haematology*, **30** (suppl.), 45–50.

Forbes, C.D., Craig, J.A., Prentice, C.R. and McNichol, G.R. (1971) Rupture of the ureter due to crush injury in a boy with severe haemophilia. *British Journal of Surgery*, **58**, 931–934.

Forbes, C.D., Barr, R.D., Prentice, C.R.M. and Douglas, A.S. (1973) Gastrointestinal bleeding in haemophilia. *Quarterly Journal of Medicine, New Series*, **42**, 503–511.

Furie, B., Limentani, S.A. and Rosenfield, C.G. (1994) A practical guide to the evaluation and treatment of hemophilia. *Blood*, **84**, 3–9.

Garcia-Pagan, J.C., Pique, J.M., Monteagudo, J. *et al.* (1988) Massive lower gastrointestinal hemorrhage caused by cytomegalovirus colitis in a hemophiliac patient with acquired immunodeficiency syndrome. *Medical Clinics of Barcelona*, **91**, 741–743.

Gomperts, E.D., Malekzadeh, M.H. and Fine, R.N. (1981) Dialysis and renal transplant in a hemophiliac. *Thrombosis and Haemostasis*, **46**, 626–628.

Gordon, R.A., d'Avignon, M.B., Storch, A.E. and Eyster, M.E. (1981) Intramural gastric hematoma in a hemophiliac with an inhibitor. *Pediatrics*, **67**, 417–419.

Gourdeau, R. and Denton, R.L. (1970) Steroids and hemophilia. *Bibliotheca Hematologica*, **34**, 65–69.

Griffin, P.H., Schnure, F.W., Chopra, S. *et al.* (1986) Intramural gastrointestinal hemorrhage. *Journal of Clinical Gastroenterology*, **8**, 389–394.

Hampton, K.K., Grant, P.J., Johnston, D. and Prentice, C.R. (1990) Pelvic haemophilic pseudotumour occurring in a patient with mild haemophilia: a brief report. *Blood Coagulation and Fibrinolysis*, **1**, 747–748.

Harrison, H.C., Lord, R.S., Chesterman, C.N. *et al.* (1972) Spontaneous intramural haematoma in the sigmoid colon of a haemophiliac. *Australian and New Zealand Journal of Surgery*, **42**, 69–70.

Heim, M., Horoszowski, H., Seligsohn, U. *et al.* (1982) Iliopsoas hematoma – its detection and treatment with special reference to hemophilia. *Archives of Orthopaedic and Traumatic Surgery*, **99**, 195–197.

Ingram, G.I.C. (1976) The history of haemophilia. *Journal of Clinical Pathology*, **29**, 3–113.

Inwood, M.J., Killackey, B. and Startup, S. (1983) The use and safety of ibuprofen in the hemophiliac. *Blood*, **61**, 709–711.

Jones, P; (1974) *Living with Hemophilia*, 1st edn, F.A. Davies, Philadelphia, p. 177.

Jones, J.J. and Kitchens, C.S. (1984) Spontaneous intra-abdominal hemorrhage in hemophilia. *Archives of Internal Medicine*, **144**, 297–300.

Klamut, M., Szczerbo-Trojanowska, M., Kowalewski, J. and Nowakowski, A. (1979) Transcatheter embolization in a haemophiliac with post-traumatic renal haemorrhage. Report of a case. *Acta Radiologica Diagnostica, Stockholm*, **20**, 606–608.

Lazerson, J. (1976) Renal disease in hemophilia, in *Hemophilia in Children – Progress in Pediatric Hematology/Oncology*, vol. 1 (ed. M.W. Hilgartner), Publishing Sciences Group, pp. 71–77.

Lee, T.G., Brickman, F.E. and Avecilla, L.S. (1977) Ultrasound diagnosis of intramural intestinal hematoma. *Journal of Clinical Ultrasound*, **5**, 423–424.

McCort, J.J. (1976) Intraperitoneal and retroperitoneal hemorrhage. *Radiology Clinics of North America*, **14**, 391–405.

McCoy, H.E. and Kitchens, C.S. (1991) Small bowel hematoma in a hemophiliac as a cause of pseudoappendicitis: diagnosis by CT imaging. *American Journal of Hematology*, **38**, 138–139.

Meyer, W.H., Levin, J., Ness, P.M. *et al.* (1983) Abnormalities of the spleen and liver in patients with hemophilia. *American Journal of Hematology*, **14**, 235–246.

Michel, G., Ritter, A., Gerken, G. *et al.* (1992) Anti-GOR and hepatitis C Virus infection. *Gastroenterology*, **104**, 272–277.

Mittal, R., Spero, J.A., Lewis, J.H. *et al.* (1985) Patterns of gastrointestinal hemorrhage in hemophilia. *Gastroenterology*, **88**, 515–522.

Morimoto, K., Hashimoto, T., Choi, S. *et al.* (1988) Ultrasonographic evaluation of intramural gastric and duodenal hematoma in hemophiliacs. *Journal of Clinical Ultrasound*, **16**, 108–113.

Oldenburger, D. and Gundlach, W.J. (1977) Intramural esophageal hematoma in a hemophiliac. An unusual cause of gastrointestinal bleeding. *Journal of the American Medical Association*, **237**, 800.

Patriquin, H. (1980) Ureteric hemorrhage in hemophilia with rapid healing. *Journal of the Canadian Association of Radiology*, **31**, 265–266.

Pauly, M.P., Watson-Williams, E. and Trudeau, W.L. (1987) Intussusception presenting with lower gastrointestinal hemorrhage in a hemophiliac. *Gastrointestinal Endoscopy*, **33**, 115–118.

Perrin, J.M., MacLean, W.E. and Janco, R.L. (1988) Does stress affect bleeding in 'hemophilia? A review of the literature. *American Journal of Pediatric Hematology Oncology*, **10**, 230–235.

Prentice, C.R.M., Lindsay, R.M., Barr, R.D. *et al.* (1971) Renal complications in haemophilia and Christmas Disease. *Quarterly Journal of Medicine*, **23**, 349–354.

Roy, V., Tillyer, M.L. and Colvin, B.T. (1988) Acute abdominal pain due to an acquired disorder of coagulation. *British Medical Journal*, **296**, 1460.

Salomon, H. and Tatarski, I. (1965) von Willebrand's disease in two families. Case reports with a contribution to the management of chronic intestinal hemorrhages. *Israeli Journal of Medical Science*, **1**, 866–869.

Singer, L.J. (1975) Renal and urological complications of hemophilia, in *Handbook of Hemophilia*, Part 1 (eds K.M. Brinkous and H.C. Hemker), Excerpta Medica, Amsterdam, pp. 377–388.

Singh, R., Clarkston, W.K., Zuckerman, D.A. *et al.* (1993) Transjugular intra-hepatic portosystemic shunt for palliation of bleeding esophageal varices in a patient with severe hemophilia A, advanced HIV infection and cirrhosis. *American Journal of Gastroenterology*, **88**, 2112–2114.

Sitaram, V., Booshanam, M.V., Chandy, M. and Kurian, G. (1990) Gastrointestinal haemorrhage in a haemophiliac due to a jejunal haemangioma. *British Journal of Clinical Practice*, **44**, 779–780.

Small, M., Rose, P.E., McMillan, N. *et al.* (1982) Haemophilia and the kidney: assessment after 11 year follow-up. *British Medical Journal*, **285**, 1609–1611.

Sreepada Rao, T.K. (1995) Acquired immuno-deficiency syndrome, in *Textbook of Nephrology*, vol. 1 (eds S.G. Massry and R.J. Glassock), Williams & Wilkins, Baltimore, pp. 855–859.

Tanowitz, H.B., Simon, D. and Wittner, M. (1992) Gastrointestinal manifestations. *Medical Clinics of North America*, **76**, 45–62.

Thould, A.K., Keeling, D.H and Murrell, J.S. (1982) Gastric microbleeding studies in patients with haemophilia taking benoxaprofen. *European Journal of Rheumatology and Inflammation*, **5**, 165–169.

Veltkamp, J.J. (1975) Clinical features of hemophilia, in *Handbook of Hemophilia*, vol. 1 (eds K.M. Brinkhous and H.C. Hemker), Excerpta Medica, Amsterdam, pp. 376–376.

Warrier, I., Tolia, V., Kueffler, S. and Lusher J. (1994) Spectrum of gastrointestinal and hepatic manifestations in HIV positive hemophiliacs. Abstract # 152, XXI Congress, World Federation of Hemophilia, Mexico City, April.

White, D.A. and Zaman, M.K. (1992) Pulmonary disease in medical management of AIDS patients. *Medical Clinics of North America*, **76**, 19–44.

Wright, F.W., Matthews, J.M. and Brook, L.G. (1971) Complications of haemophillac disorders affecting the renal tract. *Radiology*, **98**, 571–576.

PART THREE

Treatment and Complications

Haemophilia Treatment

- Absolute rest
- Compression
- Styptics
- Tannic acid application
- Perchloride of iron
- Purges of sulphate of soda
- Gelatin in 5% solution
- Dried suprarenal gland
- Transfusion has been employed without success

Sir William Osler, 1902

14 THE TREATMENT OF HEMOPHILIA: COMPREHENSIVE HEMOPHILIA CARE

L.M. Aledort

Most patients with an illness, who seek care from a physician, follow instructions and go on about the business at hand. However, when a child is born, and at birth, circumcision or shortly after he starts to crawl, he is recognized as a 'bleeder' – then the entire situation is altered. Although an ancient disease, well described in Victorian times, and despite the marked advances in molecular biology, genetics and available therapies, the new diagnosis of hemophilia wreaks havoc with the recipients of this information.

This rare disorder, presenting with symptoms of joint bleeds, prior to the 1940s, was frequently misdiagnosed as tuberculous arthritis. The recognition that hemophilia was due to a deficiency of a clotting factor which could be corrected by normal plasma was only made in the late 1940s. However, the fact that this disorder was predominantly in males, and could lead to life-threatening hemorrhages, was defined in the writings of the Talmud (Rosner, 1994). At that time, it was also recognized that this was an entity which was passed from mother to child, was seen in families and could skip generations. These deductions from clinical observation formed the basis of our understanding of the genetics of this disease. The impact on the family unit, i.e. attachment of the mother to the affected child, the disruption in day-to-day living due to the unpredictability of spontaneous bleeding episodes is poignantly described in the fictionalized biography of the Tszarevich in *Nicholas and Alexandra* by Robert Massie. Here, in no uncertain terms, the ravages of hemophilia and its effect on not only a family constellation, but possibly also the Russian empire are beautifully described. In addition, the earlier therapy of bleeding, immobilization and ice packs is depicted. A more innovative approach to pain management, relaxation techniques and hypnosis, are used skillfully by Rasputin, which afforded him extraordinary influence in the royal household. These early observations of hemophilia and the impact on family dynamics formed the basis of many years of investigation by Matteson and Agle on the psychosocial aspects of this disorder.

Complicated severe cases of hemophilia were seen throughout the world by individual practitioners caring for one to two such patients, or clustered at a few urban medical centers where pathologists, hematologists or orthopedists began caring for them (Van Eys *et al.*, 1974). The clinical challenges were great, but the therapeutic modalities almost non-existent. It was not until modern blood-banking technology came into its own in the Second World War that a major therapeutic modality became available – fresh frozen plasma. Factor VIII could not be distinguished from Factor IX deficiency, but infusions of plasma produced instantaneous pain relief, and many hemorrhages could be abated. Its limitations were transfusion reactions and fluid overload. Surgery and life-threatening hemorrhages could not always be effectively managed.

By virtue of an available therapy, although flawed, more patients clustered around medical centers which had available blood derivatives and coagulation laboratories which could identify deficiencies. Patients and their families would remain bound to such centers as their children could be brought to emergency rooms for treatment at any time of day or night. Job opportunities might frequently be rejected by fathers of these patients as they might be remote from centers treating hemophiliacs.

Orthopedists and radiologists had begun to describe the characteristic destructive lesions in joints and the marked morbidity that muscle wasting, contractures and joint immobility would produce (Petterson and Gilbert, 1985). Braces, splints, crutches and wheelchairs became the mainstay of supportive care for these patients. Long absences from school, because of immobility and pain,

Hemophilia. Edited by C.D. Forbes, L. Aledort and R. Madhok. Published in 1997 by Chapman & Hall, London. ISBN 0 412 63820 7

made home schooling routine for many, and hopeless futures were common.

This was the typical setting in the early 1960s when a few hemophilia clinics existed, managed in the main by a hematologist (blood banker), pathologist and an orthopedic surgeon. The programs had back-up by a coagulation laboratory, and usually the availability of blood products. These programs could offer only minimal services, and most patients spent large amounts of time in the hospital.

Several events occurred simultaneously which dramatically altered this approach to hemophilia care. Dr Judith Pool, in Palo Alto, California, serendipitously discovered cryoprecipitate (Pool, Hershgold and Pappenhagen, 1964). By rapid freezing of fresh frozen plasma and thawing of the material slowly, a precipitate, only a few milliliters in volume, contained fibrinogen and approximately 50% of the factor VIII of the unit of plasma. The material, requiring freezing at low temperatures, could maintain factor VIII stability for at least 2 years. Finally, patients could be transfused with sufficient factor VIII to achieve and maintain hemostasis so that emergency surgery and elective procedures could be carried out without fear of fluid overload. Blood banks throughout the nation could easily make and store cryoprecipitate.

This new therapeutic intervention led to further interest in the area of orthopedic reconstructive surgery. The possibility that joint mobility might be restored or that wheelchair-bound patients might walk again, fostered the interest and involvement of physical therapists as an adjunct to the group evaluating and treating patients. The availability of a treatment coincided with the relatively new field of physiatry. This medical approach to rehabilitation widened the horizons of the orthopedist to more than physical therapy, such as issues of adjustment to new physical activity and the assessment of activities of daily living.

At the same time, parent organizations, serving as ombudsman for their children, had spread throughout the USA and Europe. The frustration of parents because they were hostage to the disease, that their sons were 'crippled', pain-ridden and likely not to have received an optimal education, or attain occupations for which they had an aptitude was the driving force behind forming lay-oriented health care agencies. Clearly the psychosocial aspects of this disease for patients and families warranted attention. Strong social work departments did not exist in most hospitals in the USA and Europe, so that such services were hard to provide and, when available, could not be paid for.

In California, at Orthopedic Hospital in Los Angeles, Dr Shelby Dietrich attempted a novel experiment. Prior to that experiment, most patients when seen for outpatient surveillance, might need to make three separate visits – one to the hematologist, another to the ortho-

pedist and a third for rehabilitation. Dr Dietrich, in part because her institution was a rehabilitation center, conceived of a team approach, where the patient would come to a single place at one time and receive evaluation, diagnosis and be given a therapeutic regimen to follow. This approach formed the basis of what is now called comprehensive care. This early seed of an idea, fostered by a New York team of a hematologist and orthopedist, would germinate into an internationally accepted concept of a health care delivery system (Gilbert and Aledort, 1977). Within less than 10 years, this system would be defined, refined and financial support for it explored and acquired.

The key issue facing the patients with this disorder was that it was a genetic, lifelong disease of low density. It had special needs, in that lifelong spontaneous bleeding required continued attention, which at that time led to severe mobility problems. It required special diagnostic capabilities both to identify the type of hemophilia and to measure the presence or absence of inhibitors. A sophisticated blood bank was needed to provide plasma and cryoprecipitate. A team to provide a diagnosis and therapy was sorely needed. In addition to these challenges, the US pluralistic health care reimbursement system did not have adequate means to pay for these services. This was in sharp contrast to many countries in which health care was supported by a national system, frequently under the aegis of a social security plan.

During the nascence of comprehensive care, because of fiscal restraints, hemophilia treaters had to assess what services could be supported. The earliest addition at our center was a social worker, and the task at hand was, from the start, enormous. The issues were frequently a function of the age of the patient. The newborn presented special problems. First and foremost was the education of the parents. The issues for them were different depending upon whether or not hemophilia existed before in their families. The issues of allaying anxieties, offering a perspective on what a parent could expect, and educating them regarding such things as 'hemophilia-proofing' the house, appropriate crib bumpers, no scatter rugs, helmets during toddler years, etc. were formidable tasks. The older child raised different issues. The home room teachers who were frightened by the diagnosis, the physical education teacher who would not allow the child to participate were typical problems. The adolescent young man who on one hand struggled with his disease had also to deal with disclosure and developing independence from a usually overprotective family. Additionally, his burgeoning sexuality required special attention. The married couple required counseling regarding family planning. Family members needing to know their risks of being a carrier and then the likelihood of having an affected child made many demands. All these settings were challenging and taxed any social worker. However, few programs had one, and issues frequently went unresolved.

Many changes that take place in a health care system are based on new technologies, which are usually more costly, and therefore slow to be implemented. However, in hemophilia care, a key advance not only changed the system of care but it dramatically altered the life and outlook for the patients, and in the long run was less costly. The introduction of home care markedly altered hemophilia care and made new demands on the slowly growing comprehensive team caring for them. It also required little, if any, new technology.

In Texas, two brothers were given instructions and training in infusing cryoprecipitates at home. The family then moved to Chicago and the physician in charge of a major hemophilia program could not initially justify providing the family with the same service. The family flew regularly to Texas to procure material. Eventually, Dr Rabiner would consider home care as a research project, procure IRB approval and publish his results (Rabiner and Telfer, 1970). The results were clearly remarkable, and the National Hemophilia Foundation charged several physicians to prepare national guidelines for initiating such programs throughout the USA. These guidelines included issues such as technical skills at identifying veins and infusing, safety issues (i.e. contaminating others with needlesticks) and evaluation of the family unit to insure proper utilization and treatment of bleeding, and when to seek help (Van Eys *et al.*, 1974).

This new program made substantial demands on a program. Choosing the appropriate candidate, development of therapeutic regimens for different types of bleeding, and the training of the patient and/or his family required time and special skills. The need for a nurse clinician to be added to the team became imperative. Most centers could not find support for such personnel, and in some cities nurses were shared between institutions. Nurse training programs were initiated to introduce nurses to hemophilia and then instruct them in home care techniques. The earliest home care programs were initiated with cryoprecipitate and therefore freezers for −20°C storage were required. The standard freezer did not meet those requirements and special costly freezers were required. Fortunately, shortly after the introduction of cryoprecipitates, the fractionation technology had advanced to a point at which lyophilized factor VIII and IX concentrates were becoming readily available. It was not, however, until 1972 that material was available to meet US needs (Department of HEW-PHS, 1980).

Once this home care program began to be accepted by patients and physicians, we were left with an enormous unsolved problem. All of US health care was geared to support inpatient or hospital-based treatment and not for care at home. Third party payers, whether private or public, would without question pay for hospital stays, even if they were for bleeding episodes which could be simply treated at home. Thus, they would be paying for product plus days in the hospital. This had to be dealt with by a major lobbying effort. It was fought at local, state, and finally, at the national level. However, for years, this issue required individualized counseling and negotiations between patient and insurance company. Thus, financial counseling became an integral part of delivering comprehensive care. It took more than 10 years for most patients to receive coverage.

Parents of hemophilia patients were initially frightened by such a simple task as brushing one's teeth. Patients would bleed, not usually requiring therapy. However, for many years young hemophiliacs, by not having good dental hygiene, developed significant dental problems. The oral cavity has been and continues to be fraught with hemostatic problems. Enhanced fibrinolytic activity led to major bleeding even for common dental extractions resulting from poor hygiene. These extractions, prior to adequate blood product replacement, were the most common cause of hospital admissions, and even mortality. With scientific advances, e.g. concentrate and antifibrinolytic therapy, oral surgery was elevated to a new level of safety (Walsh, Rizza and Aledort, 1975). However, surgical bleeding was a substantial threat. The need for dentists and oral surgeons as part of the team became crucial. They educated both patients and teammates as to the importance of prevention. A dental hygienist then became a pivotal figure for our patients and needed to be added to the team. Regular examinations and X-rays of the mouth were part of each patient's evaluation. The need for constant reinforcement for good oral hygiene to patient and family continues to be a critical part of patient management.

The seminal work of Zimmerman, defining the factor VIII molecule, led to the discovery of a new way to identify the hemophilia carrier state (Klein *et al.*, 1977). The field of carrier detection for families of newly diagnosed hemophilia mothers or sisters of non-obligate carriers led to a need for genetic counseling in these programs. The field of genetic counseling was quite new, but hemophilia comprehensive care centers and similar programs such as sickle-cell anemia and cystic fibrosis encouraged people to enter the field. As molecular genetics has grown and intrauterine detection and carrier identification have matured, these counselors not only take pedigree histories, they also arrange for testing (and in some instances are running genetics laboratories) and offer counseling.

The advent of elective surgery made changes and new demands on the center. The coagulation laboratory had to be prepared to carry out numerous assays. The blood bank had to have available much larger quantities of factor than before to sustain hemostasis in the postoperative period. Coordination of the program became important, and clearly an administrative role was needed. Although elective surgery held the promise of mobility, and a chance for education and/or employment, patients facing surgery did not look forward to the procedure. Many of them have friends or relatives who did not survive surgery in the preconcentrate era. These preoperative anxieties frequently outweighed the benefit of surgery for these patients. This issue mandated significant intervention to overcome such fears. Social workers were too preoccupied with other issues to deal with this. The need for psychologists or psychiatrists became apparent and, when possible, were added to the team. They were able also to deal with the issues of substance abuse. Chronic joint pain resulted in almost 25% of our patients abusing pain medication and/or alcohol. Interaction with pain and drug abuse specialists regarding management of these patients became essential.

The addition of home care to the comprehensive approach emancipated patients and families, so that early treatment could occur. Long waits in emergency rooms were avoided by most patients. Families could be freed so that mothers could work and families need not be huddled near hospitals which knew how to care for these patients. Fewer joint deformities could be anticipated and physical and mental rehabilitation could occur. This created a natural need for vocational counseling. These counselors could guide young adults into appropriate career choices and older rehabilitated patients into fields in which they could now be successful. Thus, the team could do prevention, care, and help plan for the future.

As a program committed to comprehensive care, these patients were followed throughout their life. The center acted as primary as well as tertiary care givers. As primary care givers, it became important to identify specialists who would see our patient population, become familiar with the issues of hemophilia, and not be intimidated by their diagnosis. Obstetricians were recruited to insure that the potential high-risk delivery would go smoothly, and to insure that appropriate cord bloods would be obtained for diagnosis. Amniocentesis and other appropriate samples could also be obtained for both diagnosis and genetic studies. A surgeon, neurologist and urologist are key personnel who, over a lifetime, frequently are called upon to service our patients. One cannot expect these specialists to be available at regular team meetings, but be available for consultation. If a program is predominantly adult, a pediatrician needs to be available for those children who enter the program. The reverse is true for predominantly pediatric programs, where adults become associated with the center.

The distinction becomes complicated as our patients enter adolescence. In some parts of the world, and in particular the USA, adolescent medicine has become a recognized specialty. Issues of disclosure, sexuality, peer pressure and independence from family become an integral part of their medical management. The medical model has therefore evolved over the years to become a biopsychosocial one because of the extraordinary problems facing parents with chronic disease, their partners and family members.

In the USA, these free-standing, unconnected programs functioned with minimal staff, and essentially no fiscal support. Most personnel were volunteers who found the challenge of the disease worth their time. The need for expansion of this system of care was recognized by the author. With support of the National Hemophilia Foundation, a lobbying campaign was initiated for federal support for this health care system. Using hemophilia as a model for chronic disease, and joining forces with the community interested in genetic disorders, in 1975 a Hemophilia Act was passed in the USA by Congress, authorizing $3 million to support personnel in comprehensive care programs in the country. A decision had to be made, before the appropriation of funds, as to which federal agency should administer this program. It was clear that the National Institutes of Health would not do well with funding meant for support of the infrastructure of a disease entity, and were unfamiliar with supporting health care systems. A decision was made to have the program reside with the Maternal and Child Health Division of the Department of Health and Human Services (HHS). It has remained there ever since. The goal of the legislation was to create centers in the 10 HHS regions of the country so that the majority of hemophiliacs in the nation could receive this comprehensive approach to their care. The funds would be able to support personnel that were previously absent from the team because of lack of funding. Ten years after the implementation of this law, its success approach was published (Table 14.1), and the model generated great interest in the medical and scientific community (Aledort, 1982). The major achievements were that many more patients received comprehensive care, could avail themselves of home care, and their hospitalization declined, with a concomitant marked improvement in school and work attendance. Unemployment dropped to a lower level than the general population. Annual costs of care decreased, as did their families' out-of-pocket expense. The latter was in part achieved by the markedly increased underwriting of care for these patients that centers helped patients acquire.

By the creation of these centers, it was necessary to develop a template as to how they should function. It was felt necessary that patients should come to one place in order to receive multiple services, to insure coordination of care. Team meetings were held regularly to determine an ideal program for these patients to follow between visits and to insure that referring physicians receive appropriate instructions regarding the patient's current

Table 14.1 Change in patient outcomes since inception of primary and affiliated hemophilia centers in the USA

Outcome	Year before inception	10 Years later – 1985	Change
No. of patients at primary centers	1783	5606	+214%
No. of patients at affiliated centers	329	1641	+399%
No. of patients receiving regular comprehensive care	1333	5683	+326%
No. of patients doing self-infusion	514	2517	+390%
Average days lost from work or school	14.5	3.9	−73%
Percentage of adult patients unemployed	36	9.4	−74%
Average hospital admissions/year	1.9	0.22	−89%
Average days spent as inpatient	9.4	1.6	−83%
Overall cost of care/patient per year ($)	31600	8127	−74%

status and future plan. Patients were urged to be seen a minimum of once a year. These funded centers were intended also to have a diagnostic laboratory and an emergency service, plus to provide blood products. In addition, it was critical that these centers network with their community in order to provide access to needed services that might not be available on site. This was true for drug management, ongoing psychosocial, support, vocational rehabilitation, etc. Educational outreach to employers, teachers and primary care providers was part of the task. The involvement of the consumer was also critical. A Lay Advisory Board was formed so that patients and their families could assess the success and pitfalls of these programs. They were to provide input to issues such as the logistics of the system, waiting time in emergency rooms and the level of sophistication of the physicians and nurses who would see these patients in an emergency situation. This approach has been beneficial in trying to balance the reliance of the patients on the system, and the treaters recognition of their patients' desire for input.

A major positive fall-out from these centers was that there were now a large number of patients clustered in centers who could serve as excellent subjects for research. New drugs and concentrates could be quickly and easily evaluated. Epidemiologic studies such as the natural history of inhibitors could be carried out. Patients and their families could also feel that they were contributing to the knowledge base for the very disease for which they were being treated. This excellent natural resource has made possible the identification of almost all newborns, and thus the study of safety of the blood supply and new recombinant materials.

The funded centers grew with time and developed affiliated or satellite centers with which they collaborated. Over the last decade in the USA, there is now a regionalized network of care for hemophilia patients and almost all cases in the nation are cared for within the system. A major self-educational component exists as well, as center directors and their staffs meet regularly to discuss issues of mutual concern.

In 1982, the first case of acquired immunodeficiency syndrome (AIDS) in hemophiliacs was reported. This new retroviral disease infected almost 70% of USA hemophiliacs, and large numbers throughout the rest of the world. The pre-existing treatment centers were ideally poised to deal with this new disease. The addition of sexual counseling and infectious disease experts as new staff members was needed. Although centers had been dealing with consultants for years, the big difference now, however, was that this sexually and blood-borne disease made excessive new demands on the team, as now spouses and sexual partners sought guidance, education and, not infrequently, treatment by the team. The stress of this new disease was enormous, and staff burn-out was common. In some centers, where staff had been stable for years, there was now a large turnover rate. A key addition to the program in some centers to deal with this was group counseling for team members. Any and all issues could be discussed with anonymity. New financial support for the teams was critical and funding for human immunodeficiency (HIV) issues was provided by the Centers for Disease Control.

The comprehensive model of care and its positive results has led to the adoption of this system for many other lifelong diseases in the USA. Several centers in the world have trained their staff in some of these programs and then adapted this team approach in their countries. Similar centers now exist in such countries as Japan, Sweden, the UK and France. Many parts of the world with large clusters of hemophilia patients have not embraced this approach for a variety of reasons. In the main, lack of resources and cultural differences have been key factors.

The appearance of large numbers of HIV patients has, on the other hand, added a major burden to all programs throughout the world. Many have managed by sending patients to HIV programs, thereby fractionating care. Those centers with full comprehensive teams have now recognized that HIV is a second chronic disease with which these patients have to cope.

A comprehensive approach to a lifelong disease offers satisfaction to patients, their family, as well as team members. The ongoing education for the patient, as well as the team, makes it an exciting and most rewarding experience. The underwriting of such an effort is very demanding, both in countries such as the USA with a pluralistic health care system, as well as those with a centrally supported one. I encourage treaters and patients to explore the possibility of establishing similar programs. It is well worth it.

Acknowledgments

This study was in part supported by Health Services Administration grant MCB-360001; Health and Human Services grant HL-30567; The Regional Comprehensive Haemophilia Diagnostic and Treatment Center; the Margie Boas Fund; the International Haemophilia Training Center of the World Federation of Haemophilia; the Polly Annenberg Levee Hematology Center, Department of Medicine, Mount Sinai School of Medicine of the City University of New York; and grant 5MO1 RR00071 for the Mount Sinai General Clinical Research Center from the National Center for Research Resources, National Institutes of Health.

References

Aledort, L.M. (1982) Lessons from hemophilia. *New England Journal of Medicine*, **306**, 607–608.

Department of HEW-PHS (19) *Study to Evaluate the Supply–Demand Relationships for AHF and PTC through 1980.* DHEW publication no. (NIH) 77–1274.

Gilbert, M. and Aledort, L.M. (eds) (19T7) Comprehensive care in hemophilia: a team approach. *Mount Sinai Journal of Medicine*, **44**, 313–479.

Klein, H.G., Aledort, L.M., Bouma, B.N. *et al.* (1977) A cooperative study for the detection of the carrier state of classical hemophilia. *New England Journal of Medicine*, **196**, 959–962.

Petterson, H. and Gilbert, M. (eds) (1985) *Diagnostic Imaging in Hemophilia*, Springer-Verlag, pp. 1–147.

Pool, J.G., Hershgold, E.J. and Pappenhagen, A.R. (1964) High-potency antihaemophilic factor concentrate prepared from cryoglobulin precipitate. *Nature*, **203**, 312.

Rabiner, S.F. and Telfer, M.C. (1970) Home transfusion for patients with hemophilia A. *New England Journal of Medicine*, **283**, 1011–1015.

Rosner, F. (1994) Hemophilia in classic rabbinic texts. *Journal of the History of Medicine and Allied Sciences*, **49**, 240–250.

Van Eys, J., Agle, D.P., Hilgartner, M.W. and Lozuson, J. (1974) *Home Therapy for Hemophilia – A Physician's Manual*, National Hemophilia Foundation – Medical and Scientific Advisory Council.

Walsh, P.N., Rizza, C.R. and Aledort, L.M., (1975) The therapeutic role of epsilon amino caproic acid (EACA) for dental extractions in hemophiliacs. *Annals of the New York Academy of Science*, **240**, 267–276.

15 PRINCIPLES OF MANAGEMENT OF HEMOPHILIAC BLEEDING

S.V. Seremetis

In the 1990s approaches to the management of the congenital bleeding disorders are of course dominated by the appropriate dosing and timely use of clotting factor concentrates. The availability of these concentrates has changed dramatically the management of patients with clotting factor deficiencies. Use of these concentrates has allowed, in appropriate circumstances, for the introduction of homecare programs and self-infusion of clotting factor concentrates by affected individuals. This has virtually obviated the frequent hospital visits and admissions that once characterized this patient population. Hospitalization for the treatment of bleeding disorders is now the exception and is usually reserved for serious bleeding episodes or elective surgical, primarily orthopedic, procedures.

Adherence to a set of general principles of treatment and specific dosing guidelines allows for the most efficacious use of clotting factor concentrates in the treatment of hemophiliac bleeding episodes. Knowledge of these principles is of course essential for professionals involved in hemophilia care. Because most hemophilia care is delivered in the outpatient setting, and much of it self-administered in the home, an additional requirement for the optimal treatment of hemophilia is the diligent education of patients and families as to these principles and dosing guidelines.

General principles of therapy in hemophiliac bleeding

1. Episodes of hemophiliac bleeding must be treated promptly and specifically by administration of therapy which raises the level of the deficient clotting factor to a level sufficient to abrogate and prevent further bleeding.

2. An accurate diagnosis of the clotting factor deficiency and specifically a reliable measure of baseline (i.e. steady-state) factor VIII and factor IX levels is essential to any calculation of dosage of the factors to achieve hemostasis.

3. Appropriate screening assays for the presence of an inhibitor must be undertaken at regular intervals in all patients with hemophilia and, if an inhibitor is detected, specific infusion studies must be performed in order to determine adjustments in therapeutic regimens.

4. An accurate diagnosis of the type, location and timing (acute or chronic) of bleeding must be established in order to choose an effective treatment regimen. An important caveat here, however, is that when a bleeding episode is suspected and the diagnosis is obscure, treatment with replacement therapy should be initiated first and diagnostic testing should follow.

5. When a bleeding episode is identified or suspected, therapy must be instituted promptly and in doses adequate to control bleeding and continued for sufficient duration to ensure that hemostasis or wound healing is complete.

Pharmacokinetics and dosage calculations

Dosage of factor concentrate needed to replace a factor deficiency is calculated on the basis of the patients weight, the assumed plasma volume and the severity of the bleeding episode. The *in vivo* recovery and half-life of factor VIII and factor IX also need to be considered in dosage calculations of these products. For factor VIII the *in vivo* recovery is 90–100% and the half-life is approximately 12 hours. For factor IX the *in vivo* recovery is around 50% and the half-life is 16–20 h (Kaspar and Dietrich, 1985). The development of inhibitor antibodies

Hemophilia. Edited by C.D. Forbes, L. Aledort and R. Madhok. Published in 1997 by Chapman & Hall, London. ISBN 0 412 63820 7

to the relevant factors will of course confound and dramatically change recovery of infused factor activity; the approach to the treatment of bleeding episodes in individuals in whom inhibitors have developed is summarized elsewhere in this text (Chapter 21).

It is convenient to consider the administration in terms of international units (iu) per measure of body weight. By definition, 1.0 iu of factor VIII or factor IX is that amount of clotting activity found in 1.0 ml of fresh normal pooled plasma (and that 1.0 iu is equal to 100% clotting activity).

FACTOR VIII

Given the above considerations, administering 1 iu of factor VIII per kilogram body weight will result in an increase of factor VIII concentration in the recipient's plasma of approximately 2% (or 2 iu factor VIII/dl). A simple formula:

Factor VIII dose = $\frac{1}{2}$(% rise factor VIII desired)
(kg body weight)(dose as
calculated in iu).

To maintain the desired factor VIII level for prolonged periods, half of the original dose as calculated above is repeated at 12-h intervals.

FACTOR IX

The pharmacokinetics of factor IX translate into different dose levels and intervals from those of factor VIII. One iu of factor IX/kg body weight will result in an increase of factor IX of approximately 1% (or 1 iu factor IX/dl). A simple formula:

Factor IX dose = (% rise factor IX desired)
(kg body weight)

To maintain the desired factor IX level for prolonged periods, half of the original dose as calculated above is repeated at 24-h intervals.

Products for therapy

Choice of among the variety of therapeutic materials (including fresh frozen plasma, cryoprecipitate, clotting factor concentrates, desmopressin (DDAVP) and adjuvant therapies) is one of the most challenging therapeutic decisions facing clinicians in the management of bleeding disorders. We will summarize these options briefly here; in all cases there will be more detailed presentations elsewhere in this text with special focus on controversies regarding product choice.

FACTOR VIII CONCENTRATES

We are fortunate today in having a variety of types of factor VIII concentrates from which to choose for the treatment of hemophilia A. Concentrates differ in terms of their biologic source, the virus attenuation methods used and the level of purity achieved. A rational choice among the available clotting factor concentrates must be based not only upon the most current data relevant to safety and efficacy, but also must consider short- and long-term cost-effectiveness. While nomenclature is in evolution, the plasma-derived human factor VIII concentrates currently available can be classified based upon specific activity as intermediate-purity, high-purity and very high-purity (Schreiber, 1988; Schulman, 1989; Mannucci, Gringeri and Cattaneo, 1990; Hoyer, 1994). In addition, recombinant complementary DNA-derived factor VIII concentrates have recently become available (Schwartz, 1990; Hoyer, 1994). The dosing calculations described apply to all available factor VIII concentrates.

CONCENTRATES FOR THE TREATMENT OF FACTOR IX DEFICIENCY

Factor IX deficiency, comprising approximately 20% of the hemophilias, has been treated for the past 30 years with prothrombin complex concentrates (PCC). These concentrates are prepared by exploiting the common adsorption and elution properties of all the vitamin-K-dependent proteins on anion exchange resins (Menache et al., 1984). In over 30 years of clinical use, the hemostatic efficacy of PCC has been well-established (Kim et al., 1992); however, safety of this product has been a major issue in that its use has been associated with the transmission of viral disease (including human immunodeficiency virus (HIV) and hepatitis) and the occurrence of disseminated intravascular coagulation (DIC) and other thromboembolic phenomena (Kaspar, 1973; Campbell, Neff and Bowdler, 1978; Lusher, 1991). The availability of several new coagulation factor IX concentrates has increased the number of therapeutic options for the treatment of hemophilia B-related bleeding (Hrinda et al., 1991; Kaspar et al., 1991; Kim et al., 1992). Available evidence indicates that the Factor IX activity in these concentrates has the same pharmacokinetics as native factor IX and the factor IX contained in PCC; thus, dosing calculations as described above are unchanged when using this material.

Weighing these data and those from prior studies, there is wide consensus for use of high-purity factor IX concentrates in specific high-risk circumstances (i.e. surgical prophylaxis, prolonged immobilization, crush injuries, large intramuscular hematomas, advanced liver disease and in neonates) despite the absence of data from controlled trials to support this recommendation. In the absence of a history of thrombosis or one of these conditions, PCC use would also be appropriate. Antifibrinolytic therapy should not be used intercurrently with the usage of PCCs.

DDAVP

Finally, for many patients with mild to moderate hemophilia A, DDAVP represents sufficient treatment for most bleeding episodes.

DDAVP, a synthetic analog of vasopressin, was shown in 1977 to prevent bleeding in patients with mild or moderate hemophilia A or von Willebrand disease (Mannucci *et al.*, 1977). The intravenous infusion of DDAVP, at 0.3 µg/kg body weight, typically causes a three- to fivefold rise in the level of factor VIII activity and von Willebrand factor and can transiently correct the bleeding time in von Willebrand disease. A test infusion is recommended to assess efficacy before beginning elective treatment, as response to DDAVP is not universal. The endogenously released von Willebrand factor and associated factor VIII provoked by DDAVP are hemostatically and pharmacokinetically as effective as those obtained from exogenous infusion of plasma concentrates.

Since its licensure for use in the USA in 1983, intravenous (IV) DDAVP has been used to treat bleeding episodes and for surgical prophylaxis in many patients with hemophilia and von Willebrand disease. In many cases the need for blood products has been obviated, thus reducing the risk for transfusion-acquired diseases such as hepatitis and HIV infection. The development of a more easily administered form of DDAVP for home use has yielded intranasal (IN) and subcutaneous (SC) forms for administration. In Europe, an injectable formulation is available of high enough concentration to allow for patient acceptance of SC injection; this modality is efficacious in increasing levels of factor VIII and von Willebrand factor. IN administration of DDAVP via a simple atomizer produced a bioavailability equivalent to an IV dose of 0.2 µg/kg (Lethagen, Harris and Nilson, 1990; Rose and Aledort, 1991; Seremetis and Aledort, 1991). In both mild hemophiliacs and in patients with von Willebrand disease, this resulted in elevations of factor VIII and von Willebrand factor that were also comparable to the results of IV administration of an equivalent dose. IN-DDAVP has been shown to be efficacious in the home care setting and in surgical prophylaxis and represents a simple, convenient method for the treatment for mild hemophilia A and von Willebrand disease. DDAVP in any dosing form should be used with caution in young children and in the elderly as episodes of seizure and profound hyponatremia have been reported in such patients.

FRESH FROZEN PLASMA

Fresh frozen plasma contains all of the clotting factors in a concentration of approximately 1 unit of clotting factor activity per milliliter, but this product can be used only when small amounts of clotting factor must be delivered to the patient. The product is virtually never used for therapy of hemophilia in the developed world, but it is a useful product in developing countries. Moreover, methods of viral inactivation based upon, for example, the use of solvent-detergent methodology, are currently being developed for viral inactivation of fresh frozen plasma.

CRYOPRECIPITATE

Cryoprecipitate, the protein that precipitates in fresh frozen plasma thawed at 4°C, is rich in factor VIII, fibrinogen and factor XIII. It is easily prepared in most blood banks capable of component fractionation, and is currently used primarily in developing countries for the treatment of factor VIII deficiency; however, availability in these settings is compromised by the requirement that cryoprecipitate be stored at temperatures below −20°C. In addition, because of a current lack of methodology for control of viral contamination and difficulty in standardization of factor levels (making exact dosage calculations problematic), it is no longer considered a product of choice for treatment in developed countries, where concentrate preparations are generally available.

TREATMENT REGIMENS: GUIDELINES FOR THERAPY OF BLEEDING EPISODES

There is some difficulty in establishing precise guidelines for therapy of bleeding episodes in hemophilia. There is substantial variability of the bleeding phenotype, that is, the frequency and severity of bleeding episodes, even among those whose native clotting factor levels are identical at <1% of normal. Bleeding episodes vary in severity and in the condition of the tissue which is the target of the bleeding. Bleeding may be acute and spontaneous, or occur following trauma, surgical or dental procedures. On the other hand, bleeding may be chronic, which again may occur spontaneously, following trauma or inadequate treatment for acute bleeding. Although in all of these cases there is agreement that factor replacement therapy is necessary to control bleeding, there is considerable difference throughout the world concerning the amount of replacement material that should be used and the factor levels that should be maintained. The proposed regimens in Table 15.1 are built on experience of this author and consensus of the published literature and are meant to be utilized as a guide which the treater may modify based on the particulars of each bleeding episode as it presents. The

Table 15.1 Treatment regimens: guidelines for therapy of hemophilic bleeding

Bleeding site	Optimal factor level (%)	Dosage (iu/kg)	
		FVIII	FIX
Muscle hematoma	20–30	10–15	20–30
Hemarthrosis	30–50	15–25	30–50
Gastrointestinal tract bleeding	40–60	20–30	40–60
Retropharyngeal/tongue	60–100	30–50	60–100
Intracranial	60–100	30–50	60–100
Retroperitoneal	60–100	30–50	60–100
Hematuria*	30–50	15–25	30–50
Minor bleeding	20–30	10–15	20–30

FVIII = Factor VIII; FIX = Factor IX.
*If conservative therapy with hydration alone is unsuccessful in abrogation of hematuria.

keys to successful treatment of bleeding in hemophilia are early administration of factor replacement therapy and accurate diagnosis of the bleeding episode.

HEMATOMA

Hematomas, or hemorrhages under the skin and within muscles, very often can be controlled by conservative measures, including the application of ice and elastic bandage pressure. Those hematomas which cannot be controlled with a few hours of such measures require factor replacement therapy. When replacement therapy is necessary, a dose allowing for an optimal factor level of 20–30% given once is usually adequate for control of the bleeding episode. Hematomas are considered minor bleeding episodes and are usually easily controlled. An important caveat here applies to internal hematomas, including retroperitoneal and retropharyngeal hematomas which require more intensive therapy and are discussed in more detail below.

HEMARTHROSIS

Acute spontaneous bleeding into the joints occurs in severe hemophilia A and B and also in cases of severe von Willebrand disease; trauma may be followed by hemarthrosis in patients with all grades of severity of hemophilia. When there are synovial changes, bleeding may occur frequently in the same joint, constituting a target joint. Hemarthroses are by far the most common type of bleeding encountered in the context of hemophilia and diligent therapy of these episodes will postpone – if not altogether eliminate – chronic orthopedic complications of the disorder. It is essential therefore to treat joint bleeding aggressively and with adequate factor replacement, aiming at levels outlined in Table 15.1. Repeat dosing may be necessary in 12–48 h if bleeding is severe or if the joint has previously developed into a target joint. However, repeat doses of factor are not usually necessary, approximately 90% of hemarthroses being adequately treated with one dose of clotting factor concentrate (Schwartz, 1990). The need for further therapy should prompt consideration of the possibility of complicating issues, including the development of an inhibitor or the presence of septic arthritis. The latter is a particularly important consideration in the context of HIV infection.

HEMATURIA

Hematuria is a relatively common type of bleeding in persons with hemophilia and can originate from the upper or lower urinary tract. In the management of hematuria it is critical that high urinary output be maintained with oral or intravenous hydration, and this is often sufficient therapy, resulting in complete cessation of bleeding. If bleeding persists, replacement therapy should be given, dosing to maintain an optimal factor level of 30–50%; high urinary output should be maintained during therapy with factor replacement. Antifibrinolytic agents are contraindicated in the therapy of hemophilia-associated hematuria. Finally, an individual who has had recurrent episodes of hematuria warrants an investigation of the urinary tract in order to exclude an anatomic or infectious etiology for bleeding.

LIFE-THREATENING HEMORRHAGE

Areas in which bleeding episodes represent life-threatening events include the central nervous system (CNS), the retroperitoneum and the retropharyngeal space. Bleeding in any of these areas calls for hospitalization for therapy and observation; in all such cases factor replacement therapy must be instituted rapidly and prior to definitive diagnosis, if necessary. Each of these episodes requires intensive correction of the factor deficiency, with target levels between 60 and 100% (Table 15.1).

Any head injury should be regarded as a potential bleeding episode and treated accordingly, with the duration of therapy dependent upon the severity of the injury and subsequent objective findings (for example, the results of computed tomographic (CT) scanning or magnetic resonance imaging (MRI)). A headache of unusual severity lasting longer than 4 h should prompt suspicion of a CNS bleeding episode. Any case in which intracranial bleeding is documented should be treated with factor replacement appropriate to the target level of 60–100% for 10–14 days.

Retroperitoneal bleeding occurs as lower abdominal pain with the presence of iliopsoas muscle irritation and contraction (the straight-leg-raising sign). If findings are on the right-hand side they may mimic those of appendicitis. As with intracranial bleeding, an initial dose of factor replacement therapy should be given before any diagnostic interventions (again, the most useful are ultrasonography or CT scanning) are undertaken, and should be continued for 10–14 days if bleeding is documented. Retropharyngeal bleeding is a frequent sequela of pharyngitis and should be suspected in this or in any other case in which the patient complains either of neck swelling or difficulty swallowing. Again, prompt intervention with high-dose factor replacement should be instituted and diagnosis with CT scanning should be performed. In most cases, adequate and prompt replacement therapy will avert tracheostomy; again, therapy for a retropharyngeal bleeding episode should continue for 10–14 days.

References

Campbell, E.W., Neff, S. and Bowdler, A.J. (1978) Therapy with factor IX concentrate resulting in DIC and thromboembolic phenomena. *Transfusion*, **18**, 94–97.

Hoyer, L. (1994) Medical progress: hemophilia A (review). *N Engl J Med*, **330**, 38–47.

Hrinda, M.E., Huang, C., Tarr, G.C. *et al.* (1991) Preclinical studies of a monoclonal antibody-purified factor IX, Mononine. *Semin Hematol*, **28**, 6–14.

Kasper, C.K. (1973) Postoperative thromboses in hemophilia B. *N Engl J Med*, **289**, 160.

Kasper, C.K. and Dietrich, S.L. (1985) Comprehensive management of haemophilia, in *Clinics in Haematology: Coagulation Disorders*, W.B. Saunders, London.

Kasper, C.K., Abramson, S.B., Goldsmith, J.C. and Herring, S. (1991) *In vivo* recovery, half-life and safety of affinity purity solvent–detergent coagulation factor IX. *Blood*. **78**, 58a.

Kim, H.C., McMillan, White, G.C. *et al.* (1992) Purified factor IX using monoclonal immunoaffinity technique: clinical trials in hemophilia B and comparison to prothrombin complex concentrates. *Blood*, **79**, 568–575.

Lethagen, S., Harris, A.S. and Nilsson, I.M. (1990) Intranasal desmopressin (DDAVP) by spray in mild hemophilia A and von Willebrand's disease type I. *Blut*, **60**, 187–191.

Lusher, J.M. (1991) Thrombogenicity associated with factor IX complex concentrates. *Semin Hematol*, **28**, 3–5.

Mannucci, P.M., Ruggeri, Z.M., Pareti, F.I. and Capitano, A. (1977) 1-Deamino-8-D-arginine vasopressin: a new pharmacological approach to the management of hemophilia and von Willebrand's disease. *Lancet*, **1**, 869–872.

Mannucci, P.M., Gringeri, A. and Cattaneo, M. (1990) High-purity factor VIII concentrates produced without using monoclonal antibodies. *Res Clin Lab*, **20**, 227–238.

Menache, D., Behre, H.E., Orthner, C.L. *et al.* (1984) Coagulation factor IX concentrate. Method of preparation and assessment of potential *in vivo* thrombogenicity in animal models. *Blood*, **64**, 1220.

Rose, E. and Aledort, L.M. (1991) Nasal spray desmopression (DDAVP) for mild hemophilia A and von Willebrand disease. *Ann Intern Med*, **114**, 563–568.

Schreiber, A. (1988) The preclinical characterisation of monoclate factor VIII:C antihemophilic factor (human). *Semin Hematol*, **25** (suppl. 1), 27–32.

Schulman, S. (1989) Protein content of coagulation factor concentrates, in *Biotechnology and the Promise of Pure Factor VIII* (ed. H.H. Roberts), Baxter Healthcare Publications, Brussels, pp. 21–30.

Schwartz, R. for the Recombinant Factor VIII study group (1990) Human recombinant DNA-derived antihemophilic factor (factor VIII) in the treatment of hemophilia A. *N Engl J Med*, **323**, 1800–1805.

Seremetis, S.V. and Aledort, L.M. (1991) Nasal spray desmopressin (DDAVP) – experience in home care and surgical prophylaxis. *Blood*, **78** (suppl. 1), 275a.

16 HOME THERAPY

*M.W. Hilgartner, D. Cardi and
I. Goldberg*

Home therapy for the person with a bleeding disorder is defined today as the infusion of the deficient clotting factor or blood substitute in a setting outside of the hospital by a patient or family member or other paramedical personnel. This method of care has been called self-infusion, home infusion therapy, home care or home therapy. The history of its development, the rationale and patient selection, the education and training of the patient/family to carry out the procedure, the education at different ages and the psychosocial issues and complications which may develop will be covered in this chapter.

History

The greatest and most significant change in the management of hemophilia that fostered the independence of the patient/family from the physician and hospital has empowered the patient/family with a large control over the consequences of the bleeding disorder. This change began when, in 1961, Dr Richard Halden taught his family members to transfuse their children at home for bleeding episodes using fresh frozen plasma. One of these families moved to Chicago where Rabiner and Telfer (1970; Rabiner, Telfer and Rajardo, 1972), at the Michael Reese Hospital, developed a program to study the outcome of this innovative management using cryoprecipitate stored in special home freezers. The advantages became apparent very readily and large centers adopted the procedure with the establishment of teams of nurses and other medical and paramedical personnel to carry out the education and administration of the home care programs. The development of freeze-dried concentrates in the early 1970s simplified the home storage of clotting factor products, obviating the need for special freezers and using, instead, the usual household refrigerator freezers and using, instead, the usual household refrigerator for storage of products to extend the product life span. This allowed a greater number of families the advantage of this newly developing method of care, as the clotting factors were transportable and easily reconstituted for infusion (Levine and Britten, 1973).

Administration of treatment for bleeding episodes outside the hospital setting has become accepted today as the most efficient form of care delivery for the patient with a bleeding disorder in the socially conscious, economically advantaged countries of the world. These include the USA, UK (Le Quesne *et al.*, 1974), the Scandinavian countries, France, Germany, Italy, Greece, Spain, Israel, Australia and Japan (Ekert and Smibert, 1974).

The home therapy programs are now considered to be part of comprehensive care, as described in other parts of this book (Smith and Levine, 1984). These comprehensive care programs evolved, however, as the magnitude of the problems associated with the growth and development of a successful child and adult were perceived and addressed.

In the economically advantaged countries, use of this method of care has grown from 11.8%, reported in 1979 at the first European workshop in Luxembourg (Tantyl and Devreker, 1977), to the current figure of nearly 80%. The experience in our own center, at the New York Hospital Hemophilia Center, is listed in Table 16.1. Virtually all of the patients with severe factor VIII (FVIII) and factor IX (FIX) disease are on home care (77%): only those who are not ready or willing to learn or have a questionable family environment are treated by home care nursing companies or in the outpatient or emergency department. With the development of desmopression (DDAVP; Stimate) as a nasal spray, all the patients with mild FVIII deficiency and those patients

Hemophilia. Edited by C.D. Forbes, L. Aledort and R. Madhok. Published in 1997 by Chapman & Hall, London. ISBN 0 412 63820 7

Table 16.1 Methods of care delivery

New York Hospital experience with home care

193 patients 6 months–55 years of age

148 (77%)   Patients on home infusion therapy
Factor VIII, IX, XIII and inhibitor patients

145 (75%)   Patient/care-givers 3(2%) home care company

45 (23%)   Not on home care
17 mild Factor VIII and von Willebrand disease use desmopressin

28 mild Factor IX and other deficiencies use emergency room for infusion of cryoprecipitate and fresh frozen plasma

with von Willebrand's disease who respond to DDAVP will be able to be treated at home as well. Other centers have already advocated the use of subcutaneous injections of DDAVP in an effort to move treatment for this group of patients into the home (Gomperts and Sergis-Deavenport, 1989). Only those rare clotting factor deficiencies requiring fresh frozen plasma or cryoprecipitate remain to be treated in hospital as outpatients.

The fostering of a medically educated, responsible patient/family population has been particularly useful today when extended antibiotic therapy for sepsis or other therapies necessary for the well-being of the human immunodeficiency virus (HIV)-infected patient can be carried out in the home. The mutual cooperation of the comprehensive care team and the patient/family constellation for these additional therapies has been achieved from the simple teaching of a family member to infuse for a bleeding episode in the home.

Rationale

It has long been recognized that when bleeding episodes are controlled as soon as possible, the extent of bleeding is lessened, subsequent inflammation with surrounding tissue damage is interrupted and potential morbidity is decreased. The growth and development of a physically and psychologically disabled person can be inhibited in early childhood when bleeding is identified early and hemostasis acquired.

The major form of bleeding in the patient with severe hemophilia occurs in the joints, leading to deformities and crippling. Experimental work by Swanton (1959) with the hemophilic dog identified the cartilaginous destruction within the joint that occurred with bleeding. Proteolyic enzymes present in blood and other enzymes released by deteriorating cartilage, plus pressure within the joint due to volume expansion, is followed by bony disposition of iron and other heavy metals which contri-butes to the cartilaginous and subsequent bony destruction. These multiple factors were later found to be the cause of the orthopedic deformities (Hilgartner, 1975; Arnold and Hilgartner, 1977). The resulting pain and suffering of the patient and his family produced a profoundly abnormal state of mental health, resulting in marked dysfunction in all the family (Agle *et al.*, 1977). If the patient reached adulthood, he was usually a nonproductive member of society.

Early identification of joint-bleeding episodes with rapid administration of clot-promoting products to interrupt the destructive cycle was viewed as the ultimate treatment goal which would allow the patient/family a method of coping with this chronic illness, circumventing the hours associated with travel and wait in the outpatient treatment centers. As part of this goal was achieved, a new one has been developed to prevent bleeding with scheduled prophylactic therapy. General acceptance of this first premise and demonstration of its validity as a cost-saving procedure for the production of a functional adult awaited further studies.

The imprimatur of acceptance from the National Hemophilia Foundation with development of guidelines for home therapy programs drawn up by physicians knowledgeable about the disease associated with that organization helped to foster wide medical acceptance (Agle *et al.*, 1977). Studies conducted under the auspices of the offices of Maternal and Child Health reported by Smith and Levine in 1984 pointed out the advantages of home therapy within the context of comprehensive care. The decrease in number of days lost from work or school, days spent in the hospital and a decrease in the number of unemployed adults were addressed. These data, collated over a 10-year span, proved that early treatment of bleeding decreased the crippling handicaps that had prevented the education and the functioning of adults in the workforce. Data were also collected in different centers to demonstrate to the third-party insurance payers that treatment in the home, without the expense of physician and emergency room fees, was less costly overall and was extremely cost-beneficial for this lifelong chronic illness (Aledort, L.H., personal communication).

Patient selection

At the beginning of the home therapy programs, the criteria for patient selection were stringent and restrictive. The criteria have become more lenient with the advent of newer products, with physician and team experience and improved patient education. However, the basic guidelines as stated by Eyster (1981) and provided by the American National Hemophilia Foundation booklet, *Home Therapy for Hemophilia*, remain and are as follows:

1. *Confirmation of diagnosis.* The correct diagnosis of the coagulation deficiency FVIII, FIX, FXIII or von Willebrand's disorder – must be confirmed to choose the proper therapy and maximize the education needs.
2. *Bleeding frequency.* The frequency of bleeding must be ascertained to review the need for home therapy. If bleeding is less than every 2–3 months, irrespective of the degree of deficiency, the home care-giver will not maintain his or her skills sufficiently to be able to infuse product, and alternate infusers must be identified.
3. *Inhibitor status.* The presence or absence of an inhibitor to the transfused product must be ascertained to facilitate the proper choice of product and to evaluate efficacy of future infusions. These inhibitor studies must be repeated at least annually and more frequently, if necessary. In the early days of home infusion programs, patients with inhibitors were excluded because of lack of available hemostatic products for their bleeding. With the advent of a better understanding of the inhibitor states and the recognition of the ability to have hemostasis in the presence of an inhibitor with the use of frothrombin complex concentrates, the activated complexes, and FVIIa, reluctance to infuse the patients with inhibitors at home has been abandoned. These patients are now included in the programs.
4. *Psychosocial factors.* The patient/family who undertake home infusion must be competent, well-adjusted, mentally stable and able to accept the responsibility of the medical task and to make the decision concerning the presence of a bleeding episode and the need for infusion. The presence of mental illness, which might interfere with judgment, and factors such as alcoholism, drug abuse, emotional immaturity and severe depression, are contraindications for home care involvement.
5. *Age.* The minimum age was initially 4 years, at which time cooperation of the child and venous access could be anticipated. With additional experience, it has been found possible for some parents to infuse a child as young as 2 years. The advent of central line catheters, both Broviac and Infusaport, or Port-a-cath, has made it possible for children below 1 year of age to begin home infusions. The advocacy of prophylaxis in the very young child has been possible with these central lines used for routine home infusions. However, high infection rates in these central lines suggests the need to reconsider returning to the older-age child before initiating home infusions (Hilgartner and Kleinert, 1995).
6. *Record-keeping.* Accurate records of how much product is used and for what type of bleeding *must* be kept by the patient/family, and sent into the clinic at regular intervals. In fact, some clinics will not issue new products until records of use of previously released materials are provided (Eyster, 1981). This is necessary to monitor the use, to evaluate the bleeding episodes for the development of a target joint, to monitor the efficacy of the product and the amount used, or to discover the development of an inhibitor. Accurate record-keeping of product use will ultimately satisfy the third-party payer that the product is being used for its proper purpose.
7. *Clinic attendance* Regular clinic visits are imperative to make certain the patient remains in good physical and mental health without complications of his disease. These visits should occur every 6–12 months depending on the severity and frequency of the bleeding.

Although these criteria for patient selection are pertinent, all patients with hemophilia and most patients with other congenital bleeding disorders should be considered for home infusion programs today. However, there is still a small group of patients for whom this responsibility and type of management cannot be considered, who should not be pressured to comply. Unconscious self-assessment appears to be a valuable screening method for fitness in such a program. The 11 patient/family constellations in our clinic who are not on home care have many reasons for not being included in the program: they are not ready to learn; do not wish to learn; are unable to acquire sufficient skill; have poor venous access or may have an unsafe social environment with drug abuse in the household.

Patients and their families must continue to be monitored for safety in the home procedures, as risks for transmission of disease acquired from the product may still exist or transmission of disease from the patient to family member may occur. Stability and mental health in the home must be monitored by the social worker or other team members at the time of the annual clinic visit, and an evaluation of the efficacy of the health care management made at periodic intervals.

Education

Patient/family education is begun by the nurse practitioner in the hemophilia center starting with the first visit to the center where they are provided with books and literature developed for the layperson (see Further Reading). The goals of the education of the patient and family are to encourage an independent lifestyle away from the physician and hospital; to empower the families with knowledge to make medical decisions concerning the disease; and to form a partnership with the hemophilia center for ongoing care of the chronic disease. When the family exhibits an interest in home care, sessions are planned for their further education. The sessions are individual one-on-one and vary in length from 1–4 h depending on the prior knowledge of the patient/family member. The sessions review the types of bleeding episodes, the recognition and symptoms of bleeding episodes in the common bleeding sites and the philosophy of treatment in our center. This education about the disease is more important than the training for placement of the infusion needle because the medical judgment and subsequent decision-making that is being transferred to the patient or family member will be based on his or her knowledge of the disease, the consequence of bleeding in an area and the desired result of therapy. Finally, it will review when the patient/family member must contact the hemophilia center for continuing therapy or physician appraisal at the center.

A teaching manual has been developed by the Nursing and Psychosocial Committees of the National Hemophilia Foundation to cover a wide range of topics thought to be necessary for patient education by its education committee (Table 16.2). The information contained in

Table 16.2 National Hemophilia Foundation hemophilia patient/family educational modules

---

Basic information

Orthopedic

Genetics educational

Dental

Family guidance

Factor replacement

Home therapy training

AIDS and hemophilia

AIDS = Acquired immunodeficiency syndrome.

these modules was designed to be presented to the parents soon after the diagnosis of hemophilia is made in an effort to alleviate the fear and shock that come with the diagnosis. This education also starts the support process that is important whether hemophilia has been known in the family or not. These manuals were developed as teaching guidelines with checklists to review the patient/parent competency with understanding of the material. Educational brochures were also developed around each topic that may be given to the family for reference.

Many books have been written for patient education and support and translated into multiple languages. One of the better books compiled for the person is the *Hemophilia Handbook*, published by Hemophilia of Georgia. This is an excellent reference for the patients to have which covers the same information given in the modules in a patient-friendly manner, and can easily be referred to when needed at home. For those individuals with a limited understanding of English, a teaching guide entitled *Illustrated Hemophilia Guide* has been developed by the Nurses' Subcommittee of the World Federation of Hemophilia. This guide is a series of illustrations with visualization of the pertinent information which may be comprehended without the English language. A nurse instructor can give the basic knowledge of hemophilia, such as information concerning bleeding sites, complications of major and minor bleeding episodes, plus basic information about factor reconstitution and infusions using this guide.

The importance of a well-designed educational and training program cannot be overemphasized. As stated before, any well-meaning professional can teach an individual to place a needle for infusion, but the decision-making that must be done for the patient with hemophilia is much more complicated and requires knowledge, understanding and insight into the pathogenesis of hemophilia bleeding.

One group of investigators has used a questionnaire to quantify patients' retention of information and found that a self-assessment of knowledge rises from 21–55% postinstruction (Lazerson, Meredith and Lello, 1983). A controlled study was done by the team from Los Angeles Children's Hospital, who were able to show that those patient/families who went through structured teaching sessions increased their knowledge of hemophilia from 15–92% postinstruction and retained the information 30% better than the control group without the indepth teaching (Sergis-Deavenport and Varni, 1983). In addition, this knowledge was the basis of learning to cope with the disease.

Our own nursing staff have developed a checklist which they use at the end of teaching sessions and repeat periodically over the next few clinic visits to determine the competence and retention by the patient or family member of the material we believe important.

Training

It is difficult to separate training from education, as both are ongoing throughout life. Teaching begins with the family's first visit and is a continuous process. The child is included in training at an appropriate age, so that he may begin to learn when bleeding occurs and he can report to his parents when the joint 'feels funny, tingly, bubbly', etc. He must learn at an early age the important role that he plays in keeping himself well and when he should ask for his 'medicine.'

The training for home infusion is initiated once the principles of hemophilia and bleeding episodes are understood, and factor concentrates have been discussed. The infuser – parent or patient – must learn much of the principles of hemophilic management as presented in Chapter 15. The recognition of a bleeding episode begins with the appreciation of pain anywhere in the body. Superficial bleeding may produce a bruise that has a very firm center core specific to the hemophiliac. Muscle bleeding may be more serious and cause pain with swelling. These may be treated with ice and pressure bandages. Joint bleeding is usually recognized by the boy with a tingling, bubbly, unusual feeling long before limitation of motion and swelling occur. This recognition must be appreciated by an outside observer as the first evidence of bleeding. For the parent with a young baby, irritability or resistance to movement of an extremity may be the first sign of bleeding and should be treated as hemophilic bleeding before considering other etiology. The dictum of 'when in doubt, treat', coined by Peter Levine, has stood the test of time. Dosage calculations are presented and the optimum plasma level desired for each type of bleeding episode are reviewed for the appropriate type of deficiency, and whether treatment will be episodic or prophylactic.

The calculations depend on the weight of the patient, severity of the bleeding episode, amount of product desired for hemostasis and the half-life of the factor concentrate to be used, as presented in Chapter 15. If the bleeding episode is treated within 4 h of first presentation, it has been said that smaller amounts of product will bring about hemostasis using 15–20 u/kg to obtain a 30–40% plasma level. However, if the bleeding episode has been present for many hours or the bleeding has occurred in a chronic or target joint, then larger amounts of concentrate will be necessary up to 40 u/kg to achieve 80% plasma level should be used. The rationale for this amount of product to produce plasma levels of 30–40% for FVIII is based on the work of Abildgaard (1969), who showed that, if only plasma levels of 20% or less were achieved, at least 10% of the patients would fail to achieve hemostasis (Operalski *et al.*, 1995). Furthermore, if the bleeding is extremely severe, a follow-up infusion in 12–24 h may be necessary.

The practice in our clinic has been to use the higher dose of 40 u/kg for most hemarthroses in an effort to avoid a second infusion. The amount of product to be used for more serious bleeding in the retroperitonal area, retropharyngeal or central nervous system, or for trauma is usually calculated to achieve plasma levels of 100%. All product should be given to the nearest bottle, i.e. product is not discarded is the amount in the bottle is greater than that amount calculated for need, as infusion amounts are approximate, not exact.

When teaching factor preparation and venipuncture technique, emphasis is placed on understanding the principle of aseptic technique; what is considered sterile and not sterile; proper cleansing of the work area; cleansing of the skin; handling and disposal of syringes and needles with bottles of concentrate used for the infusion. Proper disposal of waste materials is particularly important to protect the patient's community from accidental transmission of viral diseases. The prevention of infection and preservation of the veins are of particular importance to these patients, who must depend on venous access for survival. Factor reconstitution is taught as shown in Table 16.3.

Various instructional tools are utilized in teaching the principles of venous access, including a manikin arm, as well as illustrations of common venous access sites. Although the patients are taught to rotate sites, favorite veins always develop. A local anesthetic cream can be applied to the area overlying the desired vein as all the

Table 16.3 Ten steps for factor reconstitution

1.	Remove caps from the concentrate and the sterile water diluent
2.	Using aseptic technique, remove protective covering from one end of double-sided needle (transfer needle) and insert into diluent stopper
3.	Remove protective covering from the other end of the needle and invert needle through stopper of concentrate. Diluent will flow into concentrate bottle by vacuum
4.	Withdraw needle from concentrate; discard needle and diluent bottle
5.	Gently rotate or swirl concentrate. Do not shake vigorously, as this may reduce the concentrate potency
6.	Inspect concentrate to insure all material is dissolved and solution is clear
7.	When all material is dissolved, draw up concentrate with filter needle
8.	More than one vial of concentrate can be drawn up in the same syringe
9.	Once reconstituted, infuse within 3–4 h. Do not refrigerate.
10.	Infusion can be pushed at 10 ml

equipment is being collected and the product is reconstituted. This gives sufficient depth of anesthesia to have a painless stick into vein or Infusaport and has helped abolish the needle-associated fear for children. Teaching is complete when the infuser has passed the test of a successful venipuncture and given good verbal responses on reasons for and implication of infusion, successful treatment of a bleeding episode and identification of signs of infiltration. Table 16.4 is a checklist used for home care training, which may be used in place of a written test.

EARLY YEARS: 0–4 YEARS

At each clinic visit, which may occur as often as every 3 months, the parents are introduced to the care and rearing of a child with a special problem superimposed on the rearing of a normal child. This is particularly important if the newly diagnosed hemophiliac is the first child and the disease is unknown to the family. The fear and anger must be dealt with and the family must be allowed to adjust to the diagnosis. They must also learn

Table 16.4   New York Hospital – Cornell Medical Center Comprehensive Hemophilia Treatment Center

Name _________________________________   Date ___________

Relationship to patient _____________________

Factor knowledge
_____   Demonstrates how to calculate dose
_____   Demonstrates where to find units on factor box
_____   Knows what kind of factor to use
_____   Can locate factor expiration
_____   Knows where to store factor
_____   Knows signs and symptoms of a reaction and proper treatment

Factor preparation
_____   Gathers materials needed
_____   Demonstrates sterile technique
_____   Demonstrates correct way to mix factor
_____   Knows what to do if vacuum does not work
_____   Demonstrates correct procedure for withdrawing factor into syringe
_____   Demonstrates correct disposal of needles and waste

Venipuncture
_____   Demonstrates adequate vein selection
_____   Demonstrates ability to apply tourniquet correctly
_____   Demonstrates correct cleansing of infusion site
_____   Demonstrates good technique for venipuncture
_____   Demonstrates ability to check for blood return
_____   Recognizes signs of infiltration
_____   Demonstrates ability to remove needle and correct disposal

Recording treatment
_____   Demonstrates ability to fill out infusion record correctly

Infusaport access
_____   Gathers materials needed for infusaport access
_____   Demonstrates good technique in cleansing port site
_____   Demonstrates correct technique for palpating port and locating port septum
_____   Demonstrates good sterile technique in accessing port with Huber needle
_____   Demonstrates good technique for flushing port
_____   Demonstrates good technique for removing Huber needle
_____   Can list potential problems with port and corrective measures to take
_____   Awareness

Broviac access
_____   Gathers materials needed for Broviac access
_____   Demonstrates good technique in cleansing port site
_____   Demonstrates good technique for flushing port
_____   Demonstrates knowledge of proper heparin flush

Nurse's signature _________________   Parent/patient signature _____________________ normal childhood growth and development and their role in this process. Introduction to the genetic counselor for genetic information about the disease, carrier detection and family planning is often useful. During this period, the family must learn basic information about the disease, how bleeding presents and methods of treatment. Both nurse educators and social work personnel are utilized to give emotional support to all members of the family, parents, grandparents and any other care-giver during these years. Phone contact is encouraged with the center personnel for support, outside contact with the local hemophilia organization and even parents of a somewhat older child with hemophilia for additional support.

Treatment products must be discussed with the parent and the decision made with the physician about which product will be used for this child. Blood product transmission of disease has been recognized over the last decade and is the cause of great anxiety to the patient and family. Therefore, the complete menu of available products should be reviewed, as well as the measures taken by the manufacturers of concentrate to provide a safe and efficacious product at a reasonable cost. Financial problems need to be considered at this early stage, as the payment for concentrate is the most expensive part of the care for this disease. The method of payment for concentrates may influence the decision of product choice for the child. Financial problems will vary with county and region and the manner in which health care problems are addressed in each country (see Chapter 30)

The first bleeding episode that warrants treatment is perhaps the first big hurdle – when the baby is brought to the doctor or hospital clinic, evaluated for bleeding and must be stuck for the infusion. With prior phone contact, the center may be alerted and ready to give the family support with the patient care. Hopefully, a skilled individual may give that first infusion to prevent the prolonged cries of the child and anguish of the parents. The manner in which the first bleeding episodes are dealt with may leave a haunting impression on the family and will influence the development of trust with the center personnel. It is a decision that may be different in many parts of the world today, and one that must be thoroughly understood by the family.

During these early years, both parent and child must learn how to limit bleeding episodes as much as possible. This can be done by making the home as safe as one would for any other child and considering toys that are made of wood or soft materials without edges that may cut a child; furniture that may be padded to minimize injury and clothing that may be protective. A small helmet may protect a toddler who tends to fall on his face; foam rubber sewed into jackets or pants may protect elbows and knees; and high boots may protect ankles. A

child must learn to walk, climb, jump and run as any other child, but he must also learn how to protect himself from injury.

4–7 YEARS

During these years, the child becomes more active with his peers, and develops more motor skills. This activity is accompanied by increasing bleeding episodes in ankles and knees. Both family and child become more upset by these repeat bleeding episodes and need further center personnel support to understand the illness. Independence of the family from the center is developed with home therapy during these years, as is a greater understanding by the boy of his limitations – what he can and what he cannot do. It is, perhaps, during these years that the decisions must be made for prophylactic treatment prior to sports or general prophylaxis to prevent the majority of bleeding episodes. The latter decision will change the family dynamics and the pattern of living with the disease. This decision concerning prophylaxis will have a profound effect on the way in which the child approaches school and the manner in which the school personnel accept him into a regular class. For those children with limited available factor concentrate, the center personnel must work with the family and school personnel to design programs that allow good physical and emotional growth with his peers without the hazards of risk-taking activities. The school personnel must learn how the treatment will be given should an injury occur and be reassured as to the boy's medical care when given by the parent.

7–14 YEARS

During these later childhood years, the boys will have learned how to cope with the disease, how to recognize a bleeding episode and when to seek treatment. He may even have learned how to dissolve his concentrate, how to calculate the dose for each type of bleeding episode and the purpose of the treatment. He must learn how to evaluate the gravity of an episode and whether treatment has brought the desired result with decrease in pain and the beginning of healing, or whether the treatment should be repeated. The ability to comprehend and to make decisions occurs with emotional maturity that must be fostered by the parent with center support. By late childhood and early adolescence, this maturity is critical so that the boy may be able to accept negative peer interaction, will not hide his bleeding and will continue to treat each episode as early as possible. It is commonplace for any adolescent with a chronic illness to minimize his illness in an effort to be like all of his peers. It is, therefore, critical for both child and parent to recognize that he is near normal with current therapy, but not yet entirely normal, and will never be exactly like his peers.

ADOLESCENT AND YOUNG ADULT

The pattern to cope with the illness is set by these decades of life and the young man is able to make his own decision about treating and infuse himself as necessary for his lifestyle. Bleeding episodes usually decrease in number due largely to maturity and activity. It may be hoped that appropriate goals have been set and the boy has not chosen risk-taking activities for his lifestyle. Center personnel input can still be useful for support of whatever has been chosen guidance as desired by the young man. Vocational guidance may be particularly important at this time to help direct him into higher education or a vocational choice and to direct him to the community resource that may encourage his choice.

Appropriate cultural philosophy must be observed for each family. However, current therapy makes a sense of self-esteem and independence possible, with gainful employment for every adult a reality. In spite of readily available concentrates for almost 25 years of home therapy, and the growth of a generation of men with few orthopedic problems and crippling, there are still many adults who were denied available products and are emotional and physical cripples today. They need a different type of support – perhaps even chronic analgesic support – to cope with the crippling pain. Orthopedic rehabilitation is still necessary for many of those less fortunate adults.

The advent of HIV disease has also changed the lifestyle for most of the young and older adults of the current generation. The ability to make medical decisions and maintain a dialogue with physician and medical staff has been essential for the use of home therapy to treat the opportunistic infections that come with HIV disease. Center personnel may only be a resource for emotional support as bleeding episodes decrease and become a less important phenomenon in life, but may continue to be the avenue through which medical care outside the hospital may be obtained.

Psychosocial issues

The patient/family's ability to adapt positively to living with hemophilia – which includes home infusion – can be significantly influenced by the groundwork that is established in the beginning year immediately following diagnosis. At this juncture, the comprehensive care team plays a vital role in providing ongoing support and education to the family. However, in order to maximize the patient/family's strengths in helping them learn to adapt, it is important that there be an ongoing assessment of the family unit's mental status, support systems and other environmental influences. In addition, it is important to maintain a clear understanding of the family dynamic. The more the comprehensive care team understands about the patient/family, the more the team can provide in terms of effective and empathic communication in giving information and support. Although it is ultimately the patient/family's task to adapt to living with hemophilia, the comprehensive care team's role in this process should not be underestimated.

In considering whether or not a patient/family is appropriate for home therapy, it has already been suggested that they must be able to exercise sound judgment, maintain an ability to make decisions concerning bleeding episodes and generally show characteristics of stability. Moreover, it is important continually to assess the family for risk factors (alcoholism, parent/child problems, mental instability) that may affect their ability to perform home therapy. Once a family has met the criteria, as previously stated, home therapy should be introduced to include both parents and the patient. Although the role of the patient might seem obvious, it is remarkable how often parents neglect to be attuned to the patient when diagnosing a bleeding episode. Therefore, it is important to emphasize the role of the patient when introducing home care. Although both parents may not be willing to participate in the actual infusion, they should be encouraged to be actively involved in the process. For example, the mother may be more comfortable in giving the infusion, whereas the father's role lies in his ability to assess with the patient the onset of a joint bleed.

At the New York Hospital, one of our treatment goals is to foster as much normalcy and independence as possible. As a result of successfully managing the task of providing home therapy, our younger families seem to have positively adapted to living with hemophilia. Within the process of mastering home infusion, there also appears the process of empowerment. This occurs in the patient/family's willingness to become educated, self-advocating and in their increased ability to determine the need for infusion. The patient/family is, therefore, able to gain a sense of mastery and control over hemophilia, which can increase their level of confidence. This, in turn, can develop more positive self-esteem in the patient. Some older families, however, are unwilling to develop a partnership for multiple reasons not associated with the disease, which hinders their growth and ability to cope with the disease. This tends to foster a state in which the patient/family are victims of the disease, rather than conquerors of the disease. This, in turn, can inevitably cause less positive self-esteem in the patient.

The onset of HIV infection has disrupted this positive growth, producing instead a lack of trust, with disruption of the partnership between patient and team.

Record-keeping

This is essential to follow the course of bleeding episodes and to determine whether treatment is adequate for the patient on home therapy. If a target joint is developing or synovitis has occurred, treatment patterns need to be changed; i.e. if episodic treatment is used, short-term prophylactic treatment 3 or 4 times weekly may be necessary. When logs are sent in promptly every 2–3 months for review by the nursing staff, the patient can be brought in for orthopedic and physical therapy evaluation and treatment changes instituted when it appears obvious that the usual treatment is not initiating hemostasis. Occasionally, it may be necessary to learn how the product is stored and reviewed for potential loss of potency. It may even be necessary to screen the patient's plasma for the development of an inhibitor. Accurate records of product use are necessary, should a lot be recalled or should it be necessary to test the patient for disease transmission. The patient, as well as the center, will have records to show where the product has been used and steps taken for action. Finally, the third-party payer needs to know that the product has been used for its proper purpose. See Tables 16.4 and 16.5 for examples of records.

A common problem worldwide with patients on home therapy is compliance with the submission of infusion records or logs. Over the years, we have changed the form several times in an effort to simplify and yet gain the same amount of information about site of bleeding, acute or chronic bleeding, amount, type and name of the product used, the lot number of the product, potential reactions and days lost from school or work. Simplification of the form was not always successful in obtaining compliance. Industry has developed peel-off labels for Germany to assist with the problem. A contract signed by the patient outlining his responsibility for record-keeping and clinic visit was also not particularly useful. A simple non-threatening reminder with the biannual clinic report has been more successful than other punitive incentives to improve compliance with this unpalatable record-keeping. Repeated patient education about the purpose appears to be important.

Ideally, electronic data management could replace the current system for the patient that could interface with our systems management of product in the New York buying consortium. Usage could be tracked with acquisition through such system, and may be put into place in the near future.

Complications

There may be medical, as well as psychosocial, complications associated with home therapy. The medical complications can arise in the patient due to inadequate therapy and must be dealt with at a comprehensive visit or sooner, if detected through the logs or nursing staff contact. The latter is an extremely important part of the center contact and frequently occurs with ordering of product. Patients can be brought in for a medical visit if problems with hemostasis or other health problems are detected, or if school or family problems are detected. Should they be school-associated, a visit to the school or contact with the school nurse or teacher may be sufficient to solve the problem. Should the problem be parent- or home-oriented, a visit to the home may often shed light on the problem and help towards its solution.

Medical complications may arise in the patient from the infusion itself, usually allergic in origin. Any patient with a previous history of hives, chills, fever or shortness of breath following the infusion of other blood products is given an antihistamine to use orally prior to the infusion and corticosteroids to have on hand should a more serious reaction appear afterwards. Instructions to slow the infusion often are sufficient to diminish a reaction. Those individuals who have had repeated respiratory reactions are given one dose of epinephrine for use before going to the nearest emergency room for care. Hepatitis B, C and even A, cytomegalovirus, Epstein–Barr virus and parvovirus are all known contaminants of blood that may be transmitted through the products transfused at home and are discussed elsewhere in this book.

Medical complications may arise in the parent or infusor with transmission of viral diseases from the blood products or from the blood of the infected patient by a needlestick or through abrasions on the hands. Hepatitis B has been transmitted to family members of patients with hemophilia before the use of hepatitis B vaccine in parent or family members. Hepatitis B vaccine is, therefore, recommended for the family member who is the infusor. Data collected through the Transfusion Safety Study in 1423 patients showed that hepatitis B can be easily transmitted from the patient with acute or chronic disease to sexual partners and household contacts while hepatitis C is poorly transmitted to both sexual and non-sexual household contacts. HIV has not been transmitted to an infusor or non-sexual contact in the same study, but continues to be of great concern.

Other complications may arise which may warrant the suspension of home therapy, such as deterioration in the family setting, that may lead to parent instability and inability to make decisions appropriate for the patient. When such a situation arises today, it may be necessary to find companies who service the patients at home for infusions or have the patient return to the emergency room for infusion.

Table 16.5   New York Hospital – Cornell Medical Center infusion log/record

Date: _______________

Product: _____________

Number of units per vial: _______________   Lot no.: __________

Number of vials used: _________________

Reason for infusion:

		Site		Weight
		R	L	
New bleed	____	Shoulder		____
Follow-up	____	Elbow	____	____
Postoperative	____	Arm	____	____
Physical therapy	____	Hand	____	____
Prophylaxis		Hip	____	____
Injury	____	Knee	____	____
Recurrent bleed	____	Calf	____	____
Spontaneous	____	Ankle	____	____
		Other	____	____

Total days lost from school/work because of bleed?

Reactions: Treatment:

References

Abildgaard, C.F. (1969) The management of bleeding in hemophilia. *Adv Pediatr*, **16**, 365.

Agle, D.P., Hilgartner, M.W., Lazerson, J. and Van Eys, J. (1977) *Home Care Program: A Manual for Physicians*, National Hemophilia Foundation, New York.

Arnold, W.D. and Hilgartner, M.W. (1977) Hemophilic arthropathy. *Journal of Bone Joint Surgery*, **59A**, 287–305.

Ekert, H. and Smibert, E. (1974) Homecare for hemophilia. *Medical Journal of Australia*, **2**, 802–806.

Eyster, M.E. (1981) Home therapy programs, in *Hemophilia in the Child and the Adult* (ed. M. Hilgartner), Mason Publishing, New York, pp. 219–229.

Gomperts, E.D. and Sergis-Deavenport (1989) Home therapy programs: the role of the nurse, physician, patient and family in self-directed care, in *Hemophilia in the Child and the Adult*, 2nd edn (ed. M. Hilgartner), Raven Press, New York, pp. 173–193.

Hilgartner, M.W. (1975) Hemophilic arthropathy. *Adv Pediatr*, **21**, 139-165.

Hilgartner, M.W. and Kleinert, D. (1995) Morbidity of central lines with coagulation. Submitted May, 1995. APS/SPR Abs.

Lazerson, J., Meredith, K. and Lello, C.J. (1983) Patient education in hemophilia, the consumer response (Abstr. 79). *15th Int. Cong. World Fed. Hemophilia*, Stockholm.

Le Quesne, B., Britten, M.I., Maragaki, C. and Dormandy, K.M. (1974) Home treatment for patients with hemophilia. *Lancet*, **2**, 507–510.

Levine, P. and Britten, A.F.H. (1973) Supervised patient management of hemophilia: a study of 45 patients with hemophilia A and B. *Ann Intern Med* **78**, 195–201.

Operalski, E.A. and the Transfusion Safety Study (1995) Comparison of HCV with HBV infection among sexual and non-sexual household contacts of persons with congenital clotting disorders. Presented 'Liver Disease in Hemophilia' Conference. NHF, Atlanta, March, 1995.

Rabiner, S.F. and Talfer, M.C. (1970) Home transfusions for patients with hemophilia A. *N Engl J Med* **283**, 1011–1015.

Rabiner, S.F., Telfer, M.C. and Rajardo, R. (1972) Home transfusions in hemophiliacs. *JAMA*, **221**, 885–887.

Sergis-Deavenport, E. and Varni, I. (1983) Behavioral assessment and management of adherence to factor replacement in hemophilia. *J Pediatr Psychol*, **8**, 367–377.

Smith, P.S. and Levine, P.H. (1984) Benefits of comprehensive care of hemophilia. *Am J Publ Health*, **74**, 616–617.

Swanton, M.D. (1959) Hemophilic arthropathy in dogs. *Lab Invest*, **8**, 1269.

Tantyl, J. and DeVreker, R.A. (eds) (1977) Management of the hemophilias; a system of home treatment. Part A: survey of hemophilia home treatment in participating countries. *Scand J Hematol*, **31** (suppl.), 5–33.

Further reading

Jones, P. (1974) *Living with Hemophilia*, F.A. Davis, Philadelphia, Pennsylvania.

Levine, P. and Brachmann, H.H. (1983) *Illustrated Hemophilia Guide*, World Federation of Hemophilia, Montreal, Canada.

National Hemophilia Foundation (1981) *Hemophilia Patient Family Education Model*, National Hemophilia Foundation, New York.

17 FACTOR VIII CONCENTRATES

E. Berntorp

The development of factor VIII (FVIII) concentrates has revolutionized hemophilia care. In cases of ordinary joint bleeds, the plasma concentration of the patient's deficient factor (i.e. FVIII in hemophilia A) has to be increased to about 20% (0.2 iu/ml) of normal (Rizza, 1972) and sometimes the dose has to be repeated. Larger doses are often recommended for routine treatment (Allain, 1979). In cases of severe bleeds, or as cover for surgery, it is necessary to increase the plasma concentration even more, usually to 50–100% of normal, and in conjunction with major surgery the level of the concentration has to be kept high for several weeks (Rickard, 1995). One international unit (iu) of FVIII per kg body weight will yield an increase in the recipient's plasma FVIII concentration of about 2% (0.02 iu/ml). As 1000 ml of plasma contains 1000 iu FVIII, obviously optimal hemophilia replacement therapy is impossible to achieve simply with plasma infusions. For this purpose, concentrates are required that contain considerably more FVIII per infused volume than does plasma.

The first concentrate (fraction I-O) became available in 1956 in Sweden, and was followed by cryoprecipitate in 1964. More active, lyophilized, concentrates became available during the 1970s. The problem of hepatitis transmitted by clotting factor concentrates has been known since the early 1970s and the human immuno-deficiency virus (HIV) catastrophe, which became widely recognized in 1984, struck the hemophilia population in the first years of the 1980s. These blood-borne diseases prompted the development of safer and more pure products. However, not until the second half of the 1980s, concomitantly with the introduction of the re-combinant DNA products, did plasma-derived concentrates that may be considered reasonably safe regarding transmission of blood-borne viruses become generally available for the treatment of the hemophilia population at large. Even today the problem of viruses has not been fully resolved, and other aspects of side-effects, especially the development of inhibitors, but also the impact of concentrates on the immune system, are issues that have yet to be resolved.

Early factor VIII concentrates

Fraction I produced with the Cohn method mainly contains fibrinogen but also some clotting factors, such as FVIII and prothrombin, as well as plasmin. This fraction was unstable with regard to FVIII and unsuitable for the treatment of patients. In 1956, Blombäck and Blombäck prepared their fraction I-O by eluting Cohn fraction I with glycine containing ethanol and citrate. It could be shown that FVIII was almost quantitatively recovered from plasma and remained stable (Nilsson, 1974). This fraction mainly contains fibrinogen but also, apart from FVIII, native von Willebrand factor (vWf) and factor XIII. Factor VIII in fraction I-O is purified 20–40 times, as compared to fresh human plasma. From 1956 until recently, fraction I-O (later named AHF-Kabi when commercially produced) was used in Sweden for the treatment of hemophilia A and von Willebrand's disease, and also as replacement in intensive care situations complicated by pathologic proteolysis. The product was withdrawn in the second half of the 1980s because of its low purity, inconvenience for use owing to the large reconstitution volume, and insufficient virus inactivation.

On a more global basis, the era of modern hemophilia therapy began in the mid-1960s when cryoprecipitate became available for clinical use. In 1959 Pool and Robinson discovered that cryoprecipitate from human plasma contained FVIII. When fresh frozen human plasma was slowly thawed at 4°C, the cryoprecipitate formed contained substantial amounts of FVIII which

Hemophilia. Edited by C.D. Forbes, L. Aledort and R. Madhok. Published in 1997 by Chapman & Hall, London. ISBN 0 412 63820 7

could be dissolved at 37°C and used for replacement therapy in hemophilia and in von Willebrand's disease (Pool, Hershgold and Pappenhagen, 1964; Pool and Shannon, 1965; Bennett and Dormandy, 1966). In this way FVIII is purified 8–20 times, as compared to the source plasma. Cryoprecipitate has been extensively used for replacement therapy, but its use is now limited as it cannot be reliably virus-inactivated.

FVIII can also be prepared from animal plasma and used for treatment of humans. Bidwell (1955) prepared concentrates from bovine and porcine plasma containing FVIII which was purified 100–400 times that in plasma. These products have been used for the treatment of hemophilia (Biggs and Macfarlane, 1966). The hemostatic effect was good on a short-term basis, but patients developed antibodies and sometimes manifested severe allergic reactions. As discussed below, porcine FVIII is still in use, especially for the treatment of hemophilia A complicated by high-titer inhibitors and in acquired hemophilia.

Modern human, plasma-derived factor VIII concentrates and recombinant products

At the end of the 1960s, more active lyophilized FVIII concentrates became available. Cryoprecipitate of pooled human donor plasma was used as the starting material, and the bulk of contaminating proteins, mainly fibrinogen, were removed by various methods. Since the advent of HIV and awareness of the risk of hepatitis transmission, several approaches have been tried to increase the safety of the products. Selection of low-risk donors and screening of donor blood have been implemented and are continuously improved. Concentrate purity has been increased both as a safety measure to reduce the viral burden in the final product, but also to reduce the putative risk of immune suppression. However, as infected donor blood and consequently virus particles may escape these measures, manufacturers of blood products have developed virucidal methods compatible with good yields and little loss of the biological activity of such labile proteins as coagulation factors.

The rapid development of FVIII concentrates during the last 10 years has yielded products with a high degree of safety. Both the purification and production methods and the mode of virus inactivation have changed, and there has been continual development of the products. The classification of the products has changed from time to time, and there is no current general consensus as to nomenclature, even if the broad categories can be said to be widely accepted.

CLASSIFICATION

The FVIII concentrates currently available can be classified both according to purity and to type of manufacturing procedure. The term purity often refers to specific activity – the product's content of VIII coagulation factor (VIII:C) in iu/mg protein. In many concentrates, however, specific activity is not a good measure of purity as albumin, for example, is added as protein carrier, and as it is open to question whether the von Willebrand factor is to be considered an impurity. The quantity of added albumin is often subtracted when protein content is calculated. However, this procedure raises questions with regard to extrapolation to the *in vivo* situation, and is only justified by the assumption that the added albumin, although not entirely pure, does not transmit viral disorders or have any other side-effect, for example, on the immune system. Thus, a better measure of purity is the amount of different contaminating proteins contained in the product expressed in terms of weight protein per iu VIII:C, although this is rather a complicated way of defining the general properties of concentrates.

With this background, the classification system outlined in Table 17.1, which is often used, seems practical and relevant for most purposes, and takes such issues as purity and manufacturing procedure into account (although, for the sake of clarity, specific activity is given

Table 17.1 Classification of factor VIII concentrates

Preparation	Manufacturing procedure	Specific activity (iu VIII:C/mg protein; added albumin excluded)
Intermediate-purity	Cryoprecipitate + further purification	1–50
High-purity	Protein precipitation + chromatographic separation	50–200
Monoclonal antibody purified	Affinity purified with monoclonal antibodies against factor VIII or von Willebrand factor	>1000
Recombinant	DNA technology. Purification includes an affinity step with monoclonal antibodies against factor VIII	>1000

when the amount of added albumin is subtracted). Plasma-derived products are qualified as being of intermediate-purity, high-purity or monoclonal antibody-purified (sometimes called superpure, ultrapure or very-high-purity). Low-purity products, not contained in the table, would thus refer to fraction I-O and cryoprecipitate. Intermediate-purity concentrates are prepared from cryoprecipitate and further purified with a variety of methods, including Al(OH)$_3$ adsorption, and glycine or polyethylene glycol precipitation. High-purity products are prepared by conventional chromatography, and the monoclonal antibody-purified products are prepared using affinity chromatography with monoclonal murine antibodies directed against FVIII or von Willebrand factor.

In addition to plasma-derived products, recombinant complementary DNA-derived FVIII concentrates are also widely marketed. At present, two recombinant FVIII products are available – Kogenate and Recombinate. Kogenate was initially cloned and developed by Genentec Inc. and is currently sold by Bayer. The product is prepared in a continuous cell culture process using baby hamster kidney (BHK) cells transfected with the FVIII gene. Coexpression of recombinant FVIII with vWf in the culture media is not required for stabilization of the FVIII molecule, but a special production culture medium containing, for example, insulin, transferrin and albumin is used (Giles and Tinlin, 1988; Chan and Lembach, l991; Klein, l991; Boedeker, 1992). Recombinate was cloned and developed at Genetics Institute Inc. and is marketed by Baxter. It is produced in a batch re-feed cell culture process using Chinese hamster ovary (CHO) cells transfected with the FVIII gene. Coexpression of FVIII with vWf stabilizes FVIII. In the absence of vWf, the heavy chain of FVIII expressed in CHO cells is not associated with the light chain and both are degraded (Kaufman, Wasley and Dorner, 1988; Wise *et al.*, 1991; Gomperts *et al.*, 1992; Kaufman, 1992). Both recombinant products are further purified using monoclonal antibody immunoaffinity and additional chromatographic steps. In the near future a second-generation cDNA product will probably become available.

Currently used monoclonal antibody-purified products as well as recombinant products all contain added human albumin. This is also true of some high-purity concentrates.

Virucidal methods applied to factor VIII concentrates

Improved screening of blood and plasmapheresis donors with mandatory testing for HIV-1 and 2 and hepatitis C virus (HCV) seropositivity and for hepatitis B (HB) surface antigen (HBsAg) greatly reduces the viral burden of the starting material from which FVIII preparations

are made (Watson *et al.*, 1992). However, as these measures are insufficient to abolish the risk of virus transmission, several virucidal methods have been developed and applied to clotting factor concentrates. In most countries the use of virucidal methods in the preparation of licensed FVIII concentrates is mandatory. The main methods currently used include terminal heating of the lyophilized products at 80°C (dry heating), heating in solution at 60°C in the presence of stabilizers (pasteurization), heating with hot vapor under high pressure, or adding a detergent/solvent mixture during manufacture (Kasper *et al.*, 1993; Mannucci, 1993, 1995). Some manufacturers have introduced double virus inactivation steps, and this strategy will probably become a requirement in some countries for licensing of products. Table 17.2 shows virucidal methods currently, or recently, used. The efficacy of individual methods is discussed below.

Biochemical properties of human plasma-derived factor VIII concentrates and recombinant products

As outlined above, purity of FVIII:C is best determined by analyzing the different contaminating proteins in the product. The more elaborate manufacturing procedures introduced during the 1980s and the virucidal methods applied also raise the question of possible protein denaturation during production which, at least theoretically, may have an impact on such *in vivo* properties as efficacy and immunogenicity. At our center, we have studied the biochemical properties of FVIII:C for many years (Berntorp and Nilsson, 1988, 1989; Nilsson and Berntorp, 1991). The results for currently available preparations are summarized in Table 17.3.

The intermediate-purity products in general have less FVIII activity per milliliter which means that a larger volume has to be infused to obtain a specific number of units – product purity is a factor of importance for therapy convenience. In most products similar values were obtained for VIII:C and factor VIII antigen (VIII:Ag), indicating that the FVIII molecule is not denatured by the manufacture and virucidal procedures. The content of vWf varies substantially from one product to another, and the monoclonal-purified and recombinant products contain virtually none at all. More importantly, almost native vWf, analyzed by multimeric sizing of the factor's molecular structure, was found in Haemate P and Beriate. Haemate P in particular has been useful in the treatment of von Willebrand's disease, as it exerts clinically significant vWf activity and may normalize the primary hemostatic defect in patients with this disease (Köhler, Hellstern and Wenzel, 1985; Berntorp and Nilsson, 1989; Mannucci *et al.*, 1992b). The other vWf-containing products listed lack the high-molecular-weight vWf multimers and do not correct the

Table 17.2 Virucidal methods used in the manufacture of factor VIII concentrates

Virucidal method	Principal manufacturers using the method	Principal product names
Heat		
Dry heating, 80°C, 72 h	BPL, SNBTS	8 Y, Z8
Heating in solution (pasteurization), 60°C, 10 h	Centeon (former Behring, Armour)	Haemate P (Humate P), Beriate P, Monoclate P
Vapor heating (60°C, 10 h, 1160 mbar)	Immuno	Kryobulin TIM3
Solvent/detergent		
TNBP and Tween 80, or Triton X-100 or cholate	Alpha, Bayer, Baxter, American Red Cross, Biotransfusion, Biotest	Profilate SD, Koate HP, Hemofil M, AHF M, factor VIII
Double inactivation		
Solvent/detergent plus dry heating, 80°C, 72 h	Novo Nordisk	Nordiate
Solvent/detergent plus dry heating, 100°C, 30 min	AIMA	Emoclot DI
Solvent/detergent plus heating in solution (63°C, 10 h)	Octapharma	Octavi SDPlus
Vapor heating (60°C, 10 h, 1160 mbar) plus polyglycate	Immuno	Immunate

Table 17.3 Biochemical properties of factor VIII concentrates (mean values for 2–7 batches)

	VIII:C	VIII:Ag (iu/ml)	vWF:Ag	Fibrinogen	Fibronectin (mg/iu VIII:C)	IgA	IgG	Specific activity (iu VIII:C/mg protein*)
Intermediate-purity								
Haemate P (Centeon)	28	32	71	0.09	0.07	0.01	0.05	5 7
Profilate SD (Alpha)	45	41	145	37	85	7.2	8.0	12.6
Kryobulin TIM3 (Immuno)	33	55	157	865	90	2.4	7.2	1.8
High-purity								
Octavi (Octapharma)	23	22	14	2.3	3.3	0.07	0.5	105
Koate HP (Bayer)	156	119	144	0.39	0.19	0.05	0.04	38
Immunate (Immuno)	85	184	74	1.5	1.03	0.05	0.1	20.9
Beriate (Centeon)	25	22	4.3	1.01	0.17	0.02	0.04	5 4
Monoclonal antibody-purified								
Octonativ-M (Pharmacia)	96	60	1.6	<0.001	<0.001	<0.001	<0.001	37
Hemofil M (Baxter)	97	58	1.2	<0.001	<0.001	0.001	0.008	11
Monoclate P (Centeon)	122	108	6.1	0.1	0.65	0.02	0.1	11
Recombinant								
Recombinate (Baxter)	50	55	<0.001	<0.001	<0.001	0.002	0.006	5.2
Kogenate (Bayer)	169	130	<0.001	<0.001	<0.001	<0.001	0.001	42

*Added carrier albumin included in figures. Albumin is added to high-purity products (except Octavi), monoclonal antibody-purified and recombinant products.
VIII:C = Factor VIII clotting activity; VIII:Ag = factor VIII antigen; vWF:Ag = von Willebrand factor antigen; IgA = immunoglobulin A; IgG = immunoglobulin G.

hemostatic defect in von Willebrand's disease as well as does Haemate P (Lethagen, Berntorp and Nilsson, 1992; Mannucci *et al.*, 1992b). The content of contaminating proteins such as fibrinogen, fibronectin, immunoglobulin A (IgA) and immunoglobulin G (IgG) is considerable in the intermediate-purity products. High-purity products contain small amounts of impurities, while these are lacking or present only in trace amounts in the monoclonal-purified and recombinant products. As specific activity figures do not correlate well with measured amounts of contaminating proteins, they are not a useful measure of product purity.

Continuous infusion of FVIII:C for several days, especially during surgery, is increasingly becoming the therapy of choice, not least because of the saving in cost. Therefore, the *in vitro* stability of FVIII products after reconstitution is a very important issue. The few studies that have been made of this issue (Weinstein, Bona and Rickles, 1991; Peerlinck, Arnout and Vermylen, 1992; Schulman, Gitel and Martinowitz, 1994) have shown VIII:C stability to vary widely from one concentrate to another, and to be dependent on temperature and the type of material (i.e. plastic or glass) used for storage vessels. Several concentrates, belonging to all the principal types of manufacturing procedure, maintain factor activities above 80% of baseline for as long as 4 weeks at 4–8°C or at 20–23°C. Thus, many commercially available FVIII concentrates may be used for continuous infusion.

In vivo properties of factor VIII concentrates

FVIII concentrates are heterogeneous preparations, and the dose of FVIII cannot be expressed simply in milligrams. Administration is based on biologic assays, of which the *in vivo* potency in patients with hemophilia is crucial. Potency of FVIII:C is estimated by *in vivo* pharmacokinetic studies and according to clinical efficacy – the hemostatic effect of the drug during joint bleeds or surgery.

PHARMACOKINETIC CONSIDERATIONS

Traditionally, the pharmacokinetic behavior of FVIII is defined in terms of *in vivo* recovery and half-life. This is not ideal, however. The estimate of *in vivo* recovery is dependent on the procedures used, i.e. on the sampling schedule, infusion time and method of blood volume estimation. Thus, *in vivo* recovery values obtained in different studies are not comparable. Ideally, therefore, comparison of different FVIII concentrates should be based on the area under the curve (AUC) obtained for FVIII activity versus time (Björkman *et al.*, 1992), which is the normal procedure for investigating bioequivalence (Gibaldi and Perrier, 1982) and obviates the need for intensive blood sampling to determine peak VIII:C activ-

ity. For comparison of different studies, clearance (CL = AUC/dose) can be used.

Most pharmacokinetic variables are vulnerable to differences in dose estimates. There are three types of assays commonly used for the measurement of VIII:C in plasma and in clotting factor concentrates: one- and two-stage clotting assays, and the chromogenic assay which may yield divergent results for VIII:C activity (Nilsson, Kirkwood and Barrowcliffe, 1979; Dawson, Kemball-Cook and Barrowcliffe, 1989; Mazurier, Parquet-Gernez and Goudemand, 1990). Consequently, the dose must be carefully defined in studies of FVIII concentrates if the true pharmacokinetic properties are to be estimated. In practice, pharmacokinetic calculations would normally be based on labeled potency, since routine administration of the concentrate to patients is based on it. None the less, assays of VIII:C in concentrates and in *ex vivo* plasma may not be directly comparable, even when compared in the same laboratory (Barrowcliffe, 1990). Assay methods of measuring VIII:C in concentrates may also differ from each other in the extent to which they are affected by concentrate purity and buffer used for dilutions (Berntorp, 1991).

The *in vivo* decline in VIII:C activity is often biphasic, with an early $t_{1/2}$ of 2–5 h and a late $t_{1/2}$ of at least 10 h (Aronson, 1979; Messori *et al.*, 1987; Rousell, Kasper and Schwartz, 1989). In conventional pharmacokinetics, the longest $t_{1/2}$ of a drug is attributed to elimination, and shorter values to distribution to extravascular compartments. The same explanation has often been given of the pharmacokinetic behavior of FVIII, despite the fact that extravascular distribution of FVIII has never been conclusively demonstrated (Aronson, 1979; Kjellman, 1984). Consequently, a two-compartment model is sometimes used to describe the pharmacokinetics of FVIII. A practical solution to this problem has been proposed, namely that the pharmacokinetics of FVIII should be described by a model-independent method (Matucci *et al.*, 1985; Longo *et al.*, 1986; Messori *et al.*, 1987). In this approach, the calculated values for pharmacokinetic variables are not dependent on the exact shape of the time/activity curve.

The best estimation of the $t_{1/2}$ of a drug is obtained by fitting a polyexponential function to the weighted concentration values (Björkman *et al.*, 1992). The exponential terms may be given as separate lines where the third line represents the terminal half-life of VIII:C. Clinically it is most important to maintain a certain minimum (trough) level of activity to prevent bleeds, especially during regular prophylaxis (Nilsson *et al.*, 1992), and for this purpose the estimated terminal half-life is one of the major variables used to describe VIII:C behavior *in vivo* and to predict trough concentrations. Clearance (CL) may be used to predict a steady-state concentration and the fluctuations around this level. *In vivo* recovery is often used clinically, and may be used as a potency variable provided the difficulties in estimating *in vivo* recovery as outlined above are borne in mind. The model-independent variables are excellent for comparison of FVIII preparations, but they are unsuitable for use in predicting the plasma activity curve of FVIII after repeated administration (Björkman *et al.*, 1992).

NORMAL VALUES OF VIII:C PHARMACOKINETIC VARIABLES IN HEMOPHILIACS

As outlined above, there are several difficulties in obtaining normal values, and comparative values between different FVIII concentrates, for pharmacokinetic variables of VIII:C. The values are also manifestly age-dependent, and those for children (in whom half-lives are generally shorter) are not well-established mainly because of technical problems in conjunction with frequent blood sampling in children. *In vivo* recovery has been found to be comparable among plasma-derived products – around 75–125% (Nilsson and Berntorp, 1991). The terminal $t_{1/2}$ mean values for various FVIII concentrates have been reported to be 10–14 h (Matucci *et al.*, 1985; Smith *et al.*, 1990, Björkman *et al.*, 1992); and there is no difference in $t_{1/2}$ between plasma-derived products and recombinant products (Bray, 1992; Growe, Poon and Scarth, 1992). It should be stressed that $t_{1/2}$ is very consistent for a given individual irrespective of the concentrate given, whereas the interindividual variation may be large (Nilsson and Berntorp, 1991). Thus, in comparing different concentrates, it is crucial to use the same patients.

In general, mean CL values ranging from 3.3 to 3.9 ml/kg per h are reported for VIII:C (Matucci *et al.*, 1985; Longo *et al.*, 1986; Messori *et al.*, 1987; Smith *et al.*, 1990), and the mean volume of distribution at steady state (V_{ss}) ranges from 0.044 to 0.058 l/kg (Messori *et al.*, 1987), even if higher values have been reported (Björkman *et al.*, 1992). Typical mean values for mean residence time (MRT) are 13–17 h (Matucci *et al.*, 1985). Some workers have reported plasma-derived products to have higher CL and V_{ss} values than recombinant products, but similar half-life values (Schwartz *et al.*, 1990; Morfini *et al.*, 1992).

Side-effects of factor VIII concentrates

The main issues to be discussed concerning side-effects of FVIII concentrates are viral transmission, the risk of inhibitor development and the impact of concentrates on the immune system.

VIRAL TRANSMISSION

There are at least 16 known viruses that can be transmitted via blood or blood products (Suomela, 1993).

However, the main blood-borne viruses transmitted by coagulation factor concentrates are HIV, hepatitis viruses A, B, C and D and B19 parvovirus. Of these, hepatitis A virus is solvent/detergent-resistant, and B19 parvovirus is both solvent/detergent- and heat-resistant. New virus transmission due to commercial FVIII concentrates virtually belongs to history, although isolated case reports of hepatitis C still appear and recently there was an epidemic of hepatitis A among hemophiliacs. There have been no reports of HIV transmission with the modern FVIII concentrates in current use. In the following, the efficacy of virucidal methods will be discussed mainly on the basis of findings in prospective clinical trials. Currently, or recently, used virucidal methods, and the respective manufacturers and product names are given in Table 17.2.

Product safety should always be evaluated in patients previously unexposed to blood or blood products (Schimpf *et al.*, 1987; Mannucci and Colombo, 1989). The statistical problem in these types of studies is illustrated by the so-called rule of three (Hanley and Lippman-Hand, 1983) which allows simple calculation of true risk. For example, if 20 patients are included in a study of hepatitis risk and no case of hepatitis is seen, the risk of virus transmission is 0–15%, expressed as a one-sided 95% confidence interval around the true risk. As the available number of previously unexposed patients is restricted, and as new virucidal methods are continuously being developed, the efficacy of several of the virucidal methods used today, which are modifications or developments of clinically documented methods, is based on *in vitro* experiments together with extrapolations of data derived from previous clinical trials of earlier products. Moreover, owing to improved donor selection and screening of blood donors, results in clinical trials are difficult to interpret concerning the efficacy of the virucidal method employed, as the risk of virus transmission should anyway be much less nowadays than it was during the early 1980s, for example.

Dry heat inactivation

During the 1980s dry heating was introduced into clotting factor concentrate manufacture, temperatures of 60–68°C being used for periods of between 24 and 72 h. However, these virus-inactivated products transmitted hepatitis at a high frequency (Colombo *et al.*, 1985; Blanchette *et al.*, 1991), and 18 cases of HIV transmissions were also documented (Mannucci, 1995). Accordingly, these dry-heating methods have been abandoned. Dry-heating at higher temperature (80°C for 72 h) is now being used by BioProducts Laboratory (BPL) and the Scottish National Blood Transfusion Service. No case of hepatitis has been recorded in conjunction with products virus-inactivated with this method (Study Group of the UK Hemophilia Centre Directors,, 1988; Skidmore *et al.*, 1990; Bennett *et al.*, 1993).

Pasteurization

Pasteurization, which has been used in the preparation of albumin products since 1948, has been used in clotting factor concentrate production for more than 10 years and has proved to be effective (Suomela, 1993). As shown in Table 17.2, pasteurization is used in the production of Beriate (Centeon) and Monoclate P (Centeon), for instance, and in the preparation of Hemate P (Centeon), which is used in hemophilia and in von Willebrand's disease in forms where plasma product therapy may be necessary. In prospective studies, the record of pasteurized products with regard to HIV and hepatitis safety is excellent. At least 153 patients have been studied with regard to hepatitis B or C transmission (Schimpf *et al.*, 1987; Mannucci *et al.*, 1990a; Kreuz *et al.*, 1992), and 210 patients with regard to HIV transmission (Schimpf *et al.*, 1987, 1989; Mannucci *et al.*, 1990a; Kreuz *et al.*, 1992), without any clinical or serologic signs of hepatitis being manifest. The risk of hepatitis after pasteurization is probably not entirely abolished, however, as there have been a few case reports of hepatitis B or C transmission in conjunction with pasteurized products (Brackmann and Egli, 1988; Schulman *et al.*, 1992; Gerritzen *et al.*, 1992b) and the method does not prevent transmission of parvovirus B 19 (Azzi *et al.*, 1992).

Vapor heating

The vapor heating procedure was developed and is used by Immuno. The method used for FVIII, called TIM 3, entails exposure to vapor at 60°C for 10 h at 1160 mbar. In prospective studies the method has proved highly effective against HIV and hepatitis with no seroconverters in a large number of patients studied ($n=81$ or 50; Mannucci *et al.*, 1988, 1990a,b, 1992a; Shapiro *et al.*, 1992). However, in one of the prospective studies evidence was found of hepatitis B infection in four of 28 previously untreated patients (Mannucci *et al.*, 1988), one being also coinfected with HCV (Mannucci *et al.*, 1990b). In a subsequent study no case of hepatitis was recorded (Mannucci *et al.*, 1992a).

The solvent/detergent procedure

Organic solvent/detergent mixtures disrupt membranes of viruses that have lipid envelopes. Since this virucidal method was first licensed by the US Food and Drug Administration in 1985, it has been extensively studied and is used in the preparation of many concentrates in current use. The method is simple, considered safe for the patient as only harmless trace amounts are left in the final product, and allows a high yield of clotting factor in the concentrate. The solvent/detergent mixture consists of an organic solvent, tri(n-butyl) phosphate (TNBP) and a detergent (sodium cholate, Tween 80 (polysorbate) or Triton X-100). Several studies have shown that solvent/detergent-treated concentrates do not transmit hepatitis B, HCV or HIV (Gazengel *et al.*, 1988; Horowitz *et al.*, 1988; Noel *et al.*, 1989; Gonzaga and Boneker, 1990; Addiego *et al.*, 1992; Di Paolantonio *et al.*, 1992; Mariani *et al.*, 1993). In these studies, 117 previously untreated patients were evaluated for hepatitis and 245 for HIV. In a review of reports published from 1988 to 1991, a total of more than 10 million units of solvent/detergent-treated concentrates were found to have been used without signs of non-A non-B hepatitis or HIV (Suomela, 1993). On the other hand, the solvent/detergent procedure does not prevent transmission of non-enveloped viruses such as parvovirus B19 (Azzi *et al.*, 1992) or hepatitis A virus, which recently appeared among 85 hemophiliacs in Europe treated exclusively with solvent/detergent-treated concentrates (Gerritzen *et al.*, 1992a; Mannucci, 1992; Temperley *et al.*, 1992; Peerlinck and Vermylen, 1993).

DOUBLE VIRUS INACTIVATION PROCEDURES

Clearly the virucidal methods discussed above have rendered FVIII concentrates much safer than they were only a few years ago, but it is also obvious that cases of hepatitis transmission still occur, as well as transmission of parvovirus B19. This has prompted several manufacturers to combine individual virucidal methods in procedures such as the combination of solvent/detergent and dry-heating at high temperatures (used by Novo Nordisk and AIMA), solvent/detergent plus pasteurization (Octapharma) or vapor heat plus polyglycate (Barrett *et al.*, 1994; Immuno). Although products treated with these combined methods have not yet been fully evaluated in clinical trials, it is known that parvovirus may still be a problem with such concentrates (Santagostino *et al.*, 1994).

Recombinant products

No virus transmission has been reported in conjunction with recombinant products, although there may be cause for concern, at least from a theoretic point of view. Human albumin is used to stabilize the product, and animal constituents, such as mammalian cells, bovine serum albumin and murine monoclonal antibodies are used in the manufacturing process.

Conclusions concerning the virus safety of FVIII concentrates

Although modern plasma-derived virus-inactivated FVIII concentrates possess a high degree of safety regarding blood-borne viruses, there have been isolated case reports of hepatitis transmission both in conjunction with heat-treated (vapor or pasteurization) and solvent/detergent-treated concentrates. Moreover, the problem of parvovirus B19 transmission has yet to be satisfactorily resolved, and this is an indication that similar and hitherto unknown viruses may escape current inactivation procedures. Studies carried out so far have not been able to single out one method as superior to another (Lusher, 1995). Although recombinant products seem to be virus-safe, none the less, inactivation procedures are included in the manufacturing process as an extra safety measure. Continuous efforts are required to improve product safety, with the goal of obtaining absolute safety.

INHIBITORS

A most serious sequela of replacement therapy in hemophilia A is the development of inhibitors to the deficient factor, a complication predominantly occurring among patients with severe hemophilia. It is difficult to compare different studies regarding inhibitor frequency, as they differ widely in design, especially in the frequency of plasma sampling. Transient inhibitors will easily be underestimated, for example in retrospective studies with infrequent inhibitor testing. Low-titer inhibitors may also be overlooked if recent treatment with FVIII has temporarily saturated the inhibitor. Studies in inhibitor patients treated with intermediate-purity products have shown that roughly two-thirds of the patients develop their inhibitor before the age of 20 years. Some hemophiliacs have developed inhibitors after 10–20 days of exposure, or even less, whereas others have not developed inhibitors until after exposure for several hundred days. Thus, there is probably no age or number of exposure days at which a hemophiliac is completely safe from developing an inhibitor (Gill, 1984; Lusher, 1987).

The frequency of inhibitor development was formerly thought to be approximately 10–20%, but in more recent prospective studies in cases of severe hemophilia the frequency has varied from 28 to 52% (Ehrenforth *et al.*, 1952; Addiego *et al.*, 1993), and in most series inhibitor development occurred after a median exposure of about 10 days. In studies using plasma-derived monoclonal antibody-purified concentrate, the proportion of previously untransfused hemophiliacs who developed inhibitors was 9–18% (Lusher *et al.*, 1990). Among patients on plasma derived concentrates, in most cases the inhibitors are of the so-called high-response type – the inhibitor manifests a strong anamnestic response upon exposure to FVIII, in contrast to the low-response type that manifests little or no anamnestic response. This response pattern is a factor of major importance to the choice of treatment.

There has been, and to some extent still is, fear that highly purified concentrates will cause a higher rate of inhibitor development. This has not been the case as far as plasma-derived concentrates are concerned even if the interpretation of results may be complicated by differences in the design of prospective and retrospective studies, e.g. differences in the frequency of blood sampling. Recombinant products are even more pure than the purest plasma products; and this, together with perhaps minor modifications of the FVIII molecule produced (as compared to that in plasma), raises the issue of whether the risk of developing inhibitors after treatment with recombinant products is higher than that after treatment with plasma-derived products. In studies using recombinant FVIII concentrates, 19–24% of previously untransfused patients with severe hemophilia have been found to develop inhibitors after a median exposure of 9 days, though the inhibitor titer was low in most cases (Lusher *et al.*, 1993; Bray *et al.*, 1994).

Thus, it does not appear that the recently developed very-high-purity products, made from plasma or with the recombinant technique, cause a higher frequency of inhibitor formation than did earlier products. Nor does it seem that the mode of virus inactivation is a determinant of the risk of inhibitor formation. However, it is important to follow the epidemiology of inhibitor development, especially when new concentrates are introduced. In a Dutch study in 1991 (Peerlinck *et al.*, 1993), an 'epidemic' of inhibitor development occurred among previously treated hemophilia patients who were switched to a newly introduced pasteurized factor concentrate. It was thought that the production process introduced neoantigens, and when the use of this concentrate was stopped, the inhibitor frequency dropped to ordinary levels.

THE IMPACT OF CONCENTRATES ON THE IMMUNE SYSTEM

In vitro findings

Many studies have shown that FVIII concentrates may cause abnormalities in *in vitro* testing of immuno-competent cell function (Watson and Ludlam, 1992). Thus, there is evidence of monocyte dysfunction (Eibl *et al.*, 1987; Pasi and Hill, 1990), inhibition of lymphocyte proliferation (Lederman *et al.*, 1986; Hay and McEvoy, 1992), inhibition of interleukin-2 (IL-2) secretion (Thorpe *et al.*, 1989) and lymphocyte IL-2 receptor expression (Hay *et al.*, 1990b). A clear correlation between product purity and inhibitory effect on immune function *in vitro* has been found in most of these studies.

In vivo findings: HIV-seronegative individuals

The situation *in vivo* is more complicated to study as many patients are infected with HCV and/or HIV. Abnormalities of immune function have been reported in treated hemophiliacs independently of HIV infection. In addition to changes similar to the *in vitro* changes described above, CD4 and CD8 cell counts may be altered. Most studies of immune changes in HIV-seronegative hemophiliacs have been done in patients exposed to FVIII concentrates of intermediate purity, and the study populations have to a large extent been chronically infected with HCV. It has therefore been discussed whether the immune changes may be attributed to viral infection, to liver disease or to the protein load provided by the concentrate. However, more recent studies with intermediate-purity virus-inactivated concentrates in boys who were seronegative for hepatitis and HIV showed no changes in CD4 and CD8 counts during treatment, beyond what was considered normal (Evans *et al.*, 1991; Funk *et al.*, 1993). Similar results were obtained in a series of 49 HIV-seronegative but HCV-seropositive patients who had been on continuous prophylaxis with low-purity or intermediate-purity concentrates for many years (Berntorp, 1994b). These studies indicate that exposure to foreign proteins contained in FVIII concentrates does not compromise the immune system, as reflected in CD4 or CD8 counts. Similar results have been obtained with monoclonal antibody-purified or recombinant products (Fukutake *et al.*, 1990; Mannucci *et al.*, 1994).

In vivo findings: HIV-seropositive individuals

The impact of factor purity upon the preservation of immune function is still debated, and reports of immuno-modulation have caused great concern with regard to progression of HIV infection in hemophiliacs. With the advent of concentrates of very high purity, especially monoclonal antibody purified and recombinant products, it has been claimed that these are more inert *vis-à-vis* the immune system than are less pure products. Two prospective randomized studies in HIV-infected hemophiliacs of monoclonal-purified products in comparison with intermediate-purity products (de Biasi *et al.*, 1991; Seremetis *et al.*, 1993) suggest that there is less rapid deterioration of CD4 cells in the groups treated with the more pure products, but the groups studied were small and the duration of follow-up limited. Further studies are needed to settle this issue, though such studies are difficult to perform as more and more patients are being switched to monoclonal-purified and recombinant products. In addition, many HIV-infected hemophiliacs are now treated with immunomodulating drugs, which further complicates the evaluation of study groups. In another controlled but retrospective study, using the rate of CD4 decline as the clinical end-point, a beneficial effect of monoclonal antibody-purified concentrate was seen (Hilgartner *et al.*, 1993).

The most important issue is not whether concentrate purity has an impact on the immune system variables measured, but rather whether progression to acquired immunodeficiency syndrome (AIDS) is interfered with. In none of the studies cited above was any difference in clinical end-points seen. In several other large clinical studies of the development of AIDS in hemophiliacs treated mainly with intermediate-purity concentrates, no difference in the risk of AIDS was found between hemophiliacs and other risk groups (Giesecke *et al.*, 1988; Goedert *et al.*, 1989; Jason *et al.*, 1989; Lee *et al.*, 1989).

To sum up, there is good evidence that intermediate-purity concentrates have an impact on immune system variables, especially *in vitro*, and some studies indicate a beneficial effect of monoclonal-purified concentrates in HIV-infected individuals as far as CD4 counts are concerned. However, and most importantly, there is no evidence that concentrate purity is a factor of importance to the rate of progression to AIDS.

Choice of FVIII concentrate

In many countries a variety of FVIII concentrates are now available, both plasma-derived and recombinant products. They differ in the type of virus inactivation used and in purity. In the choice of concentrate, the most important criterion is viral safety (Lusher, 1995). Other aspects to consider are efficacy, availability, purity, cost and convenience in handling. The safety of plasma-derived products treated with currently available virucidal methods is high regarding the risk of HIV and hepatitis B and C transmission, but they may still transmit other blood-borne viruses such as human parvovirus B19. Some workers therefore recommend recombinant FVIII where economy permits (Lusher, 1995).

Another safety aspect is the risk of inhibitor development and there is no available evidence to suggest any clear difference in the risk of inhibitor development between the products. This is still an area of some controversy, and results from current and future studies are awaited.

As discussed earlier, the various products seem to be very similar in efficacy, and this is no longer an issue in the choice of product. Purity is sometimes asserted to be of clinical importance and the use of immunoaffinity-purified and recombinant FVIII has been recommended in HIV-seropositive hemophiliacs (Lusher, 1995).

As the available products are comparable in quality, cost is an important issue in the choice of product. In some countries the unit price of monoclonal-purified products is two to three times that of the intermediate-purity concentrates, and the recombinant products are roughly 50% more expensive than the monoclonal antibody-purified products (Seremetis, 1995). Even small price differences may have a major impact on the total annual treatment cost per patient. In Sweden, for instance, where continuous high-dosage prophylaxis is used, the annual cost for a single patient requiring a total of 200 000 iu can be cut by more than US$50 000 by switching from one product to another (Berntorp, 1994a).

Product convenience will be a factor attracting increasing attention among patients, health care personnel and manufacturers, as this is one area where much remains to be done. In particular, the mode of administration needs to be improved, but other aspects to consider are reconstitution volume and solubility. Most products are similar in reconstitution volume (10 ml/1000 iu), but there are exceptions where the volume is considerably larger. Modern concentrates easily dissolve when reconstituted, though there are exceptions; and this is another aspect to be borne in mind when developing products.

To sum up, there are no conclusive quality differences between modem FVIII products. Price, local traditions and availability will ultimately decide the choice of concentrate.

Porcine factor VIII

Porcine and bovine FVIII preparations were used in the 1950s and 1960s, primarily in the UK, but were largely abandoned because of the high incidence of serious side-effects (Kernoff, 1984). Recently there has been renewed interest in polyelectrolyte fractionated porcine FVIII concentrates (Hyate:C, Porton Speywood Ltd, Wrexham, UK) for the treatment of FVIII inhibitors. Using cryoprecipitate as the starting material, prothrombin complex factors are adsorbed to alumina and VIII:C to polyelectrolyte. After extensive washing, VIII:C is eluted from the column using 1 mol/l sodium chloride, concentrated by polyethylene glycol precipitation and freeze-dried (Middleton, 1982). Successful treatment of patients with acquired hemophilia as well as of alloimmunized hemophilia A patients has been reported. The product is characterized by viral safety, a low level of cross-reactivity and the ease of monitoring plasma VIII:C activity which correlates with clinical efficacy (Kernoff, 1984; Lusher, 1987; Kessler and Ludlam, 1993; Lozier et al., 1993). Other treatment options in inhibitor patients, such as the bypassing agents, recombinant FVIIa and activated or non-activated prothrombin complex concentrates, have the disadvantage that there is no available test of their efficacy.

Porcine FVIII concentrates have not been shown to transmit HIV or human hepatitis viruses (Hay and Bolton-Maggs, 1991), nor do they transmit porcine virus pathogenic to humans. There are some other side-effects, however, including urticaria, low-grade fever and other allergic manifestations as well as postinfusion thrombocytopenia (Gringeri et al., 1991).

If the human FVIII inhibitor titer is high, cross-reactivity with porcine FVIII often occurs and the concentrate will not be effective. The effect may be predicted by measuring the inhibitor porcine FVIII titer (Kernoff, 1984; Lozier et al., 1993). In some cases there is an anamnestic response to porcine FVIII, and in approximately 25% of cases an anamnestic antihuman VIII:C antibody response is seen (Hay et al., 1990a; Hay and Bolton-Maggs, 1991). In acquired hemophilia, an anamnestic response is unusual (Hay and Bolton-Maggs, 1991). The efficacy of porcine FVIII in selected hemophiliacs with inhibitors as well as in acquired hemophilia is well established (Gatti and Mannucci, 1984; Kernoff, 1984; Brettler et al., 1989; Hay and Bolton-Maggs, 1991; Kessler and Ludlam, 1993; Lozier et al., 1993). In acquired hemophilia, some workers recommend that porcine FVIII should be considered as initial rather than alternative or last-resort therapy (Kessler and Ludlam, 1993), whereas in congenital hemophilia complicated with inhibitors immune tolerance should be considered as soon as possible after detection of the inhibitor (Lusher, 1995). In cases of failure to induce immune tolerance, or in a patient with inhibitors at high titer, porcine FVIII is one of several options, the selection of which has to be decided from case to case.

References

Addiego, J.E., Gomperts, E., Shu-Leu Liu et al. (1992) Treatment of hemophilia A with a highly purified factor VIII concentrate prepared by anti-FVIIIC immunoaffinity chromatography. *Thromb Haemostas*, 67, 19–27.

Addiego, J., Kasper, C., Abildgaard, C. et al. (1993) Frequency of inhibitor development in haemophiliacs treated with low purity factor VIII. *Lancet*, 342, 462–4.

Allain, J.-P. (1979) Dose requirement for replacement therapy in hemophilia A. *Thromb Haemostas*, 42, 825–831.

Aronson, D.L. (1979) Factor VIII (antihaemophilic globulin). *Semin Thromb Haemostas*, 6, 12–27.

Azzi, A., Ciappi, S., Zakvrezeska, K. et al. (1992) Human parvovirus B19 infection in hemophiliacs first infused with two high-purity virally attenuated factor VIII concentrates. *Am J Hematol*, 39, 228–230.

Barrett, N., Pölsler, G., Eibl, J. and Dorner, F. (1994) Inactivation and partitioning of HIV-1 and model viruses during the manufacture of Immunine and Immunate. *Ann Hematol*, 68 (suppl. 2), abstract 105.

Barrowcliffe, T.W. (1990) Standardization of assays of factor VIII and factor IX. *Res Clin Lab*, 20, 155–165.

Bennett, E. and Dommandy, K. (1966) Pool's cryoprecipitate and exhausted plasma in the treatment of von Willebrand's disease and factor XI-deficiency. *Lancet*, ii, 731.

Bennett, B., Dawson, A.A., Gibson, B.S. et al. (1993) Study of viral safety of Scottish National Blood Transfusion Service factor VIII/IX concentrate. *Transfusion Med*, 3, 295–298.

Berntorp, E. (1991) Kinetic aspects of ultra-pure concentrates, in *Factor VIII: Purity and Prophylaxis* (ed. C. Wood), Royal Society of Medicine Services, London, pp. 51–56.

Berntorp, E. (1994a) Which concentrate to choose in prophylaxis?, in *Prophylactic Treatment of Hemophilia A and B: Current and Future Perspectives*, Malmö, Sweden. Science of Medicine, New York, pp. 93–96.

Berntorp, E. (1994b) Impact of replacement therapy on the evolution of HIV infection in hemophiliacs. *Thromb Haemostas*, 71, 678–683.

Berntorp, E. and Nilsson I.M. (1988) Biochemical and *in vivo* properties of commercial virus-inactivated factor VIII concentrates. *Eur J Haematol*, 40, 205–214.

Berntorp, E. and Nilsson IM. (1989) Use of high-purity factor VIII concentrate (Hemate P) in von Willebrand's disease. *Vox Sang*, 56, 212–217.

Bidwell, E. (1955) The purification of bovine antihaemophilic globulin from animal plasma. *Br J Haematol*, 1, 386–387.

Biggs, R. and Macfarlane, R.G. (eds) (1966) *Treatment of Haemophilia and Other Coagulation Disorders*, Blackwell, Oxford.

Björkman, S., Carlsson, M., Berntorp, E. and Stenberg, P. (1992) Pharmacokinetics of factor VIII in humans. Obtaining clinically relevant data from comparative studies. *Clin Pharmacokinet*, **22**, 385–395.

Blanchette, V.S., Vorstman, E., Shore, A. *et al.* (1991) Hepatitis C infection in children with hemophilia A and B. *Blood*, **78**, 285–289.

Blombäck, B. and Blombäck M. (1956) Purification of human and bovine fibrinogen. *Arkiv Kemi*, **10**, 415–443.

Boedeker, B.G.D. (1992) The manufacturing of the recombinant factor VIII, Kogenate. *Transfus Med Rev*, **6**, 256–260.

Brackmann, H.H. and Egli, H. (1988) Acute hepatitis B infection after treatment with heat-inactivated factor VIII concentrate. *Lancet*, **ii**, 967.

Bray, G.L. (1992) Current status of clinical studies of recombinant factor VIII (Recombinate) in patients with hemophilia A. *Transfus Med Rev*, **6**, 252–255.

Bray, G.L., Gomperts, E.D., Courter, S. *et al.* (1994) A multicenter study of recombinant factor VIII (Recombinate): safety, efficacy and inhibitor risk in previously untreated patients with hemophilia A. *Blood*, **83**, 2428–2435.

Brettler, D.B., Fordberg, A., Levine, P.H. *et al.* (1989) The use of porcine factor VIII concentrate (Hyate C) in the treatment of patients with inhibitor antibodies to factor VIIIC: a multicenter US trial. *Arch Intern Med*, **149**, 1381–1385.

Chan, S.Y. and Lembach, K.J. (1991) Genetic characterization of recombinant BHK-21 cells expressing factor VIII. *Semin. Hematol*, **28** (suppl.), 10–16.

Colombo, M., Mannucci, P.M., Carnelli, V. *et al.* (1985) Non-A, non-B hepatitis by heat-treated factor VIII concentrates. *Lancet*, **ii**, 1–6.

Dawson, N.J., Kemball-Cook, G. and Barrowcliffe, T.W. (1989) Assay discrepancies with highly purified factor VIII concentrates. *Haemostasis*, **19**, 131–137.

de Biasi, R., Rocino, A., Miraglia, E. *et al.* (1991) The impact of a very high purity factor VIII concentrate on the immune system of human immunodeficiency virus-infected hemophiliacs: a randomized, prospective, two-year comparison with an intermediate purity concentrate. *Blood*, **78**, 1919–1922.

Di Paolantonio, T., Mariani, G., Ghiradini, A. *et al.* (1992) Low risk of transmission of the human immunodeficiency virus by a solvent-detergent-treated commercial factor VIII concentrate. *J Med Virol*, **36**, 71–74.

Ehrenforth, S., Kreutz, W., Scharrer, I. *et al.* (1992) Incidence of development of factor VIII and factor IX inhibitors in hemophiliacs. *Lancet*, **339**, 594–598.

Eibl, M.M., Ahmad, R., Wolf, H.M. *et al.* (1987) A component of factor VIII preparations which can be separated from factor VIII activity downmodulates human monocyte functions. *Blood*, **69**, 1153–1160.

Evans, J.A., Pasi, K.J., Williams, M.D. and Hill, F.G.H. (1991) Consistently normal CD4+, CD8+ levels in haemophilic boys only treated with a virally safe factor VIII concentrate (BPL 8Y). *Br J Haematol*, **79**, 457–461.

Fukutake, K., Hada, M., Ikematsu, S. *et al.* (1990) Multicenter study on the influence of long-term continuous use of ultrapurified factor VIII preparation on the immunological status of HIV infected and non-infected hemophilia A patients. *XIX International Congress of the World Federation of Hemophilia. Washington DC*, abstract no. 124.

Funk, M., Ebener, U., Kreuz, W. and Ehrenforth, S. (1993) Immune status of HIV and HCV negative haemophiliacs treated with intermediate-purity factor VIII concentrates. *Lancet*, **312**, 933–934.

Gatti, L. and Mannucci, P.M. (1984) Use of porcine factor VIII in the management of seventeen patients with factor VIII antibodies. *Thromb Haemostas*, **51**, 379–384.

Gazengel, C., Torcher, M.F. and the French Hemophilia Study Group (1988) Viral safety of solvent/detergent treated FVIII concentrate. Results of a French multicenter study. *XVIII International Congress of the World Federation of Hemophilia, Madrid, May 26–31*, Abstract book, p. 59.

Gerritzen, A., Schneweis, K.E., Brackmann, H.H. *et al.* (1992a) Acute hepatitis A in hemophiliacs. *Lancet*, **340**, 1231–1232.

Gerritzen, A., Schneweis, K.E., Scholt, B. *et al.* (1992b) Acute hepatitis C in hemophiliacs due to virus-inactivated clotting factor concentrates. *Thromb Haemost*, **68**, 781.

Gibaldi, M. and Perrier, D. (1982) *Pharmacokinetics*, 2nd edn, Marcel Dekker, New York.

Giesecke, J., Scalia-Tomba, G., Berglund, O. *et al.* (1988) Incidence of symptoms and AIDS in 146 Swedish haemophiliacs and blood transfusion recipients infected with human immunodeficiency virus. *Br Med J*, **297**, 99–102.

Giles, A.R. and Tinlin, S. (1988) *In vivo* characterization of recombinant factor VIII in a canine model of hemophilia A (factor VIII deficiency). *Blood*, **72**, 335–339.

Gill, E.M. (1984) The natural history of factor VIII inhibitors in patients with hemophilia A. *Prog Clin Biol Res*, **150**, 19–29.

Goedert, J.J., Kessler, C.M., Aledort, L.M. *et al.* (1989) A prospective study of human immunodeficiency virus type 1 infection and the development of AIDS in subjects with hemophilia. *N Engl J Med*, **321**, 1141–1148.

Gomperts, E., Lundblad, R., Adamson, R. *et al.* (1992) The manufacturing process of recombinant factor VIII, Recombinate. *Transfus Med Rev*, **6**, 247–251.

Gonzaga, A.L. and Bonecker, C. (1990) Follow-up of hemophiliacs using solvent/detergent treated FVIII and FIX concentrates. *XIX International Congress of the World Federation of Hemophilia, Washington, August 14–19*, Abstract book, p. 25.

Gringeri, A., Santagostino, E., Tradati, F. *et al.* (1991) Adverse effects of treatment with porcine factor VIII. *Thromb Haemostas*, **65**, 245–247.

Growe, G.H., Poon, M.-C. and Scarth, I. (1992) International symposium on recombinant factor VIII: report of the proceedings. *Transfus Med Rev*, **6**, 137–145.

Hanley, J.A. and Lippman-Hand, A. (1983) If nothing goes wrong, is everything all right? *JAMA*, **249**, 1743–1745.

Hay, C.R.M. and Bolton-Maggs, P. (1991) Porcine factor VIIIC in the management of patients with factor VIII inhibitors. *Transfus Med Rev*, **5**, 145–151.

Hay, C.R.M. and McEvoy, P. (1992) Purity of factor VIII concentrates. *Lancet*, **339**, 1613.

Hay, C.R.M., Laurian, Y., Verroust, F. *et al.* (1990a) Induction of immune-tolerance in patients with haemophilia A and inhibitors treated with porcine VIIIC by home therapy. *Blood*, **76**, 882–886.

Hay, C.R.M., McEvoy, P. and Duggan-Keen, M. (1990b) Inhibition of lymphocyte IL2-receptor expression by factor VIII concentrate: a possible cause of immunosuppression in haemophiliacs. *Br J Haematol*, **75**, 278–281.

Hilgartner, M.W., Buckley, J.D., Operskalski, E.A. *et al.* (1993) Purity of factor VIII concentrates and serial CD4 counts. *Lancet*, **341**, 1373–1374.

Horowitz, M.S., Rooks, C., Horowitz, B. and Hilgartner, M. (1988) Virus safety of solvent-detergent treated antihemophilic factor concentrate. *Lancet*, **ii**, 186–189.

Jason, J., Lui, K.-J., Ragni, M.V. *et al.* (1989) Risk of developing AIDS in HIV-infected cohorts of hemophilic and homosexual men. *JAMA*, **261**, 725–727.

Kasper, C.K., Lusher, J.M. and the Transfusion Practices Committee, AABB (1993) Recent evolution of clotting factor concentrates for hemophilia A and B. *Transfusion*, **33**, 422–434.

Kaufman, R.J. (1992) Expression and structure–function properties of recombinant human factor VIII. *Transfus Med Rev*, **6**, 235–246.

Kaufman, R.J., Wasley, L.C. and Dorner, A.J. (1988) Synthesis, processing, and secretion of recombinant human factor VIII expressed in mammalian cells. *J Biol Chem*, **263**, 6352–6362

Kernoff, P.B.A. (1984) Porcine factor VIII: preparation and use in treatment of inhibitor patients. *Prog Clin Biol Res*, **150**, 207–224.

Kessler, C.M. and Ludlam, C.A. for the International Acquired Hemophilia Study Group (1993) The treatment of acquired factor VIII inhibitors: worldwide experience with porcine factor VIII concentrate. *Semin Hematol*, **30**, 22–27.

Kjellman, H. (1984) Calculations of factor VIII *in vivo* recovery and half-life. *Scand J Haematol*, **33** (suppl. 40), 165–174.

Klein, U. (1991) Production and characterization of recombinant factor VIII. *Semin. Hematol*, **28** (suppl. 1), 17–21.

Köhler, M., Hellstem, P. and Wenzel, E. (1985) The use of heat-treated factor VIII-concentrates in von Willebrand's disease. *Blut*, **50**, 25–27.

Kreuz, W., Auerswald, G., Bruckmann, C. *et al.* (1992) Prevention of hepatitis C virus infection in children with hemophilia A and B and von Willebrand's disease. *Thromb Haemostas*, **67**, 184.

Lederman, M.M., Saunders, C., Toosi, Z. *et al.* (1986) Anti haemophilic factor (factor VIII) preparations inhibit lymphocyte proliferation and production of interleukin-2. *J Lab Clin Med*, **107**, 471–478.

Lee, C.A., Phillips, A.N., Elford, J. *et al.* (1989) The natural history of human immunodeficiency virus infection in a haemophilic cohort. *Br J Haematol*, **73**, 228–234.

Lethagen, S., Berntorp, E. and Nilsson, I.M. (1992) Pharmacokinetics and hemostatic effect of different factor VIII/von Willebrand factor concentrates in von Willebrand's disease type III. *Ann Hematol*, **65**, 253–259.

Longo, G., Matucci, M., Messori, A. *et al.* (1986) Pharmacokinetics of a new heat-treated concentrate of factor VIII estimated by model-independent methods. *Thromb Res*, **41**, 471–476.

Lozier, J.N., Santagostino, E., Kasper, C.K. *et al.* (1993) Use of porcine factor VIII for surgical procedures in hemophilia A patients with inhibitors. *Semin Hematol*, **30**, 10–21.

Lusher, J.M. (1987) Factor VIII inhibitors. Etiology, characterization, natural history, and management. *Ann NY Acad Sci*, **509**, 89–192.

Lusher, J.M. (1995) Considerations for current and future management of haemophilia and its complications. *Haemophilia*, **1**, 2–10.

Lusher, J.M., Salzman, P.M. and the Monoclate Study Group (1990) Viral safety and inhibitor development associated with factor VIII ultra-purified from plasma in hemophiliacs previously unexposed to factor VIIIC concentrates. *Semin Hematol*, **27** (suppl. 2), 1–7.

Lusher, J.M., Arkins, S., Aildgaard, C.F. *et al.* (1993) Recombinant factor VIII for the treatment of previously untreated patients with hemophilia. *N Engl J Med*, **328**, 453–459.

Mannucci, P.M. (1992) Outbreak of hepatitis A among Italian patients with hemophilia. *Lancet*, **i**, 819.

Mannucci, P.M. (1993) Clinical evaluation of viral safety of coagulation factor VIII and IX concentrates. *Vox Sang*, **64**, 197–203.

Mannucci, P.M. (1995) Viral safety of plasma-derived and recombinant products used in the management of haemophilia A and B. *Haemophilia*, **1** (suppl. 1), 14–20.

Mannucci, P.M. and Colombo, M. (1989) Revision of the protocol recommended for studies of safety from hepatitis of clotting factor concentrates. *Thromb Haemostas*, **62**, 532–534.

Mannucci, P.M., Zanetti, A.R. and Colombo, M. (1988) Prospective study of hepatitis after factor VIII concentrate exposed to hot vapour. *Br J Haematol,* **68,** 427–430.

Mannucci, P.M., Schimpf, K., Brettler, D.B. *et al.* (1990a) Low risk for hepatitis in hemophiliacs given a high-purity, pasteurized factor VIII concentrate. *Ann Intern Med,* **113,** 27–32.

Mannucci, P.M., Zanetti, A.R., Colombo, M. *et al.* (1990b) Antibody to hepatitis C virus after a vapour-heated factor VIII concentrate. *Thromb Haemostas,* **64,** 232–234

Mannucci, P.M., Schimpf, K., Abe, T. *et al.* (1992a) Low risk of viral infection after administration of vapour heated factor VIII concentrates. *Transfusion,* **32,** 134–138.

Mannucci, P.M., Tenconi, P.M., Castaman, G. and Rodeghiero, F. (1992b) Comparison of four virus-inactivated plasma concentrates for treatment of severe von Willebrand disease: a cross-over randomized trial. *Blood,* **79,** 3130–3137.

Mannucci, P.M., Brettler, D.B., Aledort, L.M. *et al.* (1994) Immune status of human immunodeficiency virus seropositive and seronegative hemophiliacs infused for 3–5 years with recombinant factor VIII. *Blood,* **83,** 1958–1962.

Mariani, G., Di Paolantonio, T, Baklaya, R. *et al.* (1993) Prospective study of the evaluation of hepatitis C virus infectivity in a high purity, solvent/detergent-treated factor VIII concentrate: parallel evaluation of other markers for lipid-enveloped and non-lipid enveloped virus. *Transfusion,* **33,** 814–818.

Matucci, M., Messori, A., Donati-Cori, G. *et al.,* (1985) Kinetic evaluation of four factor VIII concentrates by model-independent methods. *Scand J Haematol,* **34,** 22–28.

Mazurier, C., Parquet-Gemez, A. and Goudemand, M. (1990) Validation of a procedure for potency assessing of a high purity factor VIII concentrate – comparison of different factor VIII coagulation assays and effect of prediluent. *Thromb Haemostas,* **64,** 251–255.

Messori, A., Longo, G., Matucci, M. *et al.* (1987) Clinical pharmacokinetics of factor VIII in patients with classic haemophilia. *Clin Pharmacokin,* **13,** 365–380.

Middleton, S. (1982) Polyelectrolytes and preparation of factor VIIIC, in *Unresolved Problems in Haemophilia* (eds C.D. Forbes and G.D.O. Lowe), MTP Press, Lancaster, UK, pp. 109–120.

Morfini, M., Longo, G., Messori, A. *et al.* (1992) Pharmacokinetic properties of recombinant factor VIII compared with a monoclonally purified concentrate (Hemofil M). *Thromb Haemostas,* **68,** 433–435.

Nilsson, I.M. (1974) *Haemorrhagic and Thrombotic Diseases,* John Wiley, London.

Nilsson, I.M. and Berntorp, E. (1991) Clinical efficacy of clotting factor concentrates: survival, recovery and hemostatic capacity, in *Coagulation and Blood Transfusion* (eds C.Th. Smith Sibinga, P.C. Das and P.M. Mannucci), Kluwer Academic Publishers, Dordrecht, pp. 193–206.

Nilsson, I.M., Kirkwood, T.B.L. and Barrowcliffe, T.W. (1979) *In vivo* recovery of factor VIII: a comparison of one-stage and two-stage assay methods. *Thromb Haemostas,* **42,** 1230–1239.

Nilsson, I.M., Berntorp, E., Löfqvist, T. and Pettersson, H. (1992) Twenty-five years' experience of prophylactic treatment in severe hemophilia A and B. *J Intern Med,* **232,** 25–32.

Noel, L., Guerois, C., Maisonneuve, P. *et al.* (1989) Antibodies to hepatitis C virus in hemophilia. *Lancet,* **ii,** 560.

Pasi, K.J. and Hill, F.G.H. (1990) *In vitro* and *in vivo* inhibition of monocyte phagocytic function by factor VIII concentrates: correlation with concentrate purity. *Br J Haematol,* **76,** 88–93.

Peerlinck, K. and Vermylen, J. (1993) Acute hepatitis A in patients with hemophilia A. *Lancet,* **341,** 189.

Peerlinck, K., Arnout, J. and Vermylen, J. (1992) Factor VIII solutions in pre-filled syringes. *Lancet,* **ii,** 303–304

Peerlinck, K., Arnout, J., Gilles, J.G. *et al.* (1993) A higher than expected incidence of factor VIII inhibitors in multitransfused hemophilia A patients treated with intermediate purity pasteurized factor VIII concentrate. *Thromb Haemostas,* **69,** 115–118.

Pool, J.G. and Robinson J. (1959) Observations on plasma banking and transfusion procedures for haemophilic patients using a quantitative assay for antihemophilic globulin (AHG). *Br J Haematol,* **5,** 24–30.

Pool, J.G. and Shannon, A.E. (1965) Production of high-potency concentrates of antihaemophilic globulin in a closed-bag system. *N Engl J Med,* **273,** 1443–1447.

Pool, J.G., Hershgold, E.J. and Pappenhagen, A.R. (1964) High potency antihemophilic factor concentrate prepared from cryoglobulin precipitate. *Nature,* **203,** 312.

Rickard, K.A. (1995). Guidelines for therapy and optimal dosages of coagulation factors for treatment of bleeding and surgery in haemophilia. *Haemophilia,* **1** (suppl. 1), 8–13.

Rizza, C.R. (1972) The management of patients with coagulation factor deficiencies, in *Human Blood Coagulation, Haemostasis and Thrombosis* (ed. R. Biggs), Blackwell Scientific Publications, Oxford, pp. 336–360.

Rousell, R.H., Kasper, C.K. and Schwartz, R.S. (1989) The pharmacology of a new pasteurized antihemophilic factor concentrate derived from human plasma. *Transfusion,* **29,** 208–212.

Santagostino, E., Mannucci, P.M., Gringeri, A. *et al.* (1994) Eliminating parvovirus B19 from blood products. *Lancet,* **343,** 798.

Schimpf, K., Mannucci, P., Kreutz, W. *et al.* (1987) Absence of hepatitis after treatment with a pasteurized factor VIII concentrate in patients with hemophilia and no previous transfusions. *N Engl J Med,* **316,** 918–922.

Schulman, S., Gitel, S. and Martinowitz, U. (1994) Stability of factor VIII concentrates after reconstitution. *Am J Hematol,* **45,** 217–223.

Schimpf, K., Brackmann, H.H., Kreuz, W. *et al.* (1989) Absence of anti-human immunodeficiency virus types 1 and 2 seroconversion after the treatment of hemophilia A and B or von Willebrand's disease with pasteurized factor VIII concentrate. *N Engl J Med,* **321,** 1148–1152.

Schulman, S., Lindgren, A. Ch., Petrini, P. and Allander, T. (1992) Transmission of hepatitis C with pasteurized factor VIII. *Lancet,* **ii,** 305–306.

Schwartz, R.S. Abildgaard, C.F., Aledort, L.M. *et al.* (1990) Human recombinant DNA-derived antihemophilic factor (factor VIII) in the treatment of hemophilia A. *N Engl J Med,* **323,** 1806–1805

Seremetis, S.V. (1995) Modern treatment of haemophilia: choice of products for the treatment of haemophilia A and B. *Haemophilia,* **1,** 21–25.

Seremetis, S.V., Aledort, L.M., Bergman, G.E. *et al.* (1993) Three-year randomised study of high-purity or intermediate-purity factor VIII concentrates in symptom-free HIV-seropositive hemophiliacs: effects on immune status. *Lancet,* **342,** 700–703.

Shapiro, A. and the International Factor Safety Study Group (1992) A study to determine the safety of virus inactivated factor concentrates in hemophiliacs naive to blood product administration: factor VIII concentrate (human) Immuno, vapour heated and factor IX complex (human) Immuno, vapour heated. *XX International Congress of the World Federation of Hemophilia,* Athens, October 12–17. Abstract book, p. 25.

Skidmore, S.J., Pasi, K.J., Mawson, S.J. *et al.* (1990) Serological evidence that dry heating of clotting factor concentrates prevents transmission of non-A, non-B hepatitis. *J Med Virol,* **30,** 50–52.

Smith, K.J., Lusher, J.M., Cohen, A.R. and Salzman, P. (1990) Initial clinical experience with a new pasteurized monoclonal antibody purified factor VIII:C. *Semin Hematol,* **27** (suppl. 2), 25–29.

Study Group of the UK Haemophilia Centre Directors (1988) Effect of dry-heating of coagulation factor concentrates at 80°C for 72 hours on transmission of non-A, non-B hepatitis. *Lancet,* **ii,** 814–816.

Suomela, H. (1993) Inactivation of viruses in blood and plasma products. *Transfus Med Rev,* **7,** 42–57.

Temperley, I.J., Cotter, K.P., Walsh, T.J. *et al.* (1992) Clotting factors and hepatitis A. *Lancet,* **340,** 1466.

Thorpe, R., Dilger, P., Dawson, N.J. and Barrowcliffe, T.W. (1989) Inhibition of interleukin-2 secretion by factor VIII concentrates: a possible cause of immunosuppression in haemophiliacs. *Br J Haematol,* **71,** 387–391.

Watson, H.G. and Ludlam, C.A. (1992) Immunological abnormalities in haemophiliacs. *Blood Rev,* **6,** 26–33.

Watson, H.G., Ludlam, C.A., Rebus, S. *et al.* (1992) Use of several second-generation serological assays to determine the true prevalence of hepatitis C virus infection in haemophiliacs treated with non-virus inactivated factor VIII and IX concentrates. *Br J Haematol,* **80,** 514–518.

Weinstein, R.E., Bona, R.D. and Rickles, F.R. (1991) Continuous infusion of monoclonal antibody-purified factor VIII. *Am J Hematol,* **36,** 211–212.

Wise, R.J., Dorner, A.J., Krane, M. *et al.* (1991) The role of von Willebrand factor multimers and propeptide cleavage in binding and stabilization of factor VIII. *J Biol Chem,* **266,** 21948–21955.

18 DESMOPRESSIN (DDAVP)

S. Lethagen

For many years replacement therapy with blood products was the only treatment available for patients with bleeding disorders. Factor VIII (FVIII) concentrates have been used for patients with hemophilia A and von Willebrand's disease (vWD) and platelet concentrates for patients with platelet disorders. Several problems are associated with the use of blood products. They carry a risk of transmitting viral disease such as hepatitis B and C and acquired immunodeficiency syndrome (AIDS). The high cost of blood factor concentrates and the shortage of plasma-derived blood factor concentrates limits the treatment of patients with hemophilia and vWD, especially in the Third World.

The first reports in the mid-1970s that the synthetic vasopressin analog desmopressin acetate (1-desamino-8-D-arginine vasopressin: DDAVP) increased the plasma concentrations of FVIII and von Willebrand factor (vWF) stimulated the development of desmopressin as a therapeutic alternative to blood factor concentrates in mild cases of hemophilia A or vWD. The effect is immediate, with two to sixfold increases in the plasma concentrations of coagulation FVIII, vWF and tissue plasminogen activator (t-PA), and increases in platelet adhesiveness of comparable magnitude. Desmopressin is today a widely used hemostatic agent. Desmopressin is used not only in patients with mild hemophilia A or vWD, but also in those with congenital platelet dysfunction or acquired platelet dysfunction due to uremia or intake of drugs such as aspirin. It is an important alternative to blood products as it carries no risk of transmitting blood-borne diseases. It may also be used to reduce surgical blood loss in patients without known bleeding diathesis. Optimal hemostatic effect is achieved with a dosage of 0.3 µg/kg given intravenously. Delivered by intranasal spray, it is efficient for the home treatment of patients with bleeding disorders.

Recognition of the efficacy of desmopressin

Desmopressin was first synthesized as an analog of the native hormone vasopressin (Zaoral, Kolc and Sorm, 1967). The chemical structure, 1-desamino-8-D-arginine vasopressin, was derived by deamination of hemicystein at position 1 of the natural hormone, and substitution of D-arginine for L-arginine at position 8, resulting both in greater potency and more prolonged duration of the antidiuretic effect, and markedly decreased pressor activity. Thus, desmopressin has virtually no vasoconstrictive effect, and does not contract the uterus or the gastrointestinal tract. The main sites of metabolic inactivation are the liver and kidney (Walter, 1976). Being more resistant to enzymatic degradation, desmopressin is metabolized slower than vasopressin (Shimizu *et al.*, 1980). Desmopressin has mainly been used for its antidiuretic properties, e.g. in the treatment of diabetes insipidus and enuresis.

Desmopressin's hemostatic properties were discovered after a systematic search for hemostatically active pharmacologic agents. Other substances known to affect hemostatic factors are epinephrine (Ingram, 1961; Egeberg, 1963), vasopressin and its synthetic analog 8-lysine vasopressin, as well as different sympathomimetic amines, all of which affect vascular motility (Schneck and von Kaulla, 1961; Mannucci, Gagnatelli and D'Alonzo, 1972).

The plasma concentration of coagulation FVIII is also increased by physical exercise.

In the mid-1970s, two independent research groups (Cash, Gader and Da Costa, 1974; Mannucci *et al.*, 1975) found infusion of desmopressin to increase the plasma concentrations of FVIII coagulation activity (VIII:C), and t-PA in normal volunteers. Desmopressin-induced increases in VIII:C, vWF antigen (vWF:Ag) and

Hemophilia. Edited by C.D. Forbes, L. Aledort and R. Madhok. Published in 1997 by Chapman & Hall, London. ISBN 0 412 63820 7

ristocetin cofactor (Rcof) after desmopressin infusion were subsequently found to be dose-dependent (Aberg, Nilsson and Vilhardt, 1979), and desmopressin was shown to exert similar effects in patients with mild hemophilia A or von Willebrand's disease (vWD) (Mannucci et al., 1977; Kobayashi, 1979; Nilsson et al., 1980, 1982). Under cover of desmopressin, surgical procedures could be performed safely in patients with hemophilia A or vWD without the administration of blood products, which showed endogenously released FVIII and vWF to be functionally active in hemostasis (Mannucci et al., 1977a, 1977b). As the use of blood products is accompanied by a risk of viral transmission, desmopressin therapy is currently regarded as the treatment of choice in most patients with vWD type I and in selected patients with mild hemophilia A. Desmopressin has also been shown to reduce bleeding time in a variety of disorders where it is prolonged, such as congenital or drug-induced platelet dysfunction, uremia and liver cirrhosis, and is today the standard drug for treatment of bleedings or as cover for surgery in many of these conditions.

Effect of desmopressin

Desmopressin induces large and virtually immediate increases of FVIII, vWF and t-PA concentrations in plasma and of platelet adhesiveness. Maximum levels are usually reached about 30 min after intravenous injection. The rate of increase is usually two- to sixfold and is relatively constant in a given individual from time to time. The duration of the effect is dependent on the half-life of each specific factor.

Mode of action

RECEPTORS

Two general classes of vasopressin receptors have been characterized – V1 receptors, which mediate smooth-muscle contraction in the peripheral vasculature and glucose turnover in hepatocytes, and V2 receptors, which regulate water reabsorption in the collecting ducts of the kidney. Desmopressin is a strong V2 receptor agonist, but has no effect on V1 receptors. Desmopressin's hemostatic effect seems to be mediated by its strong V2 receptor agonist activity, as patients with nephrogenic diabetes insipidus, who lack this receptor, manifest no increase in hemostatic variables in response to desmopressin (Kobrinsky et al., 1985; Bichet et al., 1988). The effect is not mediated via V2 receptors in the kidneys, as anephric patients respond normally to desmopressin (Mannucci et al., 1975). By contrast, patients with other rare forms of nephrogenic diabetes insipidus seem to manifest normal clotting factor

response to desmopressin (Brenner, Seligsohn and Hochberg, 1988; Ohzeki et al., 1988). It is possible that desmopressin-induced release of FVIII and vWF is mediated by low-affinity extrarenal V2-like receptors, though the precise location of these putative receptors is not known. Putative sites of desmopressin action include endothelial cells, megakaryocytes, blood monocytes and mast cells (Schwartz, 1989; Hashemi et al., 1990; Johns, 1990; Macia et al., 1990; Murphy and Joran, 1992).

FACTOR RELEASE

In most studies evaluating the effect of desmopressin on coagulation factors, it has been found to be restricted to increasing the plasma concentrations of FVIII, vWF and t-PA (Nilsson, Mikaelsson and Vilhardt, 1982; Mannucci, 1986). These increases are so fast that they are probably caused by release from endogenous reservoirs and not by increased synthesis. FVIII is probably synthesized in sinusoid liver endothelial cells and hepatocytes (Stel, van der Kwast and Veerman, 1983; Wion et al., 1985; Zelechowska, van Mourik and Brodeniewica-Porba, 1985) and vWF is synthesized in endothelial cells and megakaryocytes (Howard, Montgomery and Hardisty, 1974; Nachman and Jaffe, 1975). Desmopressin would not appear to act directly on endothelial cells, as addition of desmopressin to cultured endothelial cells does not result in release of vWF into the culture medium (Booyse, Osikowicz and Feder, 1981; Tuddenham et al., 1982). This implies that desmopressin either acts via a second messenger or requires a cofactor not present in cell culture. Another explanation may be that cultured cells have lost some receptor that is present in vivo. Hashemi and coworkers (1990) found evidence suggesting that platelet-activating (PAF) released from monocytes is responsible for the vWF-releasing effect of desmopressin.

EFFECT ON PLATELET FUNCTION

The mechanism of action responsible for the marked increase of platelet adhesiveness in response to desmopressin is not fully understood. In studies using the annular perfusion chamber technique, in vitro addition of vWF was found to enhance platelet adhesion to the subendothelium (Weiss et al., 1978; Sakariassen et al., 1984), which gave rise to the speculation that the quantitative increase of vWF seen after administration of desmopressin is responsible for the increased platelet adhesion to subendothelium (Sakariassen et al., 1984). At our center we have systematically evaluated the desmopressin-induced increase of platelet adhesiveness as measured with a platelet retention test (Lethagen and Nilsson, 1992). Platelet retention was unaffected by change in the plasma vWF concentration, e.g. after intravenous infusion of vWF in patients with vWD type 3, which is characterized by a complete absence of vWF both in plasma, endothelial cells and platelets. The presence of platelet vWF and normally functioning platelet receptor glycoprotein (GP) IIb/IIIa seemed to be essential for desmopressin's effect on platelets (Lethagen and Nilsson, 1992). Desmopressin may promote an increased exposure of platelet vWF bound to GPIIb/IIIa on the platelet surface upon activation of platelets. Desmopressin's effect on platelets is independent of the arachidonate pathway (Lethagen and Rugarn, 1992) and does not seem to be mediated by thrombin or adenosine diphosphate (Lethagen and Nilsson, 1992).

Intravenous versus intranasal administration

Desmopressin can be administered parenterally, by intravenous (IV) or subcutaneous (SC) injection, or intranasally in drop or spray form. IV injection is the most common route in cases with hemostatic indications. In healthy volunteers, maximal effect of desmopressin on VIII:C and vWF, with peak levels after about 30 min, is achieved with an IV dosage of 0.3 µg/kg, even though the plasma concentration of desmopressin is dose-dependent. The ceiling limit of biological response to desmopressin may be due to saturation of receptor sites (Lethagen *et al.*, 1987).

The effect of SC administration of desmopressin on FVIII/vWF is comparable to that of IV administration, except that the plasma concentration of VIII:C does not peak until after 1–2 h (Köhler *et al.*, 1986; Köhler and Mariani, 1993).

Intranasal administration of desmopressin is of clinical interest as it is suitable for home treatment. Administration with a high-dose intranasal spray delivering a full dose of 300 µg with one squirt (i.e. a 100 µl dose of a 1.5 mg/ml solution) in each nostril has proved to be superior to drop administration (Harris *et al.*, 1986). In healthy volunteers, the effect of the spray on VIII:C and vWF concentrations in plasma is comparable to that of 0.2 µg/kg given IV, and the reproducibility of the spray effect is at least as good as that of IV, injection (Lethagen *et al.*, 1987). It is possible to improve the biological effect further by changes in dose volume of the nasal spray. Two metered doses of 50 µl (of a 1.5 mg/ml solution) in each nostril have been found to yield significantly higher plasma desmopressin concentrations, and consequently a greater increase in plasma FVIII, than a single metered dose of 100 µl of the same solution in each nostril (Harris *et al.*, 1988). The nasal spray currently in clinical use is a pressurized spray delivering a metered dose of 100 µl of a 1.5 mg/ml solution.

Indications for the use of desmopressin

EXPERIENCE WITH DESMOPRESSIN IN HEMOPHILIA A

As desmopressin temporarily increases the plasma concentration of FVIII, it has been used in patients with mild or moderate hemophilia A in order to prevent bleeding in connection with tooth extractions or major surgery (Mannucci *et al.*, 1987). Several large clinical trials involving about 100 patients treated for dental extractions or major surgical procedures or acute bleedings (e.g. hemarthroses, muscular hematomas or mucosal bleedings) have firmly established the hemostatic efficacy of intravenous desmopressin (Warrier and Lusher, 1983; Mariani *et al.*, 1984; de la Fuente *et al.*, 1985). Treatment with plasma-derived FVIII concentrates has several disadvantages, such as a risk of transmitting blood-borne infections, high costs and shortage of supply in some of the developing countries. As desmopressin has none of these disadvantages, it is an important alternative to factor concentrates in selected patients.

As not all hemophilia patients respond sufficiently, it is important to test candidate patients prior to any surgical procedure. In patients with mild or moderate hemophilia A, plasma VIII:C concentrations increase two- to sixfold after IV administration of desmopressin at 0.3 µg/kg (Fig. 18.1), which is the same mean percentage increase as in healthy subjects (Mannucci *et al.*, 1981; Nilsson and Lethagen, 1991).

FVIII is released immediately, peak plasma concentrations being obtained about 30–60 min after desmopressin administration. In patients with severe hemophilia A there is no increase of VIII:C in plasma after desmopressin. Mannucci and co-workers (1981) have reported the half-life of VIII:C after DDAVP to be 11 h in mild hemophilia A.

The magnitude of the FVIII response varies from patient to patient but as individual response is consistent from one time to another, a test dose should be given to each patient to insure that the response is sufficient. In general, a baseline VIII:C concentration of at least 0.10–0.15 iu/ml is required to achieve a post-injection VIII:C concentration of about 0.30–0.50 iu/ml. These levels are insufficient for major surgical procedures but may be sufficient for minor bleedings or lesser procedures. If a major surgical procedure is planned, the patient should attain postinjection VIII:C concentrations of at least 0.70–1.00 iu/ml.

Desmopressin may also be given subcutaneously. FVIII response to desmopressin given subcutaneously is of similar magnitude to that obtained with intravenous injection, but peak levels are reached later (Ghirardini *et al.*, 1987; Mannucci *et al.*, 1987).

VIII:C (IU/mL) after desmopressin

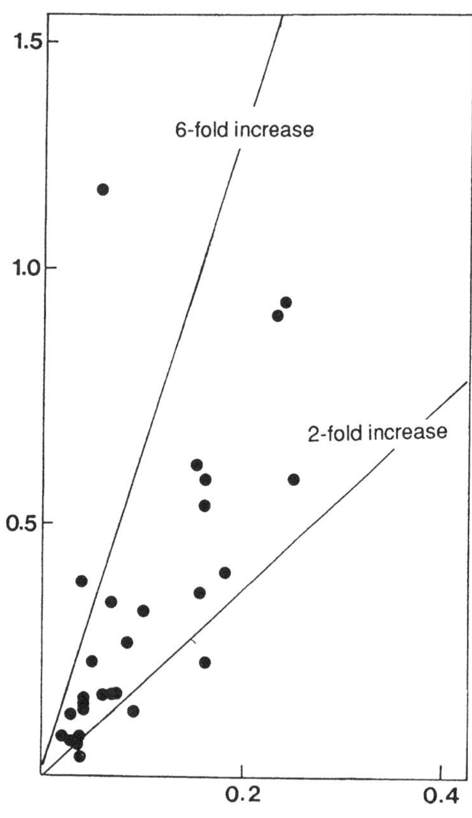

VIII:C (IU/mL) before desmopressin

Fig. 18.1 Factor VIII concentration (VIII:C) before and after desmopressin given intravenously at a dosage of 0.3 µg/kg to 28 patients with mild or moderate hemophilia A.

Intranasal administration of desmopressin is an attractive route as it enables patients to treat themselves at home without delay in the event of bleeding episodes. Early attempts at intranasal administration of desmopressin in drop form with a single-dose pipette or rhinyle were hampered by unpredictable and poor response (Mannucci, 1986). These delivery systems cannot be recommended for desmopressin. The effect of intranasal administration with a metered-dose spray is comparable to that of IV injection, however, and the reproducibility of the hemostatic effect of the spray at least as good as that of IV injection (Lethagen *et al.*, 1987). In a recent study the effect of intranasal administration of desmopressin by spray was compared to that of IV injection in patients with hemophilia A or vWD. In the hemophilia patients, there was no significant difference in peak VIII:C concentrations between three spray dosages, 300, 450 and 600 µg, and one intravenous dosage, 0.3 µg/kg (Lethagen *et al.* 1995). The recommended spray dose is 300 µg.

Many patients have used the spray with good effect for home treatment in connection with bleeding or before minor surgery (Lethagen and Ragnarson-Tenvall, 1993). As cover for other types of surgery or bleeding when a prompt response is required, the use of the IV desmopressin is to be recommended.

ACQUIRED HEMOPHILIA A

Desmopressin may also have a hemostatic effect and increase plasma concentrations of FVIII in patients with acquired hemophilia. We have tried both IV and intranasal treatment in non-hemophilic patients with antibodies against FVIII. In many cases it was possible to obtain a satisfactory increase in VIII:C and hemostatic effect. However, in patients with high antibody titers and no measurable VIII:C, no hemostatic effect can be expected (Nilsson and Lethagen, 1991). Mudad and Kane (1993), who reviewed 21 reported cases and a further case of their own, concluded that desmopressin has a role in the treatment of patients with acquired FVIII inhibitors at low titers (< 5 Bethesda units or > 5% FVIII:C in plasma).

VON WILLEBRAND'S DISEASE

There are three main types of vWD. In type 1, the full complement of vWF multimers are present in plasma but at reduced concentrations. In type 2, the hemostatically most active vWF multimers, the high-molecular-weight multimers, are absent. In type 3 (the severe recessive form), vWF is completely absent. There are several subtypes of types 1 and 2. Several groups have studied the response to desmopressin in patients with different types of vWD (Mannucci *et al.*, 1977a; Nilsson *et al.*, 1982; 1986; Ruggeri *et al.*, 1982; Holmberg *et al.*, 1983; Mannucci *et al.*, 1985; Gralnick *et al.*, 1986). Patients with type 1, which is by far the most common form, occurring perhaps in as many as 80% of all affected families (Holmberg and Nilsson, 1992), respond to desmopressin with a temporary normalization both of the plasma vWF concentration, the multimeric pattern of the vWF, and the bleeding time. In terms of the VIII:C concentration in plasma, response to desmopressin is greater after IV administration at 0.3 µg/kg than after 300 µg delivered by nasal spray, whereas reduction in the bleeding time is comparable with both modes of administration (Lethagen *et al.*, 1995). In type 2 vWD, the multimeric pattern of the vWF is not normalized by desmopressin, and the bleeding time is unaffected or only slightly improved. In the rare variant, type 2B, abnormal vWF multimers are released from endothelial cells, causing platelet aggregation and thrombocytopenia (Lethagen *et al.*, 1995).

Patients with vWD type 3, the severe recessive form, lack the ability to synthesize vWF, and do not respond to desmopressin with any increase in vWF, and manifest almost no increase in VIII:C (Nilsson *et al*, 1982). Therefore desmopressin cannot be used in the treatment of patients with type III.

Thus, desmopressin is the treatment of choice in type 1 vWD, as almost all patients respond well. A test dose of desmopressin is given at the time of diagnosis to insure that the patient's response is sufficient. Most patients with type 2 variants do not respond satisfactorily to desmopressin, and it is even contraindicated in those with type 2B. Desmopressin has no effect in patients with type 3 vWD.

PLATELET DYSFUNCTION

The effect of desmopressin in patients with inherited or acquired platelet dysfunction has been investigated in a number of studies. Most forms of congenital and drug-induced platelet dysfunction respond well to desmopressin, with normalization or reduction of bleeding time (Kobrinsky *et al.*, 1984; Winckelman and Augustin, 1985; Mannucci *et al.*, 1986; Marti *et al.*, 1986; Kentro, Lottenberg and Kitchens, 1987; Schulman *et al.*, 1987; DiMichele and Hathaway, 1990), but patients with Glanzmann's thrombasthenia do not respond. Kim and coworkers (1988) also found desmopressin to have a beneficial effect in patients with prolonged bleeding time of unknown etiology.

In a prospective study of 116 consecutive patients with platelet dysfunction diagnosed at our center, 105 (90%) responded with reduced bleeding time and increased platelet adhesiveness. Of the 11 patients who did not respond, one had severe Glanzmann's thrombasthenia (Nilsson and Lethagen, 1991).

Drug-induced platelet dysfunction can also be counteracted by desmopressin. Desmopressin has been shown to reduce bleeding time in subjects treated with aspirin (Kobrinsky *et al.*, 1984; Mannucci *et al.*, 1986; Lethagen and Rugarn, 1992), heparin (Schulman and Johnson, 1991) or dextran (Lethagen *et al.*, 1990).

UREMIA

Patients with uremia frequently manifest an increased bleeding tendency and prolonged bleeding time due to abnormal platelet function. The finding that cryoprecipitate could reduce the bleeding time in cases of uremia (Jansson *et al.*, 1980) prompted others to try utilizing the hemostatic effect of desmopressin in uremia (Watson and Koegh, 1982; Mannucci *et al.*, 1983; Shapiro and Kelleher, 1984). IV injection of desmopressin at 0.3–0.4 µg/kg normalizes the bleeding time in approximately 75% of patients with uremia. At 4 h after injection, bleeding time was less than 10 min in 60% of the patients, but after 8 h it had returned to baseline values in most cases.

LIVER CIRRHOSIS

In liver cirrhosis, a complex derangement of the hemostatic mechanism results in an increased bleeding tendency. Cirrhosis patients manifest prolonged bleeding time and subnormal concentrations of the coagulation factors synthesized by hepatocytes, especially the vitamin K-dependent coagulation factors. Although FVIII is thought to be synthesized in the liver, high concentrations of FVIII are frequently found in cases of advanced cirrhosis. Mild or moderate thrombocytopenia is also common. Several studies have shown desmopressin to reduce the bleeding time in liver cirrhosis (Agnelli *et al.*, 1983; Burrhougs *et al.*, 1985; Mannucci *et al.*, 1986), but, owing to the complexity of the hemostatic abnormalities, desmopressin cannot completely correct the increased bleeding tendency.

DESMOPRESSIN IN CONNECTION WITH SURGERY IN PATIENTS WITHOUT BLEEDING DISORDERS

Drugs affecting surgical blood loss in patients without a known bleeding diathesis have attracted much attention as a means of reducing the risk of side-effects associated with transfusion of erythrocytes or other blood products. The possible benefit of desmopressin in connection with surgery has been evaluated in several studies, most of them focused on open-heart surgery. Two earlier double-blind, placebo-controlled studies yielded promising results with significant reduction of blood loss when desmopressin was given prophylactically in connection with open-heart surgery (Salzman *et al.*, 1986) or scoliosis surgery (Kobrinsky *et al.*, 1987). However, later studies were unable to show a significant reduction in blood loss or transfusion requirements in the desmopressin-treated patients as compared to those given placebo. A recent review of 18 published double-blind, placebo-controlled, randomized clinical trials of desmopressin and blood loss after cardiac surgery showed a significant reduction of blood loss in desmopressin-treated patients in studies where there was a large blood loss in the placebo groups, equal to or exceeding 1180 ml. This suggests that desmopressin does reduce blood loss and transfusion requirements in a subgroup of patients undergoing cardiac surgery (Cattaneo and Mannucci, 1993).

Some workers have attempted to identify the patients who benefit from desmopressin. In one study, desmopressin significantly reduced blood loss when given postoperatively after cardiac surgery to patients with prolonged bleeding time and mediastinal bleeding (Czer *et al.*, 1987). In a double-blind, placebo-controlled study, desmopressin was effective in decreasing the volume of mediastinal chest tube drainage after cardiopulmonary bypass in patients with low maximal amplitude at post-bypass thromboelastography, whereas its effect did not differ from that of placebo in those with high maximal amplitude (Morgan and Hosking, 1992). In a controlled study of patients pretreated with aspirin within 7 days before coronary artery bypass grafting, Gratz and coworkers (1992) found that desmopressin significantly reduced postoperative blood loss, as compared to placebo.

Desmopressin should be used prophylactically before surgery in patients with a known bleeding disorder who have manifested satisfactory response to a test dose given prior to surgery. In most patients without any known bleeding disorder, desmopressin does not significantly reduce blood loss when given prophylactically. Although there may exist a subgroup of patients without known bleeding diathesis who might benefit from desmopressin, there is no general agreement on how to identify such patients before surgery. The best preoperative screening for general use is probably a carefully documented clinical history (Triplett, 1989). As desmopressin has few side-effects, it may safely be tried in most patients manifesting persistent postoperative bleedings.

THE USE OF DESMOPRESSIN IN BLOOD DONORS

The effect of desmopressin on the FVIII:C has led to its use in blood donors prior to blood collection, to increase the yield of VIII:C for the production of FVIII concentrates. An approximately twofold increase in the yield of VIII:C and vWF for both low- and intermediate-purity FVIII concentrates was obtained by using plasma from donors who had received desmopressin intranasally by rhinyle catheter or pipette 1 h before blood or plasma collection (Mickaelsson *et al.*, 1982; Palmer *et al.*, 1983). This approach to increasing the yield of FVIII and vWF might be suitable for use in developing countries dependent on cryoprecipitate, often prepared from blood donated by the hemophilia patients' relatives.

Dosage recommendations

HOSPITAL TREATMENT

Optimal hemostatic effect of desmopressin is achieved with a dosage of 0.3 µg/kg dissolved in saline to a total volume of 10 ml and injected IV over 10 min, or dissolved in 50–100 ml saline and infused slowly over 15–30 min. As hemostatic response to desmopressin is virtually instantaneous, it is given at this dosage immediately before surgery. In cases of major surgery, the dose can be repeated at 8–12-h intervals if necessary. In such cases, the FVIII response should be monitored and the patient's water balance checked, e.g. by means of weight control. In connection with minor surgery, a single dose of desmopressin is often sufficient. In connection with

tooth extractions, it is advantageous to give tranexamic acid concomitantly, owing to the high level of fibrinolytic activity in the oral mucosa. Desmopressin can also be given subcutaneously at a dosage of 0.3 µg/kg, but response is slow and peak concentrations of FVIII do not appear until after about 1–2 h.

HOME TREATMENT

Intranasal administration of 300 µg desmopressin by nasal spray has been shown to yield significant and highly reproducible increases in the plasma concentrations of FVIII and vWF (with peak levels after about 90 min) and enhanced platelet adhesiveness. The spray is suitable for self-administration at home, as it is easy to handle and does not involve the use of needles (Rose and Aledort, 1991). For some years now we have been prescribing the spray for patients with mild hemophilia A, vWD type 1 or platelet dysfunction. The patients have found the spray beneficial in connection with nose bleeds, menorrhagia, trauma, muscle hematoma, tooth extractions and minor surgery, and have reported a reduction in the number of visits to outpatient clinics, in absence from school or work, and in the use of FVIII:C (Lethaen and Ragnarson-Tenvall, 1993).

TACHYPHYLAXIS

Repeated administration of desmopressin at short intervals has been reported to cause decreasing response (tachyphylaxis) in some patients with hemophilia A (Lowe *et al.*, 1977; Mannucci *et al.*, 1977; Nilsson *et al.*, 1986) or vWD (Theiss and Schmidt, 1978). Mannucci, Bettega and Cattaneo (1992) studied tachyphylaxis in 22 patients with hemophilia A and in 15 patients with vWD type I, who were given four doses of desmopressin (0.3 µg/kg i.v.) at 24-h intervals. They found response to the second dose to be approximately 30% less than that to the first. Decreased FVIII response was more common among the hemophiliacs than among the vWD patients, and the vWD patients manifested only small reductions in bleeding time response.

In cases where it is necessary to give repeated doses of desmopressin for some time to patients with hemophilia A in connection with major surgery, it is advisable to monitor plasma concentrations of VIII:C. If the patient becomes unresponsive to desmopressin, FVIII concentrates have to be given. The response to desmopressin in such cases is usually re-established after 3–4 days.

In healthy volunteers given 10 doses of desmopressin at 12-h intervals for 5 days, response decreased progressively at the second and third administrations, but leveled out after the third dose. The increases in VIII concentrates concentrations were still approximately twofold after 10 doses. No difference was seen between three different dosage levels: 0.4 µg/kg IV, 0.2 µg/kg IV and 300 µg intranasally by spray(Nilsson and Lethagen, 1991).

Tachyphylaxis is rarely a problem in the clinical use of desmopressin as only one or a few doses are required for most bleedings or surgical procedures. Even if prolonged desmopressin treatment is given, tachyphylaxis is seldom a problem, though in such cases it is recommended that treatment be closely monitored.

Cautions and contraindications

ADVERSE EFFECTS

Desmopressin has few side-effects, the most common being a facial flush. Some patients experience a mild and transient headache. A small decrease in systolic and diastolic blood pressure and an increase in heart rate is often seen. Although desmopressin is a potent anti-diuretic, water retention is not a prominent clinical problem and very few cases of severe fluid overload have been reported. Moreover, uremic patients have been found to manifest no problems with fluid overload or congestive heart failure (Mannucci, 1988). None the less, several case reports have called attention to the risk of hyponatremia and seizures after administration of desmopressin (Lowe *et al.*, 1977; Koskimies, Pylkkänen and Vilska, 1984; Shepherd *et al.*, 1989; Smith *et al.*, 1989; 1992; Binch and Jacobsen, 1992; Yaouyanc *et al.*, 1992; Humphries and Siragy, 1993).

Some cases of thromboembolic episodes occurring in conjunction with the administration of desmopressin have been reported (Bond and Bevan, 1988; O'Brien *et al.*, 1989; van Dantzig, Duren and ten Cate, 1989). An evaluation of clinical trials of desmopressin in conjunction with cardiac surgery elicited no unequivocal evidence that desmopressin carries a risk of thrombosis (Mannucci and Lusher, 1989). In a more recent review of 31 clinical trials of desmopressin given to patients undergoing cardiac, orthopedic or other major surgery, no significant difference was found in the frequency of venous or arterial thrombosis between desmopressin-treated (*n* = 956) and placebo-treated patients (*n* = 877); Mannucci, Carlsson and Harris, 1994). Thus, desmopressin would not seem to be associated with any increase in the risk of thrombosis.

CONTRAINDICATIONS

Desmopressin is contraindicated in cases of polydipsia, unstable angina or severe congestive heart disease because of its antidiuretic effect. In vWD type 2B desmopressin is contraindicated because it causes platelet aggregation and thrombocytopenia. Desmopressin should be used with caution in very small children; and if given to pregnant women in conjunction with parturition, should preferably not be given before delivery as the drug is probably passed over to the fetus, but can be given immediately after delivery instead.

Future developments

The intranasal delivery system can be further developed. As mentioned above, the efficacy of the spray can be improved with adjustments of dose volume and concentration of the solution. A spray bottle containing fewer doses would be preferable for patients who only occasionally use the spray.

A peptide with a more specific effect is desirable. The most important improvement would be if the antidiuretic effect could be separated from the hemostatic effect. It would also be interesting to have a peptide which only stimulated the FVIII and vWF release and the increase of platelet adhesiveness and which did not release t-PA.

Conclusions

Desmopressin is an established hemostatic drug. Owing to the large and almost immediate increases of plasma concentrations of FVIII and vWF and of platelet adhesiveness and the shortening of the skin bleeding time brought about by desmopressin, it is useful in treating patients with bleeding disorders such as mild hemophilia A, vWD and congenital and acquired platelet disorders, and has reduced or abolished the need of blood products in many of these patients. Even in patients with no known bleeding diathesis, desmopressin may be of benefit in connection with invasive procedures in patients using aspirin or in those manifesting persistent postoperative bleedings of unknown cause.

References

Åberg, M., Nilsson, I.M. and Vilhardt, H. (1979) The release of fibrinolytic activator and factor VIII after injection of DDAVP, in *Progress in Chemical Fibrinolysis and Thrombolysis* (ed. J.F. Davidsson), Churchill Livingstone, Edinburgh, pp. 92–97.

Agnelli, G., Berretini, M., Cunto, M.D. and Nenci, G.G. (1983) Desmopressin-induced improvement of abnormal coagulation in chronic liver disease. *Lancet*, 1, 645.

Beach, P.S., Beach, R.E. and Smith, L.R. (1992) Hyponatremic seizures in a child treated with desmopressin to control enurcsis. A rationale approach to fluid intake. *Clin Pediatr Phila* 31, 566–569.

Bichet, D.G., Razi, M., Lonergan, M. *et al.* (1988) Hemodynamic and coagulation responses to 1-desamino[8-D-arginine]vasopressin in patients with congenital nephrogenic diabetes insipidus. *N Engl J Med*, 318, 881–887.

Binch, L.J.C. and Jacobsen, M.B. (1992) Hyponatremi ved behandling av von Willebrands sykdom. *Tidsskr Nor Laegeforen*, 112, 3670–3671.

Bond, L. and Bevan, D.U. (1988) Myocardial infarction in a patient with hemophilia treated with DDAVP. *N Engl J Med*, 318, 121.

Booyse, F.M., Osikowicz, G. and Feder, S. (1981) Effects of various agents on ristocetin-Willebrand factor activity in long-term cultures of von Willebrand and normal human umbilical vein endothelial cells. *Thromb Haemost*, 46, 668.

Brenner, B., Seligsohn, U. and Hochberg, Z. (1988) Normal response of factor VIII and von Willebrand factor to 1-deamino-8-D-arginine vasopressin in nephrogenic diabetes insipidus. *J Clin Endocrinol Metab*, 67, 191–193.

Burrhougs, A.K., Matthews, K., Quadiri, M. *et al.* (1985) Desmopressin and bleeding time in patients with cirrhosis. *Br Med J*, 291, 1377–1381.

Cash, J.D., Gader, A.M.A. and Da Costa, J. (1974) The release of plasminogen activator and factor VIII by LVP, AVP, DDAVP, AT III and OT in man. *Br J Haematol*, **27**, 363–364.

Cattaneo, M. and Mannucci, P.M. (1993) Desmopressin and blood loss after cardiac surgery. *Lancet*, **342**, 812.

Czer, L.S.C., Bateman, T.M., Gray, R.J. *et al.* (1987) Treatment of severe platelet dysfunction and hemorrhage after cardiopulmonary bypass: reduction in blood product usage with desmopressin. *JACC*, **9**, 1139–1147.

de la Fuente, B., Kasper, C.K., Rickles, F.R. and Hoyer, L.W. (1985) Response of patients with mild and moderate hemophilia A and von Willebrand's disease to treatment with desmopressin. *Ann Intern Med*, **103**, 6–14.

DiMichele, D.M. and Hathaway, W.E. (1990). Use of DDAVP in inherited and acquired platelet dysfunction. *Am J Hematol*, **33**, 39–45.

Egeberg, O. (1963) Changes in the activity of antihemophilic A factor (f.VIII) and in the bleeding time associated with muscular exercise and adrenaline infusion. *Scand J Clin Lab Invest*, **15**, 539–549.

Ghirardini, A., Mariani, G., Iacopino, G. *et al.* (1987) Concentrated DDAVP: further improvement in the management of mild factor VIII deficiencies. *Thromb Haemostas*, **58**, 896–898.

Gralnick, H.R., William, S.B., McKeown, L.P. *et al.* (1986) DDAVP in type IIa von Willebrand's disease. *Blood*, **67**, 465–468.

Gratz, I. Koehler, J., Olsen, D. *et al.* (1992) The effect of desmopressin acetate on postoperative hemorrhage in patients receiving aspiring therapy before coronary artery bypass operations. *J Thorac Cardiovasc Surg*, **104**, 1417–1422.

Guay, J., Reinberg, C., Rivard, G.E. *et al.* (1990) DDAVP does not reduce bleeding during spinal fusion for idiopathic scoliosis. *Can J Anaesth*, **37**, 14.

Hackman, T., Gascoyne, R.D., Naiman, S.C. *et al.* (1989) A trial of desmopressin (1-desamino-8-D-arginine vasopressin) to reduce blood loss in uncomplicated cardiac surgery. *N Engl J Med*, **321**, 1437–1443.

Harris, A.S., Nilsson, I.M., Wagner, Z.G. and Alkner, U. (1986) Intranasal administration of peptides: nasal deposition, biological response, and absorption of desmopressin. *J Pharm Sci*, **75**, 1085–1088.

Harris, A.S., Ohlin, M., Lethagen, S. and Nilsson, I.M. (1988) Effects of concentration and volume on nasal bioavailability and biological response to desmopressin. *J Pharm Sci*, **77**, 337–339.

Hashemi, S. *et al.* (1990) DDAVP-induced release of von Willebrand factor from endothelial cells in vitro; the effect of plasma and blood cells. *Biochim Biophys Acta*, **1052**, 63–70.

Holmberg, L. and Nilsson, I.M. (1992) von Willebrand's disease. *Eur J Haematol*, **48**, 127–141.

Holmberg, L., Nilsson, I.M., Borge, L. *et al.* (1983) Platelet aggregation induced by 1-deamino-8-D-arginine vasopressin (DDAVP) in type IIB von Willebrand's disease. *N Engl J Med*, **309**, 816–821.

Horrow, J.C., van Riper, D.F., Strong, M.D. *et al.* (1991) Hemostatic effects of tranexamic acid and desmopressin during cardiac surgery. *Circulation*, **84**, 2063–2070.

Howard, M.A., Montgomery, D.C. and Hardisty, R.M. (1974) Factor VIII-related antigen in platelets. *Thromb Res*, **4**, 617–624.

Humphries, K.E. and Siragy, H. (1993) Significant hyponatremia following DDAVP administration in a healthy adult. *Am J Hematol*, **44**, 12–15.

Ingram, G.I.C. (1961) Increase in antihaemophilic globulin activity following infusion of adrenaline. *J Physiol*, **156**, 217–224.

Jansson, P.A., Jubelirer, S.J., Weinstein, M.S. and Deykin, D. (1980) Treatment of bleeding tendency in uremia with cryoprecipitate. *N Engl J Med*, **303**, 1318–1322.

Johns, R.A. (1990) Desmopressin is a potent vasorelaxant of aorta and pulmonary artery isolated from rabbi and rat. *Anesthesiology*, **72**, 858–864.

Kentro, T.B., Lottenberg, R. and Kitchens, C.S. (1987) Clinical efficacy of desmopressin acetate for hemostatic control in patients with primary platelet disorders undergoing surgery. *Am J Hematol*, **24**, 215–219.

Kim, H.C., Salva, K.S., Fallot, P.L. *et al.* (1988) Patients with prolonged bleeding time of undefined etiology, and their response to desmopressin. *Thromb Haemostas*, **59**, 221–224.

Kobayashi, I. (1979) Treatment of hemophilia A and von Willebrand's disease patients with an intranasal dripping of DDAVP. *Thromb Res*, **16**, 775–779.

Kobrinsky, N.L., Israels, E.D., Gerrard, J.M. *et al.* (1984) Shortening of the bleeding time by 1-deamino-8-D-arginine vasopressin in various bleeding disorders. *Lancet*, **1**, 1145–1148.

Kobrinsky, N.L., Doyle, J.J., Israels, E.D.S. *et al.* (1985) Absent factor VIII response to synthetic vasopressin analogue in nephrogenic diabetes insipidus. *Lancet*, **1**, 1293–1294.

Kobrinsky, N.L., Letts, R.M., Patel, L.R. *et al.* 1-Desamino-8-D-arginine vasopressin (desmopressin) decreases operative blood loss in patients having Harrington rod spinal fusion surgery. A randomized, double-blinded, controlled trial. *Ann Intern Med*, **107**, 446–450.

Köhler, M. and Mariani, G. (1993) Intravenous and subcutaneous desmopressin: clinical results, in *Desmopressin in Bleeding Disorders* (eds G. Mariani, P.M. Mannucci and M. Cattaneo), Plenum Press, New York, pp. 309–316.

Köhler, M., Hellstern, P., Miyashita, C. *et al.* (1986) Comparative study of intranasal, subcutaneous and intravenous administration of desamino-D-arginine vasopressin (DDAVP). *Thromb Haemost*, **55**, 108–111.

Koskimies, O., Pylkkänen, J. and Vilska, J. (1984) Water intoxication in infants caused by the urine concentration test with vasopressin analogue (DDAVP). *Acta Paediatr Scand*, **73**, 131–132.

Lazenby, W.D., Russo, I., Zadeh, B.J. *et al.* (1990) Treatment with desmopressin acetate in routine artery bypass surgery to improve postoperative hemostasis. *Circulation*, **82** (suppl. IV), 413–419.

Lethagen, S. and Nilsson, J.M. (1992) DDAVP induced enhancement of platelet retention. Its dependence on platelet-von Willebrand factor and the platelet receptor GPIIb/IIIa. *Eur J Haematol*, **49**, 7–13.

Lethagen, S. and Ragnarson-Tenvall, G. (1993) Self-treatment with desmopressin intranasal spray in patients with bleeding disorders. Effect on bleeding symptoms and socio-economic factors. *Ann Hematol*, **66**, 257–260.

Lethagen, S. and Rugarn, P. (1992) The effect of DDAVP and placebo on platelet function and prolonged bleeding time induced by oral acetylsalicylic acid treatment in healthy volunteers. *Thrombos Haemostas*, **67**, 85–186.

Lethagen, S., Harris, A.S., Sjörin, E. and Nilsson, I.M. (1987) Intranasal and intravenous administration of desmopressin: effect on fVIII/vWF, pharmacokinetics and reproducibility. *Thrombos Haemostas*, **58**, 1033–1036.

Lethagen, S., Rugarn, P., Åberg, M. and Nilsson, I.M. (1990) Effects of desmopressin acetate (DDAVP) and dextran on hemostatic and thromboprophylactic mechanisms. *Acta Chir Scand*, **156**, 597–602.

Lethagen, S., Egervall, K., Berntorp, E. and Bengtsson, B. (1995) Desmopressin nasal spray. A dose finding study in patients with mild hemophilia A and von Willebrand's disease. *Haemophilia*, **1**, 97–102.

Lo Cicero, J., Massad, M. and Matano, J. (1991) Effect of desmopressin acetate on hemorrhage without identifiable cause in coronary bypass patients. *Am Surgeon*, **57**, 165–168.

Lowe, G., Pettigrew, A., Middleton, S. *et al.* (1977). DDAVP in haemophilia. *Lancet*, **2**, 614–615.

Macia, R.A., Silver, A.C., Gabel, R.A. *et al.* (1990) Hypotension induced by vasopressin antagonists in rats: role of mast cell degranulation. *Toxicol Appl Pharmacol*, **102**, 117–127.

Mannucci, P.M. (1986) Desmopressin (DDAVP) for treatment of disorders of hemostasis, in *Progress in Hemostasis and Thrombosis* (ed. B.S. Coller), Grune & Stratton, Orlando, pp. 19–45.

Mannucci, P.M. (1988) Desmopressin: a nontransfusional form of treatment for congenital and acquired bleeding disorders. *Blood*, **72**, 1449–1455.

Mannucci, P.M. and Lusher, J.M. (1989) Desmopressin and thrombosis. *Lancet*, **II**, 675–676.

Mannucci, P.M., Gagnatelli, G. and D'Alonzo, R. (1972) Stress and blood coagulation. in *Thrombosis: Risk Factors and Diagnostic Approaches* (eds K.M. Brinkhouse and S. Hinnom) Schattauer Verlag, Stuttgart, pp. 105–110.

Mannucci, P.M., Åberg, M., Nilsson, I.M. and Robertsson, B. (1975) Mechanism of plasminogen activator and factor VIII increase after vasoactive drugs. *Br J Haematol*, **30**, 81–93.

Mannucci, P.M., Åberg, M., Nilsson, I.M. and Robertsson, B. (1975) Mechanism of plasminogen activator and factor VIII increase after vasoactive drugs. *Br J Haematol*, **30**, 81–93.

Mannucci, P.M., Ruggeri, Z.M., Pareti, F.I. and Capitanio, A. (1977a) 1-Deamino-8-D-arginine vasopressin: a new pharmacological approach to the management of haemophilia and von Willebrand's disease. *Lancet*, **1**, 869–872.

Mannucci, P.M., Ruggeri, Z.M., Pareti, F.I. and Capitanio, A. (1977b) DDAVP in haemophilia. *Lancet*, **2**, 1171–1172.

Mannucci, P.M., Canciani, M.T., Rota, L. and Donovan, B.S. (1981) Response of factor VIII/von Willebrand factor to DDAVP in healthy subjects, and patients with haemophilia A and von Willebrand's disease. *Br J Haematol*, **47**, 283–293.

Mannucci, P.M., Remuzzi, G., Pusineri, F. *et al.* (1983) Deamino-8-D-arginine vasopressin shortens the bleeding time in uremia. *N Engl J Med*, **308**, 8–12.

Mannucci, P.M., Lombardi, R., Bader, R. *et al.* (1985) Heterogeneity of type I von Willebrand disease: evidence for a subgroup with an abnormal von Willebrand factor. *Blood*, **66**, 796–802.

Mannucci, P.M., Vicente, V., Vianello, L. *et al.* (1986) Controlled trial of desmopressin in liver cirrhosis and other conditions associated with prolonged bleeding time. *Blood*, **67**, 1148–1153.

Mannucci, P.M., Vicente, V., Alberca, I. *et al.* (1987) Intravenous and subcutaneous administration of desmopressin (DDAVP) to hemophiliacs: pharmacokinetics and factor VIII responses. *Thromb Haemostas*, **58**, 1037–1039.

Mannucci, P.M., Bettega, D. and Cattaneo, M. (1992) The development of tachyphylaxis in patients with haemophilia and von Willebrand disease after repeated doses of desmopressin (DDAVP). *Br J Haematol*, **82**, 87–93.

Mannucci, P.M., Carlsson, S. and Harris, S.D. (1994) Desmopressin, surgery and thrombosis. *Thrombos Haemostas*, **71**, 154–155.

Mariani, G., Ciavarella, N., Mazzucconi, M.G. *et al.* (1984) Evaluation of the effectiveness of DDAVP in surgery and bleeding episodes in haemophilia and von Willebrand's disease. A study of 43 patients. *Clin Lab Haematol*, **6**, 229–238.

Marti, G.E., Rick, M.E., Sidbury, J. and Gralnick, H.R. (1986) DDAVP infusion in five patients with type Ia glycogen storage disease and associated correction of prolonged bleeding times. *Blood*, **68**, 180–184.

Mikaelsson, M., Nilsson, I.M., Vilhardt, H. and Wiechel, B. (1982) Factor VIII concentrate prepared from blood donors stimulated by intranasal administration of a vasopressin analogue. *Transfusion*, **22**, 229–233.

Mongan, P.D. and Hosking, M.P. (1992) The role of desmopressin acetate in patients undergoing coronary artery bypass surgery. A controlled clinical trial with thromboelastographic risk stratification. *Anesthesiology*, 77, 38–46.

Mudad, R. and William, H.K. (1993) DDAVP in acquired hemophilia A: case report and review of the literature. *Am J Hematol*, 43, 295–229.

Murphy, D.J. and Joran, J.E. (1992) Respiratory and cardiovascular changes associated with toxic doses of a peptide antagonist of vasopressin in the rat. *Fundamental Appl Toxicol*, 18, 307–313.

Nachman, R.L. and Jaffe, E.A. (1975) Subcellular platelet factor VIII antigen and von Willebrand factor. *J Exp Med*, 141, 1101–1103.

Nilsson, I.M. and Lethagen, S. (1991) Current status of DDAVP formulations and their use, in *Hemophilia and von Willebrand's Disease in the 1990s* (eds J.M. Lusher and C.M. Kessler), Elsevier Science, Amsterdam, pp. 443–453.

Nilsson, I.M., Holmberg, L., Åberg, M. and Vilhardt, H. (1980) The release of plasminogen activator and factor VIII after injection of DDAVP in healthy volunteers and in patients with von Willebrand's disease. *Scand J Haematol*, 24, 351–359.

Nilsson, I.M., Mikaelsson, M. and Vilhardt, H. (1982) The effect of intranasal DDAVP on coagulation and fibrinolytic activity in normal persons. *Scand J Haematol*, 29, 70–74.

Nilsson, I.M., Vilhardt, H., Holmberg, L. and Åstedt, B. (1982) Association between factor VIII related antigen and plasminogen activator. *Acta Med Scand*, 211, 105–112.

Nilsson, I.M., Felding, P., Timberg, L. *et al.* (1986) Clinical experience with DDAVP, in *Factor VIII/von Willebrand Factor. Biological and Clinical Advances* (eds N.L. Ciavarella, Z. Ruggeri and T.S. Zimmerman), Wichtig, Milano, pp. 63–80.

O'Brien, J.R., Green, P.J., Salmon, G. *et al.* (1989) Desmopressin and myocardial infarction. *Lancet*, 1, 664.

Ohzeki, T., Sunaguchi, M., Tsunei, M. *et al.* (1988) Coagulation factor responsiveness in nephrogenic diabetes insipidus. *J Pediatr*, 113, 790.

Palmer, D.S., Harris, A.S., Tittley, P. and Rock, G. (1988) Effectiveness, specificity and safety of intranasal 1-deamino-8-D-arginine vasopressin treatment of normal blood donors. *Haemostasis*, 18, 187–196.

Rocha, E., Llorens, R., Paramo, J.A. *et al.* (1988) Does desmopressin acetate reduce blood loss after surgery in patients on cardiopulmonary bypass? *Circulation*, 77, 1319–1323.

Rose, E.H. and Aledort, L.M. (1991) Nasal spray desmopressin (DDAVP) for mild hemophilia A and von Willebrand disease. *Ann Intern Med*, 114, 563–568.

Ruggeri, Z.M., Mannucci, P.M., Lombardi, R. *et al.* (1982) Multimeric composition of factor VIII/von Willebrand factor following administration of DDAVP: Implications for pathophysiology and therapy of von Willebrand's disease subtypes. *Blood*, 59, 1272–1278.

Sakariassen, K.S., Cattaneo, M., van den Berg, A. *et al.* (1984) DDAVP enhances platelet adherence and platelet aggregate growth on human artery subendothelium. *Blood*, 64, 229–236.

Salvatoni, A., Maghnie, M., Lorini, R. and Marni, E. (1990) Hyponatremia and seizures during desmopressin acetate treatment in hypothyroidism. *J Pediatr*, 116, 835–836.

Salzman, E.W., Weinstein, M.J., Weintraub, R.M. *et al.* (1986) Treatment with desmopressin acetate to reduce blood loss after cardiac surgery. A double-blind randomized trial. *N Engl J Med*, 314, 1402–1406.

Schneck, N.L. and von Kaulla, K.N. (1961) Fibrinolysis and the nervous system. *Neurology (Minneap)* 11, 1959–1969.

Schulman, S. and Johnsson, H. (1991) Heparin, DDAVP and the bleeding time. *Thrombos Haemostas*, 65, 1242–1244.

Schulman, S., Johnsson, H., Egberg, N. and Blombäck, M. (1987) DDAVP-induced correction of prolonged bleeding time in patients with congenital platelet function defects. *Thromb Res*, 45, 165–174.

Schwartz, J. (1989) Vasodilation associated with V_2-type vasopressin activity: findings and implications. *Mol Cell Endocrinol*, 64, 133–136.

Shapiro, M.D. and Kelleher, S.P. (1984) Intranasal 1-deamino-8-D-arginine vasopressin shortens the bleeding time in uremia. *Am J Nephrol*, 4, 260–261.

Sheperd, L.L., Hutchinson, R.J., Worden, E.K. *et al.* (1989) Hyponatremia and seizures after intravenous administration of desmopressin acetate for surgical hemostasis. *J Pediatr*, 114, 470–472.

Shimizu, K., Hoshine, M., Kumagawa, J. *et al.* (1980) Mechanism of the prolonged antidiuretic action of DDAVP and its metabolic features, in *Antidiuretic Hormone* (eds L. Share, S. Yoshida and K. Yagi), University Park Press, Baltimore, pp. 271–284.

Smith, T.J., Gill, J.C., Ambruso, D.R. and Hathaway, W.E. (1989) Hyponatremia and seizures in young children given DDAVP. *Am J Hematol*, 31, 199–202.

Stel, H.V., van der Kwast, Th.H. and Veerman, E.C.I. (1983). Detection of factor VIII/coagulant antigen in human liver-tissue. *Nature*, 303, 530–532.

Theiss, W. and Schmidt, G. (1978) DDAVP and von Willebrand disease: repeated administration and the behaviour of the bleeding time. *Thromb Res*, 13, 1119–1123.

Triplett, D.A. (1989) Editorial: The bleeding time: neither pariah or panacea. *Arch Pathol Lab Med*, 113, 1207–1208.

Tuddenam, E.G.D., Lane, R.S., Rotblat, F. *et al.* (1982) Response to infusions of polyelectrolyte fractionated human factor VIII concentrate in human haemophilia A and von Willebrand's disease. *Br J Haematol*, 52, 259–267.

van Dantzig, J.M., Duren, D.R. and ten Cate, J.W. (1989) Desmopressin and myocardial infarction. *Lancet*, 1, 664.

Walter, R. (1976) Partial purification and characterization of post-proline cleaving enzyme: enzymatic inactivation of neurohypophysial hormones by kidney preparations of various species. *Biochim Biophys Acta*, 422, 138–158.

Warrier, I. and Lusher, J.M. (1983) DDAVP – a useful alternative to blood components in moderate haemophilia A and von Willebrand's disease. *J Pediatr*, 102, 228–233.

Watson, A.J.S. and Koegh, J.A.B. (1982) Effect of 1-deamino-8-D-arginine vasopressin on the prolonged bleeding time in chronic renal failure. *Nephron*, 32, 49–52.

Weinstein, R.E., Bona, R.D., Altman, A.J. *et al.* (1989) Severe hyponatremia after repeated intravenous administration of desmopressin. *Am J Hematol*, 32, 258–261.

Weiss, H.J., Baumgartner, H.R., Tschopp, T.B. *et al.* (1978) Correction by factor VIII of the impaired platelet adhesion to subendothelium in von Willebrand disease. *Blood*, 51, 267–279.

Winckelman, G. and Augustin, R. (1985) Improvement of primary hemostasis by DDAVP in patients with various platelet defects. *Thromb Haemostas*, 54, 12.

Wion, K.L., Kelly, D., Summerfield, J.A. *et al.* (1985) Distribution of factor VIII mRNA and antigen in human liver and other tissues. *Nature*, 317, 726–729.

Yaouyane, G., Jonville, A.P., Yaouyanc-Lapalle, H. *et al.* (1992) Seizure with hyponatremia in a child prescribed desmopressin for nocturnal enuresis. *J Toxicol Clin Toxicol*, 30, 637–641.

Zaoral, M., Kolc, J. and Sorm, F. (1967) Amino acids and peptides. LXXI. Synthesis of 1-deamino-8-D-amino-butyrine vasopressin, 1-deamino-8-D-lysine vasopressin and 1-deamino-8-D-arginine vasopressin. *Collection Czechoslov Chem Commun*, 32, 1250–1257.

Zelechowska, M.G., van Mourik, J.A. and Brodniewicz-Porba, T. (1985) Ultrastructural localization of factor VIII procoagulant antigen in human liver hepatocytes. *Nature*, 317, 729–730.

19 FACTOR IX CONCENTRATES

J.M. Lusher

During the 1950s and 1960s, whole plasma (either fresh or fresh frozen plasma) was the mainstay of treatment for hemophilia B. Since whole plasma contains only a miniscule amount of factor IX, the large volumes of plasma required to stop bleeding sometimes resulted in heart failure from fluid and plasma protein overload.

Factor IX is separated from plasma (or from cryo-precipitate supernatant) in close association with pro-thrombin and factors VII and X and concentrates containing these four clotting factors are called pro-thrombin complex concentrates (PCC), or factor IX complex concentrates (FIXCC). In 1959 the first PCC became available in France. Originally named PPB and later referred to as PPSB, this concentrate contained all of the vitamin K-dependent clotting factors – thus the name, PPSB (for prothrombin, proconvertin, Stuart factor and antihemophilic B factor, as they were then referred to; Blatrix and Soulier, 1959). Although the main indication for its use was to treat bleeding in persons with hemophilia B, PPSB was also used to treat persons with other coagulation deficiency states, including acquired deficiencies of the vitamin K-dependent factors. It is noteworthy that soon after its introduction, occurrences of disseminated intravascular coagulation (DIC) in persons with liver disease who were treated with PPSB were noted (Menaché, Fauvert and Soulier, 1959).

By 1968 a product similar to PPSB was licensed in the USA, with the generic name factor IX complex. Cutter's Konyne, and Hyland's Proplex (which was licensed by the US Food and Drug Administration (FDA) in 1970) quickly became the mainstay of treatment for hemophilia B. None of these early FIXCC were treated in any way to kill blood-borne viruses, and serologic testing of donated blood and plasma for hepatitis B antigen was not requir-ed in the USA until 1972 (Kasper and Lusher, 1993). Since each lot of clotting factor concentrate was produced from plasma collected from as many as 10 000 persons, the vast majority – if not all – of the recipients of these concentrates developed hepatitis. By the early 1970s, serologic markers for hepatitis B virus (HBV) were found in almost all persons with hemophilia who had received clotting factor concentrates (Hasiba, Spero and Lewis, 1976), and by the early 1990s when serologic testing for hepatitis C virus (HCV) became possible, it was found that most hemophiliacs who had received FIXCC were HCV-sero-positive as well (Bretter *et al.*, 1990; Rumi *et al.*, 1990; Allain *et al.*, 1991; Lusher *et al.*, 1991; Pistello *et al.*, 1991; Troisi *et al.*, 1993; Mauser-Bunschoten *et al.*, 1995). It now appears that the majority of persons infected with HCV remain chronically infected, as measured by a posi-tive HCV-RNA test (Mauser-Bunschoten *et al.*, 1995).

In 1982 the first two cases of acquired immunodefici-ency syndrome (AIDS) were reported in US hemophiliacs (Centers for Disease Control, 1982). As the AIDS epidemic progressed and as serologic testing for human immunodeficiency virus (HIV) became possible, large cohorts of hemophilic patients were tested. It is note-worthy that approximately 55% of persons with hemo-philia B who were treated with FIXCC produced from plasma collected in the USA between 1979 and 1984 became HIV-infected, in contrast to a much larger percentage (approximately 90%) of hemophilia A sub-jects who had received FVIII concentrates (Ragni *et al.*, 1987). The reasons for this are not entirely clear but include the possibility that an alcohol step used in the fractionation of some FIXCC may have killed some HIV.

At any rate, the recognition that not only serious but deadly discascs were being transmitted by both FVIII and FIX concentrates resulted in more rigorous donor-screening procedures, and much more vigorous attempts to inactivate and remove viruses from plasma-derived clotting factor concentrates.

Hemophilia. Edited by C.D. Forbes, L. Aledort and R. Madhok. Published in 1997 by Chapman & Hall, London. ISBN 0 412 63820 7

Viral attenuation methods used in manufacture of factor IX concentrates

DRY HEAT TREATING

By October 1984, two dry-heat-treated FIXCC were licensed for use by the US FDA (Table 19.1; Kasper and Lusher, 1993). Cutter's Konyne HT was heated in the dry state for 72 h at 68°C, while Baxter-Hyland's Proplex SX-T was heated for 144 h at 60°C. Neither of these products was ever subjected to a formal hepatitis safety trial, and there was evidence that certain other concentrates dry-heat-treated at temperatures between 60° and 68°C were transmitting hepatitis (Lusher *et al.*, 1988; Blanchette *et al.*, 1991), and even HIV infection (Mannucci, 1995). Thus, these methods of dry heating were largely abandoned. The only product currently marketed for use in hemophilia B which is dry-heat-treated at 60°C is Baxter/Hyland's Proplex T (Table 19.1). However, it should be noted that the time of exposure (144 h) to 60°C is much longer than that used for the FVIII concentrates which have transmitted HIV or hepatitis (Mannucci, 1995).

Dry heating at higher temperatures (80°C) for 72 h is being used for both FVIII and FIX concentrates manufactured by BioProducts Laboratory (BPL) and the

Table 19.1 Factor IX complex concentrates marketed for use in the USA 1968–1996

Brand name	Manufacturer	Food and Drug Administration Licence	Last release	Specific activity	Virus – inactivation	Separation method
Konyne	Cutter-Biological	12/68	5/85	N/A	None	DEAE absorption of effluent of Cohn fraction I
Konyne HT	Cutter Biol, Miles Inc	10/84	2/92	N/A	Dry heat: 68°C, 72 h	DEAE absorption of effluent of Cohn fraction I
Konyne 80*	Bayer, Inc	4/91		N/A	Dry heat: 80°C, 72 h	DEAE absorption of effluent of Cohn fraction I
Proplex	Hyland Division, Baxter	8/70	–	N/A	None	Tri-calcium phosphate absorption, PEG precipitation
Proplex SX	Hyland Division, Baxter	10/81	–	N/A	None	DEAE Sephadex absorption, PEG precipitation
Proplex SX-T	Hyland division, Baxter	10/84	2/88	N/A	Dry heat: 60°C, 144 h	DEAE Sephadex absorption, PEG precipitation
Proplex T*	Hyland Division, Baxter	1/86		3.9†	Dry heat: 60°C, 144 h	Tri-calcium phosphate absorption, PEG precipitation
Profilnine HT	Alpha Therapeutic	10/84	–	4.5	n-heptane, 60°C, 20 h	Tri-calcium phosphate absorption, PEG precipitation
Profilnine SD*	Alpha	1995		N/A	TNBP and polysorbate 80	Ion exchange chromatography
Prothar	Armour Pharmaceutical Co.	1983	1985	N/A	None	Chromatography
Bebulin VH*	Immuno AG	8/92		2†	Vapor (steam)	DEAE absorption heated 60°C, 10 h, 1190 mbar plus 80°C, 1 h,1375 mbar

*Indicates still being marketed, as of October 1996.
†Approximate values.
DEAE = diethyl-amino-ethyl.
PEG = polyethylene glycol.
TNPB = tri(n-butyl) phosphate.

Scottish National Blood Transfusion Service, and Bayer's Konyne 80 (licensed in the USA in 1991) is similarly treated. While the latter product has not undergone a formal prospective hepatitis safety trial in previously untreated subjects, 0.51 of patients infused with BPL or Scottish concentrates developed hepatitis (Study Group of the UK Haemophilia Centre Directors, 1988; Skidmore *et al.*, 1990; Bennett *et al.*, 1993; Mannucci, 1995).

PASTEURIZATION

Pasteurization (heating in solution at 60°C for 10 h) of FVIII concentrate was first introduced by Behringwerke (Marburg, Germany) in 1978. In the early 1980s, they began clinical trials with a similarly treated FIXCC. Results of prospective hepatitis safety studies, reported in 1987 (Schimpf *et al.*, 1987), indicated that these pasteurized concentrates did not transmit hepatitis. However, pasteurization was associated with very low yields.

MOIST HEATING IN ORGANIC SOLVENT

Moist heating was introduced by Alpha Therapeutics in the USA in 1984. In that year, lyophilized FVIII and FIXCC, heated in a moist condition in organic solvent, suspended in n-heptane at 60°C for 20 h, were licensed by the FDA. However, hepatitis safety trials conducted in the mid-1980s demonstrated that hepatitis transmission was reduced but not eliminated (Carnelli *et al.*, 1987; Kasper and Lusher, 1993). It should be noted that products produced at that time may well have had much higher virus loads in the starting plasma, as alanine aminotransferase (ALT) screening of donor plasma was not introduced until 1987, and even first-generation HCV screening of plasma for fractionation was not approved in the USA until late 1991 (Finlayson and Ankersley, 1990). It is possible that the same virus inactivation method may be effective with a lower virus load. The last FIX product which was virally attenuated by this method was Alpha's Profilnine HT (Table 19.1). However, Profilnine SD has now replaced this, and other Alpha FIX products are now solvent/detergent-treated as well (see below).

HOT VAPOR TREATMENT

Steam or vapor heating was introduced by Immuno, Vienna for both FVIII and FIX concentrates. Moistened lyophilized concentrate is exposed to hot vapor at 60°C for 10 h at a pressure of 1190 mbar, followed by 80°C for 1 h at 1375 mbar. While an Italian study reported 4/28 HBV seroconversions and one instance of HCV transmission (Mannucci, 1995), a subsequent international study involving 58 patients (19 of whom had hemophilia B) recorded no case of hepatitis or HIV seroconversion (Mannucci *et al.*, 1992; Shapiro *et al.*, 1993)

SOLVENT/DETERGENT TREATMENT

Solvent detergent treatment, in which an organic solvent, tri (n-butyl) phosphate (TNBP), and a detergent (sodium cholate, polysorbate 80 or Triton X-100) are added to clotting factor concentrates, inactivates the lipid-enveloped viruses HBV, HCV and HIV with little or no loss in coagulation factor activity. As noted by Mannucci (1995), since solvent/detergent treatment is relatively simple, safe and yields are not affected, it has progressively become the virucidal method of choice among most concentrate manufacturers, for both FVIII and FIX concentrates. Alpha's Profilnine SD, Alphanine SD, Biotest's Factor IX Biotest, BPL's Replenine, Kabi Pharmacia's Nanotiv, Octapharma AG's Octanyne and Laboratoire Français du Fractionnement et des Biotechnologies' (LFB) FIX VHP are current examples of solvent/detergent-treated FIX concentrates. AIMA's AIMAFIX is solvent/detergent-treated and also undergoes end-stage superheating. While no cases of HBV, HCV or HIV infection or seroconversion have been reported (Mannucci, 1995), it should be noted that solvent/detergent treatment does not inactivate non-lipid-enveloped viruses, such as hepatitis A virus (HAV) and human parvovirus B19. The latter is also heat-resistant (Mannucci, 1995). Outbreaks of human parvovirus B19 infection have been reported and approximately 85 cases of HAV infection have occurred in hemophiliacs following treatment with solvent/detergent-treated FVIII concentrates manufactured by AIMA in Italy and Octapharma in Austria and Germany (Gerritzen *et al.*, 1992; Mannucci, 1992; Temperley *et al.*, 1992; Peerlinde and Vermylen, 1993).

NEWER APPROACHES

Other strategies, including double inactivation methods, are now being used. For example, Armour's Mononine is subjected to chemical viral attenuation with sodium thiocyanate, and also membrane ultrafiltration (Hrinda *et al.*, 1991). Formal viral safety studies in previously untreated patients (Mannucci and Colombo, 1989) with hemophilia B demonstrated in over 30 subjects no evidence of hepatitis or HIV transmission (Shapiro *et al.*, 1993). AIMA's AIMAFIX is both solvent/detergent-treated and subjected to terminal dry heating (Table 19.2).

Burnouf-Radosevich and coworkers (1994) have recently described a new approach, referred to as nanofiltration. Based on the use of multilayered cellulose membranes with mean pore sizes of 15 nm, this approach appears to be applicable to FIX preparations (due to the small size of FIX). Viruses (both lipid-enveloped and

Table 19.2 Virucidal methods currently used in production of factor IX concentrate in the USA and Europe

Virucidal method	Main manufacturers using the method	Main product names
Dry heating, 80°C, 72 h	BioProducts Laboratory (BPL), Miles, Scottish National Blood Transfusion Service	9A, Defix, Konyne 80
Dry heating, 60°C, 144 h	Baxter	Proplex T
Pasteurization	Behringwerke	Berinin HS
Vapor heating (60°C, 10 h, 1190 mbar plus 80°C, 1375 mbar)	Immuno	Bebulin, Prothromplex, Immunine
Solvent/detergent (TNBP and polysorbate 80, or Triton X-100, or cholate)	Alpha, Biotest, BPL Pharmacia and Upjohn LFB-Lille, Octapharma AG	Profilnine SD, Alphanine SD, Factor IX Biotest, Replenine, Nanotiv, F IX VHP, Octanyne
Sodium thiocyanate plus ultrafiltration	Armour	Mononine
Solvent/detergent plus dry heating 100°C, 30 min	AIMA	AIMA F IX

TNBP = Tri(n-butyl) phosphate.

non-lipid-enveloped) of different shapes and sizes (from 20 to 300 nm) are excluded from passage through the membrane pores, whereas FIX molecules would pass through. HAV and human parvovirus B19 theoretically should not be able to pass through the pores (Table 19.3), however there are no trial results in recipients to confirm this.

NEWER APPROACHES AIMED AT VIRUS ATTENUATION OF PLASMA

Since fresh frozen plasma is still used for treatment of hemophilia in many parts of the world (Lusher *et al.*, 1994; Mannucci, 1995), in recent years there have been attempts to produce safer fresh frozen plasma by using modified virucidal methods. One approach, although not licensed for use at present, is that of adding solvent/detergent to pooled plasma (Chandy, 1995). Pasteurization has also been attempted (Horowitz *et al.*, 1992 and Burnouf-Radosevich *et al.*, 1992).

While improved donor screening techniques are now available, as noted by Mannucci (1995) and by Lusher *et al.* (1994), the risk of transmission of blood-borne infectious agents is not negligible. Additionally, to date no studies have been reported in human recipients to document whether or not solvent/detergent-treated plasma, or pasteurized plasma transmit blood-borne viruses.

Donor screening and vaccination

Blood screening for hepatitis B surface antigen (HBsAg) was first required by the US/FDA in 1972; testing by an improved method was required by 1976. However, some cases of HBV continued to occur in recipients of clotting factor concentrates (Stirling *et al.*, 1983; Kasper and Lusher, 1993). Fortunately, a hepatitis B vaccine became available in the early 1980s, and it has been strongly recommended that all hepatitis B-seronegative hemophiliacs be vaccinated (now with a recombinant hepatitis B vaccine).

There was still a high prevalence of non-A non-B hepatitis (NANBH) in recipients of blood as well as in recipients of clotting factor concentrates, however.

Table 19.3 Main blood-borne viruses transmitted by coagulation factor concentrates

Virus	Genome	Lipid-enveloped	Size (nm)	Solvent/detergent-resistant	Heat-resistant
Human immunodeficiency virus, type I	RNA	Yes	80–100	No	No
Hepatitis A virus	RNA	No	27	Yes	No
Hepatitis B virus	DNA	Yes	42	No	No
Hepatitic C virus	RNA	Yes	35–65	No	No
Hepatitis D virus	RNA	Yes	35	No	No
B19 parvovirus	DNA	No	20	Yes	Yes

Reprinted from Mannucci, P.M. (1995) Viral safety of plasma-derived and recombinant products used in the management of hemophila A and B. *Haemophilia* 1 (suppl. 1), 14–20, with permission.

While screening of whole blood donations for ALT and antibody to hepatitis B core (HBc) antigen (as surrogate tests for NANBH) was introduced in the USA in 1987, plasma that was anti-HBc positive was (and still is) used for fractionation. The stated rationale is that such antibody might neutralize any HBV not detected by screening.

Soon after the identification of HCV and development of an HCV antibody test, screening of whole blood donors in the USA began (spring, 1990). However, screening of plasma to be used in fractionation was not approved by the US/FDA until late 1991, for fear of 'removing neutralizing hepatitis antibody' (Finlayson and Tankersley, 1990; Kasper and Lusher, 1993). Soon thereafter, more specific second- and now third-generation serologic tests for antibody to HCV were developed and introduced. In view of these developments, a National Institutes of Health (NIH) Consensus Development Conference on Infectious Disease Testing for Blood Transfusions (January 9–22, 1995, Bethesda, MD) considered whether there was still a need for ALT testing, as well as testing of blood donors for HBc antibody, and syphilis testing. The panel recommended that ALT testing of blood donors be eliminated, but that syphilis testing and anti-HBs testing be retained (NIH Consensus, 1995). At present it is not known how soon this recommendation to drop ALT testing might be implemented by blood collection facilities, nor whether this recommendation will be adopted by the plasmapheresis industry.

While careful donor recruitment, selection and scrutiny, plus testing for viral markers, have greatly reduced the risks of transfusion-transmitted hepatitis and HIV infection (Thomas, 1994), the fact that plasma-derived clotting factor concentrates are produced from thousands of donors' plasma dramatically multiplies the risks – thus the need for highly effective viral attenuation methods (Lusher et al., 1994) and for effective vaccines.

At present, the only available vaccines against bloodborne viruses are hepatitis B vaccine and hepatitis A vaccine.

Risk of thrombogenicity with factor IX concentrates

Shortly after the introduction of PCCs, reports of thrombogenicity associated with their use began to appear (Triantaphyllopoulos, 1972; Kasper, 1973; Blatt et al., 1974; Cederblaum, Blatt and Roberts, 1976; Campbell, Neff and Bowdler, 1978). By the early 1970s it was apparent that a potential complication of PCC use was the development of serious thromboembolic events and/or DIC. During the preparation of PCC, some activation of clotting factors may occur. Thus, in addition to the vitamin K-dependent clotting factors, II, VII, IX and X, and proteins C and S, these concentrates contain small amounts of activated clotting factors (e.g. IXa, Xa). The latter, in addition to zymogen overload (particularly of factors II and X) have been implicated as causative agents for thromboembolic complications and DIC (White et al., 1977; Hultin, 1979; White, Lundblad and Kingdon, 1979; Seligsohn et al., 1979; Menaché et al., 1984).

While reports of thrombotic complications continued to appear in the early 1970s (Stirling et al., 1983; Thomas, 1994; NIH Consensus, 1995), Kasper surveyed hemophilia treaters in 1975 and found a large number of previously unreported cases of thrombotic complications and/or DIC in recipients of PCC (Kasper, 1975). As more reports continued to accumulate, in 1974 the Factor IX Task Force of the International Society on Thrombosis and Hemostasis (ISTH) recommended that 5–10 iu of heparin be added to each milliliter of reconstituted PCC just before use, especially in high-risk situations such as orthopedic surgery (Menaché and Roberts, 1975). The Task Force reaffirmed these recommendations the following year (Menaché, 1976).

With increasing recognition of these thrombogenic risks, by the late 1970s many physicians were suspending all elective surgical procedures – or, at least, all elective orthopedic surgical procedures – in persons with hemophilia B. For necessary surgery, many also advocated giving FFP or antithrombin III concentrates, as a source of antithrombin III on the day of surgery (Lusher, 1993).

While the addition of heparin to reconstituted PCC, and providing a source of antithrombin III certainly did not eliminate this risk (Lusher, 1991), such measures, plus an increased awareness of the thrombogenic potential and thus more judicious use of PCC, probably prevented an even high rate of such complications. None the less, there was an obvious need for a non-thrombogenic FIX concentrate.

Coagulation factor IX concentrates

During the late 1980s, so-called coagulation FIX concentrates (high-purity FIX concentrates without the other vitamin K-dependent clotting factors) were developed. Three of these were licensed for use in the USA in the early 1990s: Alpha Nine (Alpha Therapeutic Corp., Los Angeles, CA), Alpha Nine SD (Alpha Therapeutic Corp.), and Mononine (Armour Pharmaceutical Co., Collegeville, PA; Table 19.4A). Other coagulation FIX concentrates which are now available in Europe include AIMA's AIMAFIX, Biotest Pharma's Factor IX Biotest, LFB's Factor IX VHP, Immuno's Immunine, Kabi Pharmacia's Nanotiv, Octapharma's Octanyne, and BPL's Replenine (Table 19.4B). These high-purity FIX concentrates contain much higher specific activity FIX (100–300 iu/mg protein) and appear to be far less thrombogenic than are FIXCC (Mannucci et al., 1991;

Table 19.4A Coagulation factor IX products marketed for use in the USA (1996)

Brand name	Manufacturer	Food and Drug Administration License	Specific activity*	Method of viral depletion	Separation method
Alpha Nine SD	Alpha Therapeutic Corporation	8/92	190	TNBP and polysorbate 80 and loss of virus through affinity chromatography	Ion exchange and dual polysaccharide ligand affinity chromatography
Mononine	Armour Pharmaceutical Co.	8/92	188	Sodium thiocyanate and loss of virus through ultrafiltration	Monoclonal antibody immunoaffinity and other chromatography

*Approximate values.
TNBP = Tri(n-butyl)phosphate.

Table 19.4B Coagulation factor IX products marketed for use in European countries (1995)

Brand name	Manufacturer	Specific activity*	Viral inactivation†	Separation method
AIMAFIX	AIMA	100	TNBP and Tween 80; end-stage heating at 100°C for 30 min	Affinity with chromatography and diafiltration and absorption on heparin sepharose
Factor IX Biotest	Biotest Pharma	100	TNBP and Tween 80	Ion exchange and affinity chromatography
Factor IX VHP	LFB	120–200	TNBP and Tween 80	Ion exchange and affinity chromatography
Immunine	Immuno	100	Vapor-heated, 10 h at 60°C, 1190 mbar plus 1 h at 80°C, 1375 mbar	Ion exchange and hydrophobic interaction chromatography
Nanotiv	Pharmacia	200	TNBP and Triton X-100	Ion exchange and affinity chromatography
Octanyne	Octapharma	60–90	TNBP and Tween 80	Ion exchange and affinity chromatography
Replenine	BPL	164	TNBP and Tween 80	Anion exchange and metal chelate affinity chromatography

*Approximate values.
†Also loss of virus through chromatographic steps.

Goldsmith *et al.*, 1992; Berntorp *et al.*, 1993; Herring *et al.*, 1993). Sensitive tests for intravascular coagulation, including such sensitive biologic markers of the *in vivo* activation of the hemostatic system as prothrombin activation fragment F1+2, have shown no elevation after infusion of these coagulation FIX products (Kim *et al.*, 1991, 1992; Mannucci *et al.*, 1991; Kasper and Lusher, 1993; Shapiro, 1994).

Bioavailability, pharmacokinetics and efficacy of the coagulation FIX concentrates appear to be identical to FIXCC (Hrinda *et al.*, 1991; Kim *et al.*, 1991, 1992; Goldsmith *et al.*, 1992). While these high-purity, far less thrombogenic FIX concentrates are considerably more expensive than FIXCC, their use in hemophilia B seems very well-justified in certain high-risk situations. They are recommended for use in neonates, in persons with hemophilia B undergoing surgery (particularly orthopedic surgery), in those with crush injuries or large intramuscular hemorrhages, in those with hepatocellular dysfunction, and in anyone with a history of thrombotic problems following FIXCC (i.e. in any high-risk situation for thrombosis or DIC; Medical and Scientific Advisory Council, 1992; Lusher, 1995). In view of a few reports of DIC and/or thrombotic problems in recipients of

FIXCC who did not appear to have any of these high-risk factors or situations, many now prefer to use coagulation FIX concentrates in all persons with hemophilia B.

Recombinant factor IX

Factor IX was successfully cloned at approximately the same time as was FVIII (Anson, Austen and Brownlee, 1985; de la Salle *et al.*, 1985). However, its commercial production proved difficult, largely due to the complex nature of the protein and the requirement for consistent reproduction of several posttranslational modifications. Scientists at Genetics Institute (Cambridge, Ma.) have now developed a recombinant (r) human (h) FIX product which began evaluation in prelicensure clinical trials in 1995. At present, however, there is no licensed rFIX product available. In producing rhFIX, the Genetics Institute uses a well-characterized Chinese hamster (CHO) cell line transfected with human FIX complementary DNA. The rhFIX cell line is grown in medium which is free of serum, and of any animal or human-derived components. The final product contains no carrier proteins or preservatives.

As with rFVIII, such recombinant FIX technology would appear to offer not only viral safety, but unlimited supply – theoretically, sufficient to meet the needs of all hemophilia B patients.

Activated prothrombin complex concentrates for use in inhibitor patients

Since the early 1970s, PCCs have been the mainstay of treatment for bleeding episodes in hemophiliacs with inhibitor antibodies to FVIII or FIX. Following initial reports by Fekete *et al.* (1972) and by Roberts (1972), which described the effectiveness of PCC in controlling bleeding in inhibitor patients, many physicians treating hemophiliacs with inhibitors began using large doses (50–75 iu FIX/kg) of PCC, despite the fact that their mechanisms of action in this setting were unknown (Lusher, 1990). Since one assumption was that the beneficial effects of PCC in controlling bleeding in inhibitor patients resulted primarily from the small amounts of activated clotting factors which they contained, two manufacturers of PCC began producing purposely activated PCCs (APCCs). These two products, Baxter/Hyland's Autoplex and Immuno's FEIBA (for Factor Eight Inhibitor Bypassing Activity), are produced for use in inhibitor patients only; they should not be used in persons with hemophilia B without inhibitors, as the risk of thrombogenicity would be increased in the latter. While many felt that these purposely activated PCCs were considerably more effective than standard PCC in controlling bleeding in inhibitor patients, especially for

surgical coverage or other open types of bleeding, others remained skeptical about the use of both PCC and APCC (Lusher, 1990). Not only was their precise mechanism of action unknown, but there were no laboratory tests for monitoring their effectiveness in inhibitor patients, and they did not always work.

In an attempt to determine whether or not PCC really were effective in controlling bleeding in inhibitor patients, a group of investigators who were participating in the US Inhibitor Study Group designed and conducted a placebo-controlled clinical trial in the late 1970s. This trial (which then served as a model for later trials comparing other products), compared three unknowns – Cutter's Konyne, Hyland's Proplex and an albumin placebo. Episodes of acute hemarthrosis were treated with a single dose of unknown product, and subjective and objective assessments of efficacy were recorded at 6 h. Trial results indicated that a single dose of either PCC (Konyne or Proplex) was effective in controlling 50% of episodes of joint bleeding, while, interestingly, the albumin placebo was judged effective 25% of the time (Lusher *et al.*, 1980).

In an attempt to determine whether or not the more expensive APCCs were more effective than standard PCC in inhibitor patients, two controlled trials were conducted, one in the Netherlands and one in the USA. The US trial compared two different doses of Hyland's Autoplex (50 and 75 u/kg) and Hyland's non-activated PCC, Proplex, in the treatment of acute hemoarthrosis. Just as in the original trial, a single dose of unknown product was given and efficacy was assessed at 6 h (Lusher *et al.*, 1983). The Dutch trial compared Immuno's FEIBA to that company's non-activated PCC, Prothromplex. While the majority of bleeding episodes in the Dutch trial were acute hemarthroses, some episodes of intramuscular bleeding were included as well. For the latter, a second dose of unknown product was permitted. Assessment of efficacy was done at 1, 6 and 24 h (Sjamsoedin *et al.*, 1981). Under the trial conditions, no difference was noted between Autoplex (at either dosage) and Proplex (Lusher *et al.*, 1983), while there was a slightly higher response to FEIBA than to the non-activated PCC (Sjamsoedin *et al.*, 1981). It is noteworthy that in each of the three controlled trials approximately 50% of episodes of acute hemarthrosis responded to a single dose of standard PCC (Lusher *et al.*, 1980, 1983; Sjamsoedin *et al.*, 1981; Lusher, 1984).

While all PCCs are now virally attenuated (and thus differ slightly from those used in the trials), and while none of the currently available PCC (Table 19.2) or APCC (Table 19.5) have been subjected to controlled trials in inhibitor patients, PCC and APCC remain the mainstay of treatment for acute hemarthroses and soft-tissue bleeding in persons with high-titer FVIII or FIX inhibitors in most hemophilia centers. Dosage generally

Table 19.5 Activated complex concentrates* currently available in north America and Europe

Brand name	Manufacturer	Food and drug administration license	Specific activity†	Methods of viral inactivation	Separation method
Autoplex T	Baxter-Hyland	January 1987	5	Dry heat, 68°C, 144 h	Tri-calcium phosphate adsorption, polyethylene glycol precipitation, then activated
FEIBA VH	IMMUNO	January 1986	0.8	Vapor-heated, 10 h 60°C, 1190 mbar plus 1 h, 80°C, 1375 mbar	Surface-activated Factor IX complex

*Note: These activated products should be used only in persons with factor VIII or factor IX inhibitors.
†Approximate values.

used is 50–100 u/kg, and most use the same dosage calculation for standard PCC, Autoplex T and FEIBA VH, even though the unit systems are not equivalent. When using standard PCCs, one is calculating dosage in terms of FIX units. For the two APCCs, it should be noted that one factor VIII inhibitor bypassing activity (FEIBA) unit, as defined by Immuno, is not the same as one factor VIII correctional unit (FECU), as defined by Hyland for Autoplex T (Lusher, 1984, 1990).

Most physicians treating persons with hemophilia and inhibitors feel that PCC and APCC are moderately effective, but not predictably so. They are certainly not as effective as FVIII in a hemophilia A patient without inhibitors. As a result, many patients with long-standing high-titer inhibitors who have been treated with PCC and/or APCC have a greater degree of progressive debilitating musculoskeletal disease than do non-inhibitor patients of similar age. Also, as a result of less than optimal response to PCC and APCC, often more than one dose is given in an attempt to control bleeding. This not only increases the cost, but increases the risk of DIC, thromboembolism and even acute myocardial infarction. Many of the predominantly young inhibitor patients who have sustained acute myocardial infarction (often fatal) had received large, repetitive doses of PCC or APCC, but had little else in common (Agrawal, Zelkowitz and Hletko, 1981; Gruppo, Bove and Donaldson, 1983; Sullivan *et al.*, 1984; Chavin *et al.*, 1988). Most who came to postmortem examination had large transmural hemorrhages of the myocardium (Chavin *et al.*, 1988). While the precise pathogenesis of this serious complication remains unclear, one should avoid frequent repeated doses of PCC or APCC. If a bleeding episode in an inhibitor patient fails to respond to two or three doses of PCC or APCC, it is unlikely that additional doses will be beneficial and they may be quite harmful. Thus, one should consider another therapeutic option. Similarly, for iliopsoas bleeding, head injury or other serious types of bleeding where several days of treatment will be required, another type of product (for example, porcine FVIII or rFVIIa) should be used.

References

Agrawal, B.K., Zelkowitz, L. and Hletko, P. (1981) Acute myocardial infarction in a young hemophiliac patient during therapy with factor IX concentrate and epsilon aminocaproic acid. *J Pediatr*, **98**, 931–933.

Allain, J.P., Dalley, S.H., Laurian, Y. *et al.* (1991) Evidence for persistent hepatitis C virus (HCV) infection in hemophiliacs. *J Clin Invest*, **88**, 1672–1679.

Anson, D.S., Austen, D.E.G. and Brownlee, G.G. (1985) Expression of active human clotting factor IX from recombinant DNA clones in mammalian cells. *Nature*, **315**, 683–685.

Bennett, B., Dawson, A.A., Gibson, B.S. *et al.* (1993) Study of viral safety of Scottish National Blood Transfusion Service factor VIII/IX concentrates. *Transfusion Med*, **3**, 295–298.

Berntorp, E., Björkman, S., Carlsson, M. *et al.* (1993) Biochemical and *in vivo* properties of high purity factor IX concentrates. *Thromb Haemostas*, **70**, 768–773.

Blanchette, V.S., Vorstman, E., Shore, A. *et al.* (1991) Hepatitis C infection in children with hemophilia A and B. *Blood*, **78**, 285–289.

Blatrix, C. and Soulier, J.P. (1959) Preparation d'une fraction riche en prothrombine, proconvertine, facteur Stuart et facteur antihemophilique B (fraction P.P.B.) *Pathol Biol (Paris)*, **7**, 2477–2486.

Blatt, P.M., Lundblad, R.L., Kingdon, H.S. *et al.* (1974) Thrombogenic materials in prothrombin complex concentrates. *Ann Intern Med*, **81**, 766–770.

Brettler, D.B., Alter, H.J., Dienstag, J.L. *et al.* (1990) Prevalence of hepatitis C virus antibody in a cohort of hemophilia patients. *Blood*, **76**, 254–256.

Burnouf-Radosevich, M., Burnouf, T. and Huart, J.J. (1992) A pasteurized therapeutic plasma. *Infusions Ther*, **19**, 91–94.

Burnouf-Radosevich, M., Appourchaux, P., Huart, J.J. and Burnouf, T. (1994) Nanofiltration, a new specific virus elimination method applied to high purity factor IX and factor XI concentrates. *Vox Sang*, **67**, 132–138.

Campbell, E.W., Neff, S. and Bowlder, A.J. (1978) Therapy with factor IX concentrate resulting in DIC and thromboembolic phenomena. *Transfusion*, **18**, 94.

Carnelli, V., Gomperts, E.D., Friedman, A. *et al.* (1987) Assessment for evidence of non-A, non-B hepatitis in patients given n-heptane suspended heat-treated clotting factor concentrates. *Thromb Res*, **46**, 827–834.

Cederbaum, A.L., Blatt, P.M. and Roberts, H.R. (1976) Intravascular coagulation association with the use of human prothrombin complex. *Ann Intern Med*, **84**, 683.

Centers for Disease Control (1982) *Pneumocystis carinii* pneumonia among persons with hemophilia A. *Morb Mortal Wkly Rep*, **31**, 365–367.

Chandy, M. (1995) Management of haemophilia in developing countries with available resources. *Haemophilia*, **1** (suppl. 1), 44–48.

Chavin, S.I., Siegel, D.M., Rocco, T.A. Jr and Olson, J.P. (1988) Acute myocardial infarction during treatment with an activated prothrombin complex concentrates in a patient with factor VIII deficiency and a factor VIII inhibitor. *Am J Med*, **85**, 245–249.

de la Salle, H., Attenburger, W., Elkaim, R. *et al.* (1985) Active gamma-carboxylated human factor IX expressed using recombinant DNA techniques. *Nature*, **316**, 268–273.

Fekete, L.F., Holst, S.L., Peetoom, F. and DeVeber, L.L. (1972) 'Auto' factor IX concentrate: a new therapeutic approach to treatment of hemophilia A patients with inhibitors. Abstract 295, presented at XIV Congress, *Int Soc Hematol, Sao Paulo, Brazil, July 16–22, 1972.*

Finlayson, J.S. and Tankersley, D.L. (1990) Anti-HCV screening and plasma fractionation: the case against. *Lancet*, **335**, 1274–1275.

Gerritzen, A., Schneweis, K.E., Brackmann, H.H. *et al.* (1992) Acute hepatitis A in hemophiliacs. *Lancet*, **340**, 1231–1232.

Goldsmith, J.C., Kasper, C.K., Blatt, P.M. *et al.* (1992) Coagulation factor IX: successful surgical experience with a purified FIX concentrate. *Am J Hematol*, **40**, 210–215.

Gruppo, R.A., Bove, K.E. and Donaldson, V. (1983) Fatal myocardial necrosis associated with prothrombin complex concentrate therapy in hemophilia A. *N Engl J Med*, **309**, 242–243.

Hasiba, U., Spero, J.A. and Lewis, J.H. (1976) Chronic liver dysfunction in multi-transfused hemophiliacs, in *Unsolved Therapeutic Problems in Hemophilia* (eds J.C. Fratantoni and D.L. Aronson), Dept of Health, Education and Welfare publication no. (NIH) 77–1089, pp. 81–87.

Herring, S.W., Abildgaard, C., Shitanishsi, K.T. *et al.* (1993) Human coagulation factor IX: assessment of thrombogenicity in criminal models and viral safety. *J Lab Clin Med*, **121**, 394–405.

Horowitz, B., Bonomo, R., Prince, A.M. *et al.* (1992) Solvent/detergent treated plasma: a virus-inactivated substitute for fresh frozen plasma. *Blood*, **79**, 826–831.

Hrinda, M.E., Huang, C., Tarr, G.C. *et al.* (1991) Preclinical studies of monoclonal antibody-purified factor IX, Moninine. *Semin Hematol*, **28** (suppl. 6), 6–14.

Hultin, M.B. (1979) Activated clotting factors in factor IX concentrates. *Blood*, **54**, 1028.

Kasper, C.K. (1973) Postoperative thromboses in hemophilia B. *N Engl J Med*, **289**, 160.

Kasper, C.K. (1975) Thromboembolic complications. *Thromb Diath Haemorrh*, **33**, 640–644.

Kasper, C.K., Lusher, J.M. and Transfusion Practices Committee (1993) Recent evolution of clotting factor concentrates for hemophilia A and B. *Transfusion*, **33**, 422–434.

Kim, H.C., Matts, L., Eisele, J. *et al.* (1991) Monoclonal antibody – purified factor IX – comparative thrombogenicity to prothrombin complex concentrate. *Semin Hematol*, **28** (suppl. 6), 15–19.

Kim, H.C., McMillan, C., White, G.C. *et al.* (1992) Purified factor IX using monoclonal immune affinity technique: clinical trials in hemophilia B and comparison to prothrombin complex concentrates. *Blood*, **79**, 568–575.

Lush, C.J., Chapman, C.S., Mitchell, V.E. and Martin, C. (1988) Transmission of hepatitis B by dry heat treated factor VIII and IX concentrates. *Br J Haematol*, **69**, 421–428.

Lusher, J.M. (1984) Controlled clinical trials with prothrombin complex concentrates. *Progr Clin Biol Res*, **150**, 277–290.

Lusher, J.M. (1990) Strategies to promote hemostasis in patients with FVIII inhibitors, in *Recent Advances in Hemophilia Care* (ed. C.K. Kasper), Alan R. Liss, New York, pp. 39–46.

Lusher, J.M. (1991) Thrombogenicity associated with factor IX complex concentrates. *Semin Hematol*, **28** (suppl. 6), 3–4.

Lusher, J.M. (1993) Prediction and management of adverse events associated with the use of FIX complex concentrates. *Semin Hematol*, **30** (suppl. 1), 36–40.

Lusher, J.M. (1995) Considerations for current and future management of haemophilia and its complications. *Haemophilia*, **1**, 2–10.

Lusher, J.M., Shapiro, S.S., Palascak, J.E. *et al.* (1980) Efficacy of prothrombin complex concentrates in hemophiliacs with antibodies to factor VIII: a multicenter therapeutic trial. *N Engl J Med*, **303**, 421–425.

Lusher, J.M., Blatt, P.M., Penner, J.A. *et al.* (1983) Autoplex vs. proplex: a controlled, double blind study of effectiveness of hemophiliacs with inhibitors to factor VIII. *Blood*, **62**, 1135–1138.

Lusher, J.M. and the Transfusion Safety Study Group (1991) Anti-HCV prevalence in relation to type and amount of clotting factor therapy in congenital clotting disorders. *Thromb Haemost*, **65**, 996.

Lusher, J.M., Kessler, C.M., Laurian, Y. and Pierce, G. (1994) Viral contamination of blood products. *Lancet*, **334**, 405–406.

Mannucci, P.M. (1992) Outbreak of hepatitis A among Italian patients with hemophilia. *Lancet*, **1**, 819.

Mannucci, P.M. (1995) Viral safety of plasma-derived and recombinant products used in the management of hemophilia A and B. *Haemophilia*, **1** (suppl. 1), 14–20.

Mannucci, P.M. and Colombo, M. (1989) Revision of the protocol recommended for studies of safety from hepatitis of clotting factor concentrates. *Thrombos Haemost*, **61**, 532–534.

Mannucci, P.M., Bauer, K.A., Gringeri, A. *et al.* (1991) No activation of the common pathway of the coagulation cascade after a highly purified factor IX concentrate. *Br J Haematol*, **79**, 606–611.

Mannucci, P.M., Schimpf, K., Abe, T. *et al.* (1992) Low risk of viral infection after administration of vapour heated factor VIII concentrates. *Transfusion*, **32**, 134–138.

Mauser-Bunschoten, E.P., Bresters, D., Reesink, H.W. *et al.* (1995) Effect and side-effects of alpha interferon treatment in haemophilia patients with chronic hepatitis C. *Hemophilia*, **1**, 45–53.

Medical and Scientific Advisory Council (1992) Statement regarding the use of coagulation factor IX products in persons with hemophilia B. *Medical Bulletin*, 29 May. The National Hemophilia Foundation, 110 Greene St, Suite 303, New York, NY 10012, USA.

Menaché, D. (1976) Report of the task force on the clinical use of factor IX concentrates. *Thrombos Haemostas*, **35**, 748–750.

Menaché, D. and Roberts, H.R. (1975) Summary report and recommendations of task force members and consultants. *Thromb Haemostas*, **33**, 645–647.

Menaché, D., Fauvert, R. and Soulier, J.P. (1959) Utilisation en hepatologie d'une fraction contenant la prothrombine, le complex proconvertine-facteur Stuart et le facteur antihemophilique B (RPB). *Pathol Biol (Paris)*, **7**, 2515–2523.

Menaché, D., Behre, H.E., Orthner, C.L. *et al.* (1984) Coagulation factor IX concentrate: method of preparation and assessment of potential *in vivo* thrombogenicity in animal models. *Blood*, **64**, 1220–1227.

NIH Consensus Statement (1995) *Infectious Disease Testing for Blood Transfusions*. National Institutes of Health, Bethesda, MD.

Peerlinck, K. and Vermylen, J. (1993) Acute hepatitis A in patients with hemophilia. *Lancet*, **341**, 189.

Pistello, M., Ceccherini-Nelli, L., Cecconi, E. *et al.* (1991) Hepatitis C virus-inactivated concentrates: five year follow-up and correlation with antibodies to other viruses. *J Med Virol*, **33**, 43–46.

Ragni, M.V., Wikelstein, A., Kingsley, L. *et al.* (1987) 1986 update of HIV seroprevalence, seroconversion AIDS incidence, and immunologic correlates of HIV infection in patients with hemophilia A and B. *Blood*, **70**, 786–790.

Roberts, H.R. (1972) Use of animal factor VIII concentrates in patients with factor VIII inhibitors. Presented at 15th annual meeting of Am. Soc. Hematol., Hollywood, Fla., Dec. 3, 1972.

Rumi, M.G., Colombo, M., Gringeri, A. and Mannucci, P.M. (1990) High prevalence of antibody to hepatitis C virus in multitransfused hemophiliacs with normal transaminase levels. *Ann Intern Med*, **112**, 379–380.

Schimpf, K., Mannucci, P.M., Kreutz, W. *et al.* (1987) Absence of hepatitis after treatment with a pasteurized factor VIII concentrate in patients with hemophilia and no previous transfusions. *N Engl J Med*, **316**, 918–922.

Seligsohn, U., Kasper, C.K., Osterud, B. and Rapaport, S.I. (1979) Activated factor VII: presence in factor IX concentrates and persistence in the circulation after infusion. *Blood*, **53**, 828.

Shapiro, A.D. (1994) New factor IX concentrates. *Int J Pediatr Hematol Oncol*, **1**, 479–490.

Shapiro, A., Bergman, G.E. and the Mononine Study Group (1993) Monoclonal antibody purified factor IX: viral safety in PUPS. *Blood*, **82** (suppl. 1), 64a.

Shapiro, A. and the International Factor Safety Study Group (1993) Vapor heated intermediate purity factor IX concentrate tested in a safety study monitoring transfusion-related viral infections in previously untreated hemophiliacs. *Thromb Haemostas*, **69**, 943.

Sjamsoedin, L.J., Heijnen, L., Mauser-Bunschoten, E.P. *et al.* (1981) The effect of activated prothrombin complex concentrate (FEIBA) on joint and muscle bleeding in patients with hemophilia A and antibodies to factor VIII. *N Engl J Med*, **305**, 717–721.

Skidmore, S.J., Pasi, K.J., Mawson, S.J. *et al.* (1990) Serological evidence that dry heating of clotting factor concentrates prevents transmission of non-A, non-B hepatitis. *J Med Virol*, **30**, 5052.

Stirling, M.L., Murray, J.A., Mackay, P. *et al.* (1983) Incidence of infection with hepatitis B virus in 56 patients with hemophilia A 1971–79. *J Clin Pathol*, **36**, 577–580.

Study Group of the UK Haemopholia Centre Directors (1988) Effect of dry heating of coagulation factor concentrates at 80°C for 72 hours on transmission of non-A, non-B hepatitis. *Lancet*, **2**, 814–816.

Sullivan, D.W., Purdy, L.J., Billingham, M. and Glader, B.E. (1984) Fatal myocardial infarction following therapy with prothrombin complex concentrates in a young man with hemophilia A. *Pediatrics*, **74**, 279–281.

Temperley, I.J., Cotter, K.P., Walsh, T.J. *et al.* (1992) Clotting factors and hepatitis. *Lancet*, **30**, 1466.

Thomas, D. (1994) Viral contamination of blood products. *Lancet*, **343**, 1583–1584.

Triantaphyllopoulos, D.C. (1972) Intravascular coagulation following injection of prothrombin complex. *Am J Clin Pathol*, **57**, 603–610.

Troisi, C.L., Hollinger, F.B., Hoots, W.K. *et al.* (1993) A multicenter study of viral hepatitis in a United States hemophilia population. *Blood*, **81**, 412–418.

White, G.C., Roberts, H.R., Kingdom, H.S. and Lundblad, R.L. (1977). Prothrombin complex concentrates: potentially thrombogenic materials and clues to the mechanisms of thrombosis *in vivo*. *Blood*, **49**, 159.

White, G.C. 2nd, Lundblad, R.L. and Kingdom, H.S. (1979) Prothrombin complex concentrates: preparation, properties and clinical uses. *Curr Topics Hematol*, **2**, 203–244.

20 INHIBITORS IN HEMOPHILIA

L.W. Hoyer

The development of an inhibitor, an antibody that blocks procoagulant function, is one of the most serious complications of hemophilia A or of hemophilia B treatment. Similar antibodies are also recognized as a rare cause of bleeding in previously healthy individuals who develop autoimmune antifactor VIII antibodies.

While the clinical impact of inhibitor development has been recognized for over half a century (Munro, 1946; Margolius, Jackson and Ratnoff, 1961), recent studies have just begun to clarify several important issues. They have focused on three areas: better understanding of the incidence of inhibitors following coagulation factor treatment and identification of patients at highest risk of inhibitor formation, characterization of the antibodies, and the development of better therapies. Almost all of these studies have been directed toward the two more common clinical presentations – hemophilia A complicated by development of an antifactor VIII and auto-antibodies to factor VIII.

Clinical features

The typical frequency or location of bleeding usually does not change in hemophilic patients when an inhibitor develops, and joint hemorrhages continue to be the major problem. However, the development of an inhibitor should be suspected if a hemophilic patient does not respond appropriately to factor VIII (or factor IX) infusions. The question usually can be resolved by demonstrating rapid factor VIII (or factor IX) disappearance from the plasma or by *in vitro* assays. The inhibitor level does not correlate well with the frequency of bleeding, but it does limit the kinds of treatment that are possible. Although uncontrolled hemorrhage is a concern for the inhibitor patient, life expectancy is only modestly shortened (Kasper, 1989).

The clinical presentation of antifactor VIII autoantibodies is, of course, quite different, for these previously healthy individuals usually seek medical attention because of large hematomas or ecchymoses. In many cases there is also considerable intramuscular bleeding after relatively trivial trauma. Immediate attention is needed if pressure due to this bleeding compromises vessels or nerves, resulting in the development of a compartment syndrome. However, brisk and uncontrollable hemorrhage may complete surgical attempts at decompression and abnormal bleeding may first be recognized during a surgical procedure. In contrast to patients with hemophilia A, patients with autoantibody factor VIII inhibitors rarely have hemarthroses.

Inhibitor incidence

INHIBITOR INCIDENCE IN HEMOPHILIA A

Inhibitors have not been recognized in hemophilia A patients before exposure to factor VIII or a blood product containing factor VIII. Although these antibodies have been detected after as few as three to five treatments (Bray, 1992; Ehrenforth *et al.*, 1992; Lusher *et al.*, 1993), the likelihood of developing an inhibitor appears to be related to the number of exposures (Strauss, 1969; Schwarzinger *et al.*, 1987; Rasi and Ikkala, 1990; Ehrenforth *et al.*, 1992). Thus, during the first 5–10 years of life, the incidence of inhibitors in severe hemophilia A increases with the number of factor VIII infusions and new inhibitors are rarely detected after 90–100 exposure days (Strauss, 1969; McMillan *et al.*, 1988).

The frequency of patient assessment is also a key issue in evaluating inhibitor incidence. For example, several studies have detected transient low titer inhibitors that were not suspected on clinical grounds and that were

Hemophilia. Edited by C.D. Forbes, L. Aledort and R. Madhok. Published in 1997 by Chapman & Hall, London. ISBN 0 412 63820 7

only identified because of routine assessment every 3–6 months (McMillan *et al.*, Bray, 1992; Ehrenforth *et al.*, 1992; 1988; Ljung *et al.*, 1992; Lusher *et al.*, 1993).

It is controversial whether the likelihood of inhibitor formation is related to the purity of the administered factor VIII or to its production process. This issue was initially raised when more highly purified factor VIII concentrates were introduced, and it has been of special concern with the introduction of recombinant factor VIII concentrates since there is the possibility that subtle differences in factor VIII synthesis and processing might affect immunogenicity. In fact, there are some differences in the carbohydrate composition of recombinant factor VIII when compared to that purified from pooled normal plasma (Hironaka *et al.*, 1992). However, it has been very uncommon for previously multitransfused patients to develop an inhibitor when treatment was changed to monoclonal antibody-purified or recombinant factor VIII (Schwartz *et al.*, 1990; Bray, 1992; Addiego *et al.*, 1992).

Since most inhibitors are known to develop during the first few years of treatment of severe hemophilia A, most efforts to determine inhibitor incidence have evaluated the response to factor VIII in previously untreated patients (PUPs). However, the interpretation of inhibitor incidence has been difficult for these new products as there are no previous prospective studies. Until the late 1980s, inhibitor assessments were retrospective, and were based on the development of resistance to factor VIII treatment – with *in vitro* confirmation that a factor VIII inhibitor was responsible.

Unfortunately, the sequential introductions of inter-mediate-purity concentrates, the monoclonal antibody-purified factor VIII concentrates and recombinant factor VIII were not systematically evaluated for possible product-related changes in inhibitor risk. Indeed, the retrospective analyses have provided a very confusing picture. For example, while inhibitor development was infrequent for patients treated with cryoprecipitate in Belgium (7%; Peerlinck, Rosendaal and Vermylen, 1993), patients treated with plasma and cryoprecipitate at one US center had a much higher incidence (35%; Strauss, 1969). In the case of intermediate-purity prod-ucts, the cumulative incidence in different reports has been from less than 20% to almost 30% (Schwarzinger *et al.*, 1987; Rasi and Ikkala, 1990; Ehrenforth *et al.*, 1992; Ljung *et al.*, 1992; Lorenzo, Garcia and Molina, 1992; Addiego *et al.*, 1993; De Biasi *et al.*, 1994). For the monoclonal antibody-purified products, the small series designed primarily to evaluate infectious disease markers identified persistent inhibitors in 7 and 18% of PUPs (Lusher *et al.*, 1990; Addiego *et al.*, 1992).

In a very useful analysis, Briët *et al.* (1994) summariz-ed the key data for eight of these studies, limiting the comparison to those patients at highest risk (severe hemophilia A) who developed a high-response inhibitor.

The cumulative incidence of high-response inhibitors reached a plateau at 20% for this group of 451 patients after 18 years of follow-up (Briët *et al.*, 1994). However, the individual studies had cumulative incidence values from 2 to 46%, demonstrating the hazard of drawing conclusions from relatively small patient groups.

Two recent reports of the recombinant factor VIII trials provide the first detailed prospective characterizations of inhibitor development in previously untreated patients with severe hemophilia A (Lusher *et al.*, 1993; Bray *et al.*, 1994). Each multi-institution study reported data for patients with severe hemophilia A who had no prior exposure to any blood products and who were tested for an inhibitor every 3 months. At the times of publication, 14 (29%) of the 49 patients treated with Kogenate had developed an inhibitor, as had 17 (24%) of the 73 patients treated with Recombinate. However, these numbers may be misleading in two quite different ways. They are proba-bly underestimates of the overall risk of inhibitor forma-tion, since the exposure to factor VIII was relatively limited in both groups of patients. The median exposure days were only 10 and 16, respectively, for the patients who had not developed an inhibitor. To address this, the cumulative inhibitor incidence was assessed as a function of factor VIII exposure, with censoring of incomplete information, i.e. by a Kaplan–Meier plot. When analyzed in this way, the risk of inhibitor formation in the Recombinate trial was 38% after 25 exposure days and 36% after 18 exposure days in the Kogenate trial. Most of the study populations had not reached that level of exposure, however, and these values may be revised with longer follow-up.

However, it is misleading simply to count the number of patients whose plasma has a detectable antifactor VIII inhibitor at one or more assessments. Transient inhibitors were recognized in both studies (5/17 and 4/14), and these patients were successfully managed by standard, on-demand factor VIII treatment for bleeding events (Lusher *et al.*, 1993; Bray *et al.*, 1994). Many low-titer, low-response inhibitors were also detected, and most children with titers below 10 Bethesda units (BU; see below) continued to receive recombinant factor VIII for the treatment or prevention of bleeding. Their clinical response was good to excellent at conventional or modestly increased doses.

When these retrospective and prospective studies of inhibitor formation in PUPs are taken together, the best tentative conclusion is that there are no consistent differences related to the factor VIII source (Briët and Rosendaal, 1994; Hoyer, 1995). However, other recent studies have established that the manufacturing process can predispose to inhibitor formation. This is clear from the 'epidemic' of at least 14 new inhibitors that were recognized in the Netherlands and in Belgium following the introduction in 1991 of a factor VIII concentrate prepared by controlled-pore glass chromatography followed by pasteurization (Peerlinck *et al.*, 1993; Rosendaal *et al.*, 1993). Inhibitor development after exposure to this particular concentrate was much greater than for comparable patients in other studies; these patients had also been treated for many years (McMillan *et al.*, 1988). Moreover, some of the patients treated with this concentrate were in a clinical trial in which half of the patients received the same concentrate treated with the solvent/detergent method of virus inactivation rather than pasteurization. Inhibitors only developed in patients receiving the pasteurized concentrate (Peerlinck *et al.*, 1993). While the production method may have increased the factor VIII immunogenicity, pasteurization itself was not necessarily responsible since other pasteurized products have not had this problem (Rosendaal *et al.*, 1993). Subsequent *in vitro* studies of the pasteurized product indicated that it had a much more rapid effect on factor Xa generation than when sterilized by dry heat (Barrowcliffe, 1993). It is not known, of course, if the small amounts of activated factor VIII influenced inhibitor development. Fortunately, the clinical outcome was good for these inhibitor patients and the antibody levels decreased rapidly after they were switched from this product to another concentrate (Mauser-Bunschoten *et al.*, 1994). Eight months later, all had <1 BU and the factor VIII recovery was normal.

Careful analysis stimulated by the Netherlands–Belgium epidemic has reinforced the concept that inhibitors are uncommon in hemophilic patients who have been treated with factor VIII for a long period of time (McMillan *et al.*, 1988; Rosendaal *et al.*, 1993). It is likely that the rare antibodies that do develop are an immunologic response to modified factor VIII molecules that have neoantigens. As Briët has suggested, secondary inhibitors recognized in patients who have been treated with factor VIII for long periods of time may have a different immunologic basis than the primary antibodies that develop after only a few exposures to factor VIII (Briët, 1995).

INCIDENCE OF FACTOR IX INHIBITORS

Inhibitors occur infrequently in hemophilia B patients following treatment with factor IX concentrates. As in hemophilia A, only patients with severe coagulation deficiency are likely to develop an inhibitor and they are less frequent in patients with severe hemophilia B than in hemophilia A; most studies suggest an incidence of no more than 5% (Briët, 1991). Most of these patients have major gene deletions and there is no detectable factor IX protein in the plasma (Giannelli, Choo Rees, 1983).

INCIDENCE OF AUTOANTIBODY INHIBITORS

Autoantibodies to factor VIII are rare ($1-5/10^6$ population per year; Lottenberg, Kentro and Kitchens, 1987) and are recognized predominantly in adults, especially in postpartum women, individuals with immunologic disorders, including systemic lupus erythematosus and rheumatoid arthritis, and older adults with no apparent underlying disease. The disorder appears to be evenly distributed between males and females. Most patients other than postpartum women are over 50 years of age, and approximately half have an associated identifiable disorder at the time the autoantibody is diagnosed (Green and Lechner, 1981).

The condition most frequently associated with formation of an autoantibody to factor VIII is recent pregnancy. Hauser, Schneider and Lechner (1995) have recently analyzed the 51 published cases of postpartum factor VIII inhibitors and they note that the risk of inhibitor development is highest after the first delivery, but that they can occur as late as after the fourth. There is considerable heterogeneity in the time interval between delivery and onset of symptoms (most being within the first 6 months), the height of the inhibitor titer (most being between 5 and 200 BU and the severity of bleeding symptoms. Three deaths from bleeding were reported, but the inhibitor disappeared in 39 of the other 48 patients. For women whose postpartum factor VIII inhibitor completely disappears, the inhibitor does not recur with subsequent pregnancies (Coller *et al.*, 1981).

The literature on autoantibody factor VIII inhibitors continues to add descriptions of newly recognized conditions associated with this bleeding problem. Reviews provide a sense of the relative frequency of the scores of conditions that have been reported (Lechner, 1974; Green and Lechner, 1981). Interesting and provocative associations include the inhibitor that developed in a patient with chronic graft-versus-host disease following allogeneic bone marrow transplantation (Seidler *et al.*, 1994), the inhibitor that preceded the development of chronic lymphocytic leukemia (Mateo *et al.*, 1993) and the association with Sjögren's syndrome (Dannhäuser *et al.*, 1994) and juvenile rheumatoid arthritis (Deinocencio, Lovell and Gabriel, 1994). This last report describes a 13-year-old boy who developed the factor VIII inhibitor 2 months after the initial onset of arthritis. It is atypical in the sense that autoantibodies to factor VIII rarely occur in children – only 18 cases had been reported previously.

Very rarely, autoantibody factor IX inhibitors have been detected in non-hemophilic patients (Largo *et al.*, 1974; Castro, Farber and Clyne, 1972; Briët, Reisner and Roberts, 1984). As with antifactor VIII, these have been associated with systemic lupus erythematosus and the postpartum state in some cases.

Predisposition to factor VIII inhibitor formation

It has been recognized for some time that patients with

severe hemophilia A are more likely to develop an inhibitor than those with a mild or moderate factor VIII deficiency. This suggests that most patients with mild and moderate disease develop tolerance to factor VIII through exposure to their endogenous (slightly modified) molecule, although they are also treated less frequently with factor VIII. For patients with severe hemophilia A, i.e. no detectable plasma factor VIII activity, large databases have identified some mutations that have been associated with inhibitor formation more frequently than others (Tuddenham *et al.*, 1994; Antonarakis, Kazazian and Tuddenham, 1995). For example, 17 of the 23 (74%) reported patients with large multidomain deletions have developed an inhibitor. In contrast, an inhibitor was detected in 11 of the 72 (15%) patients with a deletion within a single domain and in only two of 61 (3%) patients whose severe hemophilia A was due to a missense mutation. It is of interest that an inhibitor was detected with a roughly similar frequency (three of 202) in patients with a missense mutation that caused mild or moderate hemophilia A (Tuddenham *et al.*, 1994).

In the case of nonsense mutations, stop codons that terminate protein synthesis, 24 of the 79 (30%) listed patients developed an inhibitor. Of the different stop codons shown to cause factor VIII deficiency, 10 of 24 have been associated with an inhibitor in at least one patient. However, the sites of the inhibitor-related mutations do not appear to be randomly distributed through the factor VIII gene. Inhibitors have been detected in patients with eight of the 11 different light-chain sites, i.e. within the A3, C1 or C2 domains, while only two of the 13 heavy-chain (A1 and A2 domain) and B domain sites have been associated with inhibitor formation (Tuddenham *et al.*, 1994).

Recently, it has been recognized that half of the patients with severe hemophilia A have an inversion in intron 22 of the factor VIII gene (Lakich *et al.*, 1993). While only a relatively small number of patients have been tested for this defect, an inhibitor was detected in 19 of the 71 patients in the first four series reported (Naylor *et al.*, 1992; Goodeve, Preston and Peake, 1994; Ljung, 1994; Tizzano *et al.*, 1994). Thus, it appears that multidomain deletions and factor VIII light-chain nonsense mutations are most commonly associated with inhibitor formation, that there is a significant incidence of inhibitors following factor VIII treatment of patients with the intron 22 inversion, and that inhibitor formation is uncommon for missense mutations and for heavy-chain nonsense mutations.

The assumed basis for these differences is the extent to which tolerance to factor VIII develops through the synthesis of an incomplete or modified factor VIII protein. While most patients with severe hemophilia who have no detectable plasma factor VIII activity also have no detectable plasma factor VIII protein by immunoassay,

variable small amounts of factor VIII protein have been found in approximately 30% of patients (Hoyer, 1981; McMillan *et al.*, 1988). These low levels (0.01–0.09 u/ml) do not appear to protect patients from inhibitor development, for the incidence of inhibitor development after extensive factor VIII exposure is similar to that in patients with <0.01 u/ml (McMillan *et al.*, 1988). It is not known if the factor VIII gene defects in the other 70% are associated with synthesis of incomplete or modified factor VIII that is not secreted or that is rapidly cleared from plasma.

The factor VIII gene mutations are not the only inherited characteristics that can influence inhibitor formation. The fact that related hemophiliacs are often discordant for inhibitor formation indicates that patients with the same gene defect may respond differently to factor VIII treatment (Frommel and Allain, 1977; Shapiro, 1984; Frommel *et al.*, 1981), i.e. the individual's immunologic response characteristics are also important. Although no clear associations with inhibitor formation (or resistance to inhibitor formation) have been detected for either class I or class II human leukocyte antigens (HLA; Aly *et al.*, 1990; Lippert, Fisher and Schook, 1990), the studies have been small and the patient groups have been heterogeneous with regard to age, factor VIII exposure and factor VIII gene defects. Moreover, patients with different inhibitor characteristics (high responder, low responder or transient) have not been studied separately. We very much need a study in which patients with the same molecular defect are carefully followed for inhibitor formation from initial exposure to factor VIII. Since hemophilia A is caused by many different molecular defects (Tuddenham *et al.*, 1994), useful information is most likely to come from a study of hemophilia patients in which the factor VIII gene has been modified by the intron 22 inversion (Lakich *et al.*, 1993). It should be possible to determine if there is an HLA association with inhibitor formation in these patients. As precise molecular typing of HLA loci is now possible (Ng *et al.*, 1993), this approach may be informative. Of interest in this regard is the observation that a 16-residue peptide from the factor VIII light chain (amino acids 1775–1790) has been eluted from HLA-DR2 (Chicz *et al.*, 1993).

Factors other than HLA type must also influence the immune response to factor VIII. For example, discordance in factor VIII-inhibitor formation has been noted for two pairs of hemophilic homozygotic twins (European Study Group of Factor VIII Antibody, 1979). This indicates a role for non-genetic factors, e.g. treatment schedule, factor VIII product used, sepsis at the time of factor VIII infusions, or other factors that might modulate the immune response.

Immunologic characterization of factor VIII inhibitors

PROPERTIES OF THE ANTIBODIES

With rare exceptions, the inhibitors that develop in hemophilic patients after exposure to factor VIII are immunoglobulin G (IgG) antibodies. They are predominantly of the IgG_4 subclass when inhibitor neutralization assays are done using anti-heavy-chain antisera (Hoyer, Gawryl and de la Fuente, 1984). This subclass is only 4% of the total IgG in normal plasma, but it is often relatively increased in the populations of antibodies that develop after chronic immunization (Aalberse, Van der Gaag and Van Leeuwen, 1983). IgG_4 antibodies do not fix complement, which may explain why these patients do not develop serum sickness or other manifestations of immune complex disease. By immunoblotting, IgG_4 and IgG_1 antifactor VIII reactivities have been detected in most inhibitor plasmas (Fulcher, Mahoney and Zimmerman, 1987). Hemophilic antifactor VIII antibodies have had predominantly κ light chains in some inhibitor neutralization studies (Hoyer *et al.*, 1984).

The two most characteristic properties of antibodies to factor VIII are their relatively slow inhibition of factor VIII activity and their inability to form immunoprecipitates. These features are likely to be due to the very low concentration of the antigen in normal plasma (0.2µg/ml; Fulcher and Zimmerman, 1982), the small amount of antifactor VIII IgG in the inhibitor plasmas (Lazarchick and Hoyer, 1978), and the physical properties of IgG_4 subclass antibodies (Van Der Zee, Van Swieten and Aalberse, 1986).

FACTOR VIII EPITOPES

The sites of inhibitor binding to factor VIII were first determined by immunoblotting studies. Both hemophilic and autoantibody inhibitor plasmas reacted with the Mr 44 000 A2 domain of the factor VIII heavy chain, the Mr 72 000 portion of the thrombin-treated light chain, or both (Fulcher *et al.*, 1985). More precise localization has been possible using recombinant factor VIII fragments containing well-characterized deletions. These studies have demonstrated that most antifactor VIII antibodies react with a rather small segment in the amino-terminal portion of the A2 domain (Scandella *et al.*, 1989; Ware *et al.*, 1992) or with the carboxy-terminal portion of the light chain C2 domain (Scandella *et al.*, 1995).

More recently, immunoprecipitin studies using ^{35}S-labeled A2 fragments established that some inhibitor plasmas react with this factor VIII domain even though immunoblot assays do not detect the antibodies (Scandella *et al.*, 1992). Similarly, immunoprecipitation assays detect C2 fragment reactivity more commonly than is

detected by immunoblotting (Scandella, Mattingly and Prescott, 1993). With these more sensitive assays, it is clear that most inhibitor plasmas contain both antifactor VIII heavy-chain and antifactor VIII light-chain antibodies (Hoyer and Scandella, 1994). When neutralization studies are done with factor VIII fragments, the anti-A2 and anti-C2 reactivities are found to be responsible for most, if not all, of the inhibitor activity (Scandella, Mattingly and Prescott, 1993).

Although the differences in the amino acid sequences of human and porcine factor VIII are sufficiently conservative that procoagulant functions are comparable (Lollar, Parker and Tracy, 1988), they do affect their immunologic properties. This differential reactivity with most inhibitor antibodies (Brettler *et al.*, 1989; Fiks-Sigaud *et al.*, 1993; Lozier *et al.*, 1993; Morrison, Ludlam and Kessler, 1993) has made possible an effective therapy for many inhibitor patients (see below). It has also been used to characterize further antifactor VIII binding sites using recombinant factor VIII molecules in which the putative inhibitor epitope has been replaced with the homologous porcine factor VIII sequence (Lubin *et al.*, 1994; Healey *et al.*, 1995). A hybrid molecule with porcine factor residues 387–604 substituted for the homologous human sequence had factor VIII activity that was not inactivated by an A2 domain-specific antifactor VIII inhibitor, but was neutralized by an anti-C2 antibody (Lubin *et al.*, 1994). Subsequent studies refined the localization and established that the factor VIII sequence arginine^{484}–isoleucine^{508} contains a major A2 domain determinant (Healey *et al.*, 1995). While the clinical potential for this approach depends on the amount of variability in antifactor VIII binding to major epitopes, it may be possible to prepare molecules with a small number of amino acid substitutions that are not inactivated by most inhibitors.

Two other techniques have also been used to identify inhibitor epitopes. A λgt11 library has been used to express small random factor VIII fragments as fusion proteins, and immunoblotting with an inhibitor identified a 25-amino-acid heavy-chain epitope adjacent to the Arg^{372} thrombin cleavage site (Lubahn *et al.*, 1989). Synthetic factor VIII peptides have also been used to map antibody reactivity. In one study an antibody was identified that binds to a factor VIII sequence adjacent to the Arg^{372} thrombin cleavage site (Foster *et al.*, 1988). In another, three anti-C2 inhibitors bound to a peptide consisting of amino acids 2303–2332 (Scandella *et al.*, 1995).

MECHANISM OF FACTOR VIII INHIBITION

Recent studies have begun to identify the mechanisms by which inhibitor antibodies interfere with factor VIII function. Initially, it was shown that anti-C2 inhibitors prevent factor VIII binding to phospholipid, suggesting that they interfere with the membrane-dependent incorporation of factor VIII into the intrinsic factor Xase complex (Arai, Scandella and Hoyer, 1989). This was verified in studies that identified an overlap of the epitopes recognized by anti-C2 antibodies (amino acid residues 2248–2312) with the factor VIII phospholipid-binding site (amino acid residues 2303–2332; Scandella *et al.*, 1995).

Lollar and coworkers have recently demonstrated that the other major group of antifactor VIII antibodies, those that bind to the A2 domain, do not prevent the assembly of factor X, factor VIII and factor IXa on a phospholipid surface, but that they block the function of the assembled factor Xase complex (Lollar *et al.*, 1994). Our incomplete understanding of how factor VIIIa accelerates factor X cleavage has limited further definition of the mechanism by which anti-A2 inhibitors affect the complex.

Laboratory diagnosis of inhibitors

LABORATORY DIAGNOSIS OF FACTOR VIII INHIBITORS

The development of an inhibitor by a hemophilic patient is usually first suspected when there is a failure to respond to replacement therapy, while autoantibodies to factor VIII are typically recognized through the evaluation of a patient who has adult-onset bleeding and a long activated partial thromboplastin (APTT) on screening assays. In both cases, additional laboratory tests are needed to confirm the presence of an inhibitor, to establish its specificity and to quantitate it.

The slow kinetics of factor VIII inactivation by inhibitors must be kept in mind when evaluating patients suspected of having an inhibitor (Biggs *et al.*, 1972). For this reason, inhibitor screening is usually done by incubating equal volumes of patient and normal plasma for 2 h before the APTT measurement. However, this assay is not sufficiently sensitive to detect some weak factor VIII inhibitors and it has been suggested that routine assessment of hemophilic patients should be done with an increase in the patient plasma : normal plasma ratio to 4:1 to improve the sensitivity (Kasper, 1984). If an inhibitor effect is identified by such a screening assay for a hemophilic patient, the specificity of the reaction is rarely in question. This is not the case, however, when an inhibitor is suspected in a non-hemophilic patient. For these patients, it is essential that clotting factor levels should be determined and that these assays be done using several different plasma dilutions (Kasper, 1991). Assays for the missing factor will show a consistent deficiency at all dilutions if the inhibitor is specific for a clotting factor, while a variable deficiency (reduced inactivation with dilution) may be seen for assays of other clotting factors since the inhibitor may affect the assay substrate plasmas. As antiphospholipid antibodies, usually designated lupus-type anticoagulants, also prolong the APTT and may affect the apparent levels of coagulation factors tested in a one-stage APTT-based assay, tests should also be done that specifically identify lupus-type anticoagulants (Hoyer, 1994).

Quantitative inhibitor assays are also important to guide therapy and to detect changes in the inhibitor level. They are based on the measurement of the amount of factor VIII inactivated when the patient plasma is incubated with a factor VIII source, and the Bethesda method is now used by most laboratories (Kasper *et al.*, 1975). In this assay, patient plasma, undiluted or diluted with imidazole buffer, is added to an equal volume of pooled, normal plasma. After a 2 h incubation at 37°C, the factor VIII value for the mixture is compared to that of a control in which buffer replaced the patient plasma. A Bethesda unit (BU) is then defined as that plasma dilution that causes a reduction in residual factor VIII activity to 50% of the control value (Kasper *et al.*, 1975; Kasper, 1991; Kessler, 1991). In the other commonly used assay, the new Oxford method, a factor VIII concentrate is the source of factor VIII, the incubation is for 4 h at 37°C, and one inhibitor unit inactivates 0.5 units of factor VIII (Rizza and Biggs, 1973). One BU is equivalent to 1.21 New Oxford units (Austen *et al.*, 1982).

Although the Bethesda assay values calculated for different plasma dilutions are consistent for most hemophilia A inhibitor patients, some inhibitors have complex inactivation kinetics that have been designated as type II, in contrast to those with a linear, second-order type I inactivation pattern (Gawryl and Hoyer, 1982). This can lead to confusion in the coagulation laboratory, for factor VIII inactivation by type II antibodies gives different apparent inhibitor titers for each plasma dilution tested. Most investigators report the titer as that obtained with the plasma dilution that gives the closest result to 50% residual activity (Kasper, 1989, 1991). Most autoantibodies have type II inactivation kinetics and, unless of very high titer, there may be a residual low factor VIII level in the patient's plasma. Thus, a bleeding patient may have a plasma factor VIII activity level of 2–5% of normal, even though the calculated inhibitor titer is 10–500 BU. In these patients, detectable plasma factor VIII does not exclude a high-titer autoantibody factor VIII inhibitor.

Although the Bethesda assay is used to detect and quantify factor VIII inhibitors in most laboratories, the method has limitations, for it does not assure pH control during the 2 h incubation (Verbruggen *et al.*, 1995). It has been suggested that a modified assay using better buffered samples can improve the discrimination between positive and negative samples by reducing variable, low-level non-immunologic factor VIII inactivation (Verbruggen *et al.*, 1995)

The Bethesda assay is, strictly speaking, limited to tests done with pooled normal plasma as the factor VIII source. The inhibitor titer may be changed when other factor VIII sources are used, and it is usually lower when intermediate-purity factor VIII concentrates are substituted and higher if monoclonal antibody-purified factor VIII is used. Littlewood *et al.* (1991) suggested that this may be due to the presence of phospholipid in intermediate-purity concentrates, for many inhibitors react with factor VIII near its phospholipid-binding domain (Arai, Scandella and Hoyer, 1989). Alternatively, more non-functional factor VIII in the less pure concentrates may neutralize some of the antifactor VIII. This does not appear to be an issue for recombinant factor VIII concentrates, for they have comparable properties when substituted for pooled normal plasma in the Bethesda assay (Hillman-Wiseman, Vitale and Lusher, 1994). The Bethesda assay can also be used to determine the extent of cross-reactivity of inhibitors with porcine factor VIII (Kasper, 1991; Kessler, 1991) and the clinical response to porcine factor VIII treatment is consistent with predictions made from these titers (White, 1994).

Antifactor VIII antibodies can also be detected by enzyme-linked immunosorbentassays (ELISA; Mondorf *et al.*, 1994; Regnault and Stoltz, 1994). In most cases, the assay values are comparable to the inhibitor levels, but there are plasmas that have a strongly positive ELISA result even though the Bethesda assay is negative. These plasmas may contain antibodies that bind to factor VIII but that do not prevent its procoagulant function. This is not too surprising since many monoclonal antibodies to factor VIII are not inhibitory (Goodall and Meyer, 1985). While this type of antibody might influence factor VIII persistence in the circulation after transfusion, there are no well-documented instances of such effect.

IMMUNOLOGIC PROPERTIES AND LABORATORY DIAGNOSIS OF FACTOR IX INHIBITORS

Like factor VIII inhibitors, most factor IX inhibitors are IgG (Briët, Reisner and Roberts, 1984). Some have restricted light- or heavy-chain heterogeneity (Pike *et al.*, 1972; Giddings *et al.*, 1983) but most are polyclonal (Orstavik, 1981; Orstavik and Miller, 1988). They are detected in the same way as factor VIII inhibitors, using an APTT-based assay for screening and a modified Bethesda assay to quantitate the inhibitor level. However, in contrast to the kinetics factor VIII inhibitors, factor IX inactivation is rapid, with immediate loss of procoagulant activity and no additional further loss on incubation (Lechner, 1971; George, Miller and Breckenridge, 1971).

The epitope specificity of factor IX inhibitors has not yet been determined with certainty in any cases. Binding assays have suggested that three inhibitors react with factor IX between amino acid residues 155 and 176, but the relevant short (8-mer) synthetic peptides did not neutralize inhibitor activity (Takahashi *et al.*, 1994). Further studies are needed to define the range of epitope specificities and the mechanisms by which inhibitor antibodies inactivate factor IX function.

Management of inhibitors

MANAGEMENT OF PATIENTS WITH FACTOR VIII INHIBITORS

There are two distinct management issues that must be addressed for inhibitor patients (Bloom, 1987; Kasper, 1989; Macik, 1993; Nilsson, Berntorp and Freiburghaus, 1993; Morrison and Ludlam, 1995). Initially, attention is focused on the immediate treatment of acute bleeding. In most cases, the options depend on the inhibitor titer and the extent to which the patient's inhibitor cross-reacts with porcine factor VIII. The treatment choice for acute bleeding also depends on whether the patient is a high responder, in whom an amnestic response is likely to follow factor VIII infusion, or a low responder, whose titer remains in the 0.6–5 BU range after factor VIII (Allain and Frommel, 1976). Low-responder patients can be treated with factor VIII without the expectation that they will have an amnestic response that adversely affects future treatment. In some cases, a temporary reduction in the inhibitor titer can be accomplished by plasmapheresis or immunoadsorption.

The second issue that needs to be addressed is the feasibility of reducing the inhibitor titer by inducing immune tolerance or through immunosuppression. This requires some time to accomplish and is addressed after the acute bleeding episode is under control.

Treatment with factor VIII concentrates

Bleeding is most effectively controlled when sufficient factor VIII can be given to achieve a plasma level that supports normal hemostasis, i.e. above 0.25 u/ml. For low-titer low-responder patients, this can be accomplished by infusing increased amounts of a factor VIII concentrate, with the dose adjusted according to the assayed response. In general, the effects of inhibitors as high as 5–10 BU can be neutralized in this way. Kasper has suggested that such patients receive an initial dose of 40 u of factor VIII/kg for each BU (Kasper, 1989). It is essential to monitor the response with factor VIII assays to be sure that an adequate level has been achieved. Once the circulating inhibitor has been neutralized, the amount of factor VIII needed for subsequent infusions may be similar to that for uncomplicated hemophilia A treatment – or it may be impossibly large if a brisk anamnestic response leads to enhanced antibody production. Other clinicians have paid less attention to the plasma factor VIII level, and the practice at an Oxford hemophilia center has been to treat bleeding episodes with the infusion of two to three times the standard factor VIII dose, no matter what the titer might be (Rizza and Matthews, 1982).

Continuous infusion therapy may have advantages in inhibitor patients, and satisfactory hemostasis and measurable factor VIII recovery have been achieved when sufficient factor VIII has been given (Blatt *et al.*, 1977; Gordon, Al-Batniji and Goldsmith, 1994). *In vitro* studies help assess the likelihood of success in these patients, for the kinetics of factor VIII inactivation in mixtures of patient plasma and factor VIII can be used to estimate an *in vitro* saturation dose that is used to guide therapy (Gordon, Al-Batniji and Goldsmith, 1994).

Treatment with porcine factor VIII

Many factor VIII inhibitors do not inactivate porcine factor VIII to the same extent as they do the human coagulation protein, and a high-purity porcine factor VIII concentrate, Hyate:C (Lollar, Parker and Tracy, 1988) has been used effectively in many hemophilia A (Gatti and Mannucci, 1984; Kernoff *et al.*, 1984; Brettler *et al.*, 1989; Lozier *et al.*, 1993; Hay and Lozier, 1995) and autoantibody (Brettler *et al.*, 1989; Hay and Bolton-Maggs, 1991; Morrison, Ludlam and Kessler, 1993) inhibitor patients. Thus, it is important to determine if a patient's plasma has a low or negligible inhibitor titer when incubated with porcine factor VIII (Kasper, 1991).

For hemophilia A inhibitor patients, the titer with porcine factor VIII is usually 15–30% of that with human factor VIII, with a mean of 22% for the 88 plasmas tested in the five largest series (Ciavarella, Antonecchi and Ranieri, 1984; Gatti and Mannucci, 1984; Kernoff *et al.*, 1984; Brettler *et al.*, 1989; Lozier *et al.*, 1993). Cross-reactivity is even less for most autoantibodies, i.e., for 69 patients, most reported in a single large series (Morrison, Ludlam and Kessler, 1993), the mean cross-reactivity was only 8% (Gatti and Mannucci, 1984; Kernoff *et al.*, 1984; Brettler *et al.*, 1989; Morrison, Ludlam and Kessler, 1993). In fact, many autoantibody plasmas have no detectable inhibitor when tested with porcine factor VIII, even though they have a relatively high antihuman factor VIII.

For patients with hemophilia A, porcine factor VIII is an important treatment option when there is significant bleeding – or a threat of serious bleeding – and the patient's antibody has low cross-reactivity, i.e. the titer is less than 10–15 BU against porcine factor VIII (Gatti and Mannucci, 1984; Kernoff *et al.*, 1984; Brettler *et al.*, 1989; Lozier *et al.*, 1993; Hay and Lozier, 1995). The most comprehensive clinical data are derived from an international survey of treatment centers carried out by the Factor VIII and Factor IX Scientific and Standardization Subcommittee of the International Society of Thrombosis and Hemostasis (Hay *et al.*, 1994). The 154 hemophilia A inhibitor patients treated with porcine factor VIII received nearly 5000 infusions for more than 2400 bleeding episodes – plus prophylaxis and home therapy. Overall, 80% of the infusions had a good or excellent clinical effect and 13% had a fair effect. No response to porcine factor VIII was detected in 7% of the episodes. Most of the treatment failures were attributed to a high inhibitor titer in a patient who received emergency porcine factor VIII treatment without assay information. Inadequate doses of porcine factor VIII were considered to be the cause of failure in the other cases. Effective use of porcine factor VIII included emergency and elective surgical procedures, with satisfactory hemostasis in 53 of 57 operations (Lozier *et al.*, 1993).

Porcine factor VIII is considered by many to be the first-line treatment for patients with autoantibodies to factor VIII when the titer with human factor VIII is over 10 BU, since few of these antibodies have significant cross-reactivity. A satisfactory plasma factor VIII level is usually achieved in these patients, as is normal hemostasis (Morrison, Ludlam and Kessler, 1993).

Side-effects following porcine factor VIII treatment have been noted after 2–3% of infusions, usually low-grade fever, rash, hives or chills (Kernoff *et al.*, 1984; Brettler *et al.*, 1989; Hay and Bolton-Maggs, 1991). Moderate thrombocytopenia has been detected, after five of 809 infusions in one large series (Hay and Bolton-Maggs, 1991), but significant thrombocytopenia has been rare during the past decade and has not been reported for patients receiving standard doses of porcine factor VIII. The freedom from severe side-effects has made it possible to use porcine factor VIII for home therapy in some patients, i.e. for prophylaxis or for routine treatment of hemarthrosis (Hay *et al.*, 1990).

The immune response to the coagulation protein itself has been variable. Many hemophilic inhibitor patients (approximately one-third) have been successfully treated with porcine factor VIII for repeated bleeding episodes, but the others had an increasing inhibitory titer against human and porcine factor VIII that limited its further use. Ten per cent of hemophilia A inhibitor patients had a brisk anamnestic response that limited therapy to two or three infusions before they were refractory to this therapy (Hay and Lozier, 1995).

Other forms of factor VIII

Bloom and Hutton suggested that transfusions of fresh platelet concentrates may be useful in cases of severe bleeding in high titer inhibitor patients (Bloom and Hutton, 1975; Bloom, 1987). They suggested that the platelets that adhere to and accumulate at the site of vascular injury might contain clotting factors that were protected from inhibitors. While they provided suggestive evidence of a clinical response in three patients, it is certainly not established that factor VIII is present within platelets or that it is in a protected form on the platelet surface. The recognition that some factor VIII antibodies block factor VIII interaction with phospholipid suggests an alternative mechanism, i.e. a neutralization of some of the inhibitor effect by the platelet surface (Bloom, 1987).

Temporary reduction of the inhibitor level

For patients with high inhibitor titers who have serious bleeding or a need for surgery, one should consider therapies that can rapidly reduce the inhibitor level. This has been achieved by exchange plasmapheresis, a technique that is generally available (Strauss, 1969; McCullough *et al.*, 1973; Slocombe *et al.*, 1981; Erskine, 1982; Francesconi *et al.*, 1982). While multiple manual exchanges can be effective (Strauss, 1969), continuous-flow centrifugal cell separators facilitate the process (McCullough *et al.*, 1973). Large amounts of plasma – equivalent to one to two plasma volumes – can be exchanged quickly (2–4 h) and safely.

While the basic procedure does not differ from that used in therapeutic apheresis of other conditions, the choice of replacement fluid is important for inhibitor patients. It is generally agreed that the plasma should be replaced in hemophilia A inhibitor patients with albumin (or purified protein fraction) or saline to avoid immediate stimulation of further antifactor VIII production when factor VIII concentrate administration is not planned immediately after completing the procedure, e.g. when the patient is being prepared for a surgical procedure (Erskine, 1982). In the case of autoantibodies, there is no issue of anamnesis, so that partial replacement with normal plasma is feasible.

A more complex procedure, affinity chromatography, in which patient IgG is removed by protein A-sepharose, has been effective in the treatment of a number of hemophilia A and B patients as well as patients with autoantibodies to factor VIII (Nilsson *et al.*, 1981; Uehlinger *et al.*, 1991; Gjorstrup *et al.*, 1991). As both factor VIII and factor IX inhibitors are predominantly IgG_4 and IgG_1, their selective removal by protein A (with IgG_2) provides a way to decrease the inhibitor titer without removing the other plasma proteins. In one report, the mean decrease in both plasma IgG concentration and antifactor VIII titer was 82% (Uehlinger *et al.*, 1991). These seven factor VIII inhibitor patients were treated on eight occasions, with the processing of two plasma volumes daily for 1–4 days, depending on the inhibitor level. For the six hemophilic patients, the titer was reduced to less than 10 BU, making treatment with factor VIII concentrates feasible. Depletion of autoantibodies to factor VIII is often more difficult (Uehlinger *et al.*, 1991; Gjorstrup *et al.*, 1991).

Coagulation products that bypass factor VIII

When the inhibitor titer prevents the achievement of a hemostatic factor VIII level through factor VIII concentrate therapy, preparations that bypass a need for factor VIII may have utility. The factor IX concentrates used until recently for the treatment of hemophilia B patients contain significant amounts of prothrombin, factor X and, to a varying degree, factor VII. These preparations, usually designated prothrombin complex concentrates (PCC), also contain small amounts of activated factors that may be responsible for their bypass activity. Intentional activation during concentrate production recognizes this possibility, and activated PCC (APCC) concentrates, also designated anti-inhibitor coagulant complex products, have been used extensively in the treatment of inhibitor patients (Preston *et al.*, 1977; Kurczynski and Penner, 1974).

Controlled clinical trials have established that there is a modest hemostatic effect when PCC are used to treat acute hemarthroses in factor VIII inhibitor patients (Lusher *et al.*, 1980). Acute joint bleeding episodes also respond to APCC, but controlled trials have not detected a difference between PCC and APCC in effectiveness, both giving good or excellent results in 48–64% of patients (Sjamsoedin, Heijnen and Mauser-Bunschoten, 1981; Lusher, Blatt and Penner, 1983). While case reports and surveys (Blatt, Menache and Roberts, 1980) suggest that PCC and APCC are effective in controlling other types of bleeding as well, including open bleeding in surgical situations, the treatment of more serious conditions has not been evaluated in a controlled trial (Lusher, 1994).

One of the more serious limitations in the use of PCC and APCC is the lack of any coagulation test to monitor their effectiveness. The *in vitro* 'unitages' for the APCC are defined differently for the two products licensed in the USA, and these assays cannot be correlated with any *in vivo* measure. In the case of PCC, the labeled potency reflects only the factor IX content.

Another important issue in the use of PCC and APCC, especially when large doses are given, is the risk of thrombogenicity or myocardial infarction – though these complications appear to be less frequent in inhibitor patients than in hemophilia B (Lusher, 1994). Currently licensed and distributed PCC and APCC all include a virus inactivation step in their production, and the risk of human immunodeficiency virus (HIV) or hepatitis virus transmission is believed to be very small (Lusher, 1994; Kasper *et al.*, 1993).

While one would not expect an increase in the antifactor VIII inhibitor titer after treatment with PCC or APCC, this is not always the case, and one study documented a twofold inhibitor titer increase in 13.5% of 261 treatment episodes (Kasper and Hemophilia Study Group, 1979). The increase is undoubtedly due to the presence of low levels of inactive factor VIII protein in these concentrates (Laurian *et al.*, 1984; Onder and Hoyer, 1979).

Activated factor VII is one of the components in these concentrates that may be responsible for the hemostatic effect (Hedner and Kisiel, 1983). It has the therapeutic advantage of not being proteolytically active by itself. Thus, it should not induce thromboembolic events and should be limited to an effect at the site of injury where tissue factor is exposed. Moreover, as factor VIIa is not neutralized by antithrombin III in the circulation, it is expected to reach the site of injury without modification. Its persistence is still very short in plasma – an estimated $T_{1/2}$ of 90 min (Macik *et al.*, 1993) – so that frequent administration is required. While factor VIIa affects the prothrombin time and the APTT, it is not clear that these tests have value in guiding therapy.

Recombinant factor VIIa has been studied extensively in phase II clinical trials and there have been a number of additional case reports and small series. The largest clinical experience includes a group of 41 hemophilia A inhibitor patients who have been treated with recombinant factor VIIa (Hedner, Glazer and Falch, 1993). A therapeutic effect was achieved in most patients and there were no serious side-effects or evidence of systemic coagulation cascade activation. Hedner, Glazer and Falch noted that recombinant factor VIIa infusions at 2–3 h intervals are necessary, at least initially, in patients with severe bleeding. Smaller series have reported satisfactory clinical results in five patients treated for joint and muscle bleeds (Seremetis, 1994), three patients with intracranial bleeding refractory to other approaches (Majumdar and Savidge, 1993; Schmidt *et al.*, 1994) and an instance of good hemostasis during major orthopedic surgery (O'Marcaigh *et al.*, 1994).

Tolerance induction

Induction of immune tolerance has the potential for long-term benefit and many inhibitor patients have been treated with high-dose factor VIII in an effort at reducing the inhibitor titer. In early studies, frequent large factor VIII infusions (100 u/Kg factor VIII every 12 h) were combined with APCC treatment to prevent bleeding during the initial period in which an anamnestic response increased the inhibitor titer (Brackmann, 1983). The inhibitor titer then fell so that the factor VIII dose could

be reduced, and the inhibitor eventually became undetectable in most patients who were maintained on regular factor VIII infusions. While the results of this treatment schedule were quite good (the inhibitor level falling to <1 BU in 15 of 21 patients), a tremendous amount of factor VIII was required and it was felt that frequent factor VIII infusions were needed to maintain the tolerance. The effectiveness of this regimen has been confirmed in other centers (White *et al.*, 1983; Scheibel *et al.*, 1987), but cost has limited its application.

Protocols with lower factor VIII dosage have also been effective in reducing the antifactor VIII titer (Ewing *et al.*, 1988). However, high-titer patients rarely had a good response to the low-dose regimens unless it was begun soon after inhibitor development (Peerlinck *et al.*, 1994). In the Netherlands, 27 inhibitor patients received 25 u of factor VIII/kg every other day for 1–12 months and tolerance was achieved in 18 (Van Leeuwen *et al.*, 1986). Again, success was more likely if the patient had a low or moderate inhibitor titer or if the treatment was started immediately after the inhibitor was detected.

A more complex immune tolerance regimen has been employed by Nilsson and colleagues in Malmo (Nilsson, Berntorp and Zettervall, 1988; Nilsson, 1994). When the antibody level is high (>10 BU), the inhibitor titer is lowered by immunoadsorption using protein A-sepharose. Cyclophosphamide is then given orally for 8–10 days (2–3 mg/kg) and factor VIII (or factor IX) is infused daily for 3 weeks in sufficient dosage to maintain a plasma level above 0.4 u/ml. In addition, intravenous IgG is given daily (0.4 g/kg) for 5 days starting on the fourth day of the treatment protocol. This approach has been very successful in that 10 of 11 hemophilia A inhibitor patients became tolerant. Two of them required two courses of the combined treatment to eradicate the inhibitor and one required three courses (Nilsson, 1992). After tolerance induction, the *in vivo* recovery and half-life of infused factor VIII were comparable to that in non-inhibitor hemophiliacs. These boys then received factor VIII two to three times each week on a prophylaxis schedule. A similar protocol for hemophilia B patients was successful in 6 of 7 cases (Nilsson, 1994).

As no center treats a large number of patients with this extremely heterogeneous disorder, cooperative studies are essential. An international registry of immune tolerance protocols has been established and a recent report summarizes data for 204 patients treated at 40 centers in the USA, Canada, Europe and Japan (Mariani, Ghirardini and Bellocco, 1994). Of the 158 patients who had been on treatment long enough to judge the outcome, 107 (68%) achieved tolerance and 12 (8%) had a partial response. Many of the patients who appeared to be tolerant by negative *in vitro* assays also had normal factor VIII recoveries *in vivo* and could be treated for bleeding episodes with standard doses of factor VIII. The probability of success was greatest for patients given a high factor VIII dose (over 100 units/kg per day) and for patients who had an inhibitor titer less than 10 BU at the time the immune tolerance treatment was started. Tolerance, when induced, was long-lasting, with only one recurrent inhibitor. The longest documented period of tolerance after induction has been 16 years (Mariani, Ghirardini and Bellocco, 1994).

While the International Registry did not include patient age data, experience with recombinant factor VIII suggests that early efforts in immune tolerance induction are likely to be successful (Lusher *et al.*, 1993; Bray *et al.*, 1994). Supporting this concept is a report of very good success for 21 hemophilia A children with an inhibitor (Kreuz *et al.*, 1995). The inhibitor was eliminated in 19 of these patients, with a median inhibitor persistence of 4 months for the 16 high-responder patients and 1.5 months for five low-responder patients. The report emphasized that the outcome – and length of time needed to induce immune tolerance – is significantly correlated with the extent of factor VIII exposure between inhibitor detection and the start of immune tolerance therapy (Kreuz *et al.*, 1995).

One of the difficulties with this approach for very young children is limited venous access. Addressing this concern, Lilleyman has reported success in home therapy of five inhibitor patients under the age of three (Lilleyman, 1994). The five boys all recovered normal responsiveness to transfused factor VIII after treatment with conventional factor VIII doses (20–40 u/kg) two to three times each week. Four of the boys required an implanted venous access device (Porta-Cath), but this allowed the therapy to be given by parents at home. While two devices were removed because of infection, after 2 and 4 years of use, this complication rate was considered acceptable given the benefits of the approach.

Tolerance can also be induced with porcine factor VIII. Patients with inhibitor titers over 15 BU against human factor VIII have been successfully treated with porcine factor VIII until their titers fell so that treatment with human factor VIII could be resumed (Hay *et al.*, 1990).

TREATMENT OF PATIENTS WITH AUTOANTIBODY FACTOR VIII INHIBITORS

In managing autoantibody inhibitor patients, there are several differences from hemophilic antifactor VIII that should be kept in mind. Since these patients do not have an anamnestic response when they are treated with human factor VIII, they are always low responders and can be treated with factor VIII with little likelihood that this may make subsequent therapy more difficult. In addition, most patients with an autoantibody inhibitor respond to immunosuppressive therapy and some of the inhibitors are susceptible to *in vitro* and *in vivo* neutrali-

zation by intravenous immunoglobulin (IVIg) prepared from large pools of normal plasma (Sultan *et al.*, 1984; Sultan *et al.*, 1991).

Morrison and Ludlam have recently summarized the management principles for these patients (Morrison and Ludlam, 1995). They emphasize that bleeding can usually be stopped with large amounts of human factor VIII if the antibody is low-titer – and with porcine factor VIII in most other patients. As the cross-reactivity to porcine factor VIII is very low in most autoantibody patients (it averages 7%), there is rarely a limiting resistance to porcine factor VIII. In the few instances in which the titer against porcine factor VIII is more than 10 BU, or if there is a poor response to this product, bypass therapy with (A)PCC or recombinant factor VIIa provides an alternative therapeutic approach in controlling the acute bleeding episode. At the same time, immunomodulatory and/or immunosuppressive therapy can be initiated. The direct treatment of the underlying associated medical condition often leads to simultaneous elimination of the autoimmune factor VIII inhibitor.

In contrast to the consistent observation that immunosuppressive drugs do not suppress inhibitor antibody formation in hemophilia A inhibitor patients (Bloom, 1987; Kasper, 1989), there has been considerable success using corticosteroids, cyclophosphamide, azathioprine and 6-mercaptopurine in the treatment of autoantibody inhibitors (Green, 1991). For example, the combination of cyclophosphamide, vincristine and prednisone given with factor VIII and repeated every 3–4 weeks was associated with disappearance of the inhibitor in 11 of 12 patients with various associated conditions treated by Lian and colleagues (Lian, Larcada and Chiu, 1989). In the case of postpartum inhibitors, a review of published reports found no significant difference in the interval to inhibitor disappearance (12–16 months) between the 21 patients treated with corticosteroids and 10 untreated patients. However, the median time to response was only 8 months for the 18 patients given immunosuppressive treatment (cyclophosamide, azathioprine or 6-mercaptopurine; Hauser, Schneider and Lechner, 1995).

While these and smaller series suggest that cytotoxic immunosuppressive therapy is effective in a large proportion of patients, it must be kept in mind that the spontaneous remission rate may be as high as 30% (Lottenberg, Kentro and Kitchens, 1987). Survey data suggest that children or postpartum women with autoantibody inhibitors are more likely to resolve spontaneously or with corticosteroid therapy, while the inhibitor titer does not usually fall in patients with other autoimmune disorders until they are treated with an antimetabolite or an alkylating agent (Green and Lechner, 1981). Unfortunately, there is little information from prospective randomized trials that can provide guidance in the use of these potentially hazardous drugs, and the variable natural history, with fluctuation in inhibitor titers and occasional spontaneous remissions (Lottenberg, Kentro and Kitchens, 1987), makes the interpretation of most published series very difficult. The first prospective randomized trial has been underway since 1987, and a preliminary report suggests that initial treatment with prednisone is indicated – with cyclophosphamide held as a second-line therapy for patients who are steroid-resistant (Green, Rademaker and Briët, 1993). The inhibitor disappeared in 10 of 31 patients during an initial 3-week period in which they received 1 mg, prednisone/kg per day. For the other 20 who continued in the study, the inhibitor disappeared in three of four patients randomized to an additional 6 weeks of prednisone (now 2 mg/kg per day), in three of six patients receiving 2 mg cyclophosphamide/kg per day as a single agent, and in five of 10 patients treated with both prednisone and cyclophosphamide (Green, Rademaker and Briët, 1993). In spite of these encouraging results, the potential adverse effects of cyclophosphamide must be considered, including marrow suppression, hemorrhagic cystitis, infertility and increased risk of cancer.

IVIg is widely used in the treatment of a number of autoantibody disorders and a few antifactor VIII inhibitor patients have been treated with IVIg infusion, some successfully (Sultan *et al.*, 1994). While IVIg has a variable effect on autoantibodies, many high-titer inhibitors are substantially reduced when IVIg is added *in vitro* (Sultan *et al.*, 1984, 1994; Green and Kwaan). This may not have clinical benefit, however, since a significant level of antifactor VIII remains. In a few patients, especially those with low-titer autoantibodies, the inhibitor was no longer detected after the IVIg infusion and hemostasis improved. When observed, the inhibitor titer reduction occurred within a few hours of the IVIg infusion. However, the inhibitor titer may remain low for some time, suggesting an effect on antibody synthesis (Sultan *et al.*, 1994).

It is not known how IVIg causes inhibitor titer reduction in those patients in whom an effect is noted. However, the presumed mechanism is the presence of anti-idiotype antibodies in the pooled normal human plasma (Rossi, Sultan and Kazatchk, 1988). Anti-idiotype antibodies to a number of other autoantibodies can also be detected in pooled normal human IVIg (Rossi and Kazatchkine, 1989). Supporting this concept, mixing studies were consistent with the development of anti-idiotype antibodies that neutralized the pre-remission inhibitors in two autoantibody inhibitor patients who had a clinical response after treatments not involving IVIg (Sultan, Rossi and Kazatchkine, 1987; Tiarks, Pechet and Humphreys, 1989). In most hemophilic patients there is minimal or no effect of IVIg on the *in vitro* titer and no clinical benefit has been observed (Selfried *et al.*, 1984; Sultan *et al.*, 1984; Moffat, Furlong and Bloom, 1986).

Because patients who develop autoantibodies to factor VIII continue to produce, store and release both factor VIII and von Willebrand factor (vWF), patients with inhibitors of less than 3 BU have been treated successfully with desmopressin (DDAVP; de la Fuente *et al.*, 1985; Muhm *et al.*, 1990). Factor VIII released into the plasma in response to DDAVP neutralizes the inhibitor and contributes to effective hemostasis. Since the antibody–factor VIII reaction is time-dependent, there may be only a short period in which increased factor VIII activity is detected. In patients with a high-titer inhibitor, factor VIII levels are unchanged after DDAVP, reflecting the modest extent to which this drug can cause factor VIII release (Muhm *et al.*, 1990)

MANAGEMENT OF PATIENTS WITH FACTOR IX INHIBITORS

In most cases, factor IX inhibitor patients can be successfully treated by the infusion of large amounts of factor IX complex concentrates. The inhibitor is partially or completely neutralized and the non-factor IX component includes activated enzymes that may bypass the factor IX requirement (Giddings *et al.*, 1983). Immune tolerance has been induced in factor IX inhibitor patients by the Malmo protocol in which IVIg and cyclophosphamide are given in addition to the factor IX after the inhibitor titer has been reduced to less than 10 BU by immunoadsorption (Nilsson, Berntorp and Zettervall, 1986).

References

Aalberse, R.C., Van Der Gaag, R. and Van Leeuwen, J. (1983) Serologic aspects of IgG₄ antibodies. I. Prolonged immunization results in an IgG₄-restricted response. *J Immunol*, 130, 722–725.

Addiego, J.E., Jr., Gomperts, E.D., Liu, S.-L. *et al.* (1992) Treatment of hemophilia A with a highly purified factor VIII concentrate prepared by anti-FVIIIc immunoaffinity chromatography. *Thromb Haemost*, 67, 19–27.

Addiego, J., Kasper, C., Abildgaard, *et al.* (1993) Frequency of inhibitor development in haemophiliacs treated with low-purity factor VIII. *Lancet*, 342, 462–464.

Allain, J.-P. and Frommel, D. (1976) Antibodies to factor VIII. V. Patterns of Immune response to factor VIII in haemophilia A. *Blood*, 47, 973–982.

Aly, A.M., Aledort, L.M., Lee, T.D. and Hoyer, L.W. (1990) Histocompatibility antigen patterns in hemophilic patients with factor VIII antibodies. *Br J Haematol*, 76, 238–241.

Antonarakis, S.E., Kazazian, H.H. and Tuddenham, E.G.D. (1995) Molecular etiology of factor VIII deficiency in hemophilia A. *Hum Mutation*, 5, 1–22.

Arai, M., Scandella, D. and Hoyer, L.W. (1989) Molecular basis of factor VIII inhibition by human antibodies: antibodies that bind to the factor VIII light chain prevent the interaction of factor VIII with phospholipid. *J Clin Invest*, 83, 1978–1984.

Austen, D.E.G., Lechner, K., Rizza, C.R. and Rhymes, I.L. (1982) A comparison of the Bethesda and New Oxford methods of factor VIII antibody assay. *Thromb Haemost*, 47, 72–75.

Barrowcliffe, T.W. (1993) Inhibitor development and activated factor VIII in concentrates. *Thromb Haemost*, 70, 1065–1066.

Biggs, R., Austen, D.E.G., Denson, K.W.E. *et al.* (1972) The mode of action of antibodies which destroy factor VIII. I. Antibodies which have second-order concentration graphs. *Br J Haematol*, 23, 125–135.

Blatt, P.M., Menache, D. and Roberts, H.R. (1980) A survey of the effectiveness of prothrombin complex concentrates in controlling hemorrhage in patients with hemophilia and anti-factor VIII antibodies. *Thromb Haemost*, 44, 39–49.

Blatt, P.M., White, G.C. II, McMillan, C.W. and Roberts, H.R. (1977) Treatment of anti-factor VIII antibodies. *Thromb Haemost*, 38, 523.

Bloom, A.L. (1987) The treatment of factor VIII inhibitors, in *Thrombosis and Haemostasis 1987* (eds M. Verstraete, J. Vermylen, H.R. Lijnen and J. Arnout), Leuven University Press, Leuven, pp. 447–471.

Bloom, A.L. and Hutton, R.D. (1975) Fresh platelet transfusions in haemophilic patients with factor VIII antibody. *Lancet*, 369–370.

Brackmann, H.-H. (1983) Induced immunotolerance in factor VIII inhibitor patients, in *Factor VIII Inhibitors*, 150th edn (ed. L.W. Hoyer), Alan R. Liss, New York, pp. 181–195.

Bray, G.L. (1992) Current status of clinical studies of recombinant factor VIII (Recombinate) in patients with hemophilia A. *Trans Med Rev*, VI, 252–255.

Bray, G.L., Gomperts, E.D., Courter, S. *et al.* (1994) A multi-center study of recombinant factor VIII (Recombinate): Safety, efficacy and inhibitor risk in previously untreated patients with hemophilia A. *Blood*, 83, 2428–2435.

Brettler, D.B., Forsberg, A.D., Levine, P.H. *et al.* (1989) The use of porcine factor VIII concentrate (Hyate:C) in the treatment of patients with inhibitor antibodies to factor VIII. *Arch Intern Med*, 149, 1381–1385.

Briët, E. (1991) Factor IX inhibitors in haemophilia B patients: their incidence and prospects for development with high purity factor IX products. *Blood Coagulation Fibrinolysis*, 2, 47–50.

Briët, E. (1995) Tolerance and intolerance to factor VIII: a clinical perspective, in *Inhibitors to Coagulation Factor* (eds L.M. Aledort, L.W. Hoyer, J.M. Lusher, H.M. Reisner and G.C. White), Plenum, New York.

Briët, E., Reisner, H.M. and Roberts, H.R. (1984) Inhibitors in Christmas disease, in *Factor VIII Inhibitors* (ed. L.W. Hoyer), Alan R. Liss, New York, pp. 123–139.

Briët, E. and Rosendaal, F.R. (1994) Inhibitors in hemophilia A: are some products safer? *Semin Hematol*, 31, 11–15.

Briët, E., Rosendaal, F.R., Kreuz, W. *et al.* (1994) High titer inhibitors in severe haemophilia A. A meta-analysis based on eight long-term follow-up studies concerning inhibitors associated with crude or intermediate purity factor VIII products. *Thromb Haemost*, 72, 162–164.

Castro, O., Farber, L.R. and Clyne, L.P. (1972) Circulating anticoagulants against factors IX and XI in systemic lupus erythematosus. *Ann Intern Med*, 77, 543.

Chicz, R.M., Urban, R.G., Gorga, J.C. *et al.* (1993) Specificity and promiscuity among naturally processed peptides bound to HLA-DR alleles. *J Exp Med*, 178, 27–47.

Ciavarella, N., Antoncecchi, S. and Ranieri, P. (1984) Efficacy of porcine factor VIII in the management of haemophiliacs with inhibitors. *Br J Haematol*, 58, 641–648.

Coller, B.S., Hultin, M.B., Hoyer, L.W. *et al.* (1981) Normal pregnancy in a patient with a prior postpartum factor VIII inhibitor: with observations on pathogenesis and prognosis. *Blood*, 58, 619–624.

Dannhäuser, D., Casonato, A., Pietrogrande, F. *et al.* (1994) Acquired factor VIII:C inhibitor in a patient with Sjögren's syndrome: Successful treatment with steroid and immunosuppressive therapy. *Acta Haematol*, 91, 73–76.

De Biasi, R., Rocino, A., Papa, M.L. *et al.* (1994) Incidence of factor VIII inhibitor development in hemophilia A patients treated with less pure plasma derived concentrates. *Thromb Haemost*, 71, 544–547.

Deinocencio, J., Lovell, D.J. and Gabriel, C.A. (1994) Acquired factor VIII inhibitor in juvenile rheumatoid arthritis. *Pediatrics*, 94, 550–553.

de la Fuente, B., Casper, C.K., Rickles, F.R. and Hoyer, L.W. (1985) Responses of patients with mild and moderate hemophilia A and von Willebrand's disease to treatment with desmopressin. *Ann Intern Med*, 103, 6–14.

Ehrenforth, S., Kreuz, W., Scharrer, I. *et al.* (1992) Incidence of development of factor VIII and factor IX inhibitors in haemophiliacs. *Lancet*, 339, 594–598.

Erskine, J.G. (1982) Plasma exchange in patients with inhibitors to factor VIIIC. *Plasma Ther Transfus Technol*, 3, 123–130.

European Study Group of Factor VIII Antibody (1979) Development of factor VIII antibody in haemophilic monozygotic twins. *Scand J Haemost*, 23, 64–68.

Ewing, N.P., Sanders, N.L., Dietrich, S.L. and Kasper, C.K. (1988) Induction of immune tolerance to factor VIII in hemophiliacs with inhibitors. *JAMA*, 259, 65–68.

Fiks-Sigaud, M., Bendelac, L., Parquet, A. *et al.* (1993) Comparison of anti-human and anti-porcine factor VIII inhibitor levels in 63 patients with severe haemophilia A. *Vox Sang*, 64, 210–214.

Foster, P.A., Fulcher, C.A., Houghten, R.A. *et al.* (1988) Localization of the binding regions of a murine monoclonal anti-factor VIII antibody and a human anti-factor VIII alloantibody, both of which inhibit factor VIII procoagulant activity, to amino acid residues threonine[351]-serine[365] of the factor VIII heavy chain. *J Clin Invest*, 82, 123–128.

Francesconi, M., Korninger, C., Thaler, E. *et al.* (1982) Plasmapheresis: its value in the management of patients with antibodies to factor VIII. *Haemostasis*, 11, 79–86.

Frommel, D. and Allain, J.-P. (1977) Genetic predisposition to develop factor VIII antibody in classic hemophilia. *Clin Immunol Immunopathol*, 8, 34–38.

Frommel, D., Allain, J.P., Saint-Paul, E. *et al.* (1981) HLA antigens and factor VIII antibody in classic hemophilia. European study group of factor VIII antibody. *Thromb Haemost*, 46, 687–689.

Fulcher, C.A., Mahoney, S.D.G., Roberts, J.R. *et al.* (1985) Localization of human factor FVIII inhibitor epitopes to two polypeptide fragments. *Proc Natl Acad Sci USA*, 82, 7728–7732.

Fulcher, C.A., Mahoney, S.D.G. and Zimmerman, T.S. (1987) FVIII inhibitor IgG subclass and FVIII polypeptide specificity determined by immunoblotting. *Blood*, 69, 1475–1480.

Fulcher, C.A. and Zimmerman, T.S. (1982) Characterization of the human factor VIII procoagulant protein with a heterologous precipitating antibody. *Proc Natl Acad Sci USA*, 79, 1648–1652.

Gatti, L. and Mannucci, P.M. (1984) Use of porcine factor VIII in the management of 17 patients with factor VIII antibodies. *Thromb Haemost*, 51, 379–384.

Gawryl, M.S. and Hoyer, L.W. (1982) Inactivation of factor VIII coagulant activity by two different types of human antibodies. *Blood*, 60, 1103–1109.

George, J.N., Miller, G.M. and Breckenridge, R.T. (1971) Studies on Christmas disease: investigation and treatment of a familial acquired inhibitor of factor IX. *Br J Haematol*, 21, 333–342.

Giannelli, F., Choo, K.H. and Rees, D.J.G. (1983) Gene deletions in patients with haemophilia B and anti-factor IX antibodies. *Nature*, 303, 181.

Giddings, J.C., Bloom, A.L., Kelly, M.A. and Spratt, H.C. (1983) Human factor IX inhibitors: immunochemical characteristics and treatment with activated concentrate. *Clin Lab Haematol*, 5, 165–175.

Gjorstrup, P., Berntorp, E., Larsson, L. and Nilsson, I.M. (1991) Kinetic aspects of the removal of IgG and inhibitors in hemophiliacs using protein A immunoadsorption. *Vox Sang*, 61, 244–250.

Goodall, A.H. and Meyer, D. (1985) Registry of monoclonal antibodies to factor VIII and von Willebrand factor. *Thromb Haemost*, 54, 878–891.

Goodeve, A.C., Preston, F.E. and Peake, I.R. (1994) Factor VIII gene rearrangements in patients with severe haemophilia A. *Lancet*, 343, 329–330.

Gordon, E.M., Al-Batniji, F. and Goldsmith, J.C. (1994) Continuous infusion of monoclonal antibody-purified factor VIII: rational approach to serious hemorrhage in patients with allo-/autoantibodies to factor VIII. *Am J Hematol*, 45, 142–145.

Green, D. (1991) Cytotoxic suppression of acquired factor VIII:C inhibitors. *Am J Med*, 91, 5A–14S–5A–19S.

Green, D. and Kwaan, H.C. (1987) An acquired factor VIII inhibitor responsive to high-dose gamma globulin. *Thromb Haemost*, 58, 1005–1007.

Green, D. and Lechner, K. (1981) A survey of 215 non-hemophilic patients with inhibitors to factor VIII. *Thromb Haemost*, 45, 200–203.

Green, D., Rademaker, A.W. and Briët, E. (1993) A prospective, randomized trial of prednisone and cyclophosphamide in the treatment of patients with factor VIII autoantibodies. *Thromb Haemost*, 70, 753–757.

Hauser, I., Schneider, B. and Lechner, K. (1995) Post-partum factor VIII inhibitors. A review of the literature with special reference to the value of steroid and immunosuppressive treatment. *Thromb Haemost*, 73, 1–5.

Hay, C.R.M. and Bolton-Maggs, P. (1991) Porcine FVIII.C in the management of patients with FVIII inhibitors. *Trans Med Rev*, 15, 145–151.

Hay, C.R.M., Laurian, Y., Verroust, F. *et al.* (1990) Induction of immune tolerance in patients with hemophilia A and inhibitors treated with porcine VIIIC by home therapy. *Blood*, 76, 882–886.

Hay, C.R.M. and Lozier, J.N. (1995) Porcine factor VIII therapy in patients with factor VIII inhibitors, in *Inhibitors to Coagulation Factors*, (eds L.M. Aledort, L.W. Hoyer, J.M. Lusher, H.M. Reisner and G.C. White, II), Plenum, New York, pp. 143–152.

Hay, C.R.M., Lozier, J.N., Lee, C.A. *et al.* (1994) Porcine factor VIII therapy in patients with congenital hemophilia and inhibitors: efficacy, patient selection, and side effects. *Semin Hematol*, 31, 20–25.

Healey, J.F., Lubin, I.M., Nakai, H. *et al.* (1995) Residues 484–508 contain a major determinant of the inhibitory epitope in the A2 domain of human factor VIII. *J Biol Chem*, 270, 14505–14509.

Hedner, U. and Kisiel, W. (1983) Use of human factor VIIa in the treatment of two hemophilia A patients with high-titer inhibitors. *J Clin Invest*, 71, 1836–1841.

Hedner, U., Glazer, S. and Falch, J. (1993) Recombinant activated factor VII in the treatment of bleeding episodes in patients with inherited and acquired bleeding disorders. *Trans Med Rev*, 7, 78–83.

Hillman-Wiseman, C., Vitale, C. and Lusher, J. (1994) Factor VIII inhibitor assay using plasma FVIII versus recombinant FVIII – a comparative study. *Thromb Res*, 76, 221–224.

Hironaka, T., Furukawa, K., Esmon, P.C. *et al.* (1992) Comparative study of the sugar chains of factor VIII purified from human plasma and from the culture media of recombinant baby hamster kidney cells. *J Biol Chem*, 267, 8012–8020.

Hoyer, L.W. (1981) The factor VIII complex: structure and function. *Blood*, 58, 1–13.

Hoyer, L.W. (1995) The incidence of factor VIII inhibitors in patients with severe hemophilia A, in *Inhibitors to Coagulation Factors* (eds L.M. Aledort, L.W. Hoyer, J.M. Lusher, H.M. Reisner and G.C. White), Plenum, New York, pp. 35–46.

Hoyer, L.W. and Scandella, D. (1994) Factor VIII inhibitors: structure and function in autoantibody and hemophilia A patients. *Semin Hematol*, 31 (suppl. 4), 1–5.

Hoyer, L.W., Gawryl, M.S. and de la Fuente, B. (1984) Immunological characterization of factor VIII inhibitors, in *Factor VIII Inhibitors* (ed. L.W. Hoyer), Alan R. Liss, New York, pp. 73–85.

Kasper, C.K. (1984) Measurement of factor VIII inhibitors, in *Factor VIII Inhibitors* (ed. L.W. Hoyer), Alan R. Liss, New York, pp. 87–98.

Kasper, C.K. (1989) Treatment of factor VIII inhibitors, in *Progress in Hemostasis and Thrombosis,* 9th edn (ed. B.S. Coller), W.B. Saunders, Philadelphia, pp. 57–86.

Kasper, C.K. (1991) Laboratory tests for factor VIII inhibitors, their variation, significance and interpretation. *Blood Coagulation and Fibrinolysis,* **2,** 7–10.

Kasper, C.K., Aledort, L.M., Counts, R.B. *et al.* (1975) A more uniform measurement of factor VIII inhibitors. *Thromb Diath Haem,* **34,** 875–876.

Kasper, C.K. and Hemophilia Study Group (1979) Effect of prothrombin complex concentrates on factor VIII inhibitor levels. *Blood,* **54,** 1358–1368.

Kasper, C.K., Lusher, J.M. and Transfusion Practices Committee (1993) Recent evolution of clotting factor concentrates for hemophilia A and B. *Transfusion,* **33,** 422–434.

Kernoff, P.B.A., Thomas, N.D., Lilley, P.A. *et al.* (1984) Clinical experience with polyelectrolyte-fractionated porcine factor VIII concentrate in the treatment of hemophiliacs with antibodies to factor VIII. *Blood,* **63,** 31–41.

Kessler, C.M. (1991) An introduction to factor VIII inhibitors: the detection and quantitation. *Am J Med,* **91,** 5A–1S–5A–5S.

Kreuz, W., Ehrenforth, S., Funk, M. *et al.* (1995) Immune tolerance therapy in paediatric haemophiliacs with factor VIII inhibitors: 14 years follow-up. *Haemophilia,* **1,** 24–32.

Kurczynski, E.M. and Penner, J. (1974) Activated prothrombin concentrate for patients with factor VIII inhibitors. *N Engl J Med,* **291,** 164–167.

Lakich, D., Kazazian, H.H. Jr., Antonarakis, S.E. and Gitschier, J. (1993) Inversions disrupting the factor VIII gene are a common cause of severe haemophilia A. *Nature Genetics,* **5,** 236–241.

Largo, R., Sigg, P., von Felton, A. and Straub, P.W. (1974) Acquired factor IX inhibitor in a nonhaemophilic patient with autoimmune disease. *Br J Haematol,* **26,** 129.

Laurian, Y., Girma, J.P., Lambert, T. *et al.* (1984) Incidence of immune responses following 102 infusions of autoplex in 18 hemophilic patients with antibody to factor VIII. *Blood,* **63,** 457–462.

Lazarchick, J. and Hoyer, L.W. (1978) Immunoradiometric measurement of the factor VIII procoagulant antigen. *J Clin Invest,* **62,** 1048–1052.

Lechner, K. (1971) Factor IX inhibitors: report of two cases and a study of the biological, chemical, and immunological properties of the inhibitors. *Thromb Diath Haemorrh,* **25,** 447–459.

Lechner, K. (1974) Acquired inhibitors in nonhemophilic patients. *Haemostasis,* **3,** 93.

Lian, E.C.-Y., Larcada, A.F. and Chiu, A.Y.-Z. (1989) Combination immunosuppressive therapy after factor VIII infusion for acquired factor VIII inhibitor. *Ann Intern Med,* **110,** 774–778.

Lilleyman, J.S. (1994) Domiciliary desensitization therapy for young boys with haemophilia and factor VIII inhibitors. *Br J Haematol,* **86,** 433–435.

Lippert, L.E., Fisher, L.M. and Schook, L.B. (1990) Relationship of major histocompatibility complex class II genes to inhibitor antibody formation in hemophilia A. *Thromb Haemost,* **64,** 564–568.

Littlewood, J.D., Bevan, S.A., Kemball-Cook, G. *et al.* (1991) Variable inactivation of human factor VIII from different sources by human factor VIII inhibitors. *Br J Haematol,* **77,** 535–538.

Ljung, R.C.R. (1994) Intron 22 inversions and haemophilia. *Lancet,* **343,** 791.

Ljung, R., Petrini, P., Lindgren, A.-C. *et al.* (1992) Factor VIII and factor IX inhibitors in haemophiliacs. *Lancet,* **339,** 1550.

Lollar, P., Parker, C.G. and Tracy, R.P. (1988) Molecular characterization of commercial porcine factor VIII concentrate. *Blood,* **71,** 137–143.

Lollar, P., Parker, E.T., Curtis, J.E. *et al.* (1994) Inhibition of factor VIIIa by human anti-A2 subunit antibodies. *J Clin Invest,* **93,** 2497–2504.

Lorenzo, J.I., Garcia, R. and Molina, R. (1992) Factor VIII and factor IX inhibitors in haemophiliacs. *Lancet,* **339,** 1550–1551.

Lottenberg, R., Kentro, T.B. and Kitchens, C.S. (1987) Acquired hemophilia. A natural history study of 16 patients with factor VIII inhibitors receiving little or no therapy. *Arch Intern Med,* **147,** 1077–1081

Lozier, J.N., Santagostino, E., Kasper, C.K. *et al.* (1993) Use of porcine factor VIII for surgical procedures in hemophilia A patients with inhibitors. *Semin Hematol,* **30,** 10–21.

Lubahn, B.C., Ware, J., Stafford, D.W. and Reisner, H.M. (1989) Identification of a FVIII epitope recognized by a human hemophilic inhibitor. *Blood,* **73,** 497–499.

Lubin, I.M., Healey, J.F., Scandella, D. *et al.* (1994) Elimination of a major inhibitor epitope in factor VIII. *J Biol Chem,* **269,** 8639–8641.

Lusher, J.M. (1994) Use of prothrombin complex concentrates in management of bleeding in hemophiliacs with inhibitors – benefits and limitations. *Semin Hematol,* **31,** 49–52.

Lusher, J.M., Shapiro, S.S., Palascak, J.E. and Hemophilia Study Group (1980) Efficacy of prothrombin complex concentrates in hemophiliacs with antibodies to factor VIII: a multicenter therapeutic trial. *N Engl J Med,* **303,** 421–425.

Lusher, J.M., Blatt, P.M. and Penner, J.A. (1983) Autoplex vs Proplex: a controlled double blind study of effectiveness in acute hemarthrosis in hemophiliacs with inhibitors to factor VIII. *Blood,* **62,** 1135–1138.

Lusher, J.M., Salzman, P.M. and Monoclate Study Group (1990) Viral safety and inhibitor development associated with factor VIIIC ultra-purified from plasma in hemophiliacs previously unexposed to factor VIIIC concentrates. *Semin Hematol,* **27,** 1–7.

Lusher, J.M., Arkin, S., Abildgaard, C.F. *et al.* (1993) Recombinant factor VIII for the treatment of previously untreated patients with hemophilia A. *N Engl J Med,* **328,** 453–459.

McCullough, J., Fortuny, I.E., Kennedy, B.J. *et al.* (1973) Rapid plasma exchange with the continuous flow centrifuge. *Transfusion,* **13,** 94–99.

McMillan, C.W., Shapiro, S.S., Whitehurst, D. *et al.* (1988) The natural history of factor VIII:C inhibitors in patients with hemophilia A: a national cooperative study. II. Observations on the initial development of factor VIII:C inhibitors. *Blood,* **71,** 344–348

Macik, B.G. (1993) Treatment of factor VIII inhibitors: products and strategies. *Semin Thromb Hemost,* **19,** 13–24.

Macik, B.G., Lindley, C.M., Lusher, J. *et al.* (1993) Safety and initial clinical efficacy of three dose levels of recombinant activated factor VII (rFVIIa): results of a phase I study. *Blood Coagulation Fibrinolysis,* **4,** 521–527. 4

Majumdar, G. and Savidge, G.F. (1993) Recombinant factor VIIa for intracranial haemorrhage in a Jehovah's Witness with severe haemophilia A and factor VIII inhibitors. *Blood Coagulation Fibrinolysis,* **4,** 1031–1033.

Margolius, A. Jr, Jackson, D.P. and Ratnoff, O.D. (1961) Circulating anticoagulants: a study of 40 cases and a review of the literature. *Medicine,* **40,** 145–202.

Mariani, G., Ghirardini, A. and Bellocco, R. (1994) Immune tolerance in hemophilia – principal results from the international registry. *Thromb Haemost,* **72,** 155–158.

Mateo, J., Martino, R., Borrell, M. *et al.* (1993) Acquired factor VIII inhibitor preceding chronic lymphocytic leukemia. *Ann Hematol,* **67,** 309–311.

Mauser-Bunschoten, E.P., Rosendaal, F.R., Nieuwenhuis, H.K. *et al.* (1994) Clinical course of factor VIII inhibitors developed after exposure to a pasteurised Dutch concentrate compared to classic inhibitors in hemophilia A. *Thromb Haemost,* **71,** 703–706.

Moffat, E.H., Furlong, R.A. and Bloom, A.L. (1986) *In vitro* studies of factor VIII antibody anti-idiotype reagents. *Br J Haematol,* **64,** 818–819.

Mondorf, W., Ehrenforth, S., Vigh, Z. *et al.* (1994) Screening of FVIII:C antibodies by an enzyme-linked immunosorbent assay. *Vox Sang,* **66,** 8–13.

Morrison, A.E. and Ludlam, C.A. (1995) Acquired haemophilia and its management. *Br J Haematol,* **89,** 231–236.

Morrison, A.E., Ludlam, C.A. and Kessler, C. (1993) Use of porcine factor VIII in the treatment of patients with acquired hemophilia. *Blood,* **81,** 1513–1520.

Muhm, M., Grois, N., Kier, P. *et al.* (1990) 1-Deamino-8-D-arginine vasopressin in the treatment of non-haemophilic patients with acquired factor VIII inhibitor. *Haemostasis,* **20,** 15–20.

Munro, F.L. (1946) Properties of an anticoagulant formed in the blood of a hemophiliac. *J Clin Invest,* **25,** 422–427.

Naylor, J., Green, P.M., Rizza, C.R. and Giannelli, F. (1992) Analysis of factor VIII mRNA reveals defects in every one of 28 haemophilia A patients. *Hum Mol Genetics,* **2,** 11–17.

Ng, J., Hurley, C.K., Milford, E. *et al.* (1993) The specificity of large-scale oligonucleotide typing for HLA-DR and HLA-DQ. *Tissue Antigens,* **42,** 473–479.

Nilsson, I.M. (1992) The management of hemophilia patients with inhibitors. *Trans Med Rev,* **VI,** 285–293.

Nilsson, I.M. (1994) Immune tolerance. *Semin Hematol,* **31,** 44–48.

Nilsson, I.M., Berntorp, E. and Freiburghaus, C. (1993) Treatment of patients with factor VIII and IX inhibitors. *Thromb Haemost,* **70,** 56–59.

Nilsson, I.M., Berntorp, E. and Zettervall, O. (1986) Induction of split tolerance and clinical cure in high-responding hemophiliacs with factor IX antibodies. *Proc Natl Acad Sci USA,* **83,** 9169–9173.

Nilsson, I.M., Berntorp, E. and Zettervall, O. (1988) Induction of immune tolerance in patients with hemophilia and antibodies to factor VIII by combined treatment with intravenous IgG, cyclophosphamide and factor VIII. *N Engl J Med,* **318,** 947–950.

Nilsson, I.M., Jonsson, S., Sundqvist, S.-B. *et al.* (1981) A procedure for removing high titer antibodies by extracorporeal protein-A-Sepharose adsorption in hemophilia: substitution therapy and surgery in a patient with hemophilia B and antibodies. *Blood,* **58,** 38–44.

O'Marcaigh, A.S., Schmalz, B.J., Shaughnessy, W.J. and Gilchrist, G.S. (1994) Successful hemostasis during a major orthopedic operation by using recombinant activated factor VII in a patient with severe hemophilia A and a potent inhibitor. *Mayo Clin Proc,* **69,** 641–644.

Onder, O. and Hoyer, L.W. (1979) Factor VIII coagulant antigen in factor IX complex concentrates. *Thromb Res,* **15,** 569–572.

Orstavik, K.H. (1981) Alloantibodies to factor IX in haemophilia B characterized by crossed immunoelectrophoresis and enzyme-conjugated antisera to human immunoglobulins. *Br J Haematol,* **48,** 15–23.

Orstavik, K.H. and Miller, C.H. (1988) IgG subclass identification of inhibitors to factor IX in haemophilia B patients. *Br J Haematol,* **68,** 451–454.

Peerlinck, K., Rosendaal, F.R. and Vermylen, J. (1993) Incidence of inhibitor development in a group of young hemophilia A patients treated exclusively with lyophilized cryoprecipitate. *Blood,* **81,** 3332–3335.

Peerlinck, K., Arnout, J., Gilles, J.G. *et al.* (1993) A higher than expected incidence of factor VIII inhibitors in multitransfused haemophilia A patients treated with an intermediate purity pasteurized factor VIII concentrate. *Thromb Haemost,* **69,** 115–118.

Peerlinck, K., Goubau, P., Coppens, G. *et al.* (1994) Is the apparent outbreak of hepatitis A in Belgian hemophiliacs due to a loss of previous passive immunity? *Vox Sang,* **67,** 14–17.

Pike, I.M., Yount, W.J., Puritz, E.M. and Roberts, H.R. (1972) Immunochemical characterization of a monoclonal GammaG4, gamma human antibody to factor IX. *Blood,* **40,** 1–10.

Preston, F.E., Dinsdale, R.C.W., Sutcliffe, D.J. *et al.* (1977) Factor VIII inhibitor by-passing activity (FEIBA) in the management of patients with factor VIII inhibitors. *Thromb Res,* 11, 643–651.

Rasi, V. and Ikkala, E. (1990) Haemophiliacs with factor VIII inhibitors in Finland: prevalence, incidence and outcome. *Br J Haematol,* **76,** 369–371.

Regnault, V. and Stoltz, J.-F. (1994) Quantitation of factor VIII antibodies by an enzyme-linked immunoassay method. *Blood,* **83,** 1155–1158.

Rizza, C.R. and Biggs, R. (1973) The treatment of patients who have factor-VIII antibodies. *Br J Haematol,* **24,** 65–82.

Rizza, C.R. and Matthews, J.M. (1982) Effect of frequent factor VIII replacement on the level of factor VIII antibodies in haemophiliacs. *Br J Haematol,* **52,** 13–24.

Rosendaal, F.R., Nieuwenhuis, H.K., van den Berg, H.M. *et al.* (1993) A sudden increase in factor VIII inhibitor development in multitransfused hemophilia A patients in the Netherlands. *Blood,* **81,** 2180–2186.

Rossi, F. and Kazatchkine, M.D. (1989) Antiidiotypes against autoantibodies in pooled normal human polyspecific IgI. *J Immunol,* 143, 4104–4109.

Rossi, F., Sultan, Y. and Kazatchk, M.D. (1988) Anti-idiotypes against autoantibodies and alloantibodies to VIII-C (anti-hemophilic factor) are present in therapeutic polyspecific normal immunoglobulins. *Clin Exp Immunol,* **74,** 311–316.

Scandella, D., Mattingly, M. and Prescott, R. (1993) A recombinant factor VIII A2 domain polypeptide quantitatively neutralizes human inhibitor antibodies that bind to A2. *Blood,* **82,** 1767–1775.

Scandella, D., Mattingly, M., de Graaf, S. and Fulcher, C.A. (1989) Localization of epitopes for human factor VIII inhibitor antibodies by immunoblotting and antibody neutralization. *Blood,* **74,** 1618–1626.

Scandella, D., Timmons, L., Mattingly, M. *et al.* (992) A soluble recombinant factor VIII fragment containing the A2 domain binds to some human anti-factor VIII antibodies that are not detected by immunoblotting. *Thromb Haemost,* **67,** 665–671.

Scandella, D., Gilbert, G.E., Shima, M. *et al.* (1995) Some factor VIII inhibitor antibodies recognize a common epitope corresponding to C2 domain amino acids 2248–2312 which overlap a phospholipid binding site. *Blood,* **86,** 1811–1819.

Scheibel, E., Ingerslev, J., Dalsgaard-Nielsen, J. *et al.* (1987) Continuous high-dose factor VIII for the induction of immune tolerance in haemophilia A patients with high responder state: a description of 11 patients treated. *Thromb Haemost,* **58,** 1049–1052.

Schmidt, M.L., Gamerman, S., Smith, H.E. *et al.* (1994) Recombinant activated factor VII (rFVIIa) therapy for intracranial hemorrhage in hemophilia A patients with inhibitors. *Am J Hematol,* **47,** 36–40.

Schwartz, R.S., Abildgaard, C.F., Aledort, L.M. *et al.* Human recombinant DNA-derived antihemophilic factor (factor VIII) in the treatment of hemophilia A. *N Engl J Med,* **323,** 1800–1805.

Schwarzinger, I., Pabinger, I., Korninger, C. *et al.* (1987) Incidence of inhibitors in patients with severe and moderate hemophilia A treated with factor VIII concentrates. *Am J Hematol,* **24,** 241–245.

Seidler, C.W., Mills, L.E., Flowers, M.E.D. and Sullivan, K.M. (1994) Spontaneous factor VIII inhibitor occurring in association with chronic graft-versus-host disease. *Am J Hematol,* **45,** 240–243.

Seifried, E., Gaedicke, G., Pindur, G. and Rasche, H. (1984) The treatment of haemophilia A inhibitor with high dose intravenous immunoglobulin. *Blut,* **48,** 397–401.

Seremetis, S.V. (1994) The clinical use of factor VIIa in the treatment of factor VIII inhibitor patients. *Semin Hematol,* **31,** 53–55.

Shapiro, S.S. (1984) Genetic predisposition to inhibitor formation, in *Factor VIII Inhibitors* (ed L.W. Hoyer), Alan R. Liss, New York, pp. 45–55.

Sjamsoedin, L.J., Heijnen, L. and Mauser-Bunschoten, E.P. (1981) The effect of activated prothrombin complex concentrate (FEIBA) on joint and muscle bleeding in patients with hemophilia A and antibodies to factor VIII: a double-blind clinical trial. *N Engl J Med,* **305,** 717–721.

Slocombe, G.W., Newland, A.C., Colvin, M.P. and Colvin, B.T. (1981) The role of intensive plasma exchange in the prevention and management of haemorrhage in patients with inhibitors to factor VIII. *Br J Haematol,* **47,** 577–585.

Strauss, H.S. (1969) Acquired circulating anticoagulants in hemophilia A. *N Engl J Med,* **281,** 866–873.

Sultan, Y., Maisonneuve, P., Kazatchkine, M.D. and Nydegger, U.E. (1984) Anti-idiotypic suppression of autoantibodies to factor VIII (antihaemophilic factor) by high-dose intravenous gammaglobulin. *Lancet,* **2,** 765–768.

Sultan, Y., Rossi, F. and Kazatchkine, M.D. (1987) Recovery from anti-VIII:C (antihemophiic factor) autoimmune disease is dependent on generation of antiidiotypes against anti-VIII:C autoantibodies. *Proc Natl Acad Sci USA,* **84,** 828–831.

Sultan, Y., Kazatchkine, M.D., Nydegger, U. *et al.* (1991) Intravenous immuno-globulin in the treatment of spontaneously acquired factor VIII:C inhibitors. *Am J Med,* **91,** 5A–35S–5A–39S.

Sultan, Y., Kazatchkine, M.D., Algiman, M., *et al.* (1994) The use of intravenous immunoglobulins in the treatment of factor VIII inhibitors. *Semin Hematol,* **31,** 65–66.

Takahashi, I., Mizumo, S., Kamiya, T. *et al.* (1994) Epitope mapping of human factor IX inhibitor antibodies. *Br J Haematol,* **88,** 166–173.

Tiarks, C., Pechet, L. and Humphreys, R.E. (1989) Development of anti-idiotypic antibodies in a patient with a factor VIII autoantibody. *Am J Hematol,* **32,** 217–221.

Tizzano, E.F., Domenech, M., Altisent, C. *et al.* (1994) Inversions in the factor VIII gene in Spanish hemophilia A patients. *Blood,* **83,** 3826–3831.

Tuddenham, E.G.D., Schwaab, R., Seehafer, J. *et al.* (1994) Haemophilia A: database of nucleotide substitutions, deletions, insertions and rearrangements of the factor VIII gene, second edition. *Nucl Acids Res,* **22,** 3511–3533.

Uehlinger, J., Button, G.R., McCarthy, J. *et al.* (1991) Immunoadsorption for coagulation factor inhibitors. *Transfusion,* **31,** 265–269.

Van Der Zee, J.S., Van Swieten, P. and Aalberse, R.C. (1986) Serologic aspects of IgG$_4$ antibodies. II. IgG$_4$ antibodies form small, nonprecipitating immune complexes due to functional monovalency. *J Immunol,* **137,** 3566–3571.

Van Leeuwen, E.F., Mauser-Bunschoten, E.P., Van Dijken, P.J. *et al.* (1986) Disappearance of factor VIII:C antibodies in patients with haemophilia A upon frequent administration of factor VIII in intermediate or low dose. *Br J Haematol,* **64,** 291–297.

Verbruggen, B., Novakova, I., Wessels, H. *et al.* (1995) The Nijmegen modification of the Bethesda assay for factor VIII:C inhibitors: improved specificity and reliability. *Thromb Haemost,* **73,** 247–251.

Ware, J., MacDonald, M.J., Lo, M. *et al.* (1992) Epitope mapping of human factor VIII inhibitor antibodies by site-directed mutagenesis of a factor VIII polypeptide. *Blood Coagulation Fibrinolysis,* **3,** 703–716.

White, G.C. (1994) Factor VIII inhibitor assay quantitative and qualitative assay limitations and development needs. *Semin Hematol,* 31, 6–10.

White, G.C., Taylor, R.E., Blatt, P.M. and Roberts, H.R. (1983) Treatment of a high titer anti-factor-VIII antibody by continuous factor VIII administration: report of a case. *Blood,* **62,** 141–145.

21 BLEEDING IN THE HEMOPHILIA CARRIER

I.A. Greer and I.D. Walker

Changes in the factor VIII complex and factor IX in association with normal pregnancy

Normal pregnancy is associated with a substantial alteration in hemostasis. In general the concentration of many coagulation factors increases while plasma fibrinolytic activity decreases. Both factor VIII coagulant (VIII:C) and von Willebrand factor antigen and activity increase progressively through pregnancy with increases being seen from the first trimester (Stirling *et al.*, 1984). The increase in factor VIII coagulant activity is substantial, rising from a mean of 130 iu/dl in the first trimester to a mean of 212 iu/dl at term. The increase in von Willebrand factor antigen concentrations is more variable. However, first-trimester values are around 130 iu/dl with mean values at term of around 375 iu/dl (Hathaway and Bonnar, 1987). von Willebrand factor activity rises to a mean of around 170 iu/dl in the second and third trimester (Hathaway and Bonnar, 1987). Hemophilia carriers and most women with von Willebrand's disease also have an increase in the components of the factor VIII complex during pregnancy and in the majority these components will increase sufficiently to avoid excessive bleeding. However, in von Willebrand's disease the responses are variable and von Willebrand factor activity may show a lesser rise during pregnancy than factor VIII:C activity, particularly if the initial level of factor VIII:C is low (<15 iu/dl; Hill, George and Enayat, 1982; Adashi, 1986; Ramsahoye *et al.*, 1993). Bleeding time shortens significantly in pregnancy in a minority of von Willebrand's disease (Adashi, 1986; Conti *et al.*, 1986; Ramsahoye *et al.*, 1993). Furthermore, measurement of bleeding time factor VIII:C, von Willebrand factor antigen and von Willebrand factor activity will not always identify those patients that will bleed (Lipton, Eyromlooi and Coller, 1982; Greer *et al.*, 1991).

Hemophilia carriers

The majority of carriers inherit the abnormal gene for factor VIII or factor IX from their parents. In the case of the hemophiliac father, the daughter will be an obligate carrier. If the mother is a carrier, then half her daughters will be carriers. Sporadic new mutations can also occur. Usually the carrier will have a normal gene on the other X chromosome, and because of this, they will usually have coagulation factor activity >50 iu/dl (Chediak *et al.*, 1980). This is usually sufficient for normal hemostatic function. As normal hemostatic function is present the majority of such carriers do not have significant bleeding problems and many will remain undetected unless specifically studied on the basis of a family history. Bleeding problems can, however, develop in the small number of carriers who have clotting factor activities <40 iu/dl. Some carriers will have very low coagulation factor activities due to extreme lyonization or coinheritance of a variant von Willebrand factor allele such as vWD Normandy or in conjunction with an additional chromosomal abnormality such as Turner's syndrome, where no second X chromosome is present and the woman demonstrates features compatible with hemophilia. Women homozygous for the hemophilias are extremely rare.

Bleeding problems in carriers of hemophilia A and hemophilia B

There have been few detailed assessments of the bleeding problems in carriers of hemophilia A or hemophilia B. Bunschoten *et al.* (1988) studied 148 known carriers of hemophilia A and B by way of a self-administered questionnaire with 135 responses from 94 obligate carriers defined as daughters of hemophiliacs, mothers

Hemophilia. Edited by C.D. Forbes, L. Aledort and R. Madhok. Published in 1997 by Chapman & Hall, London. ISBN 0 412 63820 7

with two or more sons with hemophilia, mothers with one affected son and a brother, grandfather or maternal uncle with hemophilia and mothers with one affected son or one or more daughters who were carriers. The other 41 women were those closely related to hemophilia patients who were classified as carriers by laboratory assay (World Health Organization, 1977). Two reference groups were also studied for comparison: first, 25 women with relatives suffering from hemophilia but who were classified as non-carriers on laboratory testing, and second, 60 women with no family history but matched for age and social class with the carrier group.

Compared to the two reference groups, the hemophilia carriers had a statistically significant tendency to bruise and reported prolonged bleeding after tooth extraction, tonsillectomy and other operations. For example, 45% of carriers reported prolonged bleeding after tonsillectomy, while only 11% reported this in each of the reference groups. Prolonged bleeding after operation was noted in 30% of the carriers and in less than 12% of each of the non-carrier reference groups. Bleeding following delivery was also increased, being reported in 22% of the carrier group and in <7% of the reference groups. To control for other factors which may influence these findings a matched pair analysis was performed on these groups and prolonged bleeding after operation and delivery and from small wounds was still found to be significant in the hemophilia carrier group. Logistic regression analysis suggested that the tendency to bleed was completely explained by the plasma concentrations of factor VIII:C and IX:C. These findings substantiate earlier studies where increased incidence of bleeding after delivery or operation had been reported (Wahlberg, Blomback and Brodin, 1982), and emphasizes the importance of assaying clotting factor activity not only in potential carriers of hemophilia but in obligate carriers and in those diagnosed as carriers using molecular biologic techniques.

A further study has focused on the obstetric and gynecologic problems of obligate carriers of hemophilia A (Greer *et al.*, 1991). This study reviewed the obstetric and gynecologic problems of 18 obligate carriers of hemophilia A and five obligate carriers of hemophilia B, including 34 pregnancies in the obligate carriers of hemophilia A and 11 pregnancies in the obligate carriers of hemophilia B. These excluded first-trimester losses and ectopic pregnancies, assessed as part of the gynecologic assessment of these women. In addition, laboratory assessment of coagulation parameters was obtained in the third trimester in four of the five hemophilia B carriers and 13 of the 18 obligate carriers of hemophilia A. In those women who were carriers of hemophilia A, the majority showed a substantial increase in plasma activities for factor VIII:C by 28–36 weeks' gestation,

with all but two attaining normal concentrations greater than 45 iu/dl (Fig. 21.l). One patient had a very low concentration of factor VIII:C in the non-pregnant state (13 iu/dl) and during pregnancy this rose to only 19 iu/dl.

The increase in factor VIII:C activity was similar in each pregnancy which the carriers had. Twenty-three of the pregnancies resulted in spontaneous vaginal delivery, seven required forceps deliveries and four needed Cesarean section. No antepartum hemorrhage occurred, three carriers had secondary postpartum hemorrhage, of which two were associated with retained products of

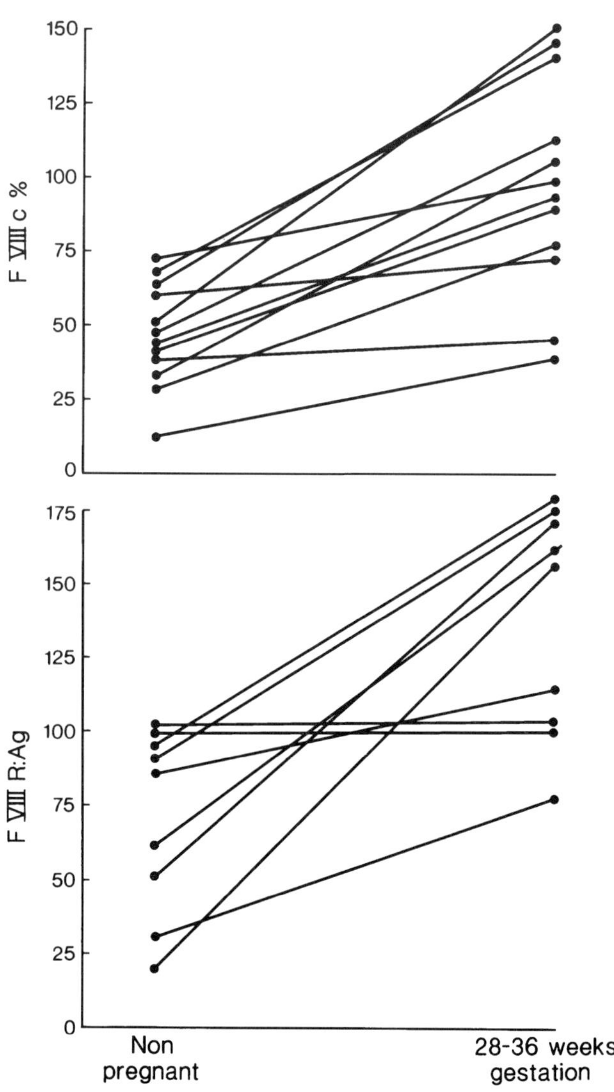

Fig. 21.1 Changes in von Willebrand factor antigen (vWF:Ag; VIIIR:Ag) and Factor VIII coagulant (VIII:C) in obligate carriers of hemophilia A during pregnancy. Where carriers have had more than one pregnancy, only the changes occurring in their first pregnancy are illustrated. From Greer, I.A., Lowe, G.D.O., Walker, J.J. and Forbes, C.D. (1991) Haemorrhagic problems in obstetrics and gynaecology in patients with congenital coagulopathies. *British Journal of Obstetrics and Gynaecology*, 98, 909–918, with permission.

conception following vaginal delivery. These required evacuation of the uterus and blood transfusion. Both these carriers had concentrations of factor VIII:C >45 iu/dl in the third trimester (76 and 97 iu/dl, respectively). The third secondary postpartum hemorrhage occurred after an elective Cesarean section in the patient with the low concentration of factor VIII:C of 19 iu/dl in the third trimester. Since this event occurred in the early 1980s she was given planned cryoprecipitate prophylaxis for 7 days after delivery and allowed home 10 days after delivery without complication. However, 4 weeks after delivery she presented with a secondary postpartum hemorrhage in excess of 1 liter, thought to be due to endometritis. She was successfully treated with cryoprecipitate, antibiotics and tranexamic acid.

Four of the 18 obligate carriers of hemophilia A had sought gynecologic advice for menorrhagia and all had had a diagnostic curettage performed without complications. Three of these women went on to have abdominal hysterectomy and one with a factor VIII:C concentration of 40 iu/dl developed a vault hematoma and was treated with factor VIII:C infusions for 1 week.

Other gynecologic problems included an ectopic pregnancy associated with major intra-abdominal hemorrhage in a patient with a factor VIII:C activity of 40 iu/dl, four spontaneous abortions with subsequent uterine evacuations which were not associated with any hemorrhagic complications and a sterilization and hysterotomy for termination of pregnancy which were uncomplicated.

The risk of postpartum hemorrhage in hemophilia carriers with reduced clotting factor activity has previously been noted (Wahlberg, Blomback and Brodin, 1982; Briet, Reisher and Blatt, 1982; Bunschoten *et al.*, 1988). The incidence of menorrhagia in this study did not appear to be excessive and indeed the study by Bunschoten *et al.* (1988) found that the incidence of menorrhagia was not significantly different from the reference groups. Clearly the majority of carriers of hemophilia A are unlikely to have problems during pregnancy, particularly. as the levels of factor VIII:C and von Willebrand factor increase significantly during pregnancy. However, it is essential that values are monitored as a small number of patients will show a very minimal change in factor VIII:C and these are usually those with baseline levels of the VIII:C. In this situation blood product cover will be required to cover the risk of postpartum hemorrhage.

A wide range of values for factor VIII:C is present in hemophilia A carriers with a mean value of factor VIII:C of 54 iu/dl (range 22–116) having been reported compared to a mean value of 96 iu/dl (range 44–136) for normal healthy females (Rizza *et al.*, 1975). Around 2% of hemophilia A carriers will have factor VIII:C levels of <30 iu/dl (Rapaport, Patch and Moore, 1961). In the

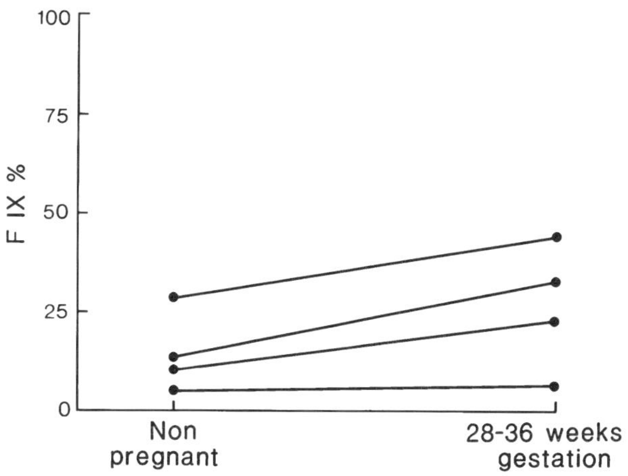

Fig. 21.2 Changes in factor IX (F IX) in obligate carriers of hemophilia B, during pregnancy. Where carriers have had more than one pregnancy, only the changes occurring in their first pregnancy are illustrated.

study reported by Greer *et al.* (1991), the carriers of hemophilia B showed much less of an increase in factor IX activity during pregnancy compared to the increase in factor VIII:C activity seen in hemophilia A carriers. All but one of the deliveries in the group of carriers of hemophilia B was covered with fresh/frozen plasma given immediately postpartum. Only one secondary postpartum hemorrhage occurred and one perineal hematoma, the latter arising prior to fresh-frozen plasma treatment. It is noteworthy that only one of the hemophilia B carriers reported in this review had factor IX activities within or around the normal range (>45 iu/dl) prior to delivery (Fig. 21.2). This was a woman with non-pregnant factor IX activity of 30 iu/dl increasing to 43, 46 and 45 iu/dl in the third trimester in her three pregnancies where levels were assessed. This had previously been noted by Briet, Reisher and Blatt (1982), who reported a single case of a carrier whose factor IX activity remained low and who had prolonged bleeding postpartum. Again it is important to monitor factor IX activity levels in these women during pregnancy and in the puerperium. However, as with hemophilia A, the increase in factor IX was consistent between pregnancies in hemophilia B carriers.

Specific measures may be required to ensure hemostasis. Two of the obligate carriers of hemophilia B had menorrhagia and underwent diagnostic curettage with prophylactic administration of fresh frozen plasma. Other procedures carried out on these women included oophorectomies and abdominal hysterectomy. None of these gynecologic procedures was complicated by peri-operative hemorrhage. However, the hysterectomy was covered with fresh frozen plasma.

Management of hemophilia carriers in pregnancy

All known and potential hemophilia carriers should ideally be seen for preconceptual genetic counseling. This counseling should include information about the availability, advantages and limitations of prenatal diagnosis (discussed elsewhere in this volume), the management of pregnancy and also the possible complications in pregnancy. Specific measures which can be taken prior to conception include the immunization of women who may require blood products against hepatitis B. Immunization against hepatitis A is also currently recommended because of recent reports of outbreaks of this form of hepatitis in some hemophiliacs.

Management of pregnancy with heritable bleeding disorders, including carriers of hemophilia A and B, should always be in conjunction with their regional hemophilia center. Coagulation factor activity should be monitored, particularly in the third trimester close to delivery, to ascertain whether or not a satisfactory increase has occurred in the activities of factor VIII:C or IX. As noted above, the activity of factor IX may not show a significant rise during pregnancy. Invasive procedures during pregnancy which may result in maternal, fetal or placental hemorrhage require careful consideration on an individual basis. The risk of hemorrhage must be taken into account when considering prenatal diagnosis by chorionic villus sampling or amniocentesis. Balancing the potential risk of hemorrhage and/or pregnancy loss against the estimated benefit of confirming or excluding a genetic bleeding disorder must form an integral part of the decision-making process when prenatal diagnosis is being considered. Where prenatal diagnosis is not performed, sexing of the fetus by ultrasound at around 18 weeks' gestation is a valuable non-invasive method of diagnosing the great majority of male fetuses. Carriers with low activities of factor VIII:C or factor IX may be at particular risk of obstetric bleeding problems in the first or second trimester (such as with miscarriage). Carriers of Hemophilia B appear to be at particular risk as the levels of factor IX do not increase as much as those of factor VIII, as discussed above. Should a patient have any bleeding episode during pregnancy, immediate assessment of the patient's coagulation status and specific clotting factor assay should be instigated so that therapy to raise clotting factor activity can be given, if necessary.

Uncomplicated vaginal delivery is the usual goal in carriers of hemophilia A or B. However, if a carrier has a male fetus and the chance of straightforward vaginal delivery is significantly compromised, early recourse to Cesarean section is preferable to a potentially traumatic instrumental vaginal delivery. It is prudent to insure that an experienced obstetrician is involved in the delivery of such patients. In addition, it is important to minimize trauma to the genital tract and perineum to reduce the risk of postpartum hemorrhage. Fetal scalp electrodes and fetal scalp sampling can cause significant problems if the fetus is affected by hemophilia and if possible these should be avoided in male fetuses which may be affected, or if the sex of the fetus is unknown. In addition, ventouse extraction should be avoided in a potentially affected fetus. The importance of atraumatic delivery is emphasized by the report of Yoffe and Buchanan (1988). This is a 10-year retrospective study of 150 newborn and young patients with hemophilia, in which eight of the infants developed central nervous system hemorrhage in the neonatal period. Other series have reported similar problems with intracranial bleeding (Bray and Lubon, 1989; Klatzel *et al.*, 1989), with traumatic vaginal delivery being implicated as the precipitant in the majority of infants with central nervous system hemorrhage.

At delivery a cord sample should be collected for assessment of the neonate. However, some hemostatic factors are physiologically present at relatively reduced levels in neonates and others are elevated. It may therefore be difficult to diagnose or exclude a mild to moderate inherited bleeding defect at birth. Repeat examination at 3–6 months may be necessary, although earlier genetic assessment would clearly be possible for some families. Intramuscular injection should be avoided in male offspring of hemophilia A and B carriers unless it has been clearly established that the baby is unaffected. Prophylactic vitamin K should be administered orally to these neonates and the general practitioner should be asked to ensure that when they receive their routine immunizations, these are either given subcutaneously or intradermally, with the intramuscular route being avoided. Furthermore, neonatal immunization against hepatitis B should be considered if the fetus is affected. Immunization against hepatitis A should also be given but delayed until the child is a year old. It is crucial that following delivery, mother and child are reviewed by the regional hemophilia center.

Blood product therapy

Where factor VIII:C activity is in excess of 40 iu/dl in the third trimester, the carrier is unlikely to bleed excessively during normal delivery, thus, blood product therapy is usually unnecessary in the event of an uncomplicated vaginal delivery. Where Cesarean section is planned or becomes necessary, factor VIII:C activity should be in excess of 50 iu/dl. Some carriers may not have reached this level in the third trimester and may require the infusion of high-purity factor VIII concentrate to obtain satisfactory levels for hemostasis. Where factor VIII:C levels are lower than 40 iu/dl then blood product therapy is required, even in the event of an uncomplicated vaginal delivery to raise factor VIII:C activity to at least 40 iu/dl.

Carriers of hemophilia B not infrequently have levels of factor IX coagulant activity at term inadequate for hemostatis function (Briet, Reisher and Blatt, 1982; Greer *et al.*, 1991). Again, it is important to review all known or potential carriers of hemophilia B in the middle part of the third trimester – around 34–36 weeks' gestation – to review their factor IX levels. These women more frequently require blood product therapy to cover even normal delivery than do carriers of hemophilia A. For vaginal delivery, factor IX activity should be $\geqslant$40 iu/dl. High-purity factor IX concentrate should be used, as factor IX concentrates (Prothrombin complex concentrates) containing in addition factors II, VII and X are potentially thrombogenic and may add to the established risk of thrombosis in the puerperium. From the above discussion it is clear that hemophilia carriers are at risk of postpartum hemorrhage and therefore levels of factor VIII:C and factor IX should be maintained at at least 40 iu/dl for 4–5 days: this period may require to be prolonged if there is evidence of continued bleeding or of wound infection. It is essential in such cases to avoid or at least minimize the use of drugs interfering with platelet function, such as non steroidal anti-inflammatory agents for postpartum analgesia.

DDAVP infusion

In non-pregnant carriers of hemophilia A or patients with the more common variants of von Willebrand's disease, the synthetic vasopressin analog desmopressin (DDAVP) is frequently used to cover procedures such as dental or minor surgery as intravenous infusion of this agent will provoke an increase in factor VIII complex components. However, in the obstetric situation, DDAVP should be used cautiously because of its mildly oxytocic effect. While this may be a relative contraindication during pregnancy, particularly in the third trimester where there would at least theoretically be a risk of precipitating preterm labour, it can be used immediately prior to or after delivery or following miscarriage or therapeutic abortion where a moderate rise in factor VIII activity is required for a few days only. A further problem with DDAVP is the risk of water retention and hyponatremia (Lowe *et al.*, 1977). Maternal water retention provoking a grand mal seizure has been reported with repeated therapy (Chediak, Albon and Maxe, 1986). Thus, where DDAVP is used, particularly in a repeated manner, it is recommended that urea and electrolytes are monitored carefully and excessive fluid input, particularly intravenously, is avoided.

With regard to pregnancy, it should also be noted that the response to DDAVP is greater in terms of the increase of von Willebrand factor and factor VIII:C in normal pregnant women than in normal non-pregnant women (fourfold versus twofold; Davison *et al.*, 1993). It has not been established, however, whether a greater response to DDAVP occurs during pregnancy in hemophilia A carriers than when these carriers are in the non-pregnant state.

Obstetric analgesia

As in any patient with defective hemostasis, intramuscular injections should be avoided. Parenteral analgesia should be administered either subcutaneously or intravenously. As noted above, antiplatelet agents should be used cautiously, if at all. The use of epidural anesthesia in hemophilia carriers is clearly highly controversial, although it has been suggested that, provided the coagulation screen is normal, the Simplate bleeding time <10 min and the platelet count $>100 \times 10^9$/l, there should in general be no contraindication to inserting an epidural catheter (Letsky, 1991). It may also be worthwhile repeating the coagulation screen and the platelet count before removing the epidural catheter. Spinal anesthesia may carry less risk.

Non-obstetric surgical procedures

For hemophilia carriers undergoing surgical procedures it is important that they are aware of any potentially increased risk of bleeding that they may have and alert the surgeon to this. Their management should be in conjunction with the regional hemophilia center. Their history of bleeding complications, level of factor VIII or IX activity and the type of procedure, along with the duration of the risk of hemorrhage, all require to be taken into account. If the carrier normally has a level of factor VIII or factor IX activity in excess of 50 iu/dl, then there is usually no need for blood product or DDAVP therapy. However, with levels below 50 iu/dl, hemostatic support may be required. For hemophilia A carriers, DDAVP infusion may be sufficient to cover minor procedures for a few days, but in hemophilia A carriers with variable levels of factor VIII:C activity and in hemophilia B carriers with baseline levels <50 iu/dl, high-potency factor VIII or IX concentrate will be required. The anesthetist should also be made aware of the hemostatic defect with regard to any regional anesthesia which is planned and intramuscular injections should be avoided, with parenteral analgesia being given by subcutaneous or intravenous injection. Again it would appear prudent to be cautious with regard to the use of non-steroidal anti-inflammatory agents or any other antiplatelet agent in the postpartum course.

Other issues for the hemophilia carrier

INVESTIGATION OF CARRIER STATUS

Female relatives of hemophiliacs often only consider investigation or raise the question of the possibility of their being a carrier when they are already pregnant or are in a relationship which is likely to lead to pregnancy. Clearly it is best if carriers are detected in advance of pregnancy and carrier testing should be avoided in pregnancy if possible. Optimal management would insure that carrier status is identified when the girl is in her early teens before she becomes sexually active and therefore before any planned or unplanned pregnancy arises. This may require that the parents of possible carriers should themselves be counseled and advised of the importance of encouraging their daughters to attend early for investigation. It is likely that women whose close male relatives are severely affected by one of the hemophilias may be more willing to seek investigation themselves than those with relatives with mild disease or whose relatives are distant. Of interest is a questionnaire survey of first-degree female relatives of 167 Finnish hemophilia A patients (Ranta *et al.*, 1994). These considered hemophilia a serious disease. The majority of these women were aware of the risk of carriership and of having an affected son. Sixteen per cent said they would definitely terminate a pregnancy where the fetus was a male and known to have hemophilia.

Varekamp *et al.* (1990) further evaluated the experience of attitudes to carrier detection and prenatal diagnosis in 549 potential and obligate carriers of hemophilia. Almost all those studied considered carrier testing to be of value. Almost 50% had been assessed for carrier status but, interestingly, 41% had not been tested and had not received information regarding the inheritance of hemophilia. Women with severely affected relatives were more likely to have been tested for carriership. The important factors for those women not having been tested was a lack of knowledge of possible carriership and a lack of awareness of carrier testing being available. Almost a third of those surveyed favored prenatal diagnosis with the subsequent possibility of termination of pregnancy if the fetus was affected. In women who objected to prenatal diagnosis, the main factor was that they did not consider that hemophilia was a disorder serious enough to justify termination of pregnancy. Clearly these surveys highlight the need for counseling with regard to carriership, pregnancy and prenatal diagnosis, as well as appropriate contraception, and every opportunity should be taken when carriers present themselves to insure that all such issues are adequately addressed.

The principles of contraception are essentially unchanged in hemophilia carriers with the method of contraception being tailored to the patient's requirements. Because of the possibility of a pregnancy resulting in an affected child, the reliability of the contraceptive method may be of fundamental importance to the carrier. The range of contraceptive aids available include barrier methods, the combined estrogen and progesterone oral contraceptive pill, the progesterone-only pill, depot preparations such as Depo-Provera and Norplant, the intrauterine contraceptive device and male and female sterilization. No technique is absolutely contraindicated and the choice will largely be governed by factors other than the bleeding disorder itself. Because, unfortunately, in the past many hemophiliacs have been infected with human immunodeficiency virus (HIV) or hepatitis viruses, hemophilia centers strongly encourage the use of condoms and advice on safe sex is usually given not only to hemophiliacs but also to their partners and female relatives. However, where contraception is a high priority it may be advisable to consider additional contraception, for example, the combined oral contraceptive pill if the couple feel that a pregnancy in this situation may be disastrous in the event of a failure of barrier contraception.

In contrast to women with von Willebrand disease, the incidence of heavy menstrual bleeding does not appear excessively high in women who are carriers of the hemophilias. In these women menorrhagia can often be dealt with by the use of appropriate contraception, where the oral contraceptive pill or the progestagen-impregnated intrauterine contraceptive device may be of value. The latter will virtually abolish heavy menstrual bleeding and also provide contraception. Depot progesterone preparations can be used but clearly intramuscular administration of such a preparation should be avoided if possible in women with low levels of factor VIII or factor IX activity. In the event that such a technique is used, there may be a need for DDAVP or blood product cover. If sterilization is performed in a carrier, again it is important to check the factor VIII or factor IX activity prior to surgery and cover this procedure with DDAVP or blood products as appropriate for a minor to intermediate surgical procedure, as discussed above.

Conclusions

Management of hemophilia carriers depends on accurate determination of carrier status. This fundamental knowledge can only be achieved if every opportunity is taken to identify potential carriers and educate them to the potential problems and the benefits from establishing carrier status. With the advent of molecular biologic techniques, our ability positively to diagnose or exclude carrier status is improving rapidly. All potential recipients of blood product therapy should be immunized for hepatitis B and currently also hepatitis A. Carriers may require DDAVP or blood product cover for elective or emergency surgery. Preconception counseling with regard to the hemostatic problems and management of pregnancy as well as genetic counseling about the disease and counseling with regard to prenatal diagnosis should also be offered. During pregnancy, there should be regular clinical and hemostatic assessment of factor VIII or IX activities. Sexing of the fetus by ultrasound may be useful, risks and benefits of invasive procedures should be carefully weighed up by obstetrician and patient along with the hematologist involved with her hemostatic management. Blood products or DDAVP may be required to cover delivery if activities of factor VIII or IX are not increased to adequate levels.

The delivery should be as atraumatic as possible in order to avoid not only maternal hemostatic problems but the potential problems with fetal trauma should the fetus suffer from hemophilia. In hemophilia A an umbilical cord blood sample should be taken from the fetus in order to help establish whether it suffers from hemophilia. Neonates with known or potential inherited bleeding defects should receive oral vitamin K and for routine immunization, any affected infant or where the infant's status with regard to hemophilia has not been established should be given intradermally. The mother should avoid intramuscular injections for analgesia in the postpartum period and levels should be maintained at a level sufficient to provide hemostasis for at least 4–5 days after delivery to minimize the risk of postpartum hemorrhage.

References

Adashi, E.Y. (1986) Lack of improvement in von Willebrand's disease during pregnancy. *New England Journal of Medicine*, 303, 1178.

Bray, G.L. and Lubon, N.L. (1989) Haemophilia presenting with intracranial haemorrhage. *American Journal of Diseases of Childhood*, 141, 1215–1217.

Briet, E., Reisher, H.M. and Blatt, P.M. (1982) Factor IX levels during pregnancy in a woman with haemophilia B. *Haemostasis*, 11, 87–89.

Bunschoten, E.P.M., van Houwelingan, J.C., Visser, E.J.M.S. *et al.* (1988) Bleeding symptoms in carriers of haemophilia A and B. *Thrombosis and Haemostasis*, 59, 349–352.

Chediak, J.R., Albon, G.N. and Maxe, B.Y. (1986) Von Willebrand's disease in pregnancy: management during delivery and outcome of offspring. *American Journal of Obstetrics and Gynecology*, 155, 618–624.

Chediak, J.R., Telfer, M.C., Jaojaroekul, T. and Green, D. (1980) Lower factor VIII coagulant activity in daughters of subjects with haemophilia A compared to other obligate carriers. *Blood*, 55, 552–558.

Conti, M., Mori, D., Conti, E. *et al.* (1986) Pregnancy in women with different types of von Willebrand's disease. *Obstetrics and Gynecology*, 68, 282–285.

Davison, J.M., Shiells, E.A., Phillips, P.R. *et al.* (1993) Metabolic clearance of vasopressin and an analogue resistant to vasopressin in human pregnancy. *American Journal of Physiology*, 264, F348–F353.

Greer, I.A., Lowe, G.D.O., Walker, J.J. and Forbes, C.D. (1991) Haemorrhagic problems in obstetrics and gynaecology in patients with congenital coagulopathies. *British Journal of Obstetrics and Gynaecology*, 98, 909–918.

Hathaway, W.E. and Bonnar, J. (1987) *Physiology of Coagulation in Pregnant Women and Newborn Infants*. John Wiley, New York, pp. 39–56.

Hill, F.G.H., George, J. and Enayat, M.S. (1992) Changes in VIII:C R:Ag, VIII:vWf and ristocetin induced platelet aggregation during pregnancy in women with von Willebrand's disease. *British Journal of Haematology*, 50, 691.

Klatzel, M., Miller, C.H., Beaton, D.L. *et al.* (1989) Post-delivery head bleeding in haemophilic neonates: causes and management. *American Journal of Diseases of Childhood*, 143, 1107–1110.

Letsky, E.A. (1991) Haemostasis and epidural anaesthesia. *International Journal of Obstetric Anaesthesia*, 1, 51–54.

Lipton, R.A., Eyromlooi, J. and Coller, B.S. (1982) Severe von Willebrand's disease during labor and delivery. *Journal of the American Medical Association*, 248, 1355–1357.

Lowe, G.D.O., Pettigrew, A., Middleton, S. *et al.* (1977) DDAVP in haemophilia. *Lancet*, ii, 614.

Ramsahoye, B.H., Dasani, H., Davies, S.V. and Pearson, J.F. (1993) Pregnancy and von Willebrand's disease. *Journal of Clinical Pathology*, 47, 569–571.

Ranta, S., Lehesjoki, A.E., Peippo, M. and Kaariaianen, H. (1994) Haemophilia A: experiences and attitudes of mothers, sisters and daughters. *Paediatric Haematology and Oncology*, 11, 387–397.

Rapaport, J.J., Patch, M.J. and Moore, F.J. (1961) Antehaemophiliac globulin levels in carriers of Haemophilia A. *Journal of Clinical Investigation*, 39, 1619–1625.

Rizza, C.R., Rhymes, J.L., Austen, D.E.G. *et al.* (1975) Detection of carriers of haemophilia. A "blind" study. *British Journal of Haematology*, 30, 447–456.

Stirling, Y., Woolf, L., North, W.R.S. *et al.* (1984) Haemostasis is normal pregnancy. *Thrombosis and Haemostasis*, 52, 176–182.

Varekamp, I., Saurmeijer, T.P., Brooker-Vriends, A.H. *et al.* (1990) Carrier testing and pre-natal diagnosis for haemophilia: experiences and attitudes of 549 potential and obligate carriers. *American Journal of Medical Genetics*, 37, 147–154.

Wahlberg, T., Blomback, M. and Brodin, U. (1982) Carriers and non-carriers of haemophilia A: I multivariate analysis of pedigree data screening, blood coagulation test and factor VIII variables. *Thrombosis Research*, 25, 401–414.

World Health Organization (1977) Methods for the detection of haemophilia carriers: a memorandum. *Bulletin of the World Health Organization*, 55, 675–702.

Yoffe, G. and Buchanan, G.R. (1988) Intracranial haemorrhage in newborn and young infants with haemophilia. *Journal of Paediatrics*, 113, 333–336.

22 MANAGEMENT OF HEMOPHILIA DURING SURGERY

N.L. Kobrinsky and D.A. Stegman

The surgical management of hemophilia has a long history (Ratnoff, 1980). The Babylonian Talmud records that the son of a woman whose three previous sons had bled to death after circumcision should be excused from this religious obligation (Slotki, 1936). Although the inherited nature of hemophilia was clearly recognized, the mechanism of bleeding was poorly understood. Until the beginning of the 18th century, it was thought that hemorrhage was entirely controlled by the contraction of blood vessels. At this time, Jean Louis Petit (1731), a leading French surgeon, recognized the role played by the clotting of blood 'within and around a severed artery, plugging the wound.' In 1819, Mr Ward, also a surgeon, suggested that hemophilia was due to a defect in blood clotting. Toward the end of the century, Georges Hayem (1956) reiterated this view.

The role of blood coagulation in normal hemostasis and in the pathogenesis of hemophilia was not generally accepted until the beginning of the 20th century. In 1901 William Henry Howell, professor of physiology at Johns Hopkins University, wrote: 'One of the most striking properties of blood is its power of clotting or coagulating shortly after it escapes from the blood vessels.' Since that time, advances in the understanding and treatment of hemophilia in industrialized countries have been explosive. Regrettably, these advances have not been enjoyed worldwide. Even today, the approach to surgery in patients with hemophilia in most Third World countries remains one of avoidance (Chandy, 1995).

Preoperative care

INDICATIONS FOR SURGERY

For hemophiliacs without factor VIII or IX inhibitors surgery can be performed with the same risks as in hemostatically normal subjects. Indications for surgery and the principles of surgical management in these patients are the same as in the non-hemophiliac (Lusher, 1995).

For patients with low-titer/low-responder inhibitors, the benefits of surgery must be carefully weighed against the potential risks of bleeding, particularly late bleeding associated with an anamnestic rise in the inhibitor titer. The high cost of factor concentrates in this setting must also be considered.

For patients with high-titer/high-responder inhibitors, elective surgery should not be considered unless a predictably hemostatic agent, such as factor VIIa, is available. Even with this agent, late postoperative bleeding remains a theoretic concern. In patients with high-titer/high-responder inhibitors, surgery without factor VIIa should be performed **in life-threatening situations only**. Activated or unactivated prothrombin complex concentrates are unpredictably hemostatic and carry a high risk of thrombotic complications. An alternative approach, using plasmapheresis with or without an immunoglobulin adsorption column followed by high doses of factor concentrate, requires technology that is unavailable in many treatment centers, carries a high risk of late postoperative bleeding and is often prohibitively expensive.

PLANNING ELECTIVE SURGERY

Surgery in patients with hemophilia is a complex endeavor and, wherever possible, should be planned well in advance. A coordinated effort is required by the surgeon, hematologist, coagulation technologist, blood bank, pharmacy, operating room, ward and physiotherapy staff (Rudowski, 1981; Willert *et al.*, 1983; Brown *et al.*, 1985; Kasper *et al.*, 1985; Lachiewicz *et al.*, 1985; Kitchens, 1986; Rudowski, Scharf and Ziemski, 1987; Rickard, 1995).

Hemophilia. Edited by C.D. Forbes, L. Aledort and R. Madhok. Published in 1997 by Chapman & Hall, London. ISBN 0 412 63820 7

PREOPERATIVE EVALUATION

The preoperative evaluation performed by the hematologist should include a complete hemostatic history, particularly past dental and surgical experiences, recent and/or current drug exposures, allergies and adverse drug reactions and other medical problems, including hepatitis and human immunodeficiency virus (HIV) status. The laboratory evaluation should include a biochemical screening profile, hepatitis B, hepatitis C and HIV serology (if not done within the preceding 6 months), an inhibitor screen and urine analysis.

SCREENING FOR COEXISTENT BLEEDING DISORDERS

Whereas hemophilia is rare, bleeding disorders characterized by a long bleeding time are common, identified in as many as 5% of the population and in 15% of the population after aspirin exposure (Fiore *et al.*, 1990). Combined defects may therefore occur; the diagnosis of hemophilia does not preclude the coexistence of another bleeding disorder characterized by a long bleeding time.

For patients over 2 years of age, a template bleeding time should therefore be considered, if not previously performed. Indications may include a history of chronic iron deficiency (not a typical feature of hemophilia), excessive blood loss with previous surgery despite adequate factor replacement and exogenous blood loss due to epistaxis, hematuria, menorrhagia or gastrointestinal bleeding. If the bleeding time is long, studies for von Willebrand disease and platelet function defects should be considered.

Patients should be reminded that aspirin-containing drugs are contraindicated in hemophilia. Patients with chronic joint disease should be advised that non-steroidal anti-inflammatories should be discontinued for at least 2 days prior to surgery. Pain can be controlled in the interim with narcotic analgesics.

SCHEDULING SURGERY

Surgery should be scheduled for a time when the attending hematologist and all ancillary staff are available. The hematologist should be prepared to go to the operating room if problems with hemostasis arise. The coagulation laboratory technologist should be advised that urgent factor determinations will be required before and at specified times following surgery. For this reason, surgery should not be scheduled as a 'first case' if preoperative factor determinations are required.

The surgeon and operating room staff should be informed that surgery must not be delayed after preoperative factor replacement has been given or the patient's plasma may not be hemostatic.

FACTOR CONCENTRATE REQUIREMENTS FOR SURGERY

As soon as surgery is scheduled, the hematologist should inform the pharmacy or blood bank of the specific type and quantity of factor concentrate to be used for perioperative and postoperative management. The inpatient stock should then be documented, with particular attention paid to product expiry date. Additional product should be ordered as needed. For example, for major surgery in a patient with hemophilia A to be maintained at a factor VIII level of 50% for 3 days (continuous infusion), 30% for 4 days (continuous infusion) and 35% peak and 5% trough for 7 days, factor VIII should be ordered as follows (Table 22.1): 35 u/kg load + 0.5 × 3.8 u/kg per h × 72 h + 0.3 × 3.8 u/kg per h × 96 h + 25 u/kg per day × 7 days = 35 + 136.8 + 109.4 + 175 = 450 u/kg.

IN-SERVICE TRAINING OF STAFF PRIOR TO SURGERY

Prior to surgery, in-service training should be arranged, particularly for staff not familiar with hemophilia. The details of drawing blood samples for factor determinations and administering factor concentrates, cryoprecipitate and desmopressin should be reviewed. Blood samples must be taken from a clean venipuncture site. If a venous access device is used, the line must be cleared, particularly if heparinized, before samples are obtained.

Blood samples should be drawn in 'blue-top', citrate anticoagulant tubes and filled to specified capacity (to

Table 22.1 Guidelines for continuous infusion factor VIII (FVIII) and IX (FIX) administration for major surgical procedures in patients with moderate and severe hemophilia A and B

	Steady-state level		Factor infusion rate	
	FVIII	FIX	FVIII	FIX
Preoperatively	50%*	40%*	35 u/kg bolus	50 u/kg bolus
Days 1–3	50%	40%	1.90 u/kg per h	3.00 u/kg per h
Days 4–7	30%	25%	1.14 u/kg per h	1.88 u/kg per h
Days 7–14	35%/5%	20%/5%†	20 u/kg bolus	20 u/kg bolus

*Postinfusion peak factor level.

†Postinfusion peak and 24-h trough factor level.

maintain consistency in the amount of citrate added to each sample). Blood samples must be taken to the coagulation laboratory and processed immediately. The pharmacy, blood bank and ward staff should be aware of the high cost of factor concentrates. Partial vials should never be discarded. Vials with adequate but not excessive factor content should be used.

Perioperative and postoperative care

MILD HEMOPHILIA A (FACTOR VIII >5%)

Desmopressin acetate (DDAVP)

Patients with mild hemophilia typically respond to the synthetic peptide desmopressin with a three- to 10-fold increase in their basal factor VIII level. The drug also increases von Willebrand factor in normal subjects and in subjects with von Willebrand disease. The use of desmopressin in bleeding disorders has recently been reviewed (Mariani, Mannucci and Cattaneo, 1993).

Patients with mild hemophilia should have their factor VIII response evaluated pre- and 1 h post-desmopressin 0.3 μg/kg intravenously (IV) over 20 min (maximum 24 μg). This response is reproducible in patients with hemophilia A and von Willebrand disease. Thus, there should not be a need to recheck a patient each time therapy is required (Rodeghiero *et al.*, 1989). Patients with a post-desmopressin factor VIII response of <30% should be prepared for dental work using factor VIII concentrate. Patients with a post-desmopressin factor VIII response of <50% should be prepared for surgery using factor VIII concentrate. Patients with a post-desmopressin factor VIII response of ⩾50% can usually be prepared for dental work and/or minor surgical procedures using desmopressin alone. Patients with a post-desmopressin factor VIII response of ⩾50% may be prepared for major surgery if first, they do not develop significant tachyphylaxis with repeated administrations at 24 h intervals × 3 doses and if second, the 24-h trough factor VIII level ⩾30%. There is no particular advantage to using both factor VIII concentrate and desmopressin. The combination in most instances will make monitoring complicated. Therefore, if desmopressin alone is not expected to be sufficient for a surgical procedure, use factor VIII concentrate from the outset (Table 22.2).

Desmopressin-stimulated plasma

Desmopressin-stimulated plasma obtained by plasmapheresis from a limited donor pool has been used to treat patients with mild and moderate hemophilia (Nilsson, 1993; Sassetti and McLeod, 1993). This approach could theoretically be taken for patients with mild hemophilia scheduled for major surgical procedures in whom tachyphylaxis to repeated doses of desmopressin would otherwise limit the use of demopressin. Desmopressin-stimulated plasma could be 'harvested' by plasmapheresis prior to surgery, frozen and administered postoperatively at intervals to maintain a hemostatic factor VIII level in the postoperative period.

Desmopressin contraindications and adverse effects

Contraindications to desmopressin include:

1. Age <1 year (because of the risk of hyponatremic seizures; Shepherd *et al.*, 1989).
2. Cyanotic congenital heart disease (because of risk of hypoxic crisis e.g. 'Tet spell' in Tetralogy of Fallot. Israels and Kobrinsky, 1989).
3. History of previous adverse reaction to desmopressin, e.g. significant hyponatremia and/or hypotension.
4. History of cardiovascular disease, e.g. ischemic heart disease, myocardial infarction, transient ischemic attacks and/or stroke (Lusher, 1993).
5. Pre-existing hyponatremia.

Pregnancy, use of the birth control pill, renal failure and hypertension are relative but not absolute contraindications to the use of desmopressin (Table 22.3).

When desmopressin is used preoperatively for hemostasis, the significant risk of hyponatremia must be recognized. Excessive intraoperative and postoperative free water must be avoided to prevent iatrogenic hyponatremia. Oliguria is a direct physiologic and pharmacologic effect of desmopressin. Urine output should therefore not be used as an indicator of the adequacy of fluid replacement and renal perfusion after desmopressin has been given. Repeated doses of desmopressin may be associated with severe hyponatremia. Electolyte monitoring is therefore essential if more than a single dose of the drug is required (Weinstein *et al.*, 1989).

Table 22.2   Desmopressin for surgery in patients with mild hemophilia

| | *Desmopressin factor VII response* | | | | | *Tachyphylaxis* | |
| | *1 h post* | | | *24 h post* | | | |
	<30%	*30–50%*	*>50%*	*<30%*	*>30%*	*Yes*	*No*
Dental	No	Yes	Yes	Yes	Yes	Yes	Yes
Minor surgery	No	Yes	Yes	Yes	Yes	Yes	Yes
Major surgery	No	No	Yes	No	Yes	No	Yes

Table 22.3 Contraindication to the use of desmopressin for surgery in patients with mild hemophilia

Absolute

Age < 1 year
Cyanotic congenital heart disease
Previous adverse reaction to desmopressin
History of cardiovascular disease
Type IIb von Willebrand disease
Hyponatremia

Relative

Pregnancy
Type IIa von Willebrand disease
Use of birth control pill

VON WILLEBRAND DISEASE

As for mild hemophilia, patients with von Willebrand disease should have their response to desmopressin evaluated before proceeding with dental and/or surgical procedures. Pre- and post-desmopressin bleeding time, factor VIII, von Willebrand antigen and ristocetin cofactor should be evaluated (Cameron and Kobrinsky, 1990; Aledort, 1991; Logan, 1992).

Most patients with type I von Willebrand disease will be desmopressin-responders (Ruggeri *et al.*, 1982). Some, but not all, patients with type IIa von Willebrand disease respond to desmopressin, usually with a shortening but incomplete correction of the bleeding time, a normal von Willebrand antigen response, but a blunted ristocetin cofactor response. Non-responders should be treated with von Willebrand factor concentrates (e.g. Humate-P, Armour Pharmaceuticals) if available or cryoprecipitate (1 bag/5–6 kg, maximum 8 bags). von Willebrand factor concentrates are less likely to transmit hepatitis C virus and other potential blood borne viruses because of virucidal processing (Berntorp and Nilsson, 1988; Mannucci *et al.*, 1992).

Patients with type IIb von Willebrand disease develop moderate to severe thrombocytopenia (platelet count less than 50×10^9/l) following desmopressin. Although the bleeding time may shorten, desmopressin should not be used for these patients (Ruggeri *et al.*, 1982; Kyrle *et al.*, 1988). Patients with type IIb disease should be treated with von Willebrand factor concentrate, if available, or cryoprecipitate.

Patients with type III von Willebrand disease do not respond to desmopressin. Such patients should receive von Willebrand factor concentrates, if available, or cryoprecipitate. Of note, the bleeding time may not correct in patients with type III von Willebrand disease despite an increase in factor VIII, von Willebrand antigen and ristocetin cofactor $\geqslant 100\%$. This is likely to be due to the importance of platelet von Willebrand factor in platelet–vessel wall adhesion.

Of interest in this regard, correction of the bleeding time in type III von Willebrand disease has been reported with the use of normal platelet transfusions (Castillo *et al.*, 1991). The use of desmopressin has also been shown further to shorten the bleeding time of patients with type III von Willebrand disease after partial correction with cryoprecipitate (Cattaneo *et al.*, 1989). Synergistic shortening of the bleeding time by desmopressin and von Willebrand factor concentrates has also been demonstrated (Table 22.4). The mechanism of the synergistic shortening of the bleeding time observed with desmopressin and cryoprecipitate or von Willebrand factor concentrates must be independent of released von Willebrand factor and implies an effect on platelet-associated von Willebrand factor.

PLATELET FUNCTION DEFECTS AND DISORDERS WITH A LONG BLEEDING TIME

In addition to its use in von Willebrand disease, desmopressin has been found to be effective in a variety of congenital and acquired platelet function defects and other bleeding disorders, including cirrhosis of the liver and uremia, characterized by a long bleeding time (Mariani, Mannucci and Cattaneo, 1993). It is therefore recommended that patients with a prolonged bleeding time be evaluated for response to desmopressin before blood products such as platelets or cryoprecipitate (Gerritsen, Akkerman and Sixma, 1978) are considered. If the bleeding time does not correct with desmopressin alone, the combination of desmopressin and ethamsylate (10–20 mg/kg IV), a derivative of the dye Congo red, may be effective (Kobrinsky, Israels and Bickis, 1991).

Table 22.4 Synergistic shortening of the bleeding time with desmopressin and Humate-P in a patient with type III von Willebrand disease

	Baseline	Desmopressin	Humate-P	Desmopressin/ Humate-P
Bleeding time (min)	24.0	24.0	19.0	11.0
Factor VIII	23%	73%	114%	316%
von Willebrand antigen	0%	18%	330%	
Ristocetin cofactor	7%	30%	315%	

Alternatively, high doses of conjugated estrogens (0.6 mg/kg per day orally or IV for 5 days) may be effective in correcting a markedly prolonged bleeding time in patients scheduled for surgery. Conjugated estrogens have been reported to correct the bleeding time in patients with uremia prior to renal biopsy (Liu, Kosfeld and Marcum, 1984).

MODERATE AND SEVERE HEMOPHILIA A AND B (<5%)

Despite the use of cryoprecipitate and factor VIII and factor IX concentrates for the past 35 years and the tremendous cost of these products, the minimal levels of factor VIII and factor IX needed to maintain hemostasis in medical and surgical situations have not been rigorously studied. Bleeding complications have been reported to occur in 4–23% of procedures, usually in the postopera-tive period rather than during operations (Rudowski, 1981; Willert *et al.*, 1983; Brown *et al.*, 1985; Kasper *et al.*, 1985; Lachiewicz *et al.*, 1985; Kitchens, 1986; Rudowski, Scharf and Ziemski, 1987). Continued factor replacement until complete wound healing has been achieved is therefore necessary. Factor replacement should also be continued with postoperative rehabilita-tion, particularly following orthopedic procedures.

INTERMITTENT FACTOR CONCENTRATE REPLACEMENT THERAPY

Guidelines for intermittent factor VIII and factor IX treatment, i.e. peak factor VIII/IX level, treatment interval and duration for major surgery, minor surgery and dental work have been based on clinical experience but have not for the most part been validated in a clinical trial setting (Rickard, 1995; Tables 22.5–22.7).

Table 22.5 Guidelines for factor VIII (FVIII) and IX (FIX) administration for major surgical procedures in patients with moderate and severe hemophilia A and B

	Peak factor level desired (u/dl)		Dosage (u/kg)		Interval (h)	
	FVIII	*FIX*	*FVIII*	*FIX*	*FVIII*	*FIX*
Preoperatively	80–100	50–80	40–50	50–80	Stat	Stat
Days 1–3	80–100	50–80	20–25	25–40	8–12	12–18
Days 4–6	60–80	40–50	15–20	20–25	8–12	12–18
Days 7–10	30–60	30–40	20–40	15–20	12	18
Days 10–12	20–40	20–30	10–20	20–30	24	24

From Rickard K.A. (1995) Guidelines for therapy and optimal dosages of coagulation factors for treatment of bleeding and surgery in hemophilia. *Hemophilia*, **1** (suppl. 1), 8–13, with permission.

Table 22.6 Guidelines for factor VIII and IX (FIX) administration for minor surgical procedures in patient with moderate and severe hemophilia A and B

	Peak factor level desired (u/dl)		Dosage (u/kg)		Interval (h)	
	FVIII	*FIX*	*FVIII*	*FIX*	*FVIII*	*FIX*
Preoperatively	50–60	30–40	20–30	30–40	Stat	Stat
Days 1–3	40–50	20–30	20–25	20–30	12	12–18
Days 4–9	20–30	20–30	15–30	20–30	24	24

From Rickard K.A. (1995) Guidelines for therapy and optimal dosages of coagulation factors for treatment of bleeding and surgery in hemophilia. *Hemophilia*, **1** (suppl. 1), 8–13, with permission.

Table 22.7 Guidelines for factor VIII (FVIII) and IX(FIX) administration for invasive dental procedures, extractions and surgery in patients with moderate and severe hemophilia A and B

	Peak factor level desired (u/dl)		Dosage (u/kg)		Interval (h)	
	FVIII	*FIX*	*FVIII*	*FIX*	*FVIII*	*FIX*
Preoperatively	70–80	50–60	35–40	50–60	Stat	Stat
Days 1–2	50–60	30–40	25–30	30–40	12	12–18

From Rickard K.A. (1995) Guidelines for therapy and optimal dosages of coagulation factors for treatment of bleeding and surgery in hemophilia. *Hemophilia*, **1** (suppl. 1), 8–13, with permission.

Continuous infusion factor replacement therapy

Recently, there has been a move to administering factor VIII and factor IX by continuous infusion for severe bleeding episodes and for surgery (McMillan *et al.*, 1970; Bona *et al.*, 1989; Martinowitz *et al.*, 1992). This approach prevents excessive peaks and troughs in factor levels, allows the monitoring of factor levels at any time (not just by extrapolating from peak and trough determinations), is much simpler for nursing staff to manage, and is considerably less expensive (Noe *et al.*, 1985). Considerable variability in factor recovery and half-life is noted in different subjects and with different products. Guidelines for achieving steady-state levels are summarized in Table 22.8. For patients with hemophilia A undergoing major surgery managed by continuous infusion factor replacement, factor VIII levels should be maintained at 50% for the first 72 h and 30% for the next 96 h. Single daily infusions to maintain a peak of 35% and a trough of 5% should then be maintained for the second postoperative week. (Table 22.1). A more conservative infusion schedule using 50 u/kg per h preoperatively and a continuous infusion of 2–4 u/kg per h has been suggested by some investigators (Harrison *et al.*, 1993; Manco-Johnson, Geraghty and Nuss, 1993; Rickard, 1995). Increased requirements for factor VIII in the perioperative period may be encountered in children in some surgical settings, presumably because of increased consumption (Noe *et al.*, 1985).

Choice of factor concentrate

A wide choice of factor concentrates is available for surgical management. Issues of viral safety, risk of inhibitor development, effects on the immune system and cost are complex and not restricted to management of surgical procedures and will not be considered further here. If factor concentrates are not available, surgery in hemophilia A can be managed using cyroprecipitate. The factor VIII content of cryoprecipitate is approximately 80 u/bag.

Close monitoring of factor VIII levels in the perioperative period is often difficult because of turnaround times of at least 90 min in most centers. Recently, use of a bedside whole blood factor VIII assay has been reported. This device provides a turnaround time of 5–7 min. Assay results correlated well with conventional assay results (Kessler *et al.*, 1993). The use of such a device offers definite advantages to surgical management of hemophilia and will undoubtedly become more widely used in the near future.

SPECIFIC CONSIDERATIONS FOR HEMOPHILIA B

For patients with hemophilia B, lower levels of factor IX are required to maintain hemostasis. For major surgery, factor IX levels should be maintained at 40% for the first 72 h and 25% for the next 96 h. Intermittent (single daily) infusions to maintain a peak of 20% and a trough of 5% should then be maintained for the second postoperative week (Table 22.1).

Prothrombin complex concentrates

Patients with hemophilia B have historically been treated with prothrombin complex concentrates. For many years prothrombin complex concentrates have been implicated in the development of deep venous thrombosis, pulmonary embolism, disseminated intravascular coagulation, myocardial infarction and stroke (Lusher, 1991; Kasper *et al.*, 1993). These complications are believed to be associated with activated factors VII, IX, X and II and with zymogen excess (Gray *et al.*, 1992).

Risk factors for the development of these complications include surgery, particularly orthopedic surgery, pre-existing liver disease, duration of treatment greater than 2–3 days, doses of prothrombin complex concentrates greater than 75 u/kg per 24 h and treatment of infants.

Purified factor IX concentrates

Because of the risk of thrombotic complications, there has been an increasing interest in the use of highly purified factor IX preparations, devoid of contaminating activated and unactivated factors II, VII and X for the treatment of patients with hemophilia B. These products have been found to provide effective hemostasis and to be free of thrombotic complications – even in high-risk clinical situations – in several recent clinical trials (Kim *et al.*, 1992; Oates *et al.*, 1993; Pabinger *et al.*, 1993; Rickard and Holman, 1993; Thomas *et al.*, 1995).

Table 22.8 Factor VIII and IX pharmacokinetics in patients with moderate and severe hemophilia A and B

	Factor VIII	*Factor IX*
Recovery	1.5–2.0%/u per kg	0.8–1.0%/u per kg
Half-life	8–12 h	12–18 h
Steady state (at 100%)	3.8 u/kg per h	7.5 u/kg per h

Based on these findings, it is recommended that purified factor IX products be used wherever possible for patients with hemophilia B, particularly in the perioperative and postoperative period.

Fresh frozen plasma

Surgery without factor concentrates in hemophilia B is extremely difficult to manage. The amount of plasma required to achieve hemostatic levels of factor IX cannot be administered by rapid intravenous infusion because of fluid overload considerations. Frozen or fresh frozen plasma (50 ml/kg) should be thawed 1 u at a time and infused continuously over 8–12 h prior to surgery with concomitant diuretic therapy. Continuous infusion of plasma should be continued during and following surgery at a rate of 3 ml/kg per h for 3 days and then reduced to 2 ml/kg per h for the next 4 days. This approach is obviously less than ideal and carries the risks of fluid overload, electrolyte imbalance, allergic and anaphlyactic reactions to plasma proteins and suboptimal hemostasis.

MODERATE AND SEVERE HEMOPHILIA A AND B (<5%) WITH INHIBITORS

Patients with inhibitors to factor VIII and, rarely, factor IX are extremely difficult management problems, particularly for surgery. Ideally, an inhibitor should be eliminated before surgery is contemplated. For urgent and emergency surgical procedures this is often not possible. Also, surgical placement of a central venous access device is usually necessary before an inhibitor immune tolerance program can be initiated. Many different immune tolerance programs have been used, with varying degrees of success over the past 20 years. This complex issue has been recently reviewed (Nilsson, Berntorp and Freiburghaus, 1993; Brettler, 1995).

Low-titer (<5 Bethesda Units; BU) inhibitors

High-dose factor replacement therapy. Patients with low-titer factor VIII inhibitors (less than 5 BU) can often be managed by overwhelming the inhibitor with high doses of factor VIII.

The required dose of factor VIII (as a first approximation) is:

inhibitor titer (BU) × plasma volume (ml) + 50 u/kg

or

$$\text{inhibitor titer (BU)} \times \text{weight (kg)} \times 70 \times$$
$$(1 - \text{hematocrit}) + 50 \text{ u/kg}$$

For example, a man with severe hemophilia A weighing 75 kg with a hematocrit of 0.40 l/l and a factor VIII

inhibitor of 4 BU would require:

$$4 \times 75 \times 70 \times (1 - 0.40) + 50 \times 75$$
$$= 12\ 600 + 3\ 750 = 16\ 350 \text{ u}$$

to achieve 100% factor VIII activity. Subsequent doses would be calculated assuming a normal factor VIII recovery and half-life but would require close monitoring of actual factor levels.

Patients with low-level inhibitors may be low-responders or high-responders. In the case of low-responders, the factor VIII antibody remains at a low level despite factor VIII treatment. Low-responder patients can usually be managed with factor VIII throughout the perioperative and postoperative period.

In the case of high-responders, the factor VIII antibody titer markedly increases within 3–4 days of factor VIII exposure. Patients can be managed with factor VIII throughout the perioperative period; however, 2–3 days postoperatively, the factor VIII inhibitor titer rises and alternative treatment strategies are necessary to maintain hemostasis. **For this reason, elective surgical procedures should not be performed on hemophiliacs with high-responder inhibitors unless alternative therapies are available (e.g. recombinant factor VIIa) for when the anamnestic antibody response occurs.**

Porcine factor VIII concentrate. An alternative treatment strategy for patients with low to moderate inhibitor titers is to use polyelectrolyte fractionated porcine factor VIII concentrate (Hyate-C; Brettler *et al.*, 1989). Potential candidates for this therapy should be screened for porcine factor VIII antibodies. If the porcine factor VIII titer is low (generally, <5 BU), porcine factor VIII concentrate may be used. Again, the possibility of an anamnestic response must be considered, particularly in patients who have previously demonstrated an anamnestic response to human factor VIII concentrates. Thrombocytopenia due to contamination by small quantities of porcine von Willebrand factor and allergic reactions have been reported with the use of this product. Porcine factor VIII concentrate has been particularly effective in the surgical and non-surgical management of acquired factor VIII inhibitors.

High-titer (>5 BU) inhibitors

Recombinant human factor VIIa. The surgical management of patients with high-titer factor VIII and IX inhibitors was a major problem until the recent development of recombinant human factor VIIa (Hedner and Kislel, 1983; Hedner, Glazer and Falch, 19000; Hedner *et al.*, 1988; Macik *et al.*, 1989; Hedner, 1990; Ingerslev, Fledstedt and Sindey-Petersen, 1991; O'Marcaigh *et al.*, 1994). At a dose of 90 u/kg IV every 4 h, factor VIIa has been very effective for both surgical and non-surgical bleeding events in patients with high-titer inhibitors. Thrombotic complications have not been observed. A cautionary note is, however, warranted. Experience with factor VIIa is still limited and there has been at least one report where adequate surgical hemostasis was not achieved (Gringeri, Santagostino and Mannucci, 1991). Undoubtedly, the development of an *in vitro* assay which predicts *in vivo* hemostatic activity will lead to more appropriate dosing, scheduling and quality assurance with the use of this agent (Jacobsen, Nielsen and Nielsen, 1993; Johansen *et al.*, 1993). Other innovative inhibitor-bypassing therapies, including activated factor X combined with phospholipids and human recombinant tissue factor, are in development (Giles, Mann and Nesheim, 1988; Gomperts *et al.*, 1991).

Factor VIIa is not yet generally available out of the context of a clinical trial. Without this product, elective surgery in hemophiliacs with high-titer antibodies is not recommended: Although prothrombin complex concentrates and activated prothrombin complex concentrates are of value in the management of non-surgical bleeds (such as hemarthroses), efficacy in general is poor and not predictable (Lusher *et al.*, 1980; Sjamsoedin *et al.*, 1981; Usher *et al.*, 1983). An assay predicting the adequacy of surgical hemostasis (as for factor VIIa) is not available. Furthermore, as previously discussed, the use of prothrombin complex concentrates and activated prothrombin complex concentrates particularly in surgical settings, is associated with a high risk of thromboembolism, myocardial infarction and disseminated intravascular coagulation.

Emergency surgery in patients with high-titer inhibitors

The management of patients with high-titer inhibitors who require emergency surgery is extremely difficult. If available, factor VIIa should be used. If factor VIIa is not available, and if time and resources allow, high-titer factor VIII and IX antibodies can be temporarily decreased or eliminated by plasmapheresis, thereby allowing the use of factor VIII or IX to achieve surgical hemostasis. The use of a Staphylococcus protein A absorption column (specifically to remove immunoglobulin) may allow more efficient antibody removal than plasmapheresis alone (Gjorstrup *et al.*, 1991; Nilsson, Sundqvist and Freiburghaus, 1991). Steroids and high-dose γ-globulin, administered after plasmapheresis, may blunt the anamnestic inhibitor response following plasmapheresis and factor replacement, though this remains a significant concern (Nilsson *et al.*, 1983; Azhar *et al.*, 1984; Sultan *et al.*, 1984).

The Malmö regimen, a very effective regimen used for inducing immune tolerance in patients with low- and high-titer factor VIII and IX inhibitors, includes the use of plasmapheresis with Staphylococcus protein A immunoadsorption, high-dose intravenous γ-globulin, methylprednisolone, cyclophosphamide and high doses of factor VIII or IX (Nilsson and Hay 1995; Nilsson, Berntorp and Freiburghaus, 1993). The use of immunoadsorption, intensive immunosuppression and factor replacement with this regimen allows the rapid removal of inhibitors with a delayed and blunted anamnestic antibody response. The Malmö regimen therefore may be an effective regimen to prepare hemophiliacs with high-titer inhibitors for urgent, if not emergency surgery.

If emergency surgery is necessary, and plasmapheresis and factor VIIa are not available, prothrombin complex concentrates or activated prothrombin complex concentrates should be used. The risk of inadequate hemostasis and/or thrombosis with this approach is significant. Preoperatively, patients should receive prothrombin complex concentrates or activated prothrombin complex concentrates at a dose of 75 u/kg by slow intravenous infusion (not greater than 100 u/min). Heparin (100 u/1000 u of prothrombin complex concentrates or activated prothrombin complex concentrates) should be added to the infused factor concentrate. Postoperatively, prothrombin complex concentrates or activated prothrombin complex concentrates should be administered at a dose of 75 u/kg every 8 hours. Heparin should be administered by continuous infusion to maintain the thrombin time at 1.5–2.0 times normal.

Specific surgical considerations

DENTAL AND OROPHARYNGEAL SURGERY

Delayed bleeding after dental surgery is a well-recognized presentation of hemophilia (Humphries and Baker, 1992). This observation underscores the need for hemostatic treatment before and after dental procedures.

Factor replacement for patients undergoing dental extractions and oral surgery is summarized in Table 22.7. Because of the high fibrinolytic activity of saliva, antifibrinolytic agents such as ε-amino-caproic acid (Amicar) and tranexamic acid (Cyklokapron) should be used in conjunction with factor replacement therapy to prevent rapid clot dissolution. Amicar should be administered before and for 3–4 days after dental work at a dose of 50 mg/kg per dose per 6 h.

GENITOURINARY SURGERY

As for dental and oropharyngeal surgery, the high fibrinolytic activity of urokinase in urine may result in clot dissolution in patients with hemophilia undergoing bladder and/or prostate surgery. Fibrinolytic inhibitor therapy, administered either systemically or by bladder irrigation is therefore recommended in addition to appropriate factor replacement therapy.

Antifibrinolytic therapy should not be administered for renal surgery (including renal biopsy) because of the risk of clot formation within the renal tubules, resulting in urinary obstruction.

ORTHOPEDIC SURGERY

Delayed bleeding following orthopedic surgery, particularly with postoperative physiotherapy, has been reported (Willert *et al.*, 1983; Lachiewicz *et al.*, 1985). Daily factor replacement should therefore be continued until complete wound healing has been achieved. Prophylactic factor replacement should also be continued prior to physiotherapy sessions.

As in patients without hemophilia, orthopedic surgical procedures are associated with a significant risk of thromboembolic complications. Therefore, in addition to factor replacement, standard approaches to the prevention of thrombotic complications e.g. low-dose heparin, should be used. Patients with hemophilia B should not receive prothrombin complex concentrates; they should receive only purified factor IX concentrates.

CARDIOTHORACIC SURGERY

Cardiothoracic surgery can be performed safely on patients with hemophilia A or B. Patients should receive factor VIII or IX before surgery (Tables 22.5). As for other surgical procedures, the use of pure factor IX concentrates is preferable to the use of prothrombin complex concentrates. If purified factor IX is not available, the addition of heparin (approximately 100 u of heparin/1000 u of prothrombin complex concentrate) may decrease but not eliminate the risk of thrombotic complications (Scharfman *et al.*, 1993). Postoperatively, continuous infusion of factor VIII or IX is recommended (Table 22.1).

CHOLECYSTECTOMY, LIVER BIOPSY AND LIVER TRANSPLANTATION

For hemophiliacs without inhibitors or significant liver disease, the principles of surgery are the same as for normal subjects. By example, successful laparoscopic cholecystectomy has recently been reported in a patient with hemophilia B (Matzsch *et al.*, 1992).

For hemophiliacs with liver disease the situation is more complex. For example, the risks and benefits of liver biopsy in patients with hemophilia and chronic liver disease due to hepatitis C and/or B are controversial. In addition to their underlying factor deficiency, such patients may also have a prolonged bleeding time and/or a coagulopathy related to cirrhosis. Patients scheduled for liver biopsy should have baseline liver functions performed in addition to a platelet count, template bleeding time, fibrinogen and factors V, IX and VII/X. If the fibrinogen is low, a D-dimer (to exclude a low-grade consumptive coagulopathy), plasminogen and euglobulin lysis time (to exclude a hyperlytic state) should also be performed. An open procedure rather than a closed liver biopsy is recommended.

Liver transplantation has been performed successfully in patients with hemophilia who have end-stage liver disease. In addition to treatment of the underlying liver disease, the procedure is curative for hemophilia. Factor VIII or IX typically reaches normal hemostatic levels within 24 h and remains normal postoperatively (Delorme *et al.*, 1990).

SPLENECTOMY

HIV-infected hemophiliacs frequently develop idiopathic thrombocytopenic purpura. This complication does not imply HIV progression but may significantly increase the risk of potentially life-threatening bleeding. As in other cases of chronic idiopathic thrombocytopenic purpura medical therapy, e.g. chronic steroid use, is for the most part disappointing and associated with significant morbidity. Splenectomy is curative in over 80% of patients. When performed early in the course of HIV disease, the procedure may be associated with improved immune function (McKernan and Hay, 1995; Tsoukas *et al.*, 1996). Patients may be prepared for surgery with immunoglobulin G (1 g/kg) or with steroids if IgG is not available. A preoperative platelet count of $50-100 \times 10^9/l$ can usually be obtained.

INSERTION OF VENOUS ACCESS DEVICE

Central venous access devices are being used with increasing frequency in patients with hemophilia for immune tolerance of an inhibitor and/or prophylaxis. For immune tolerance, an external venous access device, e.g. Hickman catheter, is recommended. A subcutaneous port is not recommended for patients with inhibitors because of inevitable bleeding and hematoma formation at the port needle access site, often leading to infection. Further, the need for daily access, necessary for immune tolerance, is more than the tissues overlying a subcutaneous port can tolerate for long periods of time. For prophylactic factor infusion in the absence of an inhibitor, venous access three times per week is generally adequate. The subcutaneous port is recommended for this situation. Patient selection and 'hands-on' patient education of catheter management are important factors in minimizing the risk of catheter-associated infection. As with other foreign bodies, antibiotic prophylaxis is recommended prior to dental work.

Infectious complications of surgery in hemophilia

Information concerning the infectious complications of surgery in hemophiliacs is limited. The cumulative incidence of postoperative wound infections in three series has been reported at 0–1% (Willert *et al.*, 1983; Brown *et al.*, 1985; Kitchens, 1986). This figure suggests that hemophiliacs are not at increased risk of postoperative wound infections; however, a higher incidence of infections related to implanted venous access devices in hemophiliacs compared with cancer patients has been recently reported (Warrier *et al.*, 1993). Whether this difference is due to relative complacency in hemophilia as compared to cancer patients is not known. Of interest, however, is the observation that factor concentrates, particularly concentrates of intermediate purity compared with high purity, have been reported to inhibit monocyte function *in vitro* and *in vivo* (Pasi and Hill, 1990). At least theoretically, this acquired monocyte dysfunction may predispose to an increased risk of postoperative infection.

A higher incidence of postoperative infections has been observed in hemophiliacs with compared with without inhibitors. This observation may reflect excessive peri- and postoperative bleeding with hematoma formation and secondary infection. Patients with inhibitors receiving steroids and immunosuppressive therapies as part of an immune tolerance program are particularly at an increased infectious risk.

In HIV-1-seropositive hemophiliacs who have not progressed to acquired immunodeficiency syndrome (AID), an increased incidence of postoperative wound infections was not observed when compared with HIV-1-seronegative hemophiliacs (Bruehrer *et al.*, 1990). In patients with full-blown AIDS there may be an increased risk of opportunistic infection related to nosocomial exposure and the increased immunosuppression associated with surgery.

Considerations for the future

Major advances have been made in the surgical management of hemophilia. Several basic clinical problems none the less remain. For patients with hemophilia A and B without inhibitors, the minimum concentration of factor VIII and IX required for hemostasis in the perioperative and postoperative period, both for intermittent and continuous intravenous administration, has not yet been clearly defined. For patients with inhibitors, assay systems that will predict surgical hemostasis with the use of activated and non-activated prothrombin complex concentrates and factor VIIa are clearly required.

In most but not all instances, surgery in hemophilia can be performed with normal hemostasis and minimal risk.

A coordinated effort by the surgeon, hematologist, coagulation laboratory, blood bank, pharmacy, operating room and ward staff is necessary. In view of this complexity, surgery should not be performed in centers where appropriate expertise and resources are not available. Patients should be referred to centers able to deliver state-of-the-art surgical care for hemophiliacs. Regrettably, such centers do not exist in the majority of Third World countries (Chandy, 1995). The thrust of the World Federation of Hemophilia Decade Plan is to make effective treatment available to people with hemophilia throughout the world (Jones, 1995). This, more than anything else, remains the challenge for the future.

Acknowledgments

The authors would like to thank Eileen A. Chamberlain, librarian, Meritcare Medical Center and Diane E. Sjolander, CRA, for her assistance with preparation of the manuscript.

References

Aledort, L.M. (1991) Treatment of von Willebrand's disease. *Mayo Clin Proc*, **66**, 841–846.

Aznar, J.A., Jorquera, J.I., Piero, A. and Garcia, I. (1984) The importance of corticoids added to continued treatment with factor VIII concentrates in the suppression of inhibitors in hemophilia A. *Thromb Haemostas*, **51**, 217–221.

Berntorp, E. and Nilsson, I.M. (1988) Biochemical and *in vivo* properties of commercial virus-inactivated factor VIII concentrates. *Eur J Haematol*, **40**, 205–214.

Bona, R.D., Weinstein, R.A., Weisman, S.J. *et al.* (1989) The use of continuous infusion of factor concentreates in the treatment of hemophilia. *Am J Hematol*, **32**, 8–13.

Brettler, D.B. (1995) Inhibitors of factor VIII and IX. *Hemophilia*, **1** (suppl. 1), 35–39.

Brettler, D.B., Forsberg, A.D., Levine, P.H. (1989) The use of porcine factor VIII concentrate (Hyate:C) in the treatment of patients with inhibitor antibodies to factor VIII. A multicenter US experience. *Arch Intern Med*, **149**, 1381–1385.

Brown, B., Steed, D.L., Webster, M.W. *et al.* (1985) Surgery in adult hemophiliacs. *Surgery*, **99**, 154–159.

Buehrer, J.L., Weber, D.L., Meyer, D.L., Meyer, A.A. *et al.* (1990) Wound infection rates after invasisve procedures in HIV-1 seropositive versus HIV-1 seronegative hemophiliacs. *Ann Surg*, **211**, 492–498.

Cameron, C.B. and Kobrinsky, N. (1990) Perioperative management of patients with von Willebrand's disease. *Can J Anaesth*, **37**, 341–347.

Castillo, R., Monteagudo, J., Escolar, G. *et al.* (1989) DDAVP shortens the prolonged bleeding times of patients with severe von Willebrand disease treated with crypprecipitate: evidence for a mechanism of action independent of released von Willebrand factor. *Blood*, **74**, 1972–1975.

Chandy, M. (1995) Management of hemophilia in developing countries with available resources. *Hemophilia*, **1** (suppl. 1), 44–48.

Delorme, M.A., Adams, P.C., Grant, D. *et al.* (1990) Orthotopic liver transplantation in a patient with combined hemophilia A and B. *Am J Hematol*, **33**, 136–138.

Fiore, L.D., Brophy, M.T., Lopez, A. *et al.* (1990) The bleeding time response to aspirin. Identifying the hyperresponder. *Am J Clin Pathol*, **94**, 292–296.

Gerritsen, S.W., Akkerman, J.W.N. and Sixma, J.J. (1978) Correction of the bleeding time in patients with storage-pool deficiency by infusion of cryoprecipitate. *Br J Haematol*, **40**, 153–160.

Giles, A.R., Mann, K.G. and Nesheim, M.E. (1988) A combination of factor Xa and phosphatidycholine-phosphatidylserine vesicles bypasses factor VIII *in vivo*. *Br J Haematol*, **69**, 491–497.

Gjorstrup, P., Bertrop, E., Larsson, L. and Nilsson, I.M. (1991) Kinetic aspects of the removal of IgG and inhibitors in hemophiliacs using protein A immunoadsorption. *Vox Sang*, **61**, 244–250.

Gomperts, E., Lawrence, J., Liu S.-L. *et al.* (1991) Safety and efficacy studies of recombinant tissue factor. *Thromb Haemostas*, **65**, 677.

Gray, E., Tubbs, J., Cesmeli, S. and Barrowcliffe, T.W. (1992) Thrombogenicity of factor IX concentrates: *in vitro* and *in vivo* results. *Br J Haematol*, **80** (suppl. 1), 20.

Gringeri, A., Santagostino, E. and Mannucci, P.M. (1991) Failure of recombinant activated factor VII during surgery in a hemophiliac with high titer factor VIII antibodies. *Haemostasis*, 21, 1–4.

Harrison, J.A., Powell, J.S. and Abilgard, C.F. (1993) Constant infusion of recombinant factor VIII (Kogenate) for surgery in hemophilia. *Thromb Haemostas*, 69, 1099.

Hayem, G. (1956) quoted by Dreyfuss, C. in *Some Milestones in The History of Hematology*, Grune-Stratton, New York, p. 87.

Hedner, U. (1990) Factor VIIa in the treatment of haemophilia. *Blood Coagul Fibrinol*, 1, 307–317.

Hedner, U. and Kisiel, W. (1983) Use of human factor VIIa in the treatment of two hemophilia A patients with high-titer inhibitors. *J Clin Invest*, 71, 1836–1841.

Hedner, U., Glazer, S. and Falch, J. (1993) Recombinant activated factor VII in the treatment of bleeding episodes in patients with inherited and acquired bleeding disorders. *Transfus Med Rev*, 7, 78–83.

Hedner, U., Glazer, S., Pingel, K. *et al.* (1988) Successful use of recombinant factor VIIa in a patient with severe haemophilia A during synovectomy. *Lancet*, 2, 1193.

Howell, W.H. (1901) Blood and lymph, in *An American Textbook of Physiology*, (ed. W.H. Howell), Saunders, Philadelphia, pp. 54–63.

Humphries, J.E. and Baker, R.C Jr. (1992) Occult hemophilia: prolonged bleeding follows extraction. *JADA*, 123, 69–70.

Ingerslev, J., Fledstedt, M. and Sindey-Petersen, S. (1991) Control of haemostasis with recombinant factor VIIa in patient with inhibitor to factor VIII. *Lancet*, 338, 831–832.

Israels, S.J. and Kobrinsky, N.L. (1989) Serious reaction to desmopressin in a child with cyanotic heart disease. *N Engl J Med*, 320, 1563.

Jacobsen, J.K., Nielsen, G.G. and Nielsen, F.E. (1993) Measuring coagulant activity in activated factor VII concentrates using a one-stage clotting assay calibrated with recombinant activated factor VII. *Thromb Haemostas*, 69, 866.

Johansen, L., Bucher, D., Hansen, L.L. *et al.* (1993) Relation between factor VIIa coagulant activity and APTT in human plasma. *Thromb Haemostas*, 69, 1125.

Jones, P. (1995) Haemophilia: a global challenge. *Haemophilia*, i, 11–13.

Kasper, C.K., Boylen, A.L., Ewing, N.P. *et al.* (1985) Hematologic management of hemophilia A for surgery. *JAMA*, 253, 1279–1283.

Kasper, C.K., Lusher, J.M. and the Transfusion Practises Committee, AABB (1993) Recent evolution of clotting factor concentrates for hemophilia A and B. *Transfusion*, 33, 422–434.

Kessler, C., Bernstein, Z., Ghesani, S. *et al.* (1993) Bedside measurement of factor VIII activity in hemophilia patients. *Thromb Haemostas*, 69, 854.

Kim, H.C., McMillan, C.W., White, G.C. *et al.* (1992) Purified factor IX using monoclonal immunoaffinity technique: clinical trials in hemophilia B and comparison to prothrombin complex concentrates. *Blood*, 79, 568–575.

Kitchens, C.S. (1986) Surgery in hemophilia and related disorders. *Medicine*, 65, 34–45.

Kobrinsky, N.L., Israels, E.D. and Bickis, M.G. (1991) Synergistic shortening of the bleeding time by desmopressin and ethamsylate in patients with various constitutional bleeding disorders. *Am J Pediatr Hematol Oncol*, 13, 437–441.

Kyrle, P.A., Niessner, H., Dent, J. *et al.* (1988) IIB von Willebrand's disease: pathogenic and therapeutic studies. *Br J Haematol*, 69, 55.

Lachiewicz, P.F., Inglis, A.E., Insall, J.N. *et al.* (1985) Total knee arthroplasty in hemophilia. *J Bone Joint Surg*, 67-A, 1361–1366.

Liu, Y.K., Kosfeld, R.E. and Marcum, S.G. (1984) Treatment of uraemic bleeding with conjugated oestrogen. *Lancet*, 2, 887–890.

Logan, L.J. (1992) Treatment of von Willebrand's disease, in *Coagulation Disorders I, Hematology Clinics of North America*, vol. 6 (eds J.A. Penner and H.I. Hassouna), W.B. Saunders, Philadelphia, pp. 1079–1094.

Lusher, J.M. (1991) Thrombogenicity associated with factor IX complex concentrates. *Semin Hematol*, 28, 3–5.

Lusher, J.M. (1993) Myocardial infarction and stroke – is the risk increased by desmopressin? in *Desmopressin in Bleeding Disorders NATO ASI Series A: Life Sciences*, vol. 242 (eds G. Mariani, P.M. Mannucci and M. Cattaneo), Plenum, New York, pp. 347–353.

Lusher, J.M. (1995) Consideration for current and future management of haemophilia and its complications. *Haemophilia*, 1, 2–10.

Lusher, J.M., Shapiro, S.S., Palascka, J.E. *et al.* (1980) Efficacy of prothrombin complex concentrates in hemophiliacs with antibodies to factor VIII. *N Engl J Med*, 303, 421–425.

Lusher, J.M., Blatt, P.M., Penner, J.A. *et al.* (1983) Autoplex vs. proplex: a double controlled double blind study of effectiveness in acute hemarthrosis in hemophiliacs with inhibitors to factor VIII. *Blood*, 62, 1135–1138.

McKernan, A.M. and Hay, C.R.M. (1995) Early rapid decline in CD4 count reversed by splenectomy in HIV infection. *Hemophilia*, 1, 67–69.

McMillan, C.W., Webster, W., Roberts, H.R. and Blythe, W.B. (1970) Continuous infusion of FVIII in classic hemophilia. *Br J Haematol*, 18, 659–667.

Macik, B.G., Hohnekr, J., Roberts, H.R. and Griffen, A.M. (1989) Use of recombinant activated factor VII for treatment of retropharyngeal hemorrhage in a hemophilic patient with high titer inhibitor. *Am J Hematol*, 32, 232–234.

Manco-Johnson, M.J., Geraght, S. and Nuss, R. (1993) Factor VIII (FVIII) requirements in children with hemophilia are double for the first 24 hours post-operatively. *Thromb Haemostas*, 69, 1100.

Mannucci, P.M., Tenconi, P.M., Castaman, G. and Rodeghiero, F. (1992) Comparison of four virus-inactivated plasma concentrate for treatment of severe von Willebrand disease: a cross-over randomized trial. *Blood*, 79, 3130–3137.

Mariani, G., Mannucci, P.M. and Cattaneo, M. (eds) (1993) *Desmopressin in Bleeding Disorders, NATO ASI Series A: Life Sciences*, vol. 242, Plenum, New York.

Martinowitz, U., Shulman, S., Gitel, S. *et al.* (1992), Adjusted dose continuous infusion of factor VIII in patients with hemophilia A. *Br J Haematol*, 82, 729–734.

Matzsch, T., Almqvist, P., Berntorp, E. *et al.* (1992) Brief clinical report. Laparoscopic cholecystectomy in a patient with hemophilia B. *Surg Laparos Endosc*, 2, 339–340.

Nilsson, I.M. (1993) The use of DDAVP in blood donors to increase the yield of factor VIII in the preparation of factor VIII concentrates, in *Desmopressin in Bleeding Disorders, NATO ASI Series A: Life Sciences*, vol. 242 (eds G. Mariani, P.M. Mannucci and M. Cattaneo), Plenum, New York, pp. 227–232.

Nilsson, I.M. and Hay, C.R.M. (1995) Results in three Australian haemophilia B patients with high-responding inhibitors treated with the Malmo model. *Haemophilia*, 1, 59–66.

Nilsson, I.M., Jonsson, S., Sunquist, S., Ahlerg, A., Bergentz, S.C. (1981) A procedure for removing high titer antibodies by extracorporeal protein A Sepharose absorption in hemophilia. *Blood*, 58, 38–44.

Nilsson, I.M., Bertorp, E., and Freiburghaus, C. (1993) Treatment of patients with factor VIII and IX inhibitors. *Thromb Haemostas*, 70, 56–59.

Nilsson, I.M., Sundqvist, S.B., Ljung, R. *et al.* (1983) Suppression of secondary antibody by intravenous immunoglobulin in a patient with hemophilia B and antibodies. *Scand J Haemtol*, 30, 458–464.

Noe, D.A., Bell, W.R., Ness, P.M. and Levin, J. (1985) Plasma clearance rates of coagulation factors VIII and IX in factor deficient individuals. *Blood*, 67, 969–972.

Oates, A., Hughes, E., Kupczyk, G. *et al.* (1993) Monocomponent factor IX: a high purity factor IX concentrate for the treatment of patients with hemophilia B. *Thromb Haemostas*, 69, 1284.

O'Marcaigh, A.S., Schmalz, B.J., Shaughnessy, W.J. and Gilchrist, G.S. (1994) Successful hemostasis during a major orthopedic operation by using recombinant activated factor VII in a patient with severe hemophilia A and a potent inhibitor. *Mayo Clin Proc*, 69, 641–644.

Pabinger, I., Kyrle, P., Lack, W., and Funovics, J. (1993) Perioperative bleeding prophylaxis using purified factor IX concentrate during surgery on two patients with hemophilia B. *Thromb Haemostas*, 69, 1284.

Pasi, K.J. and Hill, F.G.H. (1990) *In vitro* and *in vivo* inhibition of monocyte phagocytic function by factor VIII concentrates: correlation with concentrate purity. *Br J Haematol*, 76, 88–93.

Petit, J.L. (1731) Dissertation sur la manniere d'arrester le sang dans les hemorrhagies. *Mem Acad R Sci*, 1, 85–102.

Ratnoff, O.D. (1980) Why do people bleed? in *Blood, Pure and Eloquent* (ed. M.M. Wintrobe), McGraw-Hill, New York, pp. 601–657.

Rickard, K.A. (1995) Guidelines for therapy and optimal dosages of coagulation factor for treatment of bleeding and surgery in hemophilia. *Hemophilia*, 1 (suppl. 1), 8–13.

Rickard, K.A. and Holman, P. (1993) 'Immunine' therapy for total knee replacement in Christmas disease: an Australian experience. *Thromb Haemostas*, 69, 1284.

Rodeghiero, F., Castaman, G., Di Bona, E. and Ruggeri, M. (1989) Consistency of responses to repeated DDAVP infusions in patients with von Willebrand's disease and hemophilia A. *Blood*, 74, 1997–2000.

Rudowski, W.J. (1981) Major surgery in hemophilia. *Ann R Coll Surg Engl*, 63, 111–117.

Rudowski, W.J., Scharf, R. and Ziemski, J.M. (1987) Is major surgery in hemophiliac patients safe? *World J Surg*, 11, 378–386.

Ruggeri, Z.M., Mannucci, P.M., Lombardi, R. *et al.* (1982) Multimeric composition of factor VII/von Willebrand factor following administration of DDAVP: implication for pathophysiology and therapy of von Willebrand's disease subtypes. *Blood*, 59, 1272–1278.

Sassetti, R.J. and McLeod, B.C. (1993) Effects of desmopressin on normal donors in plasma exchange donations, in *Desmopressin in Bleeding Disroders, NATO ASI Series A: Life Sciences*, vol. 242 (eds G. Mariani, P.M. Mannucci and M. Cattaneo), Plenum, New York, pp. 213–225.

Scharfman, W.B., Rauch, A.E., Ferraris, V. and Burkart, P.T. (1993) Treatment of a patient with factor IX deficiency (hemophilia B) with coronary artery bypass surger. *J Thorac Cardiovas Surg*, 105, 765–766.

Shepherd, L.L., Hutchinson, R.J., Worden, E.K. *et al.* (1989) Hyponatremia and seizures after intravenous administration of desmopressin acetate for surgical hemostasis. *J Pediatr*, 114, 470–472.

Sjamsoedin, L.J., Heijen, L., Mauser-Bunschoten, E.P. *et al.* (1981) The effect of activated prothrombin complex concentrate (FEIBA) on joint and muscle bleeding in patients with hemophilia A and antibodies to factor VIII. A double blind clinical trial. *N Engl J Med*, 305, 717–721.

Slotki, W.I. (trans) (1936) discourse by Rabbi Judah, in *The Babylonian Talmud, Yebamoth*, section 64B, vol. 1 (ed. I. Epstein), Soncino Press, London, p. 431.

Sultan, Y., Kaztchkine, M.D., Maisonneuve, O. and Nydegger, U.R. (1984) Anti-idiotypic suppression of autoantibodies to factor VIII (anti-hemophilic factor) by high-dose intravenous gammaglobulin. *Lancet*, **1**, 765–768.

Thomas, D.P., Lee, C.A., Colvin, B.T. *et al.* (1995) Clinical experience with a highly purified factor IX concentrate in patients undergoing surgical operations. *Hemophilia*, **1**, 17–23.

Tsoukas, C.M., Bernard, N.F., Sampalis, J. *et al.* Longitudinal study of patients with HIV disease – observations on effects of splenectomy (submitted for publication).

Ward, Mr. (1837) quoted by Wardrop, J., in *On the Curative effects of the Abstraction of Blood*. (ed. A.Waldie), Philadelphia.

Warrier, I., Baird-Cox, K., Cygan, L.M. *et al* (1993) Experience with central venous catheter (CVC) in children with hemophilia. *Thromb Haemostas*, **69**, 854.

Weinstein, R.E., Bona, R.D., Altman, A.J. *et al.* (1989) Severe hyponatremia after repeated intravenous administration of desmopressin. *American Journal of Hemophilia*, **32**, 258–261.

Willert, H.G., Horrig, C., Ewald, W. and Scharrer, I. (1983) Orthopaedic surgery in hemophilic patients. *Arch Orthop Trauma Surg*, **101**, 121–132.

23 INFECTIOUS COMPLICATIONS OF BLOOD PRODUCTS

B.L. Evatt and W.C. Hooper

The human immunodeficiency virus (HIV) epidemic has brought into sharp focus the vulnerability of the blood supply to infectious agents. This vulnerability was not only highlighted by HIV transmission through blood transfusions, but greatly accentuated the need for safer plasma derivatives when up to 50% of hemophiliacs became infected with HIV through the use of virally contaminated plasma concentrate. The era of the HIV epidemic also witnessed the identification of hepatitis C viruses (HCV) as the major etiologic agent responsible for non-A non-B hepatitis, a virus which has infected approximately 90% of persons with hemophilia and is associated with significant mortality and morbidity. These findings, together with prior knowledge that other infectious agents such as hepatitis B virus (HBV) could be transmitted through blood products, initiated vast improvements in blood product safety.

In contrast to most blood product recipients, the hemophilia patient receives clotting factors derived from cell-free plasma and consequently is most susceptible to infectious agents transmitted in plasma. Because of plasma pooling, individuals with hemophilia (IWH) are also at significant risk of an infection even if the agent has a low prevalence rate in the blood donor population. Infectious organisms such as those associated with red cells (babesiosis, malaria) or with leukocytes (cytomegalovirus, Epstein–Barr virus or toxoplasmosis) are generally less of a threat to the IWH (Table 23.1).

Despite modern blood product purification technologies, which include pasteurization, other heating processes, solvent/detergent treatment, as well as donor screening, not all infectious agents are eliminated and some of these agents can cause significant morbidity and mortality in hemophiliac recipients of blood products.

Table 23.1 Infectious agents that are cell-associated or present in the plasma

Infectious agent	Cell-associated	Plasma-associated
Hepatitis A	No	Yes
Hepatitis B	Yes	Yes
Hepatitis C	No	Yes
Hepatitis D	No	Yes
Hepatitis E	No	Yes
Human immuno-deficiency virus	Yes	Yes
Epstein–Barr virus	Yes	No
Cytomegalovirus	Yes	No
Toxoplasmosis	Yes	No
Malaria	Yes	No
Babesiosis	Yes	No
Parvovirus B19	No	Yes

Hemophilia. Edited by C.D. Forbes, L. Aledort and R. Madhok. Published in 1997 by Chapman & Hall, London. ISBN 0 412 63820 7

The basic biologic criteria used to determine whether or not blood products are screened for certain infectious agents are listed in Table 23.2. The intention of this chapter is to focus attention on blood-borne infectious agents and their risks to the IWH.

HIV-1, HIV-2 and other retroviruses

HIV-1

Before 1985 there were virtually no blood-screening programs for HIV and not all factor concentrates were heat-treated. The combination of these two elements was devastating to the IWH on a global basis. Approximately 80% of hemophilia patients over 10 years of age with severe hemophilia A were infected with HIV in the USA (Goedert *et al.*, 1989). However, once donor-screening programs and factor viral inactivation protocols were initiated, no cases of factor-transmitted HIV have been reported since 1986 (Lee, 1995) except by manufacturing deficiencies. Unfortunately, this success has not been seen in many underdeveloped countries where HIV and other blood-borne infections are still transmitted by blood and its products (Lee, 1995).

There have been several clinical and epidemiologic studies that identified factors in the IWH that may be involved in the transition from an HIV-seropositive status to fulminating acquired immunodeficiency syndrome (AIDS) (Eyster *et al.*, 1987, 1989; Steel *et al.*, 1988; Lee *et al.*, 1989; Phillips *et al.*, 1991a, b; Lee, 1995). These factors, which can either be markers of disease progression or biological risk factors, include severity and type of hemophilia, age of seroconversion (Eyster *et al.*, 1987, 1989; Lee, 1995), human leukocyte antigen (HLA) haplotype (Steel *et al.*, 1988), p24 antigenaemia (Phillips

et al., 1991a) and CD4 count (Phillips *et al.*, 1991a, b). Independent of all other variables, the CD4 count is the most important parameter in determining the rate of disease progression (Phillips *et al.*, 1991b). In addition to the CD4 count and HLA type, several investigators have reported that other immune markers may also determine the eventual course of HIV infection. These include levels of CD8 immunoglobulin A (IgA) and β_2-microglobulin (Phillips *et al.*, 1993).

Complications of HIV infection include opportunistic infections, immune-mediated thrombocytopenia, idiopathic thrombocytopenic purpura (ITP), thrombotic thrombocytopenia purpura (TTP), lymphoma and co-infection with other blood-transmitted viruses (i.e. hepatitis). Coinfection of HIV with the HCV has been associated with severe liver disease and a more rapid progression to liver failure (Telfer *et al.*, 1994). One recent study reported that the relative risk of developing liver failure for the HIV-infected IWH was 21.4 times greater than for the HIV-negative hemophiliac (Telfer *et al.*, 1994). It has also been reported that a decline in the CD4 count and p24 antigenemia were significant risk factors for development of liver disease (Telfer *et al.*, 1994).

Clinical recognition of ITP, accompanied by prompt treatment for the IWH is particularly important because, if not treated, significant bleeding can occur (Ragni *et al.*, 1990). Although there is increasing evidence that the incidence of TTP is increasing among patients with HIV disease (Nair *et al.*, 1988), there is little information, regardless of HIV status, concerning the association of TTP among the IWH. Similar to the general HIV population, the rate of lymphoma in the HIV-positive hemophiliac is about 24 times higher than expected and is more prevalent in older age groups (Rabkin *et al.*, 1992).

Table 23.2 Biologic criteria used to evaluate the need for testing blood donor blood for infectious agents

Prevalence
  The degree to which the agent is found in the general population
  Epidemiologic evidence of transmission

Public health
  Possibility of sexual, vertical or secondary transmission
  Severity and long-term consequences of infection
  Effect in the immunocompromised individual

Epidemiologic patterns of spread
  Increased prevalence in recipients of blood transfusion
  Increased prevalence in intravenous drug users
  Association of cases in transfusion recipients to donors with disease or evidence of infection

Available technology that can remove or inactivate the infectious agent

Adapted from Galel *et al.* (1995) Prevention of AIDS transmission through screening of the blood supply. *Ann Rev Immunol* 13, 201.

HIV-2

While HIV-2 is a cause of AIDS in West Africa, it is rare in the USA and there is no information concerning HIV-2 and IWH (O'Brien, George and Holmberg, 1992). Nevertheless, in 1992 screening donated blood for HIV-2 became mandatory in the USA and elsewhere. The emergence of new HIV strains, as evidenced by the recent identification of a subtype O HIV strain, is a concern since they may not be detected by current screening methodologies (Loussert-Ajaka et al., 1994).

Human T lymphotropic virus type I (HTLV-I) and II

HTLV-I has been associated with adult T-cell leukemia, tropical spastic paraparesis and endemic myelopathy (Sandler and Fang, 1991). While HTLV-II is not conclusively linked or associated with any specific disease, it has been reported to be endemic in certain populations (Hjelle, Scalf and Swenson, 1990; Lairmore et al., 1990). Several retrospective studies have indicated that both HTLV-I and II can be transmitted by whole blood transfusion (Okochi, Sato and Hinuma, 1984; Hjelle, Sclaf and Swenson, 1990; Sullivan et al., 1991). There is no evidence that either one of these viruses can be transmitted by factor concentrate, and this is thought to be due to the association of the virus with the cell membrane; the virus probably does not exist in the cell-free plasma in significant amounts.

Hepatitis

Liver disease, primarily due to viral hepatitis, is a significant cause of morbidity and mortality in the hemophiliac population (Hay, Preston and Triger, 1985; Troisi et al., 1993). Recent estimates have suggested that between 10 and 20% of hemophiliacs infected with either HBV or HCV will develop cirrhosis of the liver (Hay et al., 1985, 1987; Telfer et al., 1994) and some of these will also develop hepatocellular carcinoma (Phillips et al., 1991a). A combined European–American study has estimated that a crude rate of hepato-cellular carcinoma in hemophiliacs was approximately 3.2/100 000 patients/year (Phillips

et al., 1991a). This is at least 30 times higher than the background incidence (Phillips et al., 1991a). Although today's plasma concentrate should be free of both HBV and HCV, transfusion-related hepatitis still remains the leading cause of infectious complications in recipients of blood transfusions (Randell and Holland, 1991). Table 23.3 shows the characteristics of the hepatitis virus.

HEPATITIS A VIRUS (HAV)

HAV was never seriously considered as a contaminant of plasma concentrate because it was believed that the major route of transmission was oral–fecal, and because no chronic carrier state was ever identified. Although in the last two decades there had been several case reports of transfusion-associated HAV (Hollinger et al., 1983; Sheretz, Russell and Reuman, 1984), it was not until recently that HAV transmission was documented by plasma concentrate (Gerritzen et al., 1992; Mannucci, 1992; Temperley et al., 1992; Evensen and Rollag, 1993; Peerlinck and Vermylen, 1993; Goudemand et al., 1994; Mosley et al., 1994; Peerlinck et al., 1994). In contrast to HBV and HCV, HAV does not have a lipid envelope and, therefore, is relatively resistant to current solvent/detergent viral inactivation processes (Peerlinck et al., 1994). In the past, HAV infection probably did not become clinically apparent in IWH because anti-HAV antibodies, which provided passive immunity, were infused with the virus (Nowicki et al., 1993; Peerlinck et al., 1994). However, protective immunoglobulins are currently eliminated in an attempt to manufacture a more purified concentrate.

Several outbreaks of HAV infection among IWH receiving highly purified, solvent/detergent-treated clotting factor concentrates have been documented in both Europe and in the USA (Gerritzen et al., 1992; Mannucci, 1992; Temperley et al., 1992; Evensen and Rollag, 1993; Peerlinck and Vermylen, 1993; Goudemand et al., 1994; Mosley et al., 1994; Peerlinck et al., 1994). The first outbreak was in Italy among 52 hemophilia A patients from 12 centers distributed throughout the country (Mannucci, 1992). Three outbreaks occurred in 1989, 10 in 1990, 33 in 1991, and six in 1992. All patients had received solvent/detergent-treated factor VIII from the same manufacturer 2 months before

Table 23.3   Characteristics of the hepatitis virus

Virus name	Blood donors screened	Solvent/ detergent inactivation	Found in concentrate	Associated with complications	Vaccine available
Hepatitis A	No	No	Yes	No	Yes
Hepatitis B	Yes	Yes	No	Yes	Yes
Hepatitis C	Yes	Yes	No	Yes	No
Hepatitis D	No	Yes	No	Yes	No
Hepatitis E	No	No	?	?	No

illness (Robertson *et al.*, 1994). A case-control study was conducted on 29 cases and 71 controls matched by age, type/severity of hemophilia and factor VIII exposure (Mannucci *et al.*, 1994). There was a direct correlation of attack rates with factor usage, but no relationship to age, travel, contact with known hepatitis patients or the ingestion of raw shellfish. Polymerase chain reaction (PCR) analysis of implicated factor VIII lots documented HAV sequences in five of 12 lots, and gene sequences of two of these matched HAV gene sequences obtained from two patients (Mannucci *et al.*, 1994). Similar HAV outbreaks have occurred in Ireland, Germany, Belgium and South Africa (Gerritzen *et al.*, 1992; Temperley *et al.*, 1992; Evensen and Rollag, 1993; Peerlinck and Vermylen, 1993; Brackmann *et al.*, 1994). In each case, the manufacturing process for factor concentrate was identical to the one used in the Italian HAV cases. No factor IX European cases were documented, and there was no relationship to HIV or other hepatitis viruses.

The first HAV outbreak in the USA was recorded in 1995 involving two patients with hemophilia A, one patient with von Willebrand disease, and one hemophilia B patient (Centers for Disease Control, 1996). All four patients received factor concentrate from the same plasma lot. Similar to the European outbreaks, PCR analysis detected HAV genetic material in the concentrate, and the manufacturing process included a solvent/detergent viral inactivation step.

Clinically, HAV infection generally follows a relatively benign course, with acute fulminant hepatitis being an infrequent occurrence. Complications from HAV infection are more likely to develop in pregnant women. A vaccination using inactivated HAV is now available and it has been recommended that physicians consider immunizations for hemophiliacs who are seronegative for HAV (Centers for Disease Control, 1996). Physicians also may want to consider immunizing seronegative HAV women of child-bearing age who have von Willebrand disease, and who may require treatment with factor concentrate during pregnancy. Preliminary studies have indicated that vaccination-induced immunity against HAV may last up to 20 years in healthy adults. No information is available in IWH or immuno-compromised persons.

HEPATITIS B VIRUS

HBV is the etiologic agent of one of the two major hepatitis infections transmitted by blood transfusions. HBV has a lipid envelope and can be transmitted in both cellular and cell-free products. All current blood derivatives, including clotting factors licensed in Europe and the USA, do not transmit HBV unless there is a breakdown in good manufacturing practices.

HBV does not directly injure hepatocytes, but rather cell injury is a consequence of a cell-mediated immune attack against the virus. Infection with HBV is generally associated with one of several outcomes:

1. Rapid elimination of the virus and clinical recovery.
2. Fulminant hepatitis.
3. A failed immune response which results in a clinically healthy carrier.
4. Chronic hepatitis, which is probably a consequence of an impaired immune response.

Although recovery generally occurs in approximately 90% of patients, long-term HBV infection can clinically persist either as chronic persistent hepatitis or chronic active hepatitis, and eventually may result in cirrhosis. Hepatocellular carcinoma can develop in a small number of cases.

Following the introduction of blood donor screening test for the hepatitis B surface antigen (HBsAg), the safety of the blood supply significantly improved. Unfortunately, HBV was still responsible for 5–10% of transfusion-associated hepatitis despite the improved screening methodology (Randell and Holland, 1991). However, due to both donor screening and improved factor concentrate purification protocols, clotting factors have been safe from transmission of HBV since 1985 and vaccination against HBV has routinely been used in hemophilia treatment centers since the mid to late 1980s. Although hemophiliacs are no longer at risk for HBV infection by factor concentrate, at least 50% have clinical evidence of HBV infection, with the majority of the infections occurring before 1985 (Hay *et al.*, 1985, 1987; Troisi *et al.*, 1993; Telfer *et al.*, 1994). Despite the safety of factor concentrate and the availability of HBV vaccination, it is important for the IWH and his family to understand that HBV can be efficiently transmitted by close interpersonal contacts, and that there is a high rate of transmission from HBsAg-positive hemophilia patients to sexual partners, parents and siblings. Today, in countries where there are good hemophilia treatment centers and risk-reduction education programs, there should be little risk of the IWH acquiring an HBV infection. The availability of an effective and safe vaccine, together with education for the patient and his family, should reduce the risk of infection to practically zero.

HEPATITIS C VIRUS

HCV, formerly known as non-A non-B hepatitis, was responsible for more than 90% of posttransfusion hepatitis (Sherlock, 1994). Before the development of specific HCV screening methodologies, surrogate tests for HBcAb and alanine aminotransferases (ALT) reduced the incidence of HCV by approximately 30%. Currently, using enzyme-linked immunosorbent assay (ELISA) and

RIBA for donor screening, the prevalence of HCV in donated blood is approximately 1% in both the USA and Europe (Sherlock, 1994).

However, in other countries, the prevalence may be as high as 3–4% (Sherlock, 1994). Individuals who now have the highest risk for acquiring an HCV infection are intravenous drug abusers, followed by blood-transfusion recipients. Interfamily spread and vertical transmission are rare, and sexual transmission of HCV is less frequent than with HBV (Brackmann et al., 1993). As a result of viral inactivation steps added to the end of the manufacturing process, the plasma concentrates licensed in both the USA and Europe have not been known to transmit HCV since 1988. For the IWH, the major risk for HCV comes from the transfusion of blood.

HCV has the ability to mutate rapidly, thus allowing it to escape detection by the host's immune system. As a consequence, chronic hepatitis is common in about 50% of infected persons (Telfer et al., 1994). The initial presentation of HCV infection in the IWH is generally mild and a fulminant course is rare. Although the natural history of HCV infection in the IWH has not been well-defined, several studies have provided useful clinical insights in to HCV pathogenesis. Chronic infection is generally characterized by fluctuating ALT serum enzymes and no association has been found between enzyme levels and viral load (Telfer et al., 1994; Lee, 1995). Abnormal ALT levels have been associated with increased factor usage, severity of hemophilia A and HIV-seropositivity (Telfer et al., 1994). Several studies have estimated that approximately 20% of patients with elevated ALT levels will develop liver cirrhosis within 10 years of infection (Telfer et al., 1994). One preliminary study by a single hemophilia treatment center has shown that significant liver dysfunction occurs in 10–20% of HCV-positive IWH, 20 years following the first exposure to lyophilized large donor pool clotting factor concentrate (Telfer et al., 1994). This risk was associated with age, HIV status and severe hemophilia A.

Recent virologic studies have demonstrated that HCV is comprised of a family of viruses with at least six major identified subtypes (Simmonds et al., 1993) and there is evidence that geography may define the prevalence of the subtypes within any one population (Silini et al., 1995). Although there has been some evidence that both progression to liver disease and treatment may be dependent in part on the subtype (Chambost et al., 1995; Tagariello et al., 1995), the data are currently too preliminary to reach any firm conclusions.

HEPATITIS DELTA VIRUS (HDV)

HDV, described in the mid-1970s, is a replication-defective virus which requires HBV as a helper virus (Smedile et al., 1981). However, recent evidence suggests that HDV can become infectious in the absence of HBV (Rizetto, 1990). HDV has been reported to be differentially expressed in different geographic areas, and is endemic in parts of Africa, southern Italy, northern South America, Romania and in the Middle East (Rizetto, Purcell and Gerin, 1980; Navascues et al., 1995). In the USA and the rest of Europe, HDV is restricted to HBsAg carriers (Navascues et al., 1995).

Infection with HDV can occur as a coinfection with HBV or status as a carrier, are especially at risk for HDV infection. Although there is no information on the prevalence of HDV in patients who exclusively use cryoprecipitate, it is known that approximately 40–48% of patients who used clotting factors and are HBsAg-positive are also positive for HDV. In contrast to HBV and HIV, HDV is paritally resistant to heat treatment and was probably still transmitted in early virus-attenuated factor concentrate used in the mid to late 1980s (Rizzetto, Shih and Gerin, 1980; Troisi et al., 1993). In addition, since anti-HBc screening was only used for blood but not for plasma donors, HDV was probably in the concentrate administered to hemophiliacs (Troisi et al., 1993).

Patients who have been infected with both HBV and HDV are at a higher risk of developing both cirrhosis and hepatocellular carcinoma as compared with HBV infection alone. In a multicenter study conducted in the USA, it was found that HDV infection was more common in hemophilia B patients (Troisi et al., 1993). This has been attributed in part to differences in safety between factor VIII and factor IX preparations.

HEPATITIS E VIRUS (HEV)

Similar to hepatitis A, HEV is a non-enveloped virus that is primarily spread through the oral–fecal route. It is found in tropical countries and can cause epidemics of acute hepatitis (Balayan, 1991). To date, no transmission of HEV by blood has been reported in western countries (Balayan, 1991; Zaaijer et al., 1995). Despite the apparent low prevalence of HEV in western countries, it has been recommended that HEV should be considered for patients who present with acute non-ABC hepatitis.

HEPATITIS GB

Clinical studies have suggested that 10–20% of hepatitis cases are not caused by hepatitis A, B, C, D or E (Simons et al., 1995). The GB agent, which shares some apparent homology with HCV, is different from the other characterized hepatitis viruses, and has been shown to consist of at least three possible viruses, GBV-A, GBV-B and GBV-C (Simons et al., 1995a, b). Serologic studies have found that, while the prevalence of antibodies against either GBV-A or GBV-B was <2% among volunteer blood donors, the rate among intravenous drug users was

3% for GBV-A and 11% for GBV-B (Simons *et al.*, 1995a). In West Africa, the prevalence was 8.4% for GBV-A and 14.6% for GBV-B (Simons *et al.*, 1995a). Molecular analysis of an IgM-positive plasma sample using degenerate PCR primers for GBV-A or GBV-B failed to detect GBV-A or GBV-B specific viral sequences in West African sample (Simons *et al.*, 1995a). However, the degenerate PCR primers did amplify a product distinct from GBV-A and GBV-B which was termed GBV-C. GBV-C is thought to be an RNA virus and may be responsible for some cases of idiopathic hepatitis.

Creutzfeldt–Jakob disease (CJD)

CJD is a progressive degenerative disease of the brain, characterized by dementia and eventual death (Manuelidis and Manuelidis, 1979; Manuelidis, 1994).

Despite intense investigations, the etiologic agent of CJD is poorly defined. Current hypotheses suggest that this degenerative disease is either a consequence of an unknown virus or belongs to a new class of transmissible agents known as prions (Manuelidis, 1994). It was recently proposed that prions may be the causative agent for familial CJD, while an uncharacterized viral complex is responsible for transmissible CJD. In support of this latter hypothesis was the observation that the clinical features of familial CJD were quite different from those of CJD transmitted by hormone growth factor (Esmonde *et al.*, 1993). It is clear, however, that the etiologic agent of CJD is extremely resistant to current means of viral inactivation (Manuelidis, 1994).

The occurrence of CJD in humans appears to be rare, and has a 10–30-year incubation period. Although the majority of cases that do occur in humans are spontaneous, person-to-person transmission has occurred by means of medical procedures or tissue-derived products. Several case reports have documented the transmission of CJD from infected persons by pituitary-derived human growth hormone injections (Brown, Preece and Will, 1992; Dumble and Klein, 1992), cornea (Manuelidis *et al.*, 1977) and dura mater transplantation (Richard *et al.*, 1987), and by the use of contaminated electroencephalogram electrodes (Harries-Jones *et al.*, 1988).

There are limited available epidemiologic data concerning CJD. A recent case-control study which compared 155 persons who developed CJD with hospitalized patients found that an equal percentage of both groups had previously received blood transfusion (Esmonde *et al.*, 1993). Another study investigated 27 patients who received blood between 1971 and 1991 from a donor who died from CJD in 1991 (Heye, Hensen and Muller, 1994). No evidence of CJD disease was found in the recipients, eight of whom lived more than 15 years following transfusion.

Laboratory studies have found no signs of infection when leukocytes from CJD patients were injected into primates, but when spinal cord tissue was injected in six separate animals, four became infected (Brown *et al.*, 1994). Additional small-animal studies have suggested that the blood of CJD patients probably contains the agent at low titers and at irregular intervals (Manuelidis, 1994). In one study, evidence of infection was observed in two mice when buffy coats from two CJD patients were inoculated into the brains of mice produced the disease, while no disease was transmitted from two other CJD patients (Tateishi, 1985). This information and the absence of any reports linking CJD to blood transfusion suggests that the transmission of CJD by blood products may be extremely rare.

Epstein–Barr virus (EBV)

EBV, a common virus, is a member of the herpes family with a seroprevalence rate that may be as high as 90% in some populations (Tosato and Blaese, 1985). Although normally spread through the oropharyngeal route, EBV is a cell-associated virus which can be transmitted through blood products containing cellular components (Aman, Ehlin-Henriksson and Klein, 1984; Tosato and Blaese, 1985). Although EBV is the etiologic agent for infectious mononucleosis (Tosato and Blaese, 1985), Burkitt's lymphoma (Zur Hausen *et al.*, 1970) and may be associated with B lymphocyte proliferation in immunocomprised persons (Zeigler *et al.*, 1982; Shapiro *et al.*, 1988), its clinical course following transmission by blood transfusion is generally asymptomatic. Because of the high prevalence rate in the donor population, there are no recommendations for screening and it is not transmitted by clotting factors.

Cytomegalovirus (CMV)

CMV, another common virus of the herpes family, is generally transmitted by both intimate exposure and body secretions. In the latent form, CMV resides in leukocytes and can become reactivated. As a consequence of this latency, it becomes difficult to determine when a CMV-antibody-positive person develops an infection whether it is due to reactivation or to a new infection.

In contrast to HIV-positive homosexuals, not all HIV-positive hemophiliacs are infected with CMV (Webster *et al.*, 1989; Lee, 1995). This difference has clearly demonstrated that CMV infection in an HIV-positive person can accelerate the progression from HIV disease to fulminant AIDS. Since immunocompromised persons have the highest risk of developing clinically apparent CMV infection, it is recommended that HIV-infected persons be given CMV-seronegative blood. Some investigators have suggested that immunocompromised patients should receive only leukocyte-depleted or irradiated blood (Preiksaitis, 1991). There is no evidence, however, to suggest that non-cellular blood products such as clotting concentrates are infectious.

B19 parvovirus (BPV)

BPV is the only parvovirus strain that has been identified in humans (Anderson, 1990). BPV infection can occur in all age groups and is primarily transmitted person-to-person by respiratory secretions (Anderson, 1990). Clinical manifestations of infection, which include upper respiratory infections, arthralgia, arthritis, transient anemia and erythema infections (Fifth disease), are usually relatively benign. However, certain patients with hemolytic anemia, sickle-cell anemia, hereditary spherocytosis and hemoglobin C have increased risks for complications, particularly transient anemia, while hydrodrops fetalis may be a complication of pregnancy. In addition, in the immunocompromised host, chronic BPV infection can produce chronic anemia (Koch *et al.*, 1990). Viral latency has been demonstrated (Foto *et al.*, 1993), and chronic infection does not appear to be a reservoir for community transmission (Anderson, 1990). Reinfection with BPV as well as symptomatic recurrence is possible.

Similar to HAV, BPV has no lipid envelope and is resistant to current viral inactivation protocols (Laurian *et al.*, 1994). It has been estimated that the frequency of BPV in blood donations is between 1:3300 and 1:50 000 units (Lefrere, Mariotti and Thauvin, 1994). PCR analysis has found BPV in factor concentrate and one study has found the virus in approximately 20% of batches tested (Zakizewska *et al.*, 1992; Lefrer, Mariotti and Thauvin, 1994). Several studies have documented both the transmission of BPV in hemophiliacs by concentrate, and that antibody protection can be passively acquired (Corsi *et al.*, 1988; Azzi *et al.*, 1992; Bley-Grosse *et al.*, 1994).

Bacteria and parasites

Although most of the recent attention in blood safety has been focused on viruses, sporadic cases of both bacteria and parasitic contamination have warranted increased attempts to detect and inactivate these organisms. This issue was underscored in the 1980s when an epidemic of transfusion-transmitted *Yersinia enterocolitica* occurred (Centers for Disease Control, 1988, 1991; Sazama, 1994). This organism, a Gram-negative bacillus, is the cause of enterocolitis, pseudoappendicular syndrome and postinfection sequalae such as arthritis (Corer and Aber, 1989; Sazama, 1994). The epidemic was relatively small, but the mortality rate was significant – approximately 59% (19 of 32 known cases; Sazama, 1994).

It has been estimated that bacterial contamination of whole blood ranges from 1 to 2%, while platelet bacterial contamination can range from 0 to 7% (Katz and Tilton, 1971; Hamill, 1990). There are at least two major means by which bacterial contamination can be introduced – by the donor or through product processing. Contamination can come from the donor primarily by skin fragments obtained through venipuncture or by asymptomatic bacteremia (Sazama, 1994). The other major sources of contamination are due to defective materials, poor technique and storage. In contrast to whole blood and platelets, bacterial contamination is rare in plasma and cryoprecipitate.

The probability of a parasitic infection occurring as a result of a blood transfusion has been estimated to be <1 in a million, but this may change as international travel increases and population demographics continue to shift (Shulman, 1991, 1994). Malaria, the most common transfusion-associated parasitic infection in the USA is usually transmitted by asymptomatic blood donors (Shulman, 1994). Once infected, the transfusion recipient may become symptomatic with chills, fever, headaches and hemolysis with an incubation period of days to months. The incubation period is largely dependent on the type of malaria parasite: *Plasmodium falciparum* has the shortest incubation period (Westphal, 1991; Shulman, 1994). Clinical consequences of malaria are usually more severe if the patient is asplenic. The malaria parasite can survive in stored whole blood, packed red cells and platelets and can withstand cryopreservation and subsequent thawing. Although the parasite is generally cell-associated, it has reportedly been transmitted by cryoprecipitate concentrate (Wells and Ala, 1985; Shulman, 1994).

The parasite *Trypanosoma cruzi*, the etiologic agent for Chagas disease, can be transmitted by platelets, whole blood, packed red cells (Gudino and Linares, 1990; Shulman, 1994). Although Chagas disease generally follows a mild clinical course, it can, however, lead to potentially fatal cardiac and gastrointestinal complications. Many patients are asymptomatic and may be parasitemic for life and, as a result, there is a risk that these persons may become part of a blood donor pool (Shulman, 1994).

Since *T. cruzi* is endemic to parts of Mexico, Central and South America, the risk of the parasite being transfusion-transmitted will generally vary among geographic regions. However, as immigration patterns change and international travel becomes more common, geographic boundaries may become less important when assigning risk for transmission of *T. cruzi*.

Other parasites of concern include babesiosis, leishmaniasis, toxoplasmosis and microfilariasis (Shulman, 1994). Babesiosis is generally acquired through tick bites and is the second most frequently reported cause of transfusion-transmitted parasitic infection. This parasite, which is found in red blood cells, can be packed red blood cells, platelet concentrates and deglycerolized red cells and can survive for 35 days at 4°C. Leishmaniasis, an extraerthrocytic parasite, has yet to be transmitted through blood products in the USA. Toxoplasmosis (*Toxoplasma gondii*), also an extraerythrocitic parasite, is thought to be present in approximately 50% of adults in the USA. Toxoplasmosis, which can be transmitted through both blood transfusions and organ transplants, frequently exists as an asymptomatic infection. However, transfusion-associated *Toxoplasmosis gondii* has only been documented in acute leukemia patients who received both chemotherapy and leukocyte infusions.

Microfilariasis can also be transmitted through blood transfusion. It has been reported that, although transfusion-acquired microfilariasis is self-limited, it can persist in the recipient's circulation for more than 2 years.

Addendum

Recently it has been reported that a variant of CJD (vCJD) disease can be transmitted to humans through the consumption of bovine spongiform encephalopathy (BSE)-contaminated beef. BSE which is probably caused by a single prion strain, became epidemic in British cattle in the mid to late 1980s through the probable ingestion of scrapie-infected sheep renderings. The neurological disorder caused by BSE resulted in not only the slaughter of infected cattle but in the ban of certain bovine renderings in both human and animal food preparations. Since 1990, there have been 14 confirmed cases of vCJD linked to BSE-contaminated beef in Britain. These cases differed from CJD in that the average age was 27 and the patients presented with both psychiatric symptoms and progressive neurological deficits. The neuropathological findings were distinctive in all cases with extensive prion protein plaques distribution throughout the cerebrum and cerebellum. None of the cases were reported to have any risk factors associated with CJD disease. Though controversial, recent laboratory evidence has suggested that prions responsible for CJD and vCJD may be differentiated through differences in glycosylation patterns. Although BSE and vCJD appears to be limited to Great Britain, much work is needed to better determine if and how BSE was transmitted to humans and to identify risk factors. To date there has been no evidence that BSE can be, or has been transmitted through blood products. This episode underscores the necessity for increased vigilance for the possible transmission of disease to humans through the use of animal-derived food or medical products.

References

Aman, P., Ehlin-Henriksson, B. and Klein, G. (1984) Epstein–Barr virus susceptibility of normal human B lymphocyte populations. *J Exp Med*, **159**, 208–220.

Anderson, L.J. (1990) Human parvoviruses. *J Infect Dis.*, **161**, 603–608.

Azzi, A., Ciappi, K., Zakrewska, K. *et al.* (1992) Human parvovirus B19 infection in hemophiliacs first infused with two high-purity, virally attenuated factor VIII concentrates. *Am J Hematol*, **39**, 228–230.

Balayan, M.S. (1991) HEV infection: historical perspective, global epidemiology and clinical features, in *Viral Hepatitis and Liver Disease* (ed. F.B. Hollinger), Williams & Wilkins, Baltimore, pp. 498–501.

Bley-Grosse, A., Hubinger-Eis, A.M., Kaiser, R. *et al.* (1994) Serological and virological markers of human parvovirus B19 infection in sera of hemophiliacs. *Thromb Haemost*, **72**, 503–507.

Brackman, S., Gerritzen, A., Oldenburg, J. *et al.* (1993) Search for intrafamilial transmission of hepatitis C virus in hemophilia patients. *Blood*, **81**, 1077–1082.

Brackmann, H.H., Oldenburg, J., Eis-Hubinger, A.M. *et al.* (1994) Hepatitis A virus among the hemophilia population at the Bonn hemophilia center. *Vox Sang*, **67**, 3–8.

Brown, P., Preece, M.A. and Will, R.G. (1992) Friendly fire in medicine: hormones, homografts, and Creutzfeldt–Jakob disease. *Lancet*, **340**, 24–27.

Brown, P., Gibbs, C.J., Rodgers-Johnson, P. *et al.* (1994) Human spongiform encephalopathy: the National Institutes of Health series of 300 cases of experimentally transmitted disease. *Ann Neurol*, **35**, 513–529.

Centers for Disease Control (1988) *Yersinia enterocolitica* bacteremia and endotoxin shock associated with red cell transfusion – United States, 1987–88. *Mob Mortal Wkly Rep*, **37**, 577–578.

Centers for Disease Control (1991) *Yersinia enterocolitica* bacteremia and endotoxin shock associated with red blood cell transfusion – United States, 1991. *Morb Mortal Wkly Rep*, **40**, 176–178.

Centers for Disease Control and Prevention (1996) Hepatitis A among persons with hemophilia who received clotting factor concentrate – United States, September–December 1995. *Morb Mortal Wkly Rep*, **45**, 29–32.

Chambost, H., Gerolami, V., Halfon, P. *et al.* (1995) Persistent hepatitis C virus RNA replication in haemophiliacs: role of co-infection with human immunodeficiency virus. *Br J Haematol*, **91**, 703–713.

Colombo, M., Mannuccia, P., Brettler, D. *et al.* (1991) Hepatocellular carcinoma in hemophilia. *Am J Hematol*, **37**, 243–246.

Corsi, O.B., Azzi, A., Morfini, M. *et al.* (1988) Human parvovirus infection in haemophiliacs first infused with treated clotting factor concentrates. *J Med Virol*, **25**, 165–170.

Cover, T.L. and Aber, R.C. (1989) *Yersini enterocolitica*. *N Engl J Med*, **321**, 16–24.

Dumble, L.J. and Klein, R.D. (1992) Creutzfeldt–Jakob legacy for Australian women treated with human pituitary gonadotropins. *Lancet*, **340**, 847–848.

Esmonde, T.F.G., Will, R.G., Slattery, J.M *et al.* (1993) Creutzfeldt–Jakob disease and blood transfusion. *Lancet*, **341**, 205–207.

Evensen, S.A. and Rollag, H. (1993) Solvent/detergent treated clotting factors and hepatitis A seroconversion. *Lancet*, **341**, 971–972.

Eyster, M.E., Gail, M.H., Ballard, J.O. *et al.* (1987) Natural history of human immunodeficiency virus infections in hemophiliacs: effects of T-cell subsets, platelet counts and age. *Ann Intern Med*, **107**, 1–6.

Eyster, M.E., Ballard, J.O., Gail, M.H. *et al.* (1989) Predictive markers for the acquired immunodeficiency syndrome (AIDS) in hemophiliacs: persistence of p24 antigen and low T4 cell count. *Ann Intern Med*, **110**, 963–969.

Foto, F., Saag, K.G., Scharosch, L.L. *et al.* (1993) Parvovirus B19-specific DNA in bone marrow from B19 arthropathy patients: evidence for B19 virus persistence. *J Infect Dis*, **167**, 744–748.

Gerritzen, A., Schneweis, K.E., Brackmann, H.H. *et al.* (1992) Acute hepatitis A in haemophilia. *Lancet*, **340**, 1231.

Goedert, J.J., Kessler, C.M., Aledort, L.M. *et al.* (1989) A prospective study of human immunodeficiency virus type 1 infection and the development of AIDS in subjects with hemophilia. *N Engl J Med*, **321**, 1141–1148

Goudemand, J., Parquet, A., d'Oiron, R. *et al.* (1994) Hepatitis A in French hemophiliacs. *Vox Sang*, **67** (suppl. 1), 9–13.

Gudino, M.D. and Linares, J. (1990) Chagas' disease and blood transfusion, in *Emerging Global Patterns in Transfusion Transmitted Infections* (eds R.G. Westphal, K.B. Carlson and J.M.Ture), American Association of Blood Banks, Arlington, Va, pp. 65–86.

Hamill, T.R. (1990) The 30-minute rule for reissuing blood: are we needlessly discarding units? *Transfusion*, **30**, 58–62.

Harries-Jones, R., Knight, R., Will, R.G. *et al.* (1988) Cruetzfeldt–Jakob disease in Enlgand and Wales, 1980–1984, a case control study of potential risk factors. *J Neurol Neurosurg Psychiatry*, **51**, 1113–1119.

Hay, C., Preston, F., Triger, D. and Underwood, J. (1985) Progressive liver disease in haemophilia: an understated problem. *Lancet*, **1**, 1495–1498.

Hay, C., Preston, F., Triger, D. *et al.* (1987) Predictive markers of chronic liver disease in hemophilia. *Blood*, **69**, 1595–1599.

Heye, N., Hensen, S. and Muller, N. (1994) Creutzfeldt–Jakob disease and blood transfusion. *Lancet*, **343**, 298–299.

Hjelle, B., Scalf, R. and Swenson, S. (1990) High frequency of human T-cell leukemia-lymphoma virus type II infection in New Mexico blood donors: determination by sequence-specific oligonucleotide hybridization. *Blood*, **76**, 450–454.

Hollinger, F.B., Khan, N.C., Oefinger, P.E. *et al.* (1983) Posttransfusion hepatitis Type A. *JAMA*, **250**, 2313–2317.

Katz, A.J. and Tilton, C.R. (1971) Contamination of platelet preparations. *N Engl J Med*, **285**, 1091.

Koch, W.C., Massey, G., Russell, C.E., and Adler, S.P. (1990) Manifestations and treatment of human parvovirus B19 infectin in immunocomprised patients. *J Pediatr*, **116**, 355–359.

Lairmore, M.D., Jacobson, S., Gracia, F. *et al.* (1990) Isolation of human T-cell lymphotropic virus type 2 from Guaymi Indians in Panama. *Proc Natl Acad Sci*, **87**, 8840–8844.

Laurian, Y., Dussaix, E., Parquet, A. *et al.* (1994) Transmission of human parvovirus B19 by plasma derived factor VIII concentrates. *Nouv Rev Fr Hematol*, **36**, 449–453.

Lee, C.A. (1995) Management of patients with HIV and/or hepatitis. *Haemophilia*, **1** (suppl. 1), 26–34.

Lee, C.A., Phillips, A., Elford, J. *et al.* (1989) The natural history of human immunodeficiency virus infection in a hemophiliac cohort. *Br J Haematol*, **73**, 228–234.

Lefrere, J.J., Mariotti, M. and Thauvin, M. (1994) B19 parvovirus DNA in solvent/detergent-treated anti-haemophilia concentrates. *Lancet*, **343**, 211–212.

Loussert-Ajaka, I., Ly, T.D., Chaix, M.L. *et al.* (1994) HIV-1/HIV-2 seronegativity in HIV-1 subtype O infected patients. *Lancet*, **343**, 1393–1394.

Mannucci, P.M. (1992) Outbreak of hepatitis A among Italian patients with haemophilia. *Lancet*, **339**, 819.

Mannucci, P.M., Gdovin, S., Gringeri, A. *et al.* (1994) Transmission of hepatitis A to patients with hemophilia by factor VIII concentrates treated with organic solvent and detergent to inactivated viruses. *Ann Intern Med*, **120**, 1–7.

Manuelidis, L. (1994) The dimensions of Creutzfeldt–Jakob disease. *Transfusion*, **34**, 915–928.

Manuelidis, E.E. and Manuelidis, L. (1979) Clinical and morphological aspects of transmissable Creutzfeldt–Jakob disease. *Prog Neuropathol*, **4**, 1–26.

Manuelidis, E.E., Angelo, J.N., Gorgacz, E.J. *et al.* (1977) Experimental Creutzfeldt–Jakob disease transmitted via the eye with infected cornea. *N Engl J Med*, **296**, 1334–1336.

Manuelidis, E.E., Kim, J.H., Maricangas, J.R. and Manuelidis, L. (1985) Transmission to animals of Creutzfeldt–Jakob disease from human blood. *Lancet*, **2**, 896–897.

Mosley, J.W., Nowicki, M.J., Kasper, C.K. *et al.* (1994) Hepatitis A virus transmission by blood products in the United States. *Vox Sang*, **67** (suppl. 1), 24–28.

Nair, J.M., Bellevue, R., Bertoni, M. and Dosik, H. (1988) TTP in patients with the AIDS-related complex: a report of two cases. *Ann Intern Med*, **109**, 209–212.

Navascues, C.A., Rodriguez, M., Sotorro, G. *et al.* (1995) Epidemiology of hepatitis D virus infection: changes in the last 14 years. *Am J Gastroenterol*, **90**, 1981–1984.

Nowicki, M.J., Mosely, J.W., Koerper, M.A. *et al.* (1993) Passive antibody to hepatitis A virus in US hemophiliacs. *Lancet*, **341**, 562.

O'Brien, T.R., George, J.R. and Holmberg, S.D. (1992) Human immunodeficiency virus type 2 infection in the United States. Epidemiology, diagnosis, and public health implications. *JAMA*, **267**, 2775–2779.

Okochi, K., Sato, H. and Hinuma, Y. (1984) A retrospective study on transmission of adult T cell leukemia virus by blood transfusion: seroconversion in recipients. *Vox Sang*, **46**, 245–253.

Peerlinck, K. and Vermylen, J. (1993) Acute hepatitis A in patients with haemophilia A. *Lancet*, **341**, 179.

Peerlinck, K., Goubau, P., Coppens, G. *et al.* (1994) Is the apparent outbreak of hepatitis A in Belgian hemophiliacs due to a loss of previous passive immunity? *Vox Sang*, **67** (suppl. 1), 14–17.

Phillips, A.N., Lee, C.A., Elford, J. *et al.* (1991a) p24 antigenaemia, CD4 lymphocyte counts and the development of AIDS. *AIDS*, **5**, 1217–1222.

Phillips, A.N., Lee, C.A., Elford, J. *et al.* (1991b) Serial CD4 lymphocyte counts and developments of AIDS. *Lancet*, **337**, 389–392.

Phillips, A.N., Sabin, C.A., Elford, J. *et al.* (1993) CD8 lymphocyte counts and serum immunoglobulin A levels early in HIV infection as predictors of CD4 lymphocyte depletion during 8 years of follow-up. *AIDS*, **7**, 975–980.

Preiksaitis, J.K. (1991) Indications for the use of cytomegalovirus-seronegative blood products. *Transfusion Med Rev*, **V**, 1–17.

Rabkin, C.S., Hilgartner, M.W., Hedberg, K.W. *et al.* (1992) Incidence of lymphomas and other cancers in HIV-infected and HIV-uninfected patients with hemophilia. *JAMA*, **267**, 1090–1094.

Ragni, M.V., Bontempo, F.A., Myers, D.J. *et al.* (1990) Hemorrhagic sequelae of immune thrombocytopenic purpura in human immunodeficiency virus infected hemophilics. *Blood*, **75**, 1267–1272.

Randell, R.L. and Holland, P.V. (1991) Transfusion-associated hepatitis, in *Transfusion Transmitted Infections* (eds D.M. Smith and R.Y. Dodd), ASCP Press, Chicago, p. 115.

Richard, J., Thadani, V., Kalb, R. *et al.* (1987) Rapidly progressive dementia in a patient who received a cadaveric dura mater graft. *Morb Mortal Wkly Rep*, **36**, 49–55.

Rizetto, M. (1990) Hepatitis delta: the virus and the disease. *J Hepatol*, (suppl. 1), S145–S152.

Rizzetto, M., Purcell, R.H. and Gerin, J.L. (1980) Epidemiology of HBV-associated delta agent: geographical distribution of anti-delta and prevalence in polytransfused HbsAg carriers. *Lancet*, **i**, 1215–1218.

Rizzetto, M., Shih, W.K. and Gerin, J. (1980) The hepatitis B virus-associated antigen: isolation from liver, development of solid-phase radioimmunoassays for delta antigen and anti-delta and partial characterization of delta antigen. *J Immunol*, **125**, 318–324.

Robertson, B.H., Friedberg, D., Norman, A. *et al.* (1994) Sequence variability of hepatitis A virus and factor VIII associated hepatitis A infection in hemophilia patients in Europ. *Vox Sang*, **67** (suppl. 1), 39–46.

Sandler, S.G. and Fang, C. (1991) Preventing transfusion-transmitted infections: issues related to migrating populations and increasing word travel. *Haematologia*, **24**, 197–210.

Sazama, K. (1994) Bacteria in blood transfusion; a review. *Arch Pathol Lab Med*, **118**, 350–365.

Shapiro, R.S., McClain, K., Frizzera, G. *et al.* (1988) Epstein–Barr virus associated B cell lymphoproliferative disorders following bone marrow transplantation. *Blood*, **71**, 1234–1243.

Sherertz, R.J., Russell, B.A. and Reuman, P.D. (1984) Transmission of hepatitis by transfusion of blood products. *Arch Intern Med*, **144**, 1579–1580.

Sherlock, S. (1994) Chronic hepatitis C. *Disease-a-Month Club*, **40**, 121–196.

Shulman, I.A. (1994) Parasitic infections and their impact on blood donor selection and testing. *Arch Pathol Lab Med*, **118**, 366–370.

Silini, M., Bono, F., Cividini, A. *et al.* (1995) Differential distribution of hepatitis C virus genotypes in patients with and without liver function abnormalities. *Hepatology*, **21**, 285–290.

Simmonds, P., Holmes, E.C., Cha, T.A. *et al.* (1993) Classification of hepatitis C virus into six major genotypes and a series of subtypes by philogenetic analysis of the NS-5 region. *J Gen Virol*, **74**, 2391–2399.

Simons, J.N., Leary, T.P., Dawson, G.J. *et al.* (1995a) Isolation of novel virus-like sequences associated with human hepatitis. *Nature Med*, **1**, 564–569.

Simons, J.N., Pilot-Mathias, T.J., Leary, T.P. *et al.* (1995b) Identification of two flavivirus-like genomes in the GB hepatitis agent. *Proc Natl Acad Sci*, **92**, 3401–3405.

Smedile, A., Dentico, P., Zanetti, A. *et al.* (1981) Infection with the delta agent in chronic HbsAg carriers. *Gastroenterology*, **81**, 992–997.

Steel, C.M., Ludlam, C.A., Beatson, D. *et al.* (1988) HLA haplotype A1 B8 DR3 as a risk factor for HIV-related disease. *Lancet*, **i**, 1185–1188.

Sullivan, M.T., Williams, A.E., Fang, C.T. *et al.* (1991) Transmission of human T-lymphotropic virus types I and II by blood transfusion. A retrospective study of recipients of blood components (1983 through 1988). The American Red Cross HTLV-I/II collaborative study group. *Arch Intern Med*, **151**, 2043–2048.

Tagariello, G., Pontisso, P., Davioli, P.G. *et al.* (1995) Hepatitis C virus genotypes and severity of chronic liver disease in haemophiliacs. *Br J Haematol*, **91**, 708.

Tateishi, J. (1985) Transmission of CJD from human blood and urine to mice. *Lancet*, **ii**, 1074.

Telfer, P., Sabin, C., Deverux, H. *et al.* (1994) The progression of HCV-associated liver disease in a cohort of haemophilic patients. *Br J Haematol*, **87**, 555–561.

Temperley, I.J., Cotter, K.P., Walsh, T.J. *et al.* (1992) Clotting factors and hepatitis A. *Lancet*, **340**, 1466.

Tosato, G. and Blaese, R.M. (1985) Epstein–Barr virus infection and immunoregulation in man. *Adv Immunol*, **37**, 99–149.

Troisi, C.L., Hollinger, F.B., Hoots, W.K. *et al.* (1993) A multicenter study of viral hepatitis in a United States hemophilic population. *Blood*, **81**, 412–418.

Webster, A., Lee, C.A., Cook, D.G. *et al.* (1989) Cytomegalovirus infection and progression towards AIDS in haemophiliacs with human immunodeficiency virus infection. *Lancet*, **2**, 63–66.

Wells, L. and Ala, F.A. (1985) Malaria and blood transfusion. *Lancet*, **1**, 1317–1318.

Westphal, R. (1991) Transfusion-transmitted malaria infections, in *Transfusion Transmitted Infections* (eds D.M. Smith and R.Y. Dodd), American Society of Clinical Pathologists Press, Chicago, Ill., pp. 167–180.

Zaaijer, H.L., Mauserbunschoten, E.P., Tenveen, J.H. *et al.* (1995) Hepatitis E virus antibodies among patients with hemophilia, blood donors and hepatitis patients. *J Med Virol*, **46**, 244–246.

Zakrewska, K., Azzi, A., Patou, G. *et al.* (1992) Human parvovirus B19 in clotting factor concentrates: B19 DNA detection by the nested polymerase chain reaction. *Br J Haematol*, **81**, 407–412.

Zeigler, J.L., Drew, W.L., Miner, R.C. *et al.* (1982) Outbreak of Burkitt's-like lymphoma in homosexual men. *Lancet*, **2**, 631–633.

Zur Hausen, H., Schulte-Holthausen, H., Klein, H. *et al.* (1970) EBV-DNA in Burkitt's tumor and anaplastic carcinoma of the nasopharynx. *Nature*, **228**, 1056–1058.

24 LIVER DISEASE IN HEMOPHILIA

M.E. Eyster

Historical perspective

Following the development of serologic tests to detect hepatitis A and B, it became apparent in the late 1970s that 80–90% of all cases of posttransfusion hepatitis were not due to either of these agents (Dienstag, 1983). An infectious etiology was implicated because this form of non-A non-B hepatitis (NANBH) could be reproduced in chimpanzees by serial injection of sera from transfusion recipients who developed an easily recognizable clinical disease. However, NANBH remained a diagnosis of exclusion for nearly 20 years until 1989, when the genome for hepatitis C virus (HCV) was cloned (Choo *et al.*, 1989) and a serologic assay for detection of a protein encoded by a portion of the genome was developed (Kuo *et al.*, 1989). Using this assay to detect antibody to HCV in prospectively followed transfusion recipients and their donors, it was subsequently shown that HCV accounts for at least 90% of the cases of chronic transfusion-associated NANBH (Alter *et al.*, 1989; Aach *et al.*, 1991).

Following the introduction of pooled plasma fractions, a 31% incidence of acute hepatitis was noted in first-time recipients of factor VIII (Kasper and Kipnis, 1972). Multiple descriptions followed of high rates of liver function abnormalities in recipients of clotting factor concentrates, including very young children (Preston *et al.*, 1978; Spero *et al.*, 1978; Gomperts *et al.*, 1981; Stirling, Becket and Percy-Robb, 1981; Rickard *et al.*, 1982; Cederbaum, Blatt and Levine, 1982; White *et al.*, 1982; Aledort *et al.*, 1985; Hay *et al.*, 1987). Peripheral blood hepatitis B virus (HBV) markers were common (Lewis, 1970) but histologic appearances in the few who underwent liver biopsies were not more consistent with NANBH than hepatitis B (Bamber *et al.*, 1981; Triger, 1990).

The first reports that asymptotic liver disease might be common in persons with hemophilia appeared in 1975 (Mannucci *et al.*, 1975). Initially, it appeared the disease was non-progressive (Mannucci, Colombo and Rizzetto, 1982) and little attention was paid to abnormal transaminase values, since symptoms were usually mild or self-limited and many individuals suffered no clinical illness. Over the next 10 years, however, it became increasingly apparent that liver disease was becoming a serious problem (Aledort *et al.*, 1985; Hay *et al.*, 1985; Triger, 1990) and, by 1992, liver disease had become the second leading cause of death in persons with hemophilia (Eyster *et al.*, 1992).

HCV is now believed to be the major cause of chronic liver disease in multitransfused persons (Makris *et al.*, 1990; Triger, 1990). Although the early course is usually benign, at least 50% of those infected with HCV develop biochemical evidence of chronic hepatitis with persistently elevated or fluctuating alanin aminotransferase (ALT) levels (Cederbaum, Blatt and Levine, 1982; Hay *et al.*, 1985; Alter *et al.*, 1989; Triger, 1990) and liver biopsies of those with chronic hepatitis show cirrhosis in 10–20% (Preston *et al.*, 1978; Spero *et al.*, 1979; White *et al.*, 1982; Aledort *et al.*, 1985). Progressive liver disease increases with advancing age (Hay *et al.*, 1987).

The prevalence of HCV antibodies in persons with hemophilia ranges from 64 to 86% using first-generation tests (Schramm *et al.*, 1989; Brettler *et al.*, 1990; Rumi *et al.*, 1990; Blanchette *et al.*, 1991). Using the more sensitive and specific second-generation tests, over 95% of recipients of non-heat-treated concentrates have been found to be anti-HVB-positive (Watson *et al.*, 1992; Eyster *et al.*, 1993). Those persons who received clotting factor concentrates during the 1970s and early 1980s before the advent of viral inactivation procedures were usually infected with HCV on the first exposure (Fletcher *et al.*, 1983; Kernoff *et al.*, 1985). In the vast majority, the infection is persistent (Allain *et al.*, 1991)

Hemophilia. Edited by C.D. Forbes, L. Aledort and R. Madhok. Published in 1997 by Chapman & Hall, London. ISBN 0 412 63820 7 even though many remain asymptomatic for extended periods of time. Fortunately, most of those treated with concentrates manufactured since 1987 have remained free of HCV infection (Mannucci, 1995).

Epidemiology

Although the roles of hepatotoxins such as alcohol and analgesics need to be clarified, epidemiologic, serologic, clinical and histologic studies strongly implicate HCV as the major cause of chronic liver disease among persons with hemophilia. In those who have been repeatedly exposed to non-heat-treated clotting factor concentrates, serologic evidence of hepatitis B and C infections is almost universal (Hasiba *et al.*, 1980; Tedder *et al.*, 1991; Troisi *et al.*, 1993).

Persons with severe hemophilia A or B are the recipients of periodic infusions of plasma fractions from hundreds of thousands of donors during their lifetime. Therefore, it is not surprising that hepatitis was the rule rather than the exception for those who received crude factor VIII or factor IX complex concentrates or large volumes of cryoprecipitate. Given the alternative of no treatment, hepatitis was considered an acceptable risk with this form of therapy during the 1970s. Both acute and chronic hepatitis were observed (Hruby and Schauf, 1978; Hasiba *et al.*, 1980; Gerety and Eyster, 1981; Mannucci, Colombo and Rizzetto, 1982; Thomas, Bamber and Kernoff, 1982; Triger, 1990). Sometimes multiple episodes of acute hepatitis occurred, leading to the suggestion that recurrent episodes might represent a hypersensitivity reaction to some component of clotting factor concentrates (Myers *et al.*, 1980). Some episodes occurred as early as 1–4 weeks after transfusion in anti-hepatitis B surface antigen (HBSAg)-positive individuals who had no serologic evidence of hepatitis A virus (HAV) infection (Hruby and Schauf, 1978; Thomas, Bamber and Kernoff, 1982). The majority of these individuals developed chronic hepatitis with fluctuating transaminase elevations. Other episodes occurred as long as 2–6 months after transfusion without serologic evidence of acute HBV infection.

With the implementation of viral inactivation procedures and the development of increasingly sensitive screening tests for HBV, transfusion-associated HBV infections had largely been eliminated by the mid-1980s. However, HCV RNA could still be detected by the polymerase chain reaction (PCR) in factor VIII concentrates with expiration dates as late as 1988 (Makris *et al.*, 1993), and a high rate of HCV transmission continued until 1989, when more stringent methods of viral inactivation were developed. An added measure of safety was achieved in 1991 when a sensitive screening tests for anti-HCV became available. Cumulative results of prospective hepatitis B and C safety studies involving 358 previously untreated patients indicate that the hepatitis

risk from currently available virally inactivated clotting factor concentrates is less than 1% (95% confidence interval 0–2%; Mannucci, 1995).

Etiology

Causes of hepatitis include the hepatotropic viruses HAV, HBV, HCV, hepatitis D (HDV) and E virus (HEV). HCV is a non-integrating enveloped RNA virus belonging to the Flaviridae family of viruses which are closely related to the bovine viral diarrhea and hog cholera viruses (Choo *et al.*, 1989; Houghton *et al.*, 1991; van der Poel, Cuypers and Reesink, 1994). HBV is an enveloped DNA hepadenovirus (Lau and Wright, 1993b). The delta virus (HDV) is a defective virus which requires the helper function of HBV to replicate (Lau and Wright, 1993). HBV infections are less likely than HCV infections to become chronic, but both can cause serious progressive liver disease. HAV and HEV are non-enveloped RNA enteric viruses which cause acute self-limited infections (Krawczykski, 1994; Lemon, 1994).

Transfusion-associated HAV is rare, since HAV spreads almost exclusively by the fecal–oral route, and percutaneous transmission is limited to a 1–2 week viremic period in the donor (Hollinger *et al.*, 1983; Sherertz, Russell and Reuman, 1984). However, in contrast to HBV and HCV, HAV is a non-enveloped and relatively heat-stable virus which may survive some viral inactivation procedures, and outbreaks of acute HAV infections attributed to solvent/detergent-treated concentrates have been reported in Italy, Germany, Ireland and Belgium (Mannucci, 1992, 1995). Therefore, hepatitis A must be considered as a cause of acute hepatitis in a concentrate recipient who develops jaundice with elevated transaminases. HEV has been associated with water-borne epidemics of hepatitis in Asia, Africa and Mexico, but is not endemic in North America or Europe. Like HAV, HEV has never been shown to progress to chronic hepatitis (Krawczykski, 1994; Lemon, 1994).

In immunosuppressed individuals, cytomegalovirus, Epstein–Barr virus and the herpes simplex virus must be included along with HBV, HCV and HDV as causes of chronic viral hepatitis. Other non-viral causes of chronic hepatitis, such as autoimmune hepatitis, chemical injury including drugs or alcohol, hemochromatosis, Wilson's disease and α_1-antitrypsin deficiency should always be considered before attributing liver disease in persons with hemophilia to HCV or HBV, with or without HDV infection.

Clinical features of chronic HBV and HCV

HBV

The mean incubation period of chronic HBV is about 90 days, with a range of 2–6 months. In immunocompetent adults, 90–95% of those infected recover. Fewer than 1% develop fulminant hepatitis and between 5 and 10% develop persistent infections with HBsAg carriage (Sherlock, 1989). The diagnosis depends on the identification of the appropriate serologic profile in the presence of an abnormal serum ALT levels. Commonly used assays for HBV detection include tests for HBsAg, anti-HBs, HBeAg, anti-HBe, immunoglobulin G (IgG) anti-HBc (core) and IgM anti-HBc (Centers for Disease Control, 1991).

The hallmark of an active HBV infection is the presence of HBsAg in the serum. IgM anti-HB$_C$ is found during the acute infection, and IgG anti-HB$_C$ persists in those with chronic infections. Those with HBsAg are highly infectious, as are those with circulating HBV DNA. Persistence of HBsAg for more than 6 months indicates either chronic infection or the carrier state. The appearance of anti-HBs is indicative of a resolved infection (or vaccination) and lasting immunity (Hoofnagle and Di Bisceglie, 1991).

Acute HBV infections can be asymptomatic or can cause a wide range of constitutional symptoms, including jaundice. However, the vast majority of chronic carriers are otherwise healthy and seem to be immunologically tolerant to the virus (Wright and Lau, 1993). From 20 to 40% of chronic carriers develop active hepatitis which is believed to occur when there is a loss of tolerance with the emergence of reactive T-cell clones causing hepatic inflammation and T-cell-mediated liver damage. Those with persistence of HBeAg or chronic HDV infections are at the highest risk for the development of cirrhosis. In one prospective study of 379 non-hemophiliacs with chronic HBV infections (Weissberg et al., 1984), the 5-year survival rate for patients with cirrhosis was 55%. Patients with chronic HBV with or without cirrhosis have a 10–390-fold risk for the development of hepatocellular carcinoma (HCC; Wright and Lau, 1993).

While HBV is a major cause of chronic hepatitis and cirrhosis and is an important risk factor for HCC worldwide, it is unlikely to be responsible for liver disease in persons with hemophilia in the absence of HBsAg carriage. Some patients have intrahepatic HBV infection without detectable anti-HBs, but these usually have anti-HBc. Hemophiliacs rarely exhibit these patterns of serologic abnormalities (Thomas et al., 1982).

HDV

HDV is a defective RNA virus which is dependent on the envelope proteins of HBV for its replication and causes hepatitis only in patients who are concurrently infected with HBV (Rizetto, 1983; Lau and Wright, 1993). HDV superinfection of hepatitis B carriers typically causes severe chronic hepatitis leading to cirrhosis, while acute HDV and HBV coinfection carries a high risk of fulminant hepatitis. The diagnosis is made by the finding of antibodies to HDV. In active infections, HDV RNA can be detected in the serum by PCR. In a multicenter Italian study which included 103 HBsAg carriers with hemophilia, the prevalence of antibodies to HDV was 37% overall, and 48% in those treated predominantly or exclusively with commercial concentrates (Rosina, Saracco and Rizzetto, 1985). In a recent prevalence study of viral hepatitis in 727 persons with hemophilia, evidence of active HBV infection was found in 8%; 19% of these were actively infected with HDV (Troisi et al., 1993). In a cohort study involving 99 hemophiliacs with HCV and human immunodeficiency virus (HIV) infections, active HDV infections were found in five of eight hemophiliacs who were chronic carriers of HBsAg (Eyster et al., 1994).

HCV

In the hemophilia population, transmission of HCV infection has been almost exclusively by blood products. However, HCV has a global prevalence of about 1% (Alter, 1995) and for nearly 6–7% of the general population in the USA, no source of infection can be identified (Alter et al., 1992).

HCV has a mean incubation period of 6–8 weeks after exposure, with a range from 2 to 22 weeks. Clinically, HCV resembles other forms of viral hepatitis, but is generally more insidious. Fatigue occurs in 95% of the reported cases, and anorexia, nausea, weakness or lethargy are frequently observed. Jaundice is present in only about 25% of those with acute infections (Alter, 1995). The diagnosis of acute HCV is based on elevated ALT levels and the appearance of anti-HCV in the absence of markers for acute HAV or HBV infections (Hoofnagle and Di Bisceglie, 1991). However, seroconversion may be delayed for several weeks after the onset of symptoms, and measurement of serum HCV RNA, which appears as early as 1–2 weeks after infection, may be required for early diagnosis. HCV RNA persists for at least several years in the vast majority of patients (Farci et al., 1991).

The immunodiagnosis of HCV is based on an anti-HCV enzyme-linked immunosorbent assay (ELISA). First-generation tests which depend on the C100 antigen encoded by the non-structural (NS4) region of the genome lacked specificity and had relatively low sensitivity. Sensitivity was enhanced in second-generation tests by the addition of two critical epitopes, one from the relatively conserved C22 core region and from another more variable non-structural region (NS3) of the genome, designated c33c (van der Poel, 1994; Alter, 1995). Specificity was enhanced by the development of the confirmatory recombinant immunoblot assay (RIBA-2). Third-generation ELISA-3 and RIBA-3 assays, which employ synthetic peptides from the core and NS4 regions plus recombinant antigens from the NS3 and NS5 regions of the genome, are expected to be licensed in 1995. These have 90–100% sensitivity and 99.8% specificity in low-risk populations. Some 80–90% of HCV RIBA-3-positive individuals are viremeic as detected by PCR (van der Poel, 1994).

The most serious feature of HCV is the progression to chronicity which occurs in about 80% of those with acute infections (Makris *et al.*, Alter, 1994a; Fig. 24.1). The diagnosis of chronic HCV is usually established in persons with NANB by the finding of long-standing ALT elevations in the presence of anti-HCV, after excluding other causes of liver disease, mentioned above. Antibodies remain persistently detectable with ELISA-2 assays throughout follow-up in the majority of patients. However, seroreversion mainly due to diminishing C100 reactivity has been described in 20% of anti-HCV-positive HIV-infected hemophiliacs (Hatzakis *et al.*, 1992; Ragni *et al.*, 1993). Sustained clearance of HCV RNA correlates with resolution of infection, whereas persistence of detectable HCV RNA predicts progression to chronic disease (Farci *et al.*, 1992). Although ALT levels may occasionally reach over 1000 u/l, values more typi-cally range from twice to 10 times normal (Schimpf *et al.*, Alter *et al.*, 1989). However, there is poor correlation between ALT abnormalities and severity of hepatic inflammation.

Multiple hepatitis viral infections

Multiple viral infections may interact in hemophilic patients, resulting in the phenomenon known as viral interference (Pontisso *et al.*, 1993). In individuals chronically infected with HBV and HDV, HBV DNA is usually suppressed, although HBsAg production continues. In those who are coinfected with HBV and HCV, there is a reciprocal relationship between HBV DNA and HCV RNA (Wright and Lau, 1993). In HBsAg carriers who are anti-HCV-positive, HCV RNA is often not detectable (Hanley *et al.*, 1993), and in those with HDV infections, HCV RNA is usually suppressed (Eyster *et al.*, 1994).

NATURAL HISTORY OF HCV

The natural history of HCV is only beginning to be understood, and the late consequences are not yet fully

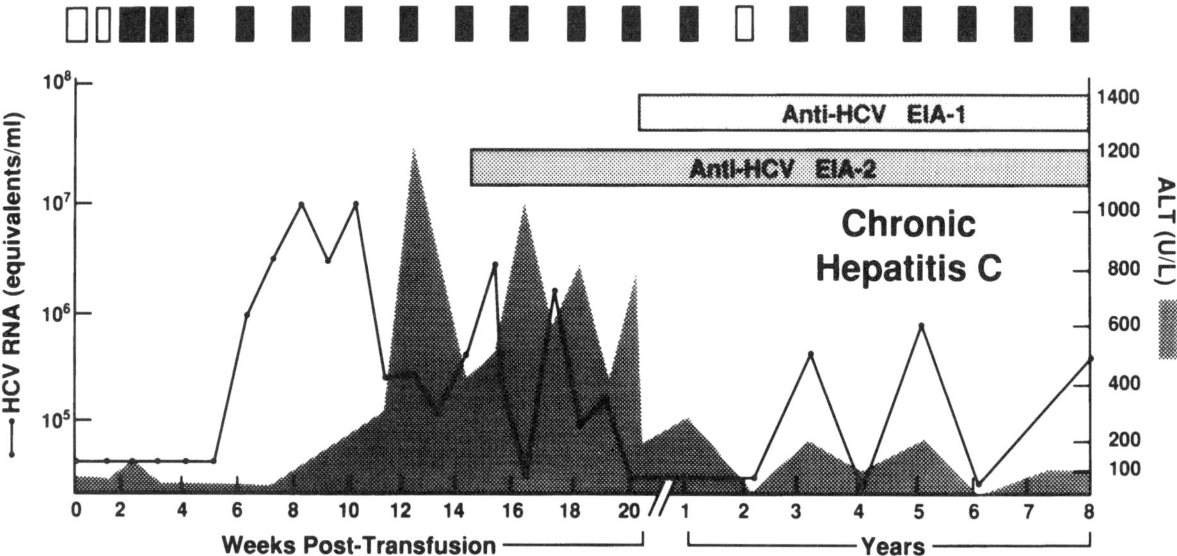

Fig. 24.1 Typical course of chronic hepatitis C in which acute infection is followed by chronic infection. Points to note are:

1. Hepatitis C virus (HCV) RNA is detectable very early after exposure. Polymerase chain reaction (PCR) was positive in the 2-week post-exposure sample, but it may become positive even sooner.
2. Viral replication, as assessed by HCV RNA level, occurs before any clinical or biochemical evidence of hepatitis.
3. The level of HCV RNA may persist, fluctuate or become non-detectable. Sometimes HCV RNA levels show a periodicity that parallels the fluctuations in alanine aminotransferase (ALT). In this case, the rise in HCV RNA shortly precedes the rise in ALT and the fall in HCV RNA precedes the fall in ALT.
4. Second-generation anti-HCV assays considerably diminish the seronegative window in HCV infection as compared with first-generation assays. None the less, anti-HCV was not detectable for 15 weeks after exposure and for 6–7 weeks after the first significant rise in ALT.
5. Antibody to HCV, as detected by second-generation assays, almost always persists; antibodies detected in the first-generation assay (anti-C100, anti-5-1-1) may disappear in some cases, particularly those who are coinfected with HIV.

Modified from Alter, H.J. (1994a) Hepatitis C: natural history, in *Viral hepatitis A to F: An Update*. American Association for the Study of Liver Diseases. Postgraduate Course. Chicago, Illinois, pp. 225–243, with permission.

defined. However, it is apparent that chronic HCV is not a benign disease in a growing number of patients who are followed over extended periods of time. In one group of 45 patients with posttransfusion NANBH undergoing 33 biopsies on one or more occasions, 20% developed cirrhosis within 1.5 and 16 years after blood transfusion. Two (6%) died of liver failure related to HCV-induced cirrhosis (Di Bisceglie *et al.*, 1991).

In a look-back study of 80 patients prospectively identified as having contracted NANB posttransfusion hepatitis between 1972 and 1980, among those who survived 15 years the probability of liver failure was about 20% (Koretz *et al.*, 1993). In a study of 333 patients with chronic HCV in whom blood transfusion was the presumed source of infection in 116, eight (7%) progressed to severe chronic hepatitis or cirrhosis in 10 years. Of the 55 who had their first biopsy more than 25 years after blood transfusion, 39 (71%) had severe chronic active hepatitis or cirrhosis (Takahasi, *et al.*, 1993). Of 100 patients from all risk groups who were followed at least 5 years, 42 developed cirrhosis and 19 developed HCC. It is well-recognized that HCV is a risk factor for HCC in patients with cirrhosis, and there may be an interaction of HCV and alcoholic liver disease in the etiology of HCC (Alter, 1994).

Although chronicity of disease was independent of risk factor, one prospective study showed that severe disease was more likely to be found in patients who acquired their infections through blood transfusion, suggesting that the size of the infectious inoculum may influence disease progression (Alter *et al.*, 1992). If confirmed, this association has serious implications for those persons with hemophilia who were exposed to massive doses of crude, untreated concentrates within the last 10–20 years. On the other hand, in a large long-term study of 568 patients with transfusion-associated NANBH and 984 control patients who had been transfused without developing hepatitis, there was no increase in mortality from all causes in the study group after an average follow-up of 18 years (Seeff *et al.*, 1992). There was, however, a statistically significant excess of liver-related mortality in the hepatitis population. Furthermore, according to data now emerging, among NANB/C cases, 35% had biochemical evidence of chronic hepatitis compared to 1% of the controls, and two-thirds of 40 patients biopsied had severe histologic lesions, including chronic active hepatitis, cirrhosis and HCC (Seef *et al.*, 1992; Alter, 1994). Since the interval from acute infection to onset of symptoms may take two to four decades, a much longer period of observation will be required to determine whether there is an overall increased mortality following transmission-associated NANBH (Alter, 1991).

Studies of the natural history of HCV in persons with hemophilia are limited. One report found that liver disease was the major cause of death in a subcohort of hemophiliacs with thrombocytopenia and leukopenia who were treated before the blood supply became contaminated with HIV in 1979 (Eyster *et al.*, 1985). Two recent reports have shown an association of age with progression of liver disease in hemophiliacs with HIV disease, but results are confounded by the presence of HIV coinfection, which appears to cause a more rapid progression of HCV disease (Eyster *et al.*, 1993; Telfer *et al.*, 1994). However, it is clear that hemophiliacs with chronic HCV face an ever-increasing risk for the development of serious liver disease throughout their lifetime. This includes the secondary development of HCC, with a crude rate of 3.2/100 000 patients/year, which is at least 30 times higher than the background incidence of this tumor in the countries of origin of the 11 801 hemophiliacs surveyed from 54 centers in the USA and Europe (Colombo *et al.*, 1991). All patients in this survey with HCC had cirrhosis. Whether HCV itself is oncogenic or whether HCC is secondary to the mitotic events accompanying rapid cellular regeneration is unclear (Simenetta *et al.*, 1992).

Pathogenesis of hepatocellular damage in HCV

The pathogenesis of hepatocullular damage by HCV is poorly understood. As with chronic HBV infection, evidence is emerging that liver damage may be mediated by a cellular immune reaction to infected hepatocytes as well as by the virus itself. Koziel *et al.* (1992, 1993) have demonstrated that HLA class I-restricted CD8+ lymphocytes which recognize core and *env* proteins specific to HCV are present in the liver of individuals with chronic HCV infections. In addition, recent studies have reported a class II-restricted CD4 lymphocyte response (Bortarelli *et al.*, 1993). However, the demonstration of HCV antigens in liver biopsies and the correlation between levels of viremia and degree of lobular inflammation and histology suggests that HCV may be directly cytopathic to hepatocytes (Krawczynski *et al.*, 1992; Lau *et al.*, 1993; Yuki, Hayashi and Kamada, 1993). Since these two mechanisms are not mutually exclusive, it is possible that they both play a role in liver cell injury.

Biochemical tests

A characteristic feature of HCV is its ability to cause repeated fluctuations of serum transaminase levels over prolonged periods of time (Alter *et al.*, 1989). Serum bilirubin and alkaline phosphatase determinations are less frequently abnormal. ALT levels roughly parallel HCV RNA levels and the degree of lobular inflammation (Lau *et al.*, 1993; Alter, 1994: Eyster *et al.*, 1994).

Transaminase elevations have been reported in more than 50% and chronic elevations in approximately 30%

of hemophiliacs treated with clotting factor concentrates before 1978 (Mannucci *et al.*, 1975; Webster *et al.*, 1976; Lesesne *et al.*, 1977; Levine *et al.*, 1977; Spero *et al.*, 1979; Hasiba *et al.*, 1980; Gerety and Eyster, 1981; Cederbaum, Blatt and Levine, 1982). In a cooperative prospective study of 1332 hemophiliacs (Cederbaum, Blatt and Levine, 1982), 72% of patients had at least one abnormal transaminase value, and 21 and 24% had persistently elevated aspartate aminotransferase (AST) and ALT levels respectively on three sets of measurements at 6-month intervals. Only 1.2% had a bilirubin >2.0 mg/dl at the time of entry, and values on these individuals remained relatively constant throughout the 3-year study. In another 1-year prospective study of 98 hemophiliacs from a single center, 68% had abnormal transaminases and none had elevated bilirubin levels (Levine *et al.*, 1977). However, ALT levels are not predictive of the severity of inflammation on liver biopsy, and serious liver disease can be present in HCV-infected individuals with minimal transaminase elevation.

Liver biopsy studies

The diagnostic paradigm for the diagnosis of chronic hepatitis includes biochemical, immunoserologic, virologic and histologic studies. While the distinction between HCV, HBV and non-viral hepatitis can often be made without liver biopsy, only biopsy can assess the extent of the injury. Features suggestive of HCV include portal lymphoid aggregates, bile duct damage and steatosis, while ground-glass hepatocytes suggest chronic HBV. The absence of these changes and the presence of moderate to severe piecemeal necrosis and/or lobular inflammation suggests autoimmune hepatitis (Czaja and Carpenter, 1993). However, there is considerable overlap, and a specific diagnosis cannot be made on histology alone.

Liver biopsies in persons with hemophilia have been limited by the underlying hemostatic defect. Published studies of liver biopsies in persons with hemophilia are summarized in Table 24.1 (Lesesne *et al.*, 1977; Preston *et al.*, 1978; Spero *et al.*, 1978; McGrath *et al.*, 1980; Schimpf *et al.*, 1981; Mannucci, Colombo and Rizzetto, 1982; White *et al.*, 1982; Aledort *et al.*, 1985; Hay *et al.*, 1985). The first to show unequivocal evidence of chronic hepatitis was carried out by Lesesne and colleagues (1977). Over the 5-year period between 1977 and 1982, 57 (98%) of 58 selected multitransfused patients with prolonged elevation of transaminases from seven centers showed evidence of chronic hepatitis ranging from mild (68%) to severe (26%). Three (6%) showed evidence of cirrhosis (Lesesne *et al.*, 1977; Preston *et al.*, 1978; Spero *et al.*, 1978; McGrath *et al.*, 1980; Mannucci, Colombo and Rizzetto, 1982; White *et al.*, 1982).

Of 32 unselected cases who underwent routine biopsy during other surgical procedures, 20 (62%) had chronic hepatitis or cirrhosis (Schimpf *et al.*, 1981). There was no evidence that chronic liver disease was a prominent cause of morbidity or death in these individuals. Furthermore, the first prospective study in 1982 of 11 hemophiliacs followed 6 years with liver biopsies every 3 years concluded that chronic liver disease was non-progressive in those who had no intrahepatic HBV markers (Mannucci, Colombo and Rizzetto, 1982). However, by 1985, cumulative data in a study by Hay *et al.* showed that 13 of 34 patients (38%) with persistently abnormal liver function tests had histologic evidence of chronic active hepatitis or cirrhosis and that chronic progressive liver disease was present in at least 21% of an unselected population of 79 who had received clotting factor concentrates.

In the largest study reported to date, biopsy or autopsy hepatic histologic materials and associated clinical data were collected from 155 hemophiliacs and analyzed retrospectively to determine the spectrum of liver disease (Aledort *et al.*, 1985). Sixty-four per cent of these individuals had trivial, mild or moderate hepatic lesions, 7% had severe lesions (chronic active hepatitis) and 15% had cirrhosis. Among 15 autopsied patients known to have received concentrates, the incidence of chronic active hepatitis and cirrhosis was 20%. No etiologic speculation was possible in this study, which was carried out before the availability of HCV tests, but histologic features suggestive of NANBH were frequently noted. In a more recent report from the hemophilia center at the Royal Free Hospital in London, there was evidence of cirrhosis in seven of 18 (39%) postmortem examinations. One patient developed HCC secondary to chronic HCV (Telfer, Watt and Lee, 1993).

Markers and cofactors of HCV disease progression

Age, HCV RNA levels, viral genotype, host factors and coinfection with HIV may all play a role in progression to serious liver disease.

Several reports suggest that there is an association of advancing age with more severe liver disease (Hay *et al.*, 1987; Di Bisceglie *et al.*, 1991; Eyster *et al.*, 1993; Takahashi *et al.*, 1994). In the study by Telfer *et al.* (1994), hepatic decompensation was more common in older patients, in heavily treated patients and in those with a diagnosis of hemophilia A. In the study by Eyster *et al.* (1993), liver failure was observed only in adults who had been infected with HCV for 10 years or more. These findings are in agreement with those of Di Bisceglie *et al.* (1991) and Takahashi *et al.* (1993), who found an association of older age with early disease progression.

Table 24.1   Liver histopathology in persons with hemophilia treated with clotting factor concentrates

Study	Number of patients	Histopathology	Comments
Lesesne *et al.* (1977)	6	3 CPH 3 CAH	All had prolonged elevations of ALTs. One was symptomatic (jaundice). Two were HBsAg+ve
Preston *et al.* (1978)	8	1 CLH 3 CPH 3 CAH 2 Cirrhosis	All had persistently elevated ALTs and were asymptomatic. Two were HBsAg+ve
Spero *et al.* (1978)	13	8 CPH 4 CPH	All had chronically elevated ALTs and were asymptomatic
McGrath *et al.* (1980)	5	4 CPH 1 CAH	Asymptotic children ages 2–9 years with persistently elevated ALTs
Schimpf *et al.* (1981)	32	10 CPH 9 CAH 1 Cirrhosis	Unselected patients biopsied during surgical procedures
White *et al.* (1982)	15	3 Mild changes 11 CPH 1 CAH	All were asymptomatic with prolonged ALTs. one was HBsAg+ve
Mannucci, Colombo and Rizzetto (1982)	11	6 CPH 4 CAH 1 Cirrhosis	Prospective study over 6 years, with repeat biopsy every 3 years. Two patients changed from CPH to CLH. Four patients with CAH had spontaneous improvement. All had persistently elevated ALTs. One was HBsAg+ve
Hay *et al.* (1985)	34	20 CPH 1 CLH 9 CAH 4 Cirrhosis	Eight-year prospective study of 79 recipients of clotting factor concentrates. Repeat biopsies in nine showed progression to cirrhosis in four. Overall 17 (21%) showed chronic progressive liver disease
Aledort *et al.* (1985)	115 biopsies 40 autopsies	75 (65%) Mild to moderate 10(9%) Severe 8(16%) Cirrhosis 24 (60%) mild to moderate 8(2%) Severe 5(13%) Cirrhosis	Histologic studies from 155 hemophiliacs collected by an *ad hoc* study group

CPH = Chronic persistent hepatitis; CAH = Chronic active hepatitis; CLH = chronic lobular hepatitis; ALT = Alanine aminotransferase; HBsAg+ve = Hepatitis B surface antigen-positive.

Sustained clearance of HCV RNA correlates with resolution of disease, whereas persistence of detectable HCV RNA predicts progression to chronic hepatitis (Farci *et al.*, 1991). Emerging data suggest that HCV RNA may also be a marker for serious liver disease (Alberti *et al.*, 1992), and that high-titer viremia correlates with lobular inflammation (Lau *et al.*, 1993) and advanced stage of disease (Gretch *et al.*, 1993; Kato *et al.*, 1993; Yuki, Hayashi and Kamada, 1993). When paired serum and liver biopsy specimens from 47 patients with confirmed chronic HCV infection and evidence of serum HCV RNA were studied, Lau *et al.* (1993) found an association with lobular inflammation, lymphoid aggregates and bile duct lesions, but not with histologic diagnosis of chronic active hepatitis or cirrhosis. However, Kato *et al.* (1993) found that the amount of HCV RNA in the serum had a tendency to increase according to the progression of histologic changes, and in a larger study of 121 viremic patients with HCV, Gretch *et al.* (1993) found significantly higher HCV RNA levels in 18 patients with end-stage liver disease than either 64 asymptomatic blood donors or 39 patients with chronic active hepatitis. Furthermore, Kato *et al.* (1993) showed that the amount of HCV RNA increased exponentially as the duration of infection increased, and in studies of 17 HIV-positive/HCV-positive haemophiliacs and 17 HIV-negative/HCV-positive age-matched controls, Eyster *et al.* (1994) reported significant increases in HCV RNA levels over time in HIV-negative as well as HIV-positive individuals. Although a longitudinal relationship between viral load and disease progression has not yet been established, these data suggest that HCV viral load increases as disease progresses.

Sequence analysis of different viral isolates has shown that multiple genotypes of HCV exist. The original classification system proposed by Okamato *et al.* (1991) described five different genotypes, designated by Roman numerals I through V. Subsequently, Simmonds *et al.* (1993) described six major groupings and a series of subtypes by phylogenetic analysis of the non-structural NS-5 region of the genome. The first genotype cloned by Choo *et al.* is type I, which corresponds to type 1a of Simmonds. Type II is 1b, type III is 2a, type IV is 2b and V is 3a. Genotype 1a (I) is most common in the USA, whereas 1b (II) and 2a (III) are most common in Japan and in Europe. Preliminary data suggest that genotype 1b may be associated with the presence of more severe liver disease, higher viral loads and poorer responses to therapy (Pozzato *et al.*, 1991; Yoshioka *et al.*, 1992; Kobayashi *et al.*, 1993). However, viral genotypes and viral load may be interrelated, since type 2a generally replicates to lower titers in plasma than does type 1b (Kobayashi *et al.*, 1993).

One of the most striking features of chronic HCV infections is the inability of the host to develop a protective immune response, even after reinfection with the identical strain of virus (Farci *et al.*, 1992; Lai *et al.*, 1994; Prince, 1994). Under pressure, HCV has a very high mutation rate, and experimental data in both chimpanzees and humans have shown that this is associated with the emergence of closely related but immunologically distinct quasi-species which are not neutralized by circulating antibodies (Mizokami, Gojobori and Lau, 1994; Alter, 1995). In serial studies, HCV RNA levels have been shown to increase over time, even in HIV-negative, HCV-infected hemophiliacs, implying that the immune response is not adequate to control the infections (Eyster *et al.*, 1994). T-cell deviations, including lower CD4+ percentages and counts and CD56+ natural killer subsets, have been previously reported in HIV-negative persons with hemophilia (Hassett *et al.*, 1993).

Multiple HCV variants have been demonstrated in hemophiliacs treated with clotting factor concentrates. Jarvis *et al.* (1994) showed that the major circulating genotype changed in nine of 29 (31%) patients studied over a 10-year period of time. In one-third of the patients, the change occurred after the introduction of virally inactivated products, implicating reactivation rather than reinfection. Those who were coinfected with HIV showed a greater tendency to change genotype.

HIV coinfection

HIV coinfection appears to accelerate progression to hepatic decompensation in HCV-infected hemophiliacs

(Eyster *et al.*, 1993; Telfer *et al.*, 1994). In a retrospective study of 255 HCV-seropositive hemophiliac by Telfer *et al.* (1994), the risk of hepatic decompensation was 10.8% at 20 years after first treatment with large donor pool clotting factor concentrate. HIV-seropositive patients were 21 times more likely to develop hepatic decompensation than HIV-seronegative patients. For HIV-seropositive patients, the rates of decline in CD4 lymphocyte count and the development of p24 antigenemia were significant risk factors for hepatic decompensation. Cirrhosis was seen in nine (49%) of 19 HIV-seropositive patients.

In a prospective cohort study of 223 hemophiliacs by Eyster *et al.* (1993), an increased frequency of liver failure was found in those who were infected with both HCV and HIV compared to those who were infected with HCV only (Eyster *et al.*, 1993). Among coinfected subjects, cumulative incidence of liver failure was 42% 27 years after the first exposure to clotting factor concentrates, and 17% 10 years after HIV infection. By comparison, cumulative acquired immunodeficiency syndrome (AIDS) incidence 10 years after HIV infection was 31%. Lymphocytopenia, decreased CD4 counts and possibly thrombocytopenia were associated with liver failure. The hypothetical progression of HCV disease and HIV disease as related to time and lymphocyte and CD4 counts in concentrate recipients is depicted in Figure 24.2.

In a subsequent report by Eyster *et al.*, (1994) involving a subcohort of HCV-positive, HIV-positive individuals and age-matched HCV-positive, HIV-negative controls, HCV load increased over time, was enhanced by HIV, and further increased as immune deficiency progressed. Over a 12-year period, HCV RNA levels increased nearly threefold in those who remained HIV-negative from a mean of 9.47×10^5 to 2.81×10^6 mmol/ml. Among those who became HIV-positive, HCV RNA levels increased 58-fold from 2.85×10^5 to 1.66×10^7 mmol/ml. The rate of increase was eightfold faster for HIV-positive subjects than for those who remained HIV-negative. Telfer *et al.* (1994) also found significantly higher HCV RNA levels in HIV-seropositive than HIV-seronegative anti-HCV-positive hemophiliacs. Although the immunopathogenesis of HCV disease is poorly understood, these findings strongly support the possibility that cellular immunity is important in controlling HCV infection and that HIV-induced immune deficiency may permit increased HCV replication.

Immunologic manifestations of chronic hepatitis

Autoimmune markers and concurrent immunologic diseases occur commonly in chronic HBV and HCV (Czaja *et al.*, 1995). Glomerulonephritis, polyarteritis nodosa,

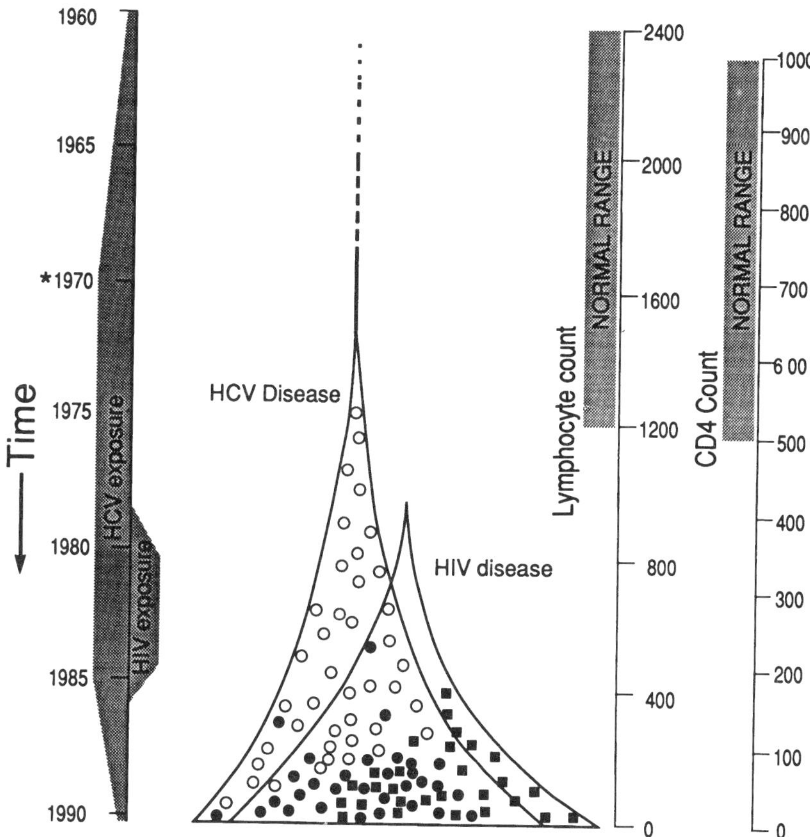

Fig. 24.2 Modified Venn diagram depicting the hypothetical progression of hepatitic C virus (HCV) and human immunodeficiency virus (HIV) disease as related to time and lymphocyte and CD4 counts in multitransfused persons with hemophilia. Almost all heavily treated persons with hemophilia have been infected with HCV. Most infections occurred in the 1970s when clotting factor concentrates were introduced (*) or earlier (left scale). HIV infections occurred between 1978 and 1986. Over the ensuing years, the total lymphocyte count and the CD4-positive lymphocyte counts have decreased, especially for the HIV-infected patients (right scale). Concurrently, over time the incidences of histologic liver disease (O), liver failure (●) and acquired immunodeficiency syndrome (AIDS)-defining illnesses (■) have increased. From Eyster, M.E., Diamondstone, L.S., Lien, J.M. *et al.* (1993) Natural history of hepatitis C virus (HCV) infection is multitransfused hemophiliacs: effect of coinfection with human immunodeficiency virus (HIV). *Journal of Acquired Immune Deficiency Syndrome*, 6, 602–610, with permission.

cutaneous vasculitis, cryoglobulinemia, antinuclear antibodies (ANA) and anti-smooth-muscle antibodies (SMA) are associated with both HBV and HCV infections, and thyroiditis, antithyroid antibodies and liver/kidney microsome type 1 (anti-LKM 1) antibodies are found with increased frequency in HCV infections. Recent studies have demonstrated an association of certain autoimmune expression reflects a genetic predisposition that is facilitated by the viral infection or whether autoimmune expression is coincidental with viral infection (Lunel, 1994). However, it is important that a definitive diagnosis of HBV or HCV be established before initiating treatment with interferon-α, since its deleterious effect on autoimmune hepatitis is well-recognized.

Other HCV-related diseases

Recent evidence suggests that HCV plays a role in the pathogenesis of essential mixed cryoglobulinaemia

(Agnello, Chung and Kaplan, 1992; Misiani *et al.*, 1992). Type II cryoglobulin is strongly associated with concomitant HCV infection and a high rate of false-negative anti-HCV antibody tests because HCV virions and HCV antigen–antibody complexes are concentrated in cryoprecipitates, often in association with rheumatoid factor (Agnello, Chung and Kaplan, 1992).

As with type II mixed cryoglobulinemia, there is now a strong association between HCV and porphyria cutanea tarda (Alter, 1995). Although the cause of the reduced hepatic uroporphyrinogen decarboxylase activity observed in this disorder is unclear, HCV infection appears to be the primary cause of the liver disease that accompanies porphyria cutanea tarda (Fargion *et al.*, 1992).

Treatment

Interferon-α is the only therapy approved for the treatment of patients with chronic HBV and HCV as of 1994 in both the USA and Europe. The best independent predictors for response to therapy are the baseline HBV DNA (Perez *et al.*, 1990; Perrillo *et al.*, 1990) and HCV RNA levels (Hagiwara *et al.*, 1993; Kobayashi *et al.*, 1993; Lau *et al.*, 1993). Those with high viral loads at initiation of treatment respond less well. Advanced histologic stage, older age, longer duration of hepatitis prior to treatment, transfusion-associated infection, HCV genotype and iron content of the liver may also affect response to therapy (Lau *et al.*, 1993; van der Poel, Cuypers and Reesink, 1994; van Thiel *et al.*, 1994). The presence of HIV infection has been associated with poor response to interferon-α in some studies (Telfer *et al.*, 1995) but not in others (Boyer *et al.*, 1992). Possible differences may relate to the degree of immune deficiency.

HBV AND HDV

Five million units of interferon-α given daily, or 10 million units three times a week for 16 weeks, increases the frequency of HBeAg loss in chronic HBV and results in a sustained loss of serum HBV DNA in 20% of cases. In a meta-analysis of 15 randomized controlled trials, including 837 HBsAg/HBeAg-positive adults, 37% versus 17% controls lost HBV DNA, and 7.8% versus 1.8% controls lost HBsAg (Wong *et al.*, 1993). Pretreatment with prednisone appears to enhance efficacy in patients with low pretreatment ALT activity (Perrillo *et al.*, 1990; Korenman *et al.*, 1991).

In about half the patients with chronic HDV treated with higher doses of interferon (9 million units three times a week for 48 weeks), there is histologic improvement with return to normal of the ALT and loss of detectable HDV RNA. However, relapse is common after treatment is stopped (Farci *et al.*, 1994).

HCV

Several studies in persons with transfusion- and community-acquired HCV have shown that a 6-month course of interferon-α 3 million units three times a week for 6 months results in biochemical and histologic responses in approximately half of the patients treated (Davis *et al.*, 1989; Causse *et al.*, 1991). Responses are associated with a loss of HCV RNA from the serum (Shindo *et al.*, 1991). HCV RNA disappears before the ALT levels become normal and reappears in patients who relapse (Hagiwara *et al.*, 1993). Unfortunately, sustained responses are difficult to achieve. Relapses occur in half of the patients who initially achieve a complete remission, for an overall sustained response rate of only 20–25%.

Published data on the results of interferon therapy in persons with hemophilia are limited (Makris *et al.*, 1991; Bresters *et al.*, 1992; Telfer *et al.*, 1995). Combined results of the 57 patients reported as of the end of 1994 show that ALT levels reverted to normal in 22 (39%), HCV RNA became undetectable in 17/41 (41%), and only 7/57 (12%) had a sustained response. HCV RNA levels were not quantitated in any of these individuals, and responses were lower in those individuals who were also HIV-infected. Increased clinical effects and side-effects of interferon-α therapy in HIV-negative persons with hemophilia and chronic HCV seem to be comparable to non-hemophilia patients with chronic HCV (Mauser-Bunschoten *et al.*, 1995; Telfer *et al.*, 1995).

PRACTICAL CONSIDERATIONS FOR INTERFERON-α TREATMENT

Over half of the patients treated with interferon-α experience unpleasant side-effects, including flu-like symptoms of myalgia, fever and headache. Leukopenia and thrombocytopenia are frequent, and depression and activation or exacerbation of autoimmune disorders such as hypothyroidism or hyperthyroidism are also seen. These side-effects occur mainly at the initiation of therapy, are dose-related and are reversible when therapy is discontinued. They are partially ameliorated with the use of ibuprofen or non-steroidal anti-inflammatory agents, by the latter are often contraindicated in persons with hemophilia. Furthermore, the cost of therapy is considerable, and there are no controlled studies on the prevention of cirrhosis. None the less, it is the only form of therapy with any proven benefit, and it seems rational to try and eradicate or reduce the viral load with interferon-α.

Liver biopsy is used to determine the extent of injury. If the diagnosis of chronic HBV or HCV can be established by the appropriate virologic, serologic and biochemical markers, and the diagnosis of autoimmune hepatitis is excluded, liver biopsy can be deferred in persons with hemophilia. Given the potential for bleeding complications and the added cost of clotting factor concentrate, we initiate interferon-α therapy without biopsy in those who are otherwise suitable candidates. This includes those with persistently elevated transaminases with positive HCV RNA assays who are well-compensated, have had no previous history of ascites and have good synthetic liver function. Because of the potential for the development of severe bacterial infections and worsening thrombocytopenia, interferon-α is generally contraindicated in those with signs of decompensating liver disease (ascites, bleeding esophageal varices, encephalopathy, progressive jaundice and muscle wasting). Those with HbsAg-positivity need additional evaluation to determine whether they are HbeAg-positive and whether they are coinfected with HDV, since the treatment of chronic HBV differs from HCV.

During treatment, it is essential to monitor the patient carefully for the development of anemia, neutropenia and thrombocytopenia, especially during the first few weeks of therapy. Thereafter, these parameters can be followed less frequently, along with the ALT levels. Tests of thyroid function and a careful history with reference to symptoms of depression are required. Decisions regarding dosing and duration of therapy are made based on ALT levels and HCV RNA levels: the goal is to obtain normal ALT and loss of detectable HCV RNA at the completion of a 6-month course of therapy. If relapse occurs following cessation of therapy, recurrent therapy should be considered, since about half of those with initial responses will respond again. The role of maintenance therapy is currently under investigation.

Patients with HCV who are coinfected with HIV pose special problems for treatment with interferon. Those with low CD4 T-lymphocyte counts tolerate treatment less well, and enhanced toxicity is common in those with late-stage HIV infections who are receiving multiple drug combinations. At present, we are treating HIV-coinfected patients only by protocols approved by our Institutional Review Board and with informed consent.

OTHER FORMS OF THERAPY UNDER INVESTIGATION

Steroids are known to enhance viral proliferation, and for patients with HBV, treatment with corticosteroids before interferon may offer a therapeutic advantage to those with lower ALT levels. Newer approaches to the experimental treatment of HBV include the use of Ampligen, interferon-β, consensus interferon-α, lymphoblastoid interferon and a cytosine analog, Lamivudine (3TC; Hoofnagle, 1993).

In patients with HCV, the guanosine analog ribavirin is associated with an ALT response, but HCV RNA remains detectable. These findings have prompted the investigation of combination ribavirin and interferon-α, higher doses of interferon-α, non-steroidal anti-inflammatory agents to enhance interferon-α therapy, N-acetyl cysteine (an antioxidant and glutathione source) to induce response to interferon, and the use of ursodeoxycholic acid to suppress the anti-inflammatory reaction (Lindsay, 1993).

LIVER TRANSPLANTATION

Liver transplantation is the only viable option for patients with decompensated end-stage liver disease. Unfortunately, for patients transplanted for HBV infection, results have been disappointing. One-year survivals are only 50%, compared to 90% for those transplanted for alcoholic liver disease (Todo *et al.*, 1991), with recurrent HBV infection in those who are HBV-DNA-positive accounting for most of the deaths. In contrast, although the graft usually becomes infected with HCV shortly after

transplantation, survival post-transplantation is not impaired (Feray *et al.*, 1992; van der Poel, Cuypers and Reesink, 1994). In persons with hemophilia, the transplant has the added benefit of restoring normal coagulation (Bontempo *et al.*, 1987). Unfortunately, coinfection with HIV is usually a contraindication to liver transplant because of high mortality and reinfection rate.

Transmission to family members

HBV is transmitted sexually, perinatally and by intimate or close personal contact. Sexual and perinatal transmission is very efficient, and household transmission is well-documented, especially when the contact has an acute infection or is a chronic carrier of HBeAg (Centers for Disease Control, 1991). Regular sexual contacts of adults with acute HBV infection have a 30% risk of infection, and persons living in the same household as an HBV carrier have a 40% or higher likelihood of current or prior HBV infection (Centers for Disease Control, 1987). The presence of HBeAg is indicative of high-levels of circulating HBV, and HBeAg-positive persons are 5–10 times more likely to transmit HBV than are HBeAg-negative individuals (Alter, 1994b). Therefore, prophylactic HBV vaccination is recommended for all household and sexual contacts of HBsAg carriers (Centers for Disease Control, 1991).

Experimental and epidemiologic studies indicate that HCV is mainly transmitted by the parenteral route. The rate of transmission after needle-stick exposure from a known HCV antibody-positive source is 3–10% (Mitsui *et al.*, 1992). However, HCV circulates in low titers in the blood of most infected persons, except during the acute infection or with coincident HIV infection, and is detected inconsistently in other body fluids (Fried *et al.*, 1993; Alter, 1994; Eyster *et al.*, 1994). These findings may explain the relatively low prevalence of sexual transmission of HCV compared to HBV in promiscuous heterosexual and homosexual populations when intravenous drug use is excluded as a risk factor.

Studies of sexual or household HCV transmission have revealed conflicting results. A small number of case-control studies demonstrate that heterosexual and household transmissions occur, but most studies employing second-generation anti-HCV and/or well-validated complementary DNA-PCR assays indicate that the risk is very low to absent (Brettler *et al.*, 1992; Bresters *et al.*, 1993; Osmond *et al.*, 1993). Studies from high endemic areas in the Far East showing higher rates of apparent sexual or household transmission may be confounded by infection of husband and wife by a common external source or may be related to geographic differences in viral subtypes (Centers for Disease Control, 1991; Bresters *et al.*, 1993; Alter, 1994).

Several studies have evaluated the risk of sexual transmission of HCV to female partners of hemophiliacs (Eyster *et al.*, 1991; Brettler *et al.*, 1992; Bresters *et al.*, 1993). Brettler *et al.* (1992) found one of 66 (2%) HIV-positive and two of 40 (5%) HIV-negative female sexual partners to be positive for anti-HCV. All had other risk factors. Brettler *et al.* found no HCV infections in 33 female sexual partners of HCV-positive hemophiliacs with mean duration of relationship 12 years (Brettler *et al.*, 1992). In a study by Eyster *et al.* (1991), involving 234 female sexual partners of 231 multitransfused hemophilic men, the prevalence of anti-HCV among female sexual partners with no other known risk factors was 5/194 (2.6%). Men who were coinfected with HIV and HCV were five times more likely to transmit both viruses than would have been expected by chance, suggesting that HIV might be a cofactor for the sexual transmission of HCV. Taken together, these studies indicate that sexual transmission of HCV is inefficient and has rarely been documented, even with long-term ongoing activity with a steady partner. However, future studies employing highly sensitive, specific standardized assays to detect and quantitate the relative infectivity of source patients are needed.

As with sexual transmission, studies examining perinatal transmission of HCV have yielded conflicting results. Evaluating the risk of maternal–infant transmission is particularly difficult because the diagnosis depends upon the detection of HCV-RNA in the neonate. The majority of studies published before 1994 have shown a 0–5% infection rate of infants born to anti-HCV-positive mothers (Giovanni *et al.*, 1990; Alvarez *et al.*, 1992; Reinus *et al.*, 1992; Lam *et al.*, 1993; Alter, 1995). A few showing higher infection rates involved mothers who were coinfected with HIV (Giovannini *et al.*, 1990; Alvarez *et al.*, 1992).

In a more recent study by Ohto *et al.* (1994), 6% (3/53) anti-HCV-positive women transmitted HCV to their infants, and the risk of transmission was directly related to the titer of HCV-RNA in the mother. Of the 37 women who were also positive for HCV-RNA, the risk of transmission was 11%, and among the infants born to mothers with titers of 10^6 or greater, the risk was 36%. There was no transmission from those with lower titers or negative HCV-RNA assays. Furthermore, nucleotide sequencing of the HCV genomes from the infected mother–infant pairs showed 97–99% homology, compared to 66–92% homology between infected infants. Taken together, these studies indicate that perinatal transmission of HCV is inefficient compared to HBV, but that transmission occurs in about 10% of HCV-RNA-positive mothers and is enhanced when maternal viral burden is high (Alter, 1994).

These findings have led to the following recommendations from the Centers for Disease Control (1991) regarding counseling to anti-HCV-positive individuals for potential infectivity:

1. Blood spills should be cleaned with soap, disinfected with bleach, and blood-stained articles should be discarded in plastic bags.
2. Household articles such as toothbrushes and razors should not be shared, and cuts or skin lesions should be covered.
3. HCV-positive individuals should be informed of the potential for sexual transmission. As of 1994, there are insufficient data to recommend changes in current sexual practices for persons with a steady sexual partner. However, for the prevention of many sexually transmitted diseases, including HBV and HIV infections, safe sex should be practiced.
4. Consideration may be given to testing exposed sexual partners for anti-HCV and, if positive, evaluating them for chronic liver disease. As of 1994, there are no recommendations advising against pregnancy, nor are there any special treatments or precautions for HCV-antibody-positive pregnant women or their offspring.

Vaccines

Plasma-derived and recombinant HBV vaccines are available. Both are safe and effective, with a 95% seroconversion rate after proper administration (Centers for Disease Control, 1991). A formalin-inactivated vaccine which is well-tolerated and effective in HAV prevention is licensed in over 30 countries and will soon be available in the USA (Lemon, 1994). The high mutation rate of HCV, the failure of infection to elicit protective immunity and the lack of *in vitro* systems for propagating HCV pose formidable challenges for the successful development of an HCV vaccine (Houghton *et al.*, 1991).

Practical considerations and guidelines for management

Although chronic liver disease is a frequent outcome in hemophiliacs, the majority remain asymptomatic for many years, even after cirrhosis has been documented. Therefore the approach to the evaluation, treatment and prevention of hepatitis and chronic liver disease in persons with hemophilia must be individualized. However, we employ the following guidelines:

1. Persons with hemophilia should undergo periodic screening for HBsAg, anti-HBs and anti-HCV. Chronic HBsAg carriers should be screened for anti-HDV. Those without HBV markers should be vaccinated, and consideration should be given to revaccination of those who lose anti-HBs positivity.

2. Treatment with interferon-α should be considered for HBsAg carriers and anti-HCV-positive individuals with elevated transaminases who are HBeAg- or HCV-RNA-positive. These individuals should also be cautioned about the use of potentially hepatotoxic medications and alcohol.

3. Health care providers should explain the necessity for regular follow-up evaluations, which should include a targeted history and physical examination looking for stigmata of liver disease such as spider nevi, icterus, splenomegaly and ascites, and a battery of liver function tests, including serum albumin and prothrombin time.

4. Yearly screening for hepatocellular carcinoma with abdominal ultrasound and α-fetoprotein for those with established cirrhosis should be considered (although this is controversial because of the unfavorable cost/benefit ratio).

5. Family members should be counseled to avoid transmission of HCV and HBV.

6. It is advisable to establish a relationship with a gastro-enterologist/hepatologist to facilitate the management of those with decompensated liver disease. Cirrhotic patients with ascites are usually treated with a low-sodium diet and spironolactone alone or in association with furosemide. Those with diuretic-resistant ascites need therapeutic paracentesis. Spontaneous bacterial peritonitis is a severe infective complication requiring early diagnosis and treatment. A cathartic such as lactulose is used for the treatment of hepatic encephalopathy.

7. Bleeding from esophageal and gastric varices constitutes a medical emergency which is treated in an intensive care unit in conjunction with a gastroenterologist skilled in endoscopic variceal sclerotherapy or ligation, and drug therapy to lower portal pressure. When hypoprothrombinemia is present, fresh frozen plasma is required to correct the clotting defects of advanced liver disease. The assistance of an interventional radiologist for the creation of a transjugular intrahepatic portosystemic shunt (TIPS procedure) may be indicated for those who fail sclerotherapy and pharmacologic measures. Long-term drug therapy may include the use of β-blockers.

8. Liver transplantation should be considered in anti-HCV-positive hemophiliacs with decompensated cirrhosis who are HBsAg- and HIV-negative. HBsAg carriers who are HBV-DNA-negative may also benefit. HIV infection is generally a contraindication to liver transplant unless CD4+ lymphocyte counts are near normal.

Conclusions

HCV is the primary cause of chronic liver disease in the vast majority of multitransfused persons with hemophilia who received non-viral inactivated clotting factor concentrates during the 1970s and early 1980s. HBV accounts for a small minority of cases. Alcohol and drugs may potentiate liver damage in susceptible individuals. Although most of those infected remain asymptomatic for many years, an increasing number are developing clinical manifestations of liver disease and dying of liver failure 20 years or more after their first exposure to concentrates. HIV appears to accelerate progression to liver failure and the associated immune deficiency state is accompanied by high-titer HCV-RNA viremia which increases over time. Interferon-α therapy to reduce HCV-RNA viral load should be considered in those with persistently elevated transaminases prior to the onset of hepatic decompensation. Liver transplant is the only viable option for those with decompensated end-stage liver disease.

Acknowledgement

We wish to acknowledge with gratitude the assistance of Ms Linda Nelson in the preparation of this manuscript.

References

Aach, R.D., Stevens, C.E., Hollinger, F.B. *et al.* (1991) Hepatitis C virus infection in post-transfusion hepatitis. An analysis with first- and second-generation assays. *New England Journal of Medicine*, **325**, 1325–1329.

Agnello, V., Chung, R.T. and Kaplan, L.M. (1992) A role for hepatitis C virus infection in type II cryoglobulinaemia. *New England Journal of Medicine*, **327**, 1490–1495.

Alberti, A., Morsica, G., Chemello, L. *et al.* (1992) Hepatitis C viraemia and liver disease in symptom-free individuals with anti-HCV. *Lancet*, **340**, 697–698.

Aledort, L.M., Levine, P.H., Hilgartner, M. *et al.* (1985) A study of liver biopsies and liver disease among hemophiliacs. *Blood*, **66**, 369–372.

Allain, J.P., Dailey, S.H., Laurian, Y. *et al.* (1991) Evidence for persistent hepatitis C virus (HCV) infection in hemophiliacs. *Journal of Clinical Investigation*, **88**, 1672–1679.

Alter, H.J. (1994a) Hepatitis C: natural history, in *Viral Hepatitis A to F: An Update*, American Association for the Study of Liver Diseases Postgraduate Course. Chicago, Illinois, November 11–12, pp. 225–243.

Alter, M.J. (1994b) Transmission of hepatitis C virus – route, dose, and titer. *New England Journal of Medicine*, **330**, 784–785.

Alter, H.J. (1995) To C or not to C: these are the questions. *Blood* (in press).

Alter, H.J., Purcell, R.H., Shih, J.W. *et al.* (1989) Detection of antibody to hepatitis C virus in prospectively followed transfusion recipients with acute and chronic non-A, non-B hepatitis. *New England Journal of Medicine*, **321**, 1494–1500.

Alter, M.J., Margolis, H.S., Krawczynski, K. *et al.* (1992) The natural history of community-acquired hepatitis C in the United States. *New England Journal of Medicine*, **327**, 1899–1905.

Alvarez, L.P., Gurbindo, Hernandez-Samelayo, T. *et al.* (1992) Mother-to-infant transmission of HIV and hepatitis C infections in children born to HIV-seropositive mothers. *AIDS*, **6**, 427–428.

Bamber, M., Murray, A.K., Weller, I.V.D. *et al.* (1981) Clinical and histological features of a group of patients with sporadic non-A non-B hepatitis. *Journal of Clinical Pathology*, **34**, 1175–1180.

Blanchette, V.S., Vorstman, E., Shore, A. *et al.* (1991) Hepatitis C infection in children with hemophilia A and B. *Blood*, **78**, 285–289.

Bontempo, F.A., Lewis, J.H., Gorenc, T.J. *et al.* (1987) Liver transplantation in hemophilia A. *Blood*, **69**, 1721–1724.

Bortarelli, P., Brunctto, M., Minutello, M. *et al.* (1993) T-lymphocyte response to hepatitis C virus in different clinical courses of infection. *Gastroenterology*, **104**, 580–587.

Boyer, N., Marcellin, P., Degott, C. *et al.* (1992) Recombinant interferon-α for chronic hepatitis C in patients positive for antibody to human immunodeficiency virus. *Journal of Infectious Diseases*, **165**, 723–726.

Bresters, D., Mauser-Bunschoten, E.P., Cuypers, H.T.M *et al.* (1992) Disappearance of hepatitis C virus RNA in plasma during interferon alpha-2b treatment in hemophilia patients. *Scandinavian Journal of Gastroenterology*, **27**, 166–168.

Bresters, D., Mauser-Bunschoten, E.P., Reesink, H.W. *et al.* (1993) Sexual transmission of hepatitis C virus. *Lancet*, **342**, 210–211.

Brettler, D.B., Alter, H.J., Dienstag, J.L. *et al.* (1990) Prevalence of hepatitis C antibody in a cohort of hemophilia patients. *Blood*, **76**, 254–256.

Brettler, D.B., Mannucci, P.M., Gringeri, A. *et al.* (1992) The low risk of hepatitis C virus transmission among sexual partners of hepatitis C-infected hemophilic males: an international multicenter study. *Blood*, **80**, 540–543.

Causse, X., Godinot, H., Chevallier, M. *et al.* (1991) Comparison of 1 or 3 MU of interferon alfa-2b and placebo in patients with chronic non-A, non-B hepatitis. *Gastroenterology*, **101**, 497-502.

Cederbaum, A.I., Blatt, P.M. and Levine, P.H. (1982) Abnormal serum transaminase levels in patients with hemophilia A. *Archives of Internal Medicine*, **142**, 481–484.

Centers for Disease Control (1987) Hepatitis B in an extended family – Alabama. *Morbidity and Mortality Weekly Report*, **36**, 744–751.

Centers for Disease Control (1991) Public health service interagency guidelines for screening donors of blood, plasma, organs, tissues and semen for evidence of hepatitis B and hepatitis C. *Morbidity and Mortality Weekly Report*, **40**, 1–17.

Centers for Disease Control (1991) Hepatitis B virus: a comprehensive strategy for eliminating transmission in the United States through universal childhood vaccination. Recommendations of the Immunization Practices Advisory Committee (ACIP). *Morbidity and Mortality Weekly Report*, **40**, 1–25.

Choo, Q.L., Kuo, G., Weiner, A.J. *et al.* (1989) Isolation of a cDNA clone derived from a blood-borne non-A, non-B viral hepatitis genome. *Science*, **244**, 359.

Columbo, M., Mannucci, P.M., Brettler, D.B. *et al.* (1991) Hepatocellular carcinoma in hemophilia. *American Journal of Hematology*, **37**, 243–246.

Czaja, A.J., and Carpenter, H.A. (1993) Sensitivity, specificity, and predictability of biopsy interpretations in chronic hepatitis. *Gastroenterology*, **105**, 1824–1832.

Czaja, A.J., Carpenter, H.A., Santrach, P.J. and Moore, S.B. (1995) Immunologic features and HLA associations in chronic viral hepatitis. *Gastroenterology*, **108**, 157–164.

Davis, G.L., Balart, L.A., Schiff, E.R. *et al.* (1989) Treatment of chronic hepatitis C with recombinant interferon alfa: a multicenter randomized, controlled trial. *New England Journal of Medicine*, **321**, 1501–1506.

Di Bisceglie, A.M., Goodman, Z.D., Ishak, K.G. *et al.* (1991) Long-term clinical and histopathological follow-up of chronic posttransfusion hepatitis. *Hepatology*, **14–6**, 969–974.

Dienstag, J.L. (1983) Non-A, non-B hepatitis. I. Recognition, epidemiology and clinical features. *Gastroenterology*, **85**, 439–462.

Eyster, M.E., Whitehurst, D.A., Catalano, P.M. *et al.* (1985) Long-term follow-up of hemophiliacs with lymphocytopenia or thrombocytopenia. *Blood*, **66**, 1317–1320.

Eyster, M.E., Alter, H., Aledort, L.M. *et al.* (1991) Heterosexual co-transmission of hepatitis C virus (HCV) and human immunodeficiency virus (HIV). *Annals of Internal Medicine*, **115**, 764–768.

Eyster, M.E., Ragni, M.V., Shapiro, S. *et al.* (1992) Changing causes of death in Pennsylvania's hemophiliacs, 1976–1991: impact of liver disease and acquired immunodeficiency syndrome (AIDS). *Blood*, **71**, 2494–2495.

Eyster, M.E., Diamondstone, L.S., Lien, J.M. *et al.* (1993) Natural history of hepatitis C virus (HCV) infection in multitransfused hemophiliacs: effect of coinfection with human immunodeficiency virus (HIV). *Journal of Acquired Immune Deficiency Syndrome*, **6**, 602–610.

Eyster, M.E., Sanders, J.C., Battegay, M. and Di Bisceglie, A.M. (1994) Suppression of hepatitis C virus (HCV) replication by hepatitis D virus (HDV) in HIV-infected hemophiliacs with chronic hepatitis B and C. *Blood*, **84**, 466a.

Eyster, M.E., Fried, M.W., Di Bisceglie, A.M., Goedert, J.J. for the Multicenter Hemophilia Cohort Study (1994) Increasing HCV RNA levels in hemophiliacs: relationship to HIV infection and liver disease. *Blood*, **84**, 1020–1023.

Farci, P., Alter, H.J., Wong, D. *et al.* (1991) A long-term study of hepatitis C virus replication in non-A, non-B hepatitis. *New England Journal of Medicine*, **325**, 98–104.

Farci, P., London, W.T., Wong, D.C. *et al.* (1992) The natural history of infection with hepatitis C virus (HCV) in chimpanzees: comparison of serologic responses measured with first- and second-generation assays and relationship to HCV viremia. *Journal of Infectious Diseases*, **165**, 1006–1011.

Farci, P., Alter, H.J., Govindarajan, S. *et al.* (1992) Lack of protective immunity against reinfection with hepatitis C virus. *Science*, **258**, 135–140.

Farci, P., Mandas A., Coiana, A. *et al.* (1994) Treatment of chronic hepatitis D with interferon alpha 2-a. *New England Journal of Medicine*, **330**, 88–94.

Fargion, S., Piperno, A., Cappellini, M.D. *et al.*, (1992) Hepatitis C virus and porphyria cutanea tarda: evidence of a strong association. *Hepatology*, **16**, 1322–1326.

Feray, C., Samuel, D., Thiers, V. *et al.* (1992) Reinfection of liver graft by hepatitis C virus after liver transplantation. *Journal of Clinical Investigation*, **89**, 1361–1365.

Fletcher, M.L., Trowell, J.M., Craske, J. *et al.* (1983) Non-A non-B hepatitis after transfusion of factor VIII in infrequently treated patients. *British Medical Journal*, **287**, 1754–1757.

Fried, M.W., Shindo, M., Fong, T.L. *et al.* (1993) Absence of hepatitis C viral RNA from saliva and semen of patients with chronic hepatitis C. *Gastroenterology*, **102**, 1306–1308.

Gerety, R.J. and Eyster, M.E. (1981) Hepatitis in hemophiliacs. in *Non-A, Non-B Hepatitis* (ed. R.J. Gerety), Academic Press, London, pp. 97–117.

Giovannini, M., Tagger, A., Ribero, M.L. *et al.* (1990) Maternal infant transmission of hepatitis C virus and HIV infections: a possible interaction. *Lancet*, **335**, 1166.

Gomperts, E.D., Lazerson, J., Berg, D. *et al.* (1981) Hepatocellular enzyme patterns and hepatitis B virus exposure in multitransfused young and very young hemophilia patients. *American Journal of Hematology*, **11**, 55–59.

Gretch, D., Corey, L., Wilson, J. *et al.* (1993) Assessment of hepatitis C virus RNA levels by quantitative competitive RNA polymerase chain reaction: high-titer viremia correlates with advanced stage of disease. *Journal of Infectious Diseases*, **169**, 1219–1225.

Hagiwara, H., Hayashi, N., Mita, E. *et al.* (1993) Quantitative analysis of hepatitis C virus RNA in serum during interferon alfa therapy. *Gastroenterology*, **104**, 877–883.

Hanley, J.P., Dolan, G., Day, S. *et al.* (1993) Interaction of hepatitis B and hepatitis C infection in haemophilia. *British Journal of Haematology*, **85**, 611–612.

Hasiba, U., Eyster, M.E., Gill, F.M. *et al.* (1980) Liver dysfunction in Pennsylvania's multitransfused hemophiliacs. *Digestive Diseases and Sciences*, **25**, 776–782.

Hassett, J., Gjerset, G.F., Mosley, J.W. *et al.* (1993) Effect on lymphocyte subsets of clotting factor therapy in human immunodeficiency virus-1-negative congenital clotting disorders. *Blood*, **82**, 1351.

Hatzakis, A., Polychronaki, H., Miriagou, V. *et al.* (1992) Antibody responses to hepatitis C virus (HCV) by second generation immunoassays in a cohort of patients with bleeding disorders. *Vox Sanguinis*, **63**, 204–209.

Hay, C.R.M., Preston, F.E., Triger, D.R. and Underwood, J.C.E. (1985) Progressive liver disease in haemophilia: an understated problem? *Lancet*, **1**, 1495–1498..

Hay, C.R.M., Preston, F.E., Triger, D.R. *et al.* (1987) Predictive markers of chronic liver disease in hemophilia. *Blood*, **6**, 1595–1599.

Hollinger, F.B., Khan, N.C., Oefinger, P.E. *et al.* (1983) Posttransfusion hepatitis type A. *Journal of the American Medical Association*, **250**, 2313–2317.

Hoofnagle, J.H. (1993) Chronic hepatitis B: prospects for new antiviral agents, in *New and Evolving Therapies for Hepatic and Biliary Diseases Postgraduate Course*, American Association for Study of Liver Diseases, Chicago, Illinois, pp. 151–160.

Hoofnagle, J.H. and Di Bisceglie, A.M. (1991) Serologic diagnosis of acute and chronic viral hepatitis. *Seminars in Liver Disease*, **11**, 73–83.

Houghton, M., Weiner, A., Han, J. *et al.* (1991) Molecular biology of the hepatitis C viruses: implications for diagnosis, development and control of viral disease. *Hepatology*, **14**, 381–387.

Hruby, M.A. and Schauf, V. (1978) Transfusion-related short-incubation hepatitis in hemophilic patients. *Journal of the American Medical Association*, **240**, 1355–1357.

Jarvis, L.M., Watson, H.G., McOmish, F. *et al.* (1994) Frequent reinfection and reactivation of hepatitis C virus genotypes in multitransfused hemophiliacs. *Journal of Infectious Diseases*, **170**, 1018–1022.

Kasper, C.K. and Kipnis, S.A. (1972) Hepatitis and clotting factor concentrates. *Journal of the American Medical Association*, **221**, 510.

Kato, N., Yokosuka, O., Hosoda, K. *et al.* (1993) Quantification of hepatitis C virus by competitive reverse transcription-polymerase chain reaction: increase of the virus in advanced liver disease. *Hepatology*, **18**, 16–20.

Kernoff, P.B.A., Lee, C.A., Karayiannis, P. and Thomas, H.C. (1985) High risk of non-A non-B hepatitis after a first exposure to volunteer or commercial clotting factor concentrates: effects of prophylactic immune serum globulin. *British Journal of Haematology*, **60**, 469–479.

Kobayashi, Y., Watanabe, S., Konishi, M. *et al.* (1993) Quantitation and typing of serum hepatitis C virus RNA in patients with chronic hepatitis C treated with interferon-β. *Hepatology*, **18**, 1319–1325.

Korenman, J., Baker, B., Waggoner, J. *et al.* (1991) Long-term remission of chronic hepatitis B after alpha-interferon therapy. *Annals of Internal Medicine*, **114**, 629–634.

Koretz, R.L., Abbey, H., Coleman, E. and Gitnick, G. (1993) Non-A, non-B posttransfusion hepatitis. Looking back in the second decade. *Annals of Internal Medicine*, **119**, 110-115.

Koziel, M.J., Dudley, D., Wong, J.T. *et al.* (1992) Intrahepatic cytotoxic T lymphocytes specific for hepatitis C virus in persons with chronic hepatitis. *Journal of Immunology*, **149**, 3339–3344.

Koziel, M.J., Dudley, D., Afdhal, N. *et al.* (1993) Hepatitis C virus (HCV) – specific cytotoxic T lymphocytes recognize epitopes in the core and envelope proteins of HCV. *Journal of Virology*, **67**, 7522–7532.

Krawczykski, K. (1994) Hepatitis E: clinical course and presentation, in *Viral Hepatitis A to F: An Update*, American Association for the Study of Liver Diseases Postgraduate Course, Chicago, Illinois, pp. 83–91.

Krawczynski, K., Beach, M.J., Bradley, D.W. *et al.* (1992) Hepatitis C virus antigen in hepatocytes. Immunomorphologic detection and identification. *Gastroenterology*, **103**, 622.

Kuo, G., Choo, Q.-L., Alter, H.J. *et al.* (1989) An assay for circulating antibodies to a major etiologic virus of human non-A, non-B hepatitis. *Science*, **244**, 362–364.

Lai, M.E., Mazzoleni, A.P., Argiolu, F. *et al.* (1994) Hepatitis C virus in multiple episodes of acute hepatitis in polytransfused thalssemic children. *Lancet*, **343**, 388-390.

Lam, J.P.H., McOmish, F., Burns, S.M. (1993) Infrequent vertical transmission of hepatitis C virus. *Journal of Infectious Diseases*, **167**, 572-576.

Lau, J.Y.N. and Wright, T.L. (1993) Molecular virology and pathogenesis of hepatitis B. *Lancet*, **342**, 1335-1339.

Lau, J.Y.N., Davis, G.L., Kniffen, J. *et al.* (1993) Significance of serum hepatitis C virus RNA levels in chronic hepatitis C. *Lancet*, **341**, 1501-1504.

Lemon, S. (1994) Hepatitis A virus: clinical course and serology, in *Viral Hepatitis A to F: An Update*, American Association for the Study of Liver Diseases Postgraduate Course (1994) Chicago, Illinois, pp. 43-53.

Lesesne, H.R., Morgan, J.E., Blatt, P.M. *et al.* (1977) Liver biopsy in hemophilia A. *Annals of Internal Medicine*, **86**, 703-707.

Levine, P.H., McVerry, B.A., Attock, B. and Dormandy, K.M. (1977) Health of the intensively treated hemophiliac, with special reference to abnormal liver chemistries and splenomegaly. *Blood*, **50**, 1-9.

Lewis, J.H. (1970) Hemophilia, hepatitis and HAA. *Vox Sanguinis*, **19**, 406-409.

Lindsay, K.L. (1993) Chronic hepatitis C: issues and problems with current therapy, in *New and Evolving Therapies for Hepatic and Biliary Disease Postgraduate Course*, American Association for Study of Liver Diseases, Chicago, Illinois, pp. 131-150.

Lunel, F. (1994) Hepatitis C virus and autoimmunity: fortuitous association or reality? *Gastroenterology*, **107**, 1550-1555.

McGrath, K.M., Lilleyman, J.S., Triger, D.R. and Underwood, J.C.E. (1980) Liver disease complicating severe haemophilia in childhood. *Archives of Disease in Childhood*, **55**, 537-540.

Makris, M., Preston, F.E., Triger, D.R. *et al.* (1990) Hepatitis C antibody and chronic liver disease in haemophilia. *Lancet*, **335**, 1117-1119.

Makris, M., Preston, F.E., Triger, D.R. *et al.* (1991) A randomized controlled trial of recombinant interferon-alpha in chronic hepatitis C in hemophiliacs. *Blood*, **78**, 1672-1677.

Makris, M., Garson, J.A., Ring, C.J.A. *et al* (1993) Hepatitis C viral RNA in clotting factor concentrates and the development of hepatitis in recipients. *Blood*, **81**, 1898-1902.

Mannucci, P.M. (1992) Outbreak of hepatitis A among Italian patients with hemophilia. *Lancet*, **1**, 819.

Mannucci, P.M. (1995) Viral safety of plasma-derived and recombinant products used in the management of haemophilia A and B. *Haemophilia*, **1**, 14-20.

Mannucci, P.M., Capitanio, A., Del Ninno, E. *et al.* (1975) Asymptomatic liver disease in haemophiliacs. *Journal of Clinical Pathology*, **28**, 620-624.

Mannucci, P.M., Colombo, M. and Rizzetto, M. (1982) Nonprogressive course of non-A, non-B chronic hepatitis in multitransfused hemophiliacs. *Blood*, **60**, 655-658.

Mauser-Bunschoten, E.P., Bresters, D., Reesink, H.W. *et al.* (1995) Effect and side-effects of alpha interferon treatment in haemophilia patients with chronic hepatitis C. *Haemophilia*, **1**, 45-53.

Misiani, R., Bellavita, P., Fenilia, D. *et al.* (1992) Hepatitis C virus infection in patients with essential mixed cryoglobulinaemia. *Annals of Internal Medicine*, **117**, 573-577.

Mitsui, T., Iwano, K., Masuko, K. *et al.* (1992) Hepatitis C virus infection in medical personnel after needle stick accident. *Hepatology*, **16**, 1109-1114.

Mizokami, M., Gojobori, T. and Lau, J.Y.N. (1994) Molecular evolutionary virology: its application to hepatitis C virus. *Gastroenterology*, **107**, 1181-1182.

Myers, T.J., Tembrevilla-Zubiri, C.L., Klatsky, A.U. and Rickles, F.R. (1980) Recurrent acute hepatitis following the use of factor VIII concentrates. *Blood*, **55**, 748-751.

Ohto, H., Terazawa, S., Sasaki, N. *et al.* (1994) Transmission of hepatitis C virus from mothers to infants. *New England Journal of Medicine*, **330**, 744-750.

Okamoto, H., Okada, S., Sugiyama, Y. *et al.* (1991) Nucleotide sequence of the genomic RNA of hepatitis C virus isolated from a human carrier: comparison with reported isolates for conserved and divergent regions. *Journal of General Virology*, **72**, 2697-2704.

Osmond, D.H., Padian, N.S., Sheppard, H.W. *et al.* (1993) Risk factors for hepatitis C virus seropositive heterosexual couples. *Journal of the American Medical Association*, **269**, 361-365.

Perez, V., Tanno, H., Villamil, F. and Fay, Q. (1990) Recombinant interferon alfa-2b following prednisone withdrawal in the treatment of chronic type B hepatitis. *Journal of Hepatology*, **11**, 5113-5117.

Perrillo, R.P., Schiff, E.R., Davis, G.L. *et al.* (1990) A randomized, controlled trial of interferon alfa-2b alone and after prednisone withdrawal for the treatment of chronic hepatitis B. *New England Journal of Medicine*, **323**, 295-301.

Pontisso, P., Ruvoletto, M.G., Fattovich, G. *et al.* (1993) Clinical and virological profiles in patients with multiple hepatitis virus infections. *Gastroenterology*, **105**, 1529-1533.

Pozzato, G., Moretti, M., Franzin, F. *et al.* (1991) Severity of liver disease with different hepatitis C viral clones. *Lancet*, **338**, 509.

Preston, F.E., Triger, D.R., Underwood, J.C.E. *et al.* (1978) Percutaneous liver biopsy and chronic liver disease in haemophiliacs. *Lancet*, **2**, 592-594.

Prince, A.M. (1994) Immunity in hepatitis C virus infection. *Vox Sanguinis*, **67**, 227-228.

Ragni, M.V., Ndimbie, O.K., Rice, E.O. *et al.* (1993) The presence of hepatitis C virus (HCV) antibody in human immunodeficiency virus-positive hemophilic men undergoing HCV "seroreversion". *Blood*, **82**, 1010-1015.

Reinus, J.F., Leikin, E.L., Alter, H.J. *et al.* (1992) Failure to detect vertical transmission of hepatitis C virus. *Annals of Internal Medicine*, **117**, 881-886.

Rickard, K.A., Batey, R.G., Dority, P. *et al.* (1982) Hepatitis and haemophilia therapy in Australia. *Lancet*, **2**, 146-148.

Rizzetto, M. (1983) The delta agent. *Hepatology*, **3**, 729-737.

Rosina, F., Saracco, G. and Rizzetto, M. (1985) Risk of post-transfusion infection with the hepatitis delta virus. A multi-center study. *New England Journal of Medicine*, **312**, 1488-1491.

Rumi, M.G., Colombo, M., Gringeri, A. and Mannucci, P.M. (1990) High prevalence of antibody to hepatitis C virus in multitransfused hemophiliacs with normal transaminase levels. *Annals of Internal Medicine*, **112**, 379-380.

Schimpf, K.L., Zimmermann, K., Bleyl, U. and Döhnert, G. (1981) Liver biopsy findings in haemophilia, in *Haemophilia* (eds U. Seligsohn *et al.*), Castlehouse Publications, pp. 149-153.

Schramm, W., Roggendorf, M., Rommel, F. *et al.* (1989) Prevalance of antibodies to hepatitis C virus (HCV) in haemophiliacs. *Blut*, **59**, 390-392.

Seeff, L.B., Buskell-Bales, Z., Wright, E.C. *et al.* (1992) Long-term mortality after transfusion-associated non-A, non-B hepatitis. *New England Journal of Medicine*, **327**, 1906-1911.

Sherertz, R.J., Russell, B.A. and Reuman, P.D. (1984) Transmission of hepatitis A by transfusion of blood products. *Archives of Internal Medicine*, **144**, 1579-1580.

Sherlock, S. (1989) Viral hepatitis, in *Diseases of the Liver and Biliary System*, 8th edn, Blackwell Scientific Publications, Boston, MA.

Shindo, M., Di Bisceglie, A.M., Cheung, L. *et al.* (1991) Decrease in serum hepatitis C viral RNA during alpha-interferon therapy for chronic hepatitis C. *Annals of Internal Medicine*, **115**, 700-704.

Simmonds, P., Holmes, E.C., Cha, T.A. *et al.* (1993) Classification of hepatitis C virus into six major genotypes and a series of subtypes by phylogenetic analysis of the NS-5 region. *Journal of General Virology*, **74**, 2391-2399.

Simonetti, R.G., Cammà, C., Fiorello, F. *et al.* (1992) Hepatitis C virus infection as a risk factor for hepatocellular carcinoma in patients with cirrhosis. *Annals of Internal Medicine*, **116**, 97-102.

Spero, J.A., Lewis, J.H., Van Thiel, D.H. *et al.* (1978) Asymptomatic structural liver disease in hemophilia. *New England Journal of Medicine*, **298**, 1373-1378.

Spero, J.A., Lewis, J.H., Fisher, S.E. *et al.* (1979) The high risk of chronic liver disease in multitransfused juvenile hemophiliac patients. *Journal of Pediatrics*, **94**, 875-878.

Stirling, M.L., Becket, G.J. and Percy-Robb, I.W. (1981) Liver function in Edinburgh Haemophiliacs: a five-year follow-up. *Journal of Clinical Pathology*, **34**, 17-20.

Takahashi, M., Yamada, G., Miyamoto, R. *et al.* (1993) Natural course of chronic hepatitis C. *American Journal of Gastroenterology*, **88**, 240-243.

Tedder, R., Briggs, M., Ring, C. *et al.* (1991) Hepatitis C antibody profile and viraemia prevalence in adults with severe haemophilia. *British Journal of Haematology*, **79**, 512-515.

Telfer, P.T., Watt, P.B. and Lee, C.A. (1993) Liver disease in hemophilia.

Telfer, P., Sabin, C., Devereux, H. (1994) The progression of HCV-associated liver disease in a cohort of haemophilic patients. *British Journal of Haematology*, **87**, 555-561.

Telfer, P.T., Brown, D., Devereux, H. *et al.* (1994) HCV RNA levels and HIV infection: evidence for a viral interaction in haemophilic patients. *British Journal of Haematology*, **88**, 397-399.

Telfer, P., Devereux, H., Colvin, B. *et al* (1995) Alpha interferon for hepatitis C virus infection in haemophilic patients. *Haemophilia*, **1**, 54-58.

Thomas, H.C., Bamber, M. and Kernoff, P.B.A. (1982) Clinical, immunological and histological aspects of non-A, non-B hepatitis in hemophiliacs, in *Unresolved Problems in Haemophilia* (eds C.D. Forbes and G.D.O. Lowe), pp. 27-37.

Todo, S., Demetris, A.J., Van Tield, D.H. (1991) Orthotopic liver transplantation for patients with hepatitis B virus-related liver disease. *Hepatology*, **13**, 619-626.

Triger, D.R. (1990) Chronic liver disease in haemophiliacs. *British Journal of Haematology*, **74**, 241-245.

Troisi, C.L., Hollinger, F.B., Hoots, W.K. *et al.* (1993) A multicenter study of viral hepatitis in a United States hemophilic population. *Blood*, **81**, 412-481.

van der Poel, C.L. (1994) Hepatitis C virus: into the fourth generation. *Vox Sanguinis*, **67**, 95-98.

van der Poel, C.L., Cuypers, H.T. and Reesink, H.W. (1994) Hepatitis C virus six years on. *Lancet*, **334**, 1475-1479.

Van Thiel, D.H., Friedlander, L., Fagiuoli, S. *et al.* (1994) Response to interferon α therapy is influenced by the iron content of the liver. *Journal of Hepatology*, **20**, 410-415.

Watson, H.G., Ludlam, C.A., Rebus, S. *et al.* (1992) Use of several second generation serological assays to determine the true prevalence of hepatitis C virus infection in haemophiliacs treated with non-virus inactivated factor VIII and IX concentrates. *British Journal of Haematology*, **80**, 514–518.

Webster, W.P., Blatt, P.M., Lesesne, H.R. and Roberts, H.R. (1976) *National Institute of Health Report 77–1089*, Department of Health, Education and Welfare, Washington, DC, pp. 41–50.

Weissberg, J.I., Andres, L.L., Smith, C.I. *et al.* (1984) Survival in chronic hepatitis B: an analysis of 397 patients. *Annals of Internal Medicine*, **101**, 613–616.

White, G.C., Zeitler, K.D., Lesesne, H.R. *et al.* (1982) Chronic hepatitis in patients with hemophilia A: histologic studies in patients with intermittently abnormal liver function tests. *Blood*, **60**, 1259–1262.

Wong, D.K.H., Cheung, A.M., O'Rourke, K. *et al.* (1993) Effect of alpha-interferon in patients with hepatitis B e antigen-positive chronic hepatitis B: a meta-analysis. *Annals of Internal Medicine*, **119**, 312–323.

Wright, T.L. and Lau, J.Y.N. (1993) Clinical aspects of hepatitis B virus infection. *Lancet*, **342**, 1340–1344.

Yoshioka, K., Kakumu, S., Wakita, T. *et al.* (1992) Detection of hepatitis C virus by polymerase chain reaction and response to interferon-alpha therapy: relationship to genotypes of hepatitis C virus. *Hepatology*, **16**, 293–299.

Yuki, N., Hayashi, N., and Kamada, T. (1993) HCV viraemia and liver injury in symptom-free blood donors. *Lancet*, **342**, 444.

25 HIV-1 INFECTION IN HEMOPHILIA

J.J. Goedert and B.L. Kroner

Background and historical aspects

Transfusion of blood, blood components, and some plasma products during the late 1970s until the mid-1980s resulted in many infections with human immunodeficiency virus type 1 (HIV-1). Persons with hemophilia were at especially high risk by virtue of their need for infusions of factor VIII or factor IX concentrate, each lot derived from the plasma of thousands of donors. This chapter reviews the early history and current knowledge of HIV-1 and acquired immunodeficiency syndrome (AIDS), with a focus on hemophilia.

INITIAL CASES – CLINICAL DISEASE AND IMMUNOLOGY

By the end of the 1970s, *Pneumocystis carinii* pneumonia was a clearly defined clinical condition that was known to occur almost exclusively in persons who had a deficiency of cell-mediated immune deficiency (Walzer *et al.*, 1974). This included children with congenital deficiencies and especially patients who were receiving corticosteroids or other drugs for cancer chemotherapy or to suppress rejection of a transplanted organ. Thus, when *Pneumocystis* pneumonia occurred in previously healthy homosexual men during 1980 and early 1981, Dr Michael Gottlieb in Los Angeles and a number of physicians in New York City reported that they probably represented a new or previously unrecognized immune deficiency disease (Centers for Disease Control (CDC), 1981a, b).

In the middle of 1981, a large group of homosexual men in New York City, San Francisco and Los Angeles was reported with Kaposi's sarcoma (Friedman-Kien, 1981; Hymes *et al.*, 1981), a malignancy that had been associated with iatrogenic immune deficiency (Gange and

Jones, 1978; Haim *et al.*, 1972; Klepp, Dahl and Stenwig, 1978; Hoshaw and Schwartz, 1980). A number of these men also had *Pneumocystis* pneumonia or other rare life-threatening opportunistic infections. The US CDC quickly established a functional definition and national surveillance for cases of Kaposi's sarcoma, *Pneumocystis* pneumonia and a few other opportunistic infections in persons with no known underlying immune deficiency (CDC, 1981c). It would be a year before these diseases were collectively known to the world as AIDS.

Immunologic assessment of these early cases noted severely impaired or even undetectable *in vitro* responses of lymphocytes following stimulation with pokeweed mitogen, concanavalin A or other antigens (Gottlieb *et al.*, 1981; Masur *et al.*, 1981). Using the newly developed technology of flow cytometry with fluorescent monoclonal antibodies, these cases were found to have reduced levels of T lymphocytes with the helper-inducer (T4, now termed CD4) phenotype and usually increased levels with the suppressor-cytotoxic (T8, now termed CD8) phenotype. Healthy adults were noted to have a $T4^+{:}T8^+$ ratio that was greater than 1.0. In contrast, the ratios for the homosexual men with *Pneumocystis* pneumonia or Kaposi's sarcoma were inverted and often well below 0.5. Levels of granulocytes, macrophages and particularly B lymphocytes and serum antibodies were generally normal or elevated in these patients.

In the first year of the AIDS epidemic, when only homosexual men appeared to be affected, three theories regarding its cause were especially popular. First, the immune system had simply been overloaded by sexually acquired and other infectious diseases and innumerable alloantigens from exposure to semen from hundreds of partners. Second, immunotoxicity occurred from nitrite inhalants or a contaminant of these drugs that were closely associated with receptive anal intercourse. Third,

Hemophilia. Edited by C.D. Forbes, L. Aledort and R. Madhok. Published in 1997 by Chapman & Hall, London. ISBN 0 412 63820 7

a known virus (particularly hepatitis B virus or cytomegalovirus) or other infectious agent had mutated or recombined to alter its tropism or virulence.

CASES WITH HEMOPHILIA AND OTHERS

The first known case of AIDS in a hemophiliac was diagnosed in October 1981 and reported by the CDC that following July (CDC, 1982a). July 1982 marked a major turning point in establishing the cause of AIDS, with a meeting called by the CDC to report the first three cases of *Pneumocystis* pneumonia in persons with hemophilia. These three males were not homosexually active, did not use nitrite inhalants or other recreational drugs and had nothing in common with each other except their coagulation disorder and its treatment with factor VIII concentrate. Almost all recipients of factor VIII concentrate had been infected with hepatitis B virus, increasing the possibility of an immunotoxic strain of hepatitis B or some other blood-borne virus. None the less, because factor VIII concentrate was derived from the plasma of tens of thousands of donors and had been in use for less than 10 years, the theory of antigenic overload persisted. There was, however, consensus that the outbreak of opportunistic infections was not limited to homosexual men, and a name for this disease must not imply a restriction to the gay community. Henceforward, any person with an opportunistic malignancy or life-threatening infection that met the CDC surveillance definition had the acquired immunodeficiency syndrome or AIDS.

During the remainder of 1982 and 1983, AIDS cases were reported among heterosexual intravenous drug users, Haitian Americans and residents of Haiti and areas of central Africa (CDC, 1982b, c; Masur *et al.*, 1982; Malebranche *et al.*, 1983; Marx, 1983; Pape *et al.*, 1983; Pitchenik *et al.*, 1983; Vieira *et al.*, 1983).

Approximately as many women as men in these groups were diagnosed with AIDS, thus focusing attention on the likelihood of an infectious AIDS agent that could be transmitted by heterosexual (vaginal) intercourse as well as by homosexual (anal) intercourse. The development of AIDS in the wife of a man with hemophilia was particularly illustrative (Pitchenik *et al.*, 1984). The magnitude of the catastrophe was presaged by the initial reports and immunologic characterization of AIDS in a young blood transfusion recipient and in infants who had been born to women who had AIDS or were otherwise in a high-risk group for AIDS, such as intravenous drug users or Haitians (CDC, 1982d, e).

THE DISCOVERY OF AND TESTING FOR HIV

In 1983, Barre-Sinoussi, Montangier and their colleagues at the Pasteur Institute reported the observation that previously unknown retroviral-like particles were seen by electron microscopy in the supernatant of a cultured lymph node from a homosexual man (Bru) who had generalized lymphadenopathy and deficiency of CD4 lymphocytes (Barre-Sinoussi *et al.*, 1983). They subsequently proposed the name lymphadenopathy-associated virus (LAV$_{Bru}$) for this new virus.

The major breakthrough came in May 1984 with the papers of Popovic, Gallo and their colleagues at the National Cancer Institute (NCI; Popovic *et al.*, 1984; Gallo *et al.*, 1984; Sarngadharan *et al.*, 1984; Schüpbach *et al.*, 1984). They reported that a new human retrovirus, initially designated human T lymphotropic virus type III (HTLV-III), could be isolated from most patients with AIDS (Gallo *et al.*, 1984). At least as important, they identified cell lines and methods for continuous long-term cultures that produced substantial quantities of viral proteins and infectious virions (Popovic *et al.*, 1984). They performed preliminary biochemical characterization of the major viral proteins and developed a prototype enzyme-linked immunosorbent assay (ELISA or EIA) and Western blot assay for antiviral antibodies (Sarngadharan *et al.*, 1984; Schüpbach *et al.*, 1984).

Academic and commercial laboratories immediately applied these techniques. In March 1985, the US Food and Drug Administration licensed the first commercial EIA for detecting anti-HIV antibodies in donated blood and plasma. The National Hemophilia Foundation (NHF) quickly followed with the recommendation that all donated blood products be screened for HIV (Ragni, 1988). Years later, the prototype of HIV from the NCI laboratory, designated HTLV-IIIB, and that from the Pasteur laboratory, designated LAV, were found to be molecularly indistinguishable strains of HIV and presumably from the same patient (Chermann *et al.*, 1991; Guo *et al.*, 1991; Chang *et al.*, 1993). Remarkably, the Pasteur strain was not that from the original patient's culture (LAV$_{Bru}$) but was a contaminant from the culture of a different French patient (Lai; Chang *et al.*, 1993). For reasons that are still unknown, the virus that was discovered in both laboratories was easily and very quickly adapted to lymphocyte cultures, such that it not only contaminated these key cultures of the NCI and Pasteur laboratories but also those of other laboratories that were attempting to identify the cause of AIDS. This strain, which has been used for most of the licensed HIV antibody assays and the initial vaccine development efforts, is now termed HIV-1$_{Lai}$.

The virus and its detection

HIV-1 has the basic structure of other retroviruses, with three major structural gene regions – *gag*, which yields the viral core proteins, *env*, which yields the envelope proteins and *pol*, which yields the reverse transcriptase

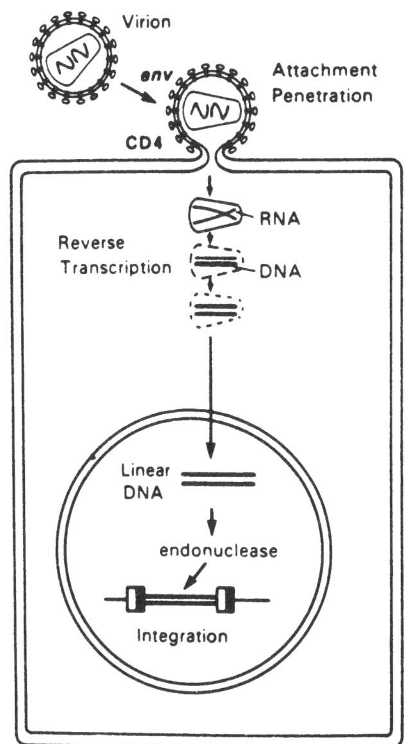

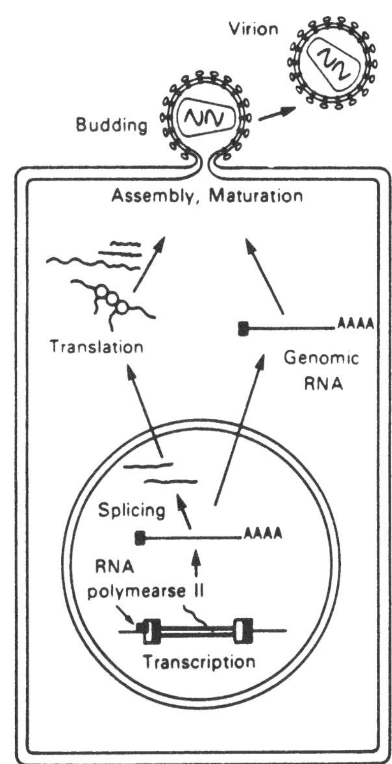

Fig. 25.1 Life cycle of human immunodeficiency virus type 1.

and integrase enzymes that are required for replication of a DNA copy of the viral RNA genome and the integration of this DNA provirus into the genome of the host cell (Fig. 25.1; Gallo, 1990). The structural proteins are the major antigens of HIV-1, particularly the major core protein p24 and its precursor p55, and the glycosylated external and transmembrane envelope proteins gp120 and gp41, respectively, and their precursor gp160 (Gallo, 1990). As such, HIV-1 antibodies are predominantely directed against these five proteins.

The prototype HIV-1 ELISA was remarkably sensitive (88%) and specific (99.4%) for the diagnosis of HIV-1 infection among normal controls and persons with AIDS (Sarngadharan *et al.*, 1984; Weiss *et al.*, 1984). Specificity was improved when sera were considered truly positive only when they had antibodies on Western blot against at least the core and envelope antigens. Licensed first-generation ELISA/EIA tests were cited as 97% sensitive and 99% specific by their manufacturers. These tests included HIV-1 proteins obtained from cultivation of the virus in human lymphocytes, which increased the chance of non-specific reactions caused by cellular contaminants. First-generation tests have also been reported to be associated with HIV-1 false-positive results in persons vaccinated with influenza virus (MacKenzie *et al.*, 1992). Subsequent improvements in the development of EIA test kits included HIV-1 proteins that were made from recombinant technology or that were chemically

synthesized. Recombinant proteins have also been applied to the Western blot confirmation test which has reduced the number of indeterminant results (Thorn *et al.*, 1987; Smith and Parks, 1990; Johnson, 1992). The sensitivity of current EIAs for antibody-positive sera is essentially 100%, and the specificities range from 99.8 to 99.95% (Dodd, 1994).

HIV-1 also has several regulatory genes that modify its rate and capacity for interference with functions of the infected cell and for its own ability to replicate and infect other cells. The characterization of these regulatory genes and their functions are complex and are beyond the scope of this chapter. This material has been reviewed elsewhere by Hahn (1992).

Overview of HIV-1 and AIDS epidemiology

AIDS AND HIV-1 IN THE WORLD

Three general patterns of AIDS have been described for the nations of the world (Blattner, 1991). Pattern I countries are those in which the preponderance of AIDS cases have occurred among homosexual men and parenteral drug users, such as the USA, Canada, Australia and western, northern and southern Europe. Pattern II countries are those in which heterosexual activity is the predominant mode of transmission, such as those in

Sub-Saharan Africa, Haiti and, more recently, Thailand and India. Pattern III countries have had approximately equal proportions of AIDS cases among homosexual men and heterosexuals, as observed in Brazil and Mexico.

Molecular sequencing of the virus has revealed at least six genotypes of HIV-1, lettered A through F (Myers *et al.*, 1992). Because the initial preventive vaccines are not expected to have cross-neutralization, genotypes are likely to affect the ability to control the epidemic. To some extent, the spread of HIV-1 can be viewed as six or more epidemics. All six genotypes have been found in Africa, although HIV-1 sequences that have been detected in east and central Africa are usually genotype A or D, whereas those detected in southern Africa are almost always genotype C. Genotype B has accounted for virtually all of the HIV-1 infections and AIDS cases in the USA and western Europe. Not surprisingly, the only preventive vaccines to have entered human trials have been based on HIV-1 genotype B. Such strategy is likely to be short-sighted. As a result of historic, economic and travel ties to southern Africa, HIV-1 genotype C is now spreading rapidly through urban areas of India. Likewise, in Thailand genotype B was originally found among parenteral drug users in Bangkok but has become over-shadowed by the heterosexual dissemination of genotype E in many regions of the country. The most recently described subtype, F, includes viruses found in Brazil (Potts *et al.*, 1993; Louwagie *et al.*, 1994) and Romania (Dumitrescu *et al.*, 1994).

EPIDEMIOLOGIC STUDIES

The early assays for HIV-1 antibodies were powerful tools for studying its prevalence, incidence and risk factors. Prevalence and incidence are key concepts. Prevalence of HIV-1 is the number of infected people divided by the number in the population. Because prevalence is usually described at one point in time, it may increase or decrease depending upon migration, mortality and birth rates that have different effects on the numerator and denominator. For example, the prevalence of HIV-1 infection in the US hemophilia population in 1988 was approximately 50% (Goedert *et al.*, 1989). Today, the prevalence is much lower than 50% because thousands of infected hemophiliacs have died of HIV-1-related diseases and are no longer included in the numerator and denominator. Likewise, new uninfected hemophiliacs continue to be diagnosed and added only to the denominator.

Incidence of HIV-1 is always a rate, that is, the number who become infected during a defined period of time, such as a month or a year. Incidence is closely related to risk, and it varies with exposures and practices. For example, the incidence or hazard of HIV-1 infection in the hemophilia population peaked in 1982 at 22 new infections per year per 100 uninfected hemophiliacs (Kroner *et al.*, 1994). The hazard today is zero because there are no new infections occurring in the uninfected hemophilia population due to HIV-1 screening of donated plasma and changes in the process of manufacturing blood products. Another epidemiologic term worth noting is the cumulative incidence, which is the proportion of individuals who became infected between the beginning and the end (or up to the present) of the HIV-1 epidemic.

HIV-1 seroprevalence estimates for various populations in the USA during the late 1980s are summarized in Table 25.1. Because HIV-1 was introduced into populations at different points in time and is predominantly spread by needle-sharing and sexual contact, there was and continues to be marked geographic variation in the

Table 25.1 Seroprevalence estimates for human immunodeficiency virus type 1 (HIV-1) in US populations during the late 1980s

Population	Seroprevalence (%)	Reference
Homosexual men	32	Centers for Disease Control (1991)
Intravenous drug users	3.9	Centers for Disease Control (1991)
Persons in treatment for tuberculosis	5.9	Centers for Disease Control (1991)
Family planning clinics	0.2	Centers for Disease Control (1991)
Non-HIV hospital patients	0.7	St. Louis *et al.* (1990)
Child-bearing women	0.07	Gwinn *et al.* (1991)
Job Corps entrants	0.23	St. Louis *et al.* (1991)
University students	0.0	Gayle *et al.* (1990)
Prisoners	0.8	Centers for Disease Control (1989)
Military applicants		
Black males	0.37	
Hispanic males	0.18	
White males	0.05	US Department of Defense (1992)
Blood donors (1985–1986)		
Males	0.04	
Females	0.01	Centers for Disease Control (1991)
Persons with hemophilia	46–55	Fricke *et al.* (1992)
		Goedert *et al.* (1989)

prevalence of HIV-1, even among those at highest risk, homosexual men and parenteral drug users. In the first 12 months of screening donated blood during 1985–1986, the American Red Cross found that 0.33% of the units were repeatedly reactive for HIV-1 antibody by ELISA. Only 0.031% of these units were HIV-1-positive with confirmatory tests, highlighting the importance of using a test with a very high specificity, such as the Western blot, in low-risk populations (Sayers, 1988).

HIV-1 epidemiology in hemophilia

Commercially manufactured factor concentrates became the treatment of choice for severely affected hemophiliacs in the early 1970s. These concentrates are derived from the plasma of 2000 to 25 000 donors and contain not only clotting factors but also other plasma proteins, including a variety of alloantigens and a number of viruses that circulate in plasma and are too small for filtration. It is therefore not surprising that the introduction of a blood-borne virus, such as HIV, into the blood donor population was quickly followed by its transmission to persons with hemophilia via these factor concentrates. In 1982, the NHF and the CDC found that there were no batches of factor concentrate that were shared among the small number of hemophiliacs with AIDS at that time (CDC, 1982f). Stored frozen serum samples, tested retrospectively for exposure to HIV-1, indicated that the first HIV-1 seroconversion in a hemophiliac, occurred in early 1978 (Evatt *et al.*, 1985; Eyster *et al.*, 1987; Ragni *et al.*, 1986). It has been estimated that 6800 hemophiliacs in the USA were eventually infected over the next 8 years (Rosenberg *et al.*, 1991).

PREVALENCE AND INCIDENCE IN US HEMOPHILIA PATIENTS

The prevalence of HIV-1 among persons with hemophilia peaked near the end of 1985, when approximately 50% of subjects at centers in the USA were infected at this time (Goedert *et al.*, 1989; Fricke *et al.*, 1992). HIV-1 seroprevalence rates were associated with the type and severity of hemophilia (Goedert *et al.*, 1989) and the type and quantity of blood products received (Ragni *et al.*, 1987; Gjerset *et al.*, 1991). As shown in Table 25.2, seroprevalence rates were higher for more severe patients presumably because they received larger and more frequent doses of concentrate. Within each severity category,

Table 25.2   Prevalence of HIV-1 seroconversion in hemophilia populations

	Seroprevalence (%)	*Reference*
By treatment type		
Cryoprecipitate only	10–14	Ragni *et al.* (1987)
Non-heat-treated factor VIII	82–88	Gjerset *et al.* (1971)
Non-heat-treated factor IX	48–59	
By type and severity		
Type A, severe	77	Goedert *et al.* (1989)
Type A, moderate	46	
Type A, mild	25	
Type B, severe	42	
Type B, moderate	27	
Type B, mild	8	
By selected country of residence		
Sweden	37	Berntorp *et al.* (1987)
Netherlands	24	Wolfs *et al.* (1988)
Denmark	59	Melbye *et al.* (1984)
Scotland	16	Melbye *et al.* (1984)
UK	34	Cheingsong-Popov *et al.* (1984)
France	42–47	AIDS–Hemophilia French Study Group (1985) Gringeri *et al.* (1988)
Germany	47–53	Gürtler *et al.* (1984) Gringeri *et al.* (1988)
Italy	31	Gringeri *et al.* (1988) Gringeri *et al.* (1988)
Israel	61	Orgad *et al.* (1987)
Spain	59	Magallon *et al.* (1992)

the hemophilia B patients (i.e. factor IX recipients) had a lower seroprevalence than the hemophilia A patients, who predominantly received factor VIII, although there were several who received factor IX due to the development of an inhibitor. Several investigators have reported a lower prevalence of HIV-1 in hemophilia B patients than in hemophilia A patients (Evatt *et al.*, 1985; Eyster *et al.*, 1985; Jason *et al.*, 1986; Ragni *et al.*, 1987; Jackson *et al.*, 1988; Goedert *et al.*, 1989). Speculation on this phenomenon has centered around the differences in the methods of manufacturing factor VIII and factor IX, since the two concentrates are usually made from the same donor pools (Aronson, 1979a, b). HIV-1 RNA has been detected in several batches of non-heat-treated factor VIII (Semple *et al.*, 1991; Zhang *et al.*, 1991; Heredia *et al.*, 1994), although comparable results for non-heat-treated factor IX concentrates have not been reported.

Cumulative HIV-1 seroincidence in an unbiased cohort of adults and children at risk for HIV-1 and attending one of five hemophilia treatment centers in the USA resembles the prevalence estimates reported above, with HIV-1 infection found in 50% of the population overall, 78% of factor VIII recipients and 37% of factor IX recipients (Kroner *et al.*, 1994). Furthermore, this study reported a strong association of mean annual dose of non-heat-treated factor VIII concentrate with the cumulative incidence of HIV-1 in hemophilia A patients. Recipients of high doses (>50 000 u/year) had a cumulative incidence of 96%, compared to 92% for recipients of moderate doses (20 001–50 000 u/year) and 56% for recipients of low doses (1–20 000 u/year). Hemophilia A patients who received only factor IX or single-donor products such as cryoprecipitate and fresh frozen plasma had a 16% cumulative incidence.

The risk of seroconversion among American subjects in the Multicenter Hemophilia Cohort Study increased gradually during the late 1970s and then increased very rapidly to peak in December 1982 (Fig. 25.2; Kroner *et al.*, 1994). It is noteworthy that the peak risk of HIV-1 seroconversion occurred 3 months after the first person with hemophilia-associated AIDS was reported (CDC, 1982a) and coincident with the recommendation by the USA NHF to limit the use of non-heat-treated factor VIII concentrate for newly diagnosed and previously untreated patients with hemophilia (Medical and Scientific Advisory Council, 1982). Although this is only a temporal association, an abrupt, steep decline in risk would have occurred with an immediate change to either cryoprecipitate or the newly developed heat-treated factor VIII concentrates for such patients. Alternatively, coincidence with depletion of the most susceptible members of the population, that is, completion of HIV-1 seroconversion among those who used factor VIII concentrate regularly, is also possible. It should be noted that additional measures taken to reduce the risk of

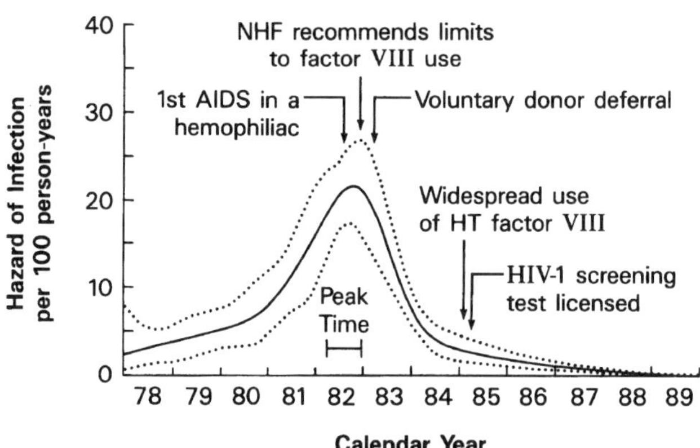

Fig. 25.2 Estimate of the human immunodeficiency virus type1 (HIV-1) hazard rate (risk among susceptibles) from 1978 to 1990 for a cohort of 636 hemophiliacs from the USA. Dotted curves represent the 95% confidence envelope. Arrows represent public health measures to reduce the risk of acquired immunodeficiency syndrome (AIDS) among persons with hemophilia, all of which occurred after the first reported case of AIDS in this population. NHF = National Hemophilia Foundation; HT = heat-treated.

blood-borne associated AIDS occurred after the peak. Thus, HIV-1 antibody screening of donated blood and other measures helped to reduce the risk of HIV-1 seroconversion among hemophiliacs to nearly zero by 1986.

The peak risk in December 1982 with use of factor VIII concentrate therapy was approximately 127 new infections per 100 person-years with more than 50 000 u/year, 107 per 100 person-years with 20 000–50 000 u/year, and 32 per 100 person-years with less than 20 000 u/year (Fig. 25.3; Kroner *et al.*, 1994). Compared to use of factor VIII concentrate, the peak risk with use of factor

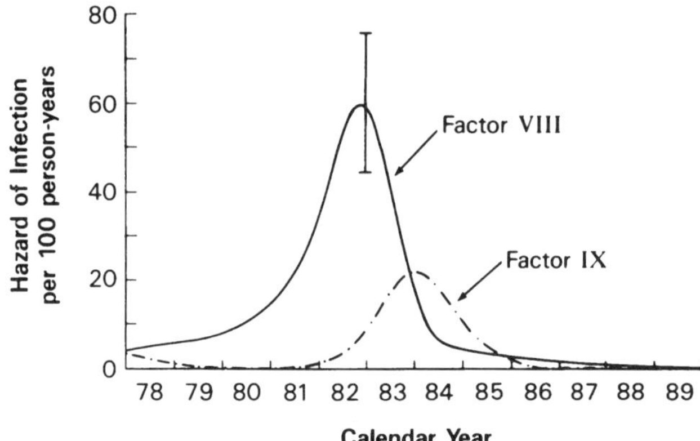

Fig. 25.3 Estimate of the human immunodeficiency virus type 1 (HIV-1) hazard rate for US hemophiliacs who used either non-heat-treated factor VIII concentrate or non-heat-treated factor IX concentrate. Error bar shows the 95% confidence interval for factor VIII at January 1983.

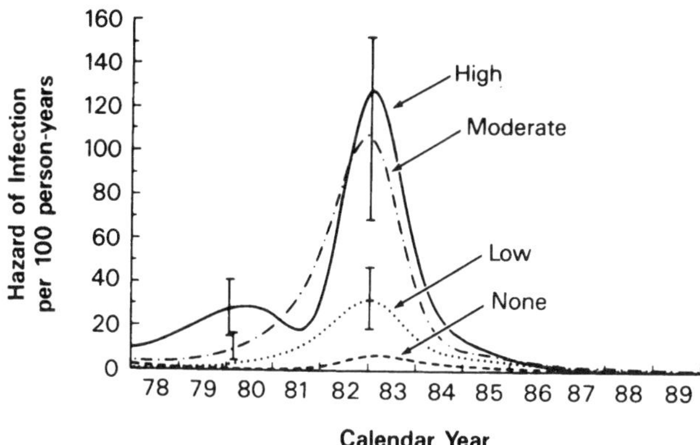

Fig. 25.4 Estimate of the human immunodeficiency virus type 1 (HIV-1) hazard rate for US type A hemophiliacs, grouped by mean annual dose of non-heat-treated factor VIII concentrate used between 1978 and 1984. Dose level was categorized as high (> 50 000 u), moderate (20 001–50 000 u), low (1–20 000 u) and none (no factor VIII). Error bars show the 95% confidence intervals for January 1980 and January 1983.

IX concentrates was lower and the risk persisted longer (Fig. 25.4; Kroner *et al.*, 1994). The reason for this later decline in risk is unknown. However, in contrast to heat-treated factor VIII concentrate, which in the USA was first licensed for use in March 1983 and entered widespread clinical practice by 1985, heat-treated factor IX concentrate was not licensed in the USA until October 1984 and was not routinely used until the middle of 1985 (Kasper *et al.*, 1993). The risk for subjects with factor VIII inhibitors appeared to reflect the plasma products they received in the respective years.

PREVALENCE AND INCIDENCE IN EUROPEAN HEMOPHILIA PATIENTS

The HIV-1 epidemic among hemophilia patients in Europe was more varied and complex, typically reflecting the source of plasma for their factor concentrates and the early introduction of heat-treated products in 1983 at some centers (Berntorp *et al.*, 1987; Orgad *et al.*, 1987; Wolfs *et al.*, 1988; Kroner *et al.*, 1994). As shown in Table 25.2, prevalence rates ranged from 16 to 61% for selected countries. Overall, the prevalence of HIV-1 seropositivity among European hemophilia A patients reflects the timing and doses of American-source factor VIII concentrate (Gürtler *et al.*, 1984; Melbye *et al.*, 1984; AIDS–Hemophilia French Study Group, 1985; Ball *et al.*, 1985; Berntorp *et al.*, 1987; Orgad *et al.*, 1987; Kroner *et al.*, 1994). This has been well-documented by Melbye and colleagues, who demonstrated a 59% prevalence in Danish hemophiliacs treated with commercial product made from US donors, compared to a 16% seroprevalence in Scottish hemophiliacs treated

almost exclusively with concentrate made from local donors (Melbye *et al.*, 1984). Remarkably, 83% of the HIV-1-positive Scottish hemophiliacs at some time had received commercial, as well as locally prepared, factor concentrate.

The Edinburgh cohort stands out as a noteworthy exception. At that center, 15 patients were thought to have been infected through a single lot of contaminated Scottish-source factor VIII concentrate (Ludlam *et al.*, 1985). Recent molecular sequencing, however, has shown that these hemophiliacs were infected with at least three different viral types (Holmes *et al.*, 1992). The source of these unrelated HIV-1 infections is unknown, but it seems likely that more than a single contamination may have occurred.

By 1985, the association between non-heat-treated factor concentrates and HIV-1 seroconversion in hemophiliacs was well-documented, and many treaters had changed to using heat-treated products that were rapidly becoming available. In February 1985, French researchers demonstrated that hemophiliacs receiving heat-treated factor concentrates were likely to be protected from infection with HIV (Rouzioux *et al.*, 1985). Officials in France changed from non-heat-treated to heat-treated factor VIII concentrates in October 1985. As part of the Multicenter Hemophilia Cohort Study (MHCS), we had the opportunity to evaluate the effect of the implementation of viral-inactivated factor concentrate in 68 HIV-infected hemophiliacs from Chambéry, France (Kroner *et al.*, 1994). Approximately 6.8% (95% confidence interval (CI), 2.4–14.5%) of these hemophiliacs were still seronegative in February 1985, and 1.9% (95% CI, 0–6.2%) seroconverted after October 1985. If these data can be generalized to the approximately 1350 hemophiliacs in France who were ultimately infected with HIV-1, between 32 and 196 hemophiliacs seroconverted after February 1985.

As in the USA, the association of HIV-1 infection in Europe with factor IX concentrate is well-documented. The reported risks are inconsistent, however, perhaps because local production of this product is often sufficient, making importation from the USA unnecessary. A consistent finding, with one notable exception, is that hemophilia A patients have a higher HIV-1 seroprevalence than hemophilia B patients (Melbye *et al.*, 1984; AIDS–Hemophilia French Study Group, 1985; Blombäck *et al.*, 1987; Orgad *et al.*, 1987; Gringeri *et al.*, 1988).

The exception is in Italy, where the cumulative incidence of HIV-1 infection for factor IX-deficient patients was 44% compared to 29% among their factor VIII-deficient counterparts (Gringeri *et al.*, 1988). These findings are intriguing, considering that Italian hemophiliacs were treated with commercially prepared factor VIII and factor IX concentrates made from American donor pools (Mannucci *et al.*, 1984).

Transmission to partners and others

HIV-1 has been transmitted by men with hemophilia through heterosexual intercourse, resulting in numerous cases of AIDS in women and, as a result of perinatal transmission of HIV-1, in cases of pediatric AIDS in their children. Hematologists, other physicians and all health practitioners have a clear obligation to warn HIV-1 infected hemophilia patients that their sexual partners are at serious risk of becoming infected with HIV-1 and developing AIDS. They are also at increased risk of transmitting other infectious agents. The extent of these risks and measures to reduce them are discussed below.

PREVALENCE AND INCIDENCE OF HIV-1

Men with hemophilia have transmitted HIV-1 to approximately 15% of their wives or other steady female sexual partners (Goedert *et al.*, 1987; Ragni *et al.*, 1989). This prevalence rate was reported shortly after the discovery of HIV-1 and has remained stable, suggesting a low incidence rate of HIV-1 transmissions during the late 1980s and early 1990s. How many children of hemophiliacs have become infected with HIV-1 or developed AIDS is unknown. National AIDS surveillance data in the USA categorize pediatric AIDS cases by whether or not they are offspring of HIV-1-infected women but do not subcategorize by the mode of infection in these mothers. The Hershey Hemophilia Center sponsors clinics for families of hemophiliacs, and blood is drawn for HIV-1 testing. Six children have been born since 1984 to three HIV-1-infected sexual partners of hemophiliacs, although the HIV-1 status of the mother was not known at the time of delivery for the child born in 1984. HIV-1 infection was transmitted to two of the unrelated children (33%). This is a minimum estimate of the number who are infected because the issue has not been specifically investigated.

RISK BY STAGE OF DISEASE: ANTIGENEMIA

Several studies have suggested that heterosexual HIV-1 transmission to female partners of hemophiliacs is related to low $CD4^+$ count, HIV-1 p24 antigenemia and progression to AIDS (Goedert *et al.*, 1987; Smiley *et al.*, 1988). This increased risk for transmission when the infected partner is symptomatic has also been found in other heterosexual couple studies of non-hemophiliacs (Johnson and Laga, 1988; Staszewski *et al.*, 1988). Interestingly, greater infectiousness of the hemophiliac may not be confined to periods late in HIV-1 infection. In a cohort of 45 female partners of 45 HIV-1 antibody-positive hemophiliacs in Western Pennsylvania, six of the female partners became infected with HIV-1 early in the course of the hemophiliac's infection when he was still asymptomatic (Ragni *et al.*, 1989). None of the partner seroconversions could be related to the presence of serum p24 antigen, clinical status or any other marker of immune dysfunction in the index hemophiliac. These findings have given rise to the belief that HIV-1 infectiousness varies over the course of infection, with a bimodal risk which corresponds to the episodes of increased viremia in the patient. Increased viremia occurs very early after seroconversion, then usually drops to low levels while the antigen is in complex with antibody, and then increases again as HIV-1 disease progresses and B-cell function declines (Allain *et al.*, 1987). Among blood transfusion recipients, O'Brien and colleagues observed that secondary sexual transmission was more common among transfusion recipients who developed AIDS quickly (O'Brien *et al.*, 1994).

SPECIFIC PRACTICES: CONDOMS

The sexual practices of HIV-discordant hemophilic couples have been studied since the mid-1980s to examine the prevalence of high-risk behavior in this group. Between 1985 and 1991, the proportion of women at low risk for HIV infection increased from 7 to 69%, primarily because more couples were using condoms during all acts of vaginal intercourse (Dublin, Rosenberg and Goedert, 1992). Abstinence from vaginal intercourse increased from 7 to 13%, while the frequency of oral and anal sex decreased. Preliminary data from a more recent inquiry into this group's sexual behavior show an increase of the proportion of women reporting low risk for HIV infection to 82% (MHCS, unpublished data). These same data indicate that 79% of sexually active women in this cohort report using condoms all the time during vaginal intercourse with their partner.

Unprotected sex has been more commonly reported among women who had less education, women who engaged in oral and anal sex with their partner and among those whose partners had not had AIDS (Dublin, Rosenberg and Goedert, 1992). Ongoing studies have shown that unprotected vaginal intercourse at the time of study enrollment was strongly associated with continued risk at follow-up. This indicates that, while changes in sexual behavior of a population over time may be dramatic, change in individual behavior may be very slow and incremental.

ATTITUDES AND BEHAVIORS AFFECTING UNSAFE SEX

In preliminary findings gathered from 57 HIV-discordant, sexually active couples, those practicing unprotected sex were only slightly more likely to report negative attitudes about condom use, e.g. that they did not enjoy sex as much when condoms were used or that they felt more intimate when they did not use condoms (MHCS, unpublished data). Compared to couples who always had sex with a condom, those who had unsafe sex were significantly more likely to agree that their hemophilic partner might feel rejected if asked to use a condom. Remarkably, one-third of the women who reported unprotected sex with their HIV-infected partner were much more likely to believe that, because they had not yet been infected with HIV-1, they were unlikely to become infected in the future. None of the women who only had sex with condoms agreed with this statement.

PROCREATION

Despite consistent recommendations against unprotected intercourse by and with seropositive hemophilic men, many HIV-discordant couples in this population have reported pregnancies. Indeed, a notable portion of these reported pregnancies were planned.

In a study designed to investigate the reasons for these pregnancies, Jason and Evatt (1990) interviewed 20 couples reporting pregnancies in which both the male hemophiliac and the female sexual partner were HIV-infected. Thirty-seven per cent of these pregnancies were reported as planned, despite at least some hemophilia treatment center counseling with recommendations to the contrary. Reasons cited for these planned pregnancies included the belief that their child would not be infected and that their religion prohibited contraception.

The MHCS examined the sexual behavior of their HIV-discordant couples and found five (11%) who engaged in unprotected intercourse for the purpose of conception despite knowledge of the hemophiliac's infection with HIV-1 (Dublin *et al.*, 1993). All five of these couples were knowledgeable about the risk of transmission to the woman and subsequently the unborn child.

Artificial insemination with sperm from an HIV-1-positive hemophilic man that was 'washed' to remove infectious HIV-1 has been performed on several occasions (CDC, 1990a). In at least one case the female partner became infected with HIV-1 and did not become pregnant. Counseling efforts aimed at reducing the risk of HIV-1 transmission between HIV-discordant couples should include educational messages which address the issue of procreational sex.

RISK OF HIV-1 IN HOUSEHOLD CONTACTS

A number of investigators have shown that transmission of HIV-1 occurs through blood, sexual activity and perinatal events. The risk of transmission through normal, routine household interaction appears to be non-existent, as has been shown in studies of household contacts of persons infected with HIV-1 (Lawrence *et al.*, 1985; McFadden, Jason and Feorino, 1986; Fischl *et al.*, 1987).

There have been two notable HIV-1 transmissions between siblings with hemophilia (CDC, 1992a, 1993b). In the first case, a 4-year-old boy with hemophilia became infected with HIV-1 following exposure to needles or syringes used to provide intravenous therapy to his 8-year-old brother, who was known to have been infected previously with HIV-1 through receipt of unscreened blood products. On 15 reported occasions, the mother of the two boys treated them with intravenous factor replacement in immediate succession but in no particular order. During these treatment sessions, the mother reported placing used needles and other infusion paraphernalia within reach of the child being treated. Because the viral strains from the two brothers were genetically similar, those investigating this transmission concluded that the younger brother was almost certainly infected with HIV-1 originating from the older brother due to inadvertent intravenous or percutaneous exposure to the older brother's blood.

The second case of HIV-1 transmission between hemophilic brothers may have occurred through the sharing of a razor when both brothers cut themselves and bled slightly while shaving. In this case, the laboratory and epidemiologic evidence indicated that the younger brother became infected with an HIV-1 strain that had previously infected his older brother through the use of unscreened blood products. The investigators were unable to determine precisely the mode of transmission in this case. However, both brothers reported the above-mentioned incident of blood contact, and researchers believe that this incident or another unrecognized or unreported incident of blood contact caused the transmission (CDC, 1993b).

At least 17 studies in the USA and Europe have investigated the risk of HIV-1 infection in non-sexual, non-needle-sharing household contacts of persons infected with HIV-1. None of these 1167 contacts who were followed for more than 1700 person-years seroconverted (Simonds and Chanock, 1993). There is overwhelming evidence to suggest that casual household contact with an HIV-infected person poses virtually no risk for infection. However, HIV-1 has been transmitted in households where percutaneous, skin or mucous membrane contact with HIV-infected blood occurred. These examples of HIV transmission in households underline the importance of adherence to infection control guidelines, particularly in settings where health care is provided. The NHF has also recommended that personal items such as razors and toothbrushes should not be shared.

RISK OF HEPATITIS AND TUBERCULOSIS IN SEXUAL AND HOUSEHOLD CONTACTS

Transmission of the hepatitis C virus (HCV) from the hemophiliac to his female sexual partner is relatively rare (about 2%) compared to the transmission rate for HIV-1 (Eyster *et al.*, 1991). In fact, the incidence of sexual transmission of HCV appears to be enhanced in the presence of HIV-1. The risks of sexual and household transmission of the hepatitis viruses from a hemophilic patient are discussed further in Chapter 24.

AIDS-related opportunistic infections are not known to be a hazard for HIV-uninfected household contacts of HIV-infected persons with hemophilia. However, the transmission of pulmonary tuberculosis (TB), one of the AIDS-defining conditions, can be a significant cause of morbidity in household contacts of affected patients. The prevalence of pulmonary TB in the HIV-1-infected population is approximately 4% (CDC, 1994), and the prevalence of multidrug-resistant strains of TB has been increasing since 1988 (CDC, 1990b). The risk of active tuberculosis in household contacts of patients with pulmonary TB is approximately 6% and does not appear to be related to the HIV-1 status of the index case (Nunn *et al.*, 1994).

Clinical manifestations, course and outcome

OVERVIEW OF NATURAL HISTORY AND SPECIFIC AIDS DIAGNOSES

As of January 1993, clinical AIDS – that is, a life-threatening opportunistic infection or malignancy – had been diagnosed in 2214 persons with hemophilia in the USA (CDC, 1993a). Of these, the initial AIDS-defining conditions have been *Pneumocystis carinii* pneumonia in 46%, *Candida* esophagitis in 24% and wasting syndrome in 20% (Table 25.3). Through 1994, 3863 persons with hemophilia in the USA had been diagnosed with AIDS (CDC, 1994): however, the CDC surveillance definition also changed during this time to include laboratory measurements of severe immunosuppression (CDC, 1992b). Since 1990, the number of cases of hemophilia-associated clinical AIDS reported each year has increased slightly and ranges from 340 to 440 (CDC, 1994). This relatively stable incidence reflects the effects of therapeutic interventions and the fact that there are no new cases of HIV-1 infection occurring in this population.

Table 25.3 Acquired immunodeficiency syndrome (AIDS)-defining clinical diseases in 2475 US hemophiliacs through 1992*

Disease	Number (%)
Pneumocystis carinii pneumonia	1133 (45.8)
Candidiasis of the esophagus or lung	593 (23.9)
Wasting syndrome	499 (20.2)
Mycobacterium avium	249 (10.0)
Cryptococcosis	195 (7.9)
HIV encephalopathy	191 (7.7)
Cytomegalovirus, including retinitis	145 (5.9)
Toxoplasmosis of brain	106 (4.3)
Chronic herpes simplex	92 (3.7)
Cryptosporidiosis	70 (2.8)
Other *Mycobacterium*	59 (2.4)
Immunoblastic lymphoma	53 (2.2)
Histoplasmosis	44 (1.8)
Extrapulmonary tuberculosis	40 (1.6)
Recurrent bacterial infections	37 (1.5)
Burkitt's lymphoma	28 (1.1)
Progressive multifocal leukoencephalopathy	27 (1.1)
Kaposi's sarcoma	24 (1.0)
Primary lymphoma of brain	19 (0.8)
Pulmonary tuberculosis	17 (0.7)
Lymphoid interstitial pneumonia	13 (0.5)
Recurrent pneumonia	11 (0.4)
Coccidiomycosis	9 (0.4)
Salmonella septicemia	5 (0.2)
Isosporiasis	2 (0.1)

*Based on cases reported to the Centers for Disease Control, adjusted for reporting delays. More than one disease per patient may have been reported.
HIV = Human immunodeficiency virus.

AGE AND OTHER DIFFERENCES IN HEMOPHILIA

Several studies have found that younger infected persons, excluding perinatally infected infants (Pizzo *et al.*, 1995), progress to AIDS more slowly than older infected ones (Eyster *et al.*, 1987; Moss *et al.*, 1988; Goedert *et al.*, 1989; Biggar and the International Registry of Seroconverters, 1990; Blaxhult *et al.*, 1990; Darby *et al.*, 1990; Schinaia *et al.*, 1991; Mariotto *et al.*, 1992; Fig. 25.5). In the MHCS we observed that youth was associated with slower rates of progression not only from seroconversion to AIDS but also from seroconversion to intermediate markers, such as depletion of $CD4^+$ lymphocytes, and also from the intermediate markers to AIDS (Eyster *et al.*, 1993). We have also observed that younger hemophilic subjects have better survival from all levels of $CD4^+$ lymphocytes to death (Ehmann *et al.*, 1994), and others have reported better post-AIDS survival among younger patients (Schinaia *et al.*, 1993; Whitmore-Overton *et al.*, 1993; Saah *et al.*, 1994).

Rosenberg, Goedert and Biggar directly compared AIDS incidence rates in hemophiliacs to homosexual men (1994). In both groups the AIDS incidence rates were approximately 4% higher per year of age at seroconversion. The trend was linear with age. Thus, no particular age group, such as adolescence or over 50 years, appeared to be at unusually high or low risk. We speculated that an intrinsic component of aging, such as the irreversible commitment of 'memory' lymphocytes, may be responsible.

After adjustment for age, homosexual men progress from HIV-1 seroconversion to AIDS at a significantly faster rate than persons with hemophilia (Rosenberg, Goedert and Biggar, 1994). For example, among persons who seroconverted at age 30, AIDS developed within 10 years in approximately 50% of the hemophiliacs and in approximately 75% of the homosexual men. However, this slower progression rate for hemophiliacs is probably unrelated to hemophilia or its treatment. Rather, it is primarily because Kaposi's sarcoma, which may occur with only mild immune deficiency, is extraordinarily rare among hemophiliacs but relatively frequent among homosexual men. Therefore, some but perhaps not all of the higher risk for homosexual men is due to their propensity to Kaposi's sarcoma.

LABORATORY MARKERS OF AIDS

The $CD4^+$ lymphocyte is the primary target of HIV-1 infection, and depletion of these cells from the peripheral blood and from lymph nodes is the principal characteristic of HIV-related immune deficiency. Measurement of CD^+ lymphocytes is the mainstay of immunologic assessment of the HIV-infected patient. A $CD4^+$ lymphocyte count below 200 cells/µl is the threshold at which the risk of opportunistic infection, particularly *Pneumocystis carinii* pneumonia, increases dramatically (CDC, 1992c). The association is so clear that in 1993 severe immune deficiency, defined as a $CD4^+$ lymphocyte count below 200 cells/µl, was added to the US surveillance definition of AIDS (CDC, 1992b). The risk of less common, more severe opportunistic infections, such as *Mycobacterium avium* complex and cytomegalovirus hepatitis, ophthalmitis and colitis, is even higher when the $CD4^+$ lymphocyte count falls below 50 cells/ µl (Horsburgh and Selik, 1989; Nightingale *et al.*, 1992; Muñoz *et al.*, 1993). Not surprisingly, the risk of death among HIV-infected hemophiliacs is directly related to the CD4 level (Phillips *et al.*, 1992; Mills and Jones, 1993; Ehmann *et al.*, 1994; Fig. 25.6).

Several studies have investigated the effect of using high-purity factor VIII concentrates to reduce the antigenic stimulation of the immune system and to slow the decline in $CD4^+$ cells in HIV-1-infected persons with hemophilia (de Biasi *et al.*, 1991; Goldsmith *et al.*, 1991; Hilgartner *et al.*, 1993; Seremetis *et al.*, 1993; Goedert *et al.*, 1994). The results showed that use of high-purity products appeared to sustain the $CD4^+$ lymphocyte level, although there was no measurable benefit in the risk reduction of AIDS or death (Goedert *et al.*, 1994).

Two important cautions about the interpretation of $CD4^+$ lymphocyte counts must be emphasized. First, prognosis is little affected by changes in the CD4 count that occur during zidovudine therapy (Choi *et al.*, 1993). Second, the counts can be highly variable, particularly at levels above 200 or 500 cells/µl. This variability can be reduced by consistently using the same laboratory, but much of it is intrinsic to *in vivo* changes in the total lymphocyte count and to the multiplication of two or three measurement errors – the total leukocyte count, the proportion of lymphocytes and the proportion of $CD4^+$ mononuclear cells.

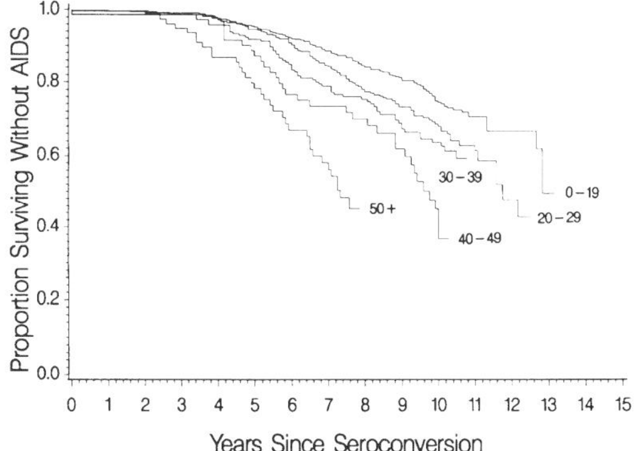

Fig. 25.5 Kaplan–Meier plots of proportion surviving without acquired immunodeficiency syndrome (AIDS) by age at seroconversion.

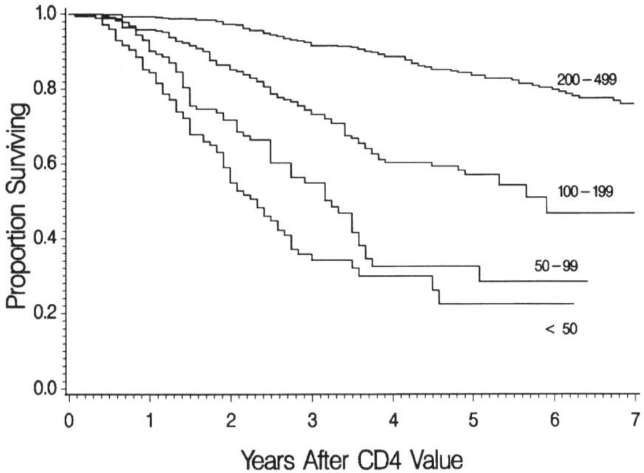

Fig. 25.6 Kaplan–Meier plots of proportion surviving by CD4 levels.

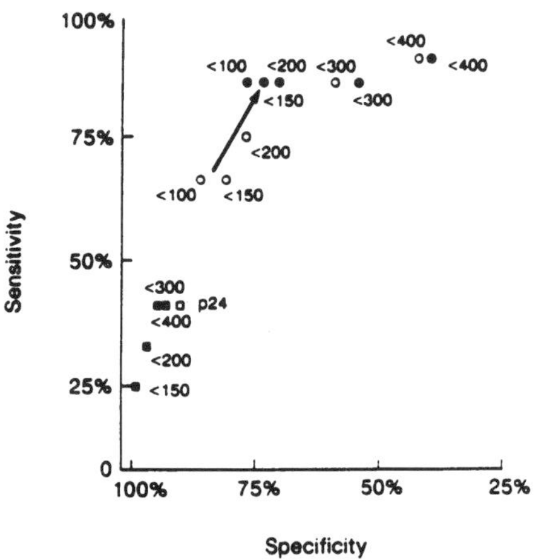

Fig. 25.7 Comparison of sensitivity and specificity of serum p24 antigen or low CD4$^+$ cell count, or both, as predictive markers for acquired immunodeficiency syndrome (AIDS). Open squares indicate p24 antigen alone; closed squares, p24 antigen and low CD4$^+$ cell count; open circles indicate low CD4$^+$ cell count alone; closed circles, p24 antigen or low CD4$^+$ cell count. The arrow shows how sensitivity is increased by using both tests, with either a positive p24 antigen or a low CD4$^+$ cell count considered abnormal.

Secondary to the depletion of CD4$^+$ lymphocytes, dysregulation of humoral immunity and other components of the immune response can lead to marked elevations in activation markers, particularly β_2-microglobulin, neopterin, α-interferon and others. There may also be unusually high antibody titers due to reactivation of herpes viruses (Croen, 1991; Safrin, 1994). Alternatively, antibodies may be rapidly lost against hepatitis C virus (discussed further in Chapter 24) or nearly absent against syphilis (Haas *et al.*, 1990; Johnson *et al.*, 1991). Loss of antibodies to factor VIII has also been observed in patients with inhibitors and advanced HIV-1 disease (Bray *et al.*, 1993). Circulating immune complexes are often detected as the dysregulated immune system attempts to cope with a myriad of new and reactivated antigenic exposures.

HIV-1 p24 antigenemia is a highly specific but relatively insensitive marker of increased AIDS risk. In a cohort of 87 HIV-infected hemophilic subjects in Hershey, Pennsylvania, who were tested approximately annually, only 21% developed p24 antigenemia and 64% developed CD4$^+$ lymphocyte counts below 200 cells/µl within 8 years of HIV-1 antibody seroconversion (Eyster *et al.*, 1989). Of the 71 subjects without p24 antigen, 64 (90%) were free of AIDS for 8 years. The sensitivity for developing AIDS was only 42% for those with p24 antigenemia. The sensitivity and specificity for AIDS were both 75% with a CD4$^+$ lymphocyte count below 200 cells/µl. With either a low CD4 count or p24 antigenemia, sensitivity for AIDS increased to 83% with specificity of 70% or higher (Fig. 25.7). Four (67%) of six subjects who were p24 antigenemic developed AIDS within 2 years of a CD4$^+$ lymphocyte count below 200 cells/µl. Some subjects have circulating immune complexes of p24 antigen and anti-p24 antibodies that may result in apparent loss of anti-p24 and apparent absence of p24 antigen. Antigen detection is slightly increased with an immune-complex dissociation (ICD)

step, but the predictive value for AIDS of the ICD-p24 and the conventional p24 EIAs appears very similar (Henrard *et al.*, 1995).

Prediction of AIDS with serologic activation markers, particularly β_2-microglobulin and neopterin, in addition to CD4 counts, has been extensively studied and found to be of value in homosexual men (Moss *et al.*, 1988; Fahey *et al.*, 1990; Krämer *et al.*, 1990). Data for hemophilic cohorts are more sparse. However, as in the male homosexual cohorts, after adjustment for CD4 counts, elevation of either β_2-microglobulin (above 3 mg/l) or neopterin (above 15 nmol/l) has been associated with a two- to fourfold increased risk of AIDS (MHCS, unpublished data). β_2-Microglobulin and neopterin levels are highly correlated, but most studies have found slightly better sensitivity and specificity with neopterin.

HOST FACTORS

The major histocompatibility complex (MHC) found on chromosome 6 consists of genes which regulate the immune system. It is therefore not surprising that many studies have shown that products of the MHC, in particular the very polymorphic human leukocyte antigen (HLA) region, play a role in HIV-1 disease progression (reviewed by Mann, Carrington and Kroner, 1994).

Alleles of the HLA genes are not randomly assorted, but typically are inherited together as a haplotype for reasons which are probably due to selection advantage. We studied HLA haplotype-sharing in 95 HIV-1-infected whole sibling pairs to investigate the concordance between the number of shared haplotypes (0, 1 or 2) and HIV-1 disease progression (Kroner *et al.*, 1995). Based on age-adjusted intraclass correlation coefficients (ICC), there was a highly significant concordance in CD4 decline to less than 20% within 5 years after seroconversion in pairs sharing one or two haplotypes (ICC = 0.99 and 0.75, respectively). Similar results were found in the two groups for the concordance in the 5-year incidence of AIDS (ICC = 0.66 and 0.63). No concordance was observed with either disease end-point in the pairs that shared zero haplotypes. Rechavi *et al.* (1987) reported the diagnosis of Burkitt's lymphoma in two hemophilic brothers who were also HLA-identical. Two other reports documented AIDS in siblings with hemophilia, although no genetic determinants were investigated (Lissen *et al.*, 1983; Meropol *et al.*, 1989).

HIV-ASSOCIATED CONDITIONS, INCIDENCE AND PREDICTIVE VALUE

Eyster *et al.* studied the pre-AIDS incidence rates of eight HIV-associated conditions – herpes zoster, thrombocytopenia, oral candidiasis, oral hairy leukoplakia, persistent fever, weight loss, TB and non-AIDS pneumonia – as well as the value of these conditions for predicting AIDS. The risks and associations differed for those who became infected before, as opposed to after, age 18 (Eyster *et al.*, 1993b). Thrombocytopenia was the most frequently observed condition, with 10-year cumulative incidences of 43% in adults and 27% in children. Other conditions more frequent in adults than in children were oral candidiasis (10-year cumulative risk 30% versus 12%), non-AIDS pneumonia (25% versus 15%), weight loss (21% versus 5%) and fever (14% versus 4%). The risks of herpes zoster, TB and hairy leukoplakia were similar in the two age groups. Except for thrombocytopenia in children, all conditions occurred at CD4$^+$ lymphocyte counts less than 350 cells/µl. In adults, the relative hazards of AIDS after persistent fever, weight loss, oral candidiasis, and non-AIDS pneumonia were 10.4, 3.2, 3.8 and 2.2, respectively. Oral candidiasis was the strongest predictor of AIDS in children, with a relative hazard of 18.3.

NON-HODGKIN'S LYMPHOMA AND OTHER MALIGNANCIES

With the advent of therapy to slow the progression of HIV-1 infection, in particular the nucleoside analogs and *Pneumocystis carinii* pneumonia (PCP) prophylaxis, survival time for infected individuals has significantly increased. Investigators have reported that, as a result, persons with HIV-1 are at an increased risk of developing cancers which are associated with immunosuppression, in particular non-Hodgkin's lymphoma (NHL; Pluda *et al.*, 1990; Rabkin *et al.*, 1992). Rabkin *et al.* showed that the incidence of NHL in a cohort of hemophiliacs averaged 0.15 cases per 100 person-years after HIV-1 seroconversion. At every age group, the risk of NHL was significantly greater than that for the general age-matched populations. The relative risk, however, was highest among adolescents and young adults for reasons that remain unexplained.

Kaposi's sarcoma which is the original AIDS-defining malignancy, occurs predominantly among homosexual men and rarely among persons with hemophilia (Beral *et al.*, 1990). In the MHCS, only three cases of Kaposi's sarcoma have occurred – one in a homosexual hemophilia patient and two in hemophiliacs from Greece, an endemic area for classic (non-AIDS) Kaposi's sarcoma (Rabkin *et al.*, 1992). No excess risk of cancers, other than NHL and Kaposi's sarcoma has been found among persons with hemophilia and with or without HIV-1 infection (Rabkin *et al.*, 1992).

SURVIVAL AFTER AIDS – ALL-CAUSE MORTALITY

Several investigators have reported factors which are associated with improved survival after the diagnosis of AIDS. These include a temporal trend toward a more recent diagnosis (Jacobson *et al.*, 1993; Schinaia *et al.*, 1993; Whitmore-Overton *et al.*, 1993; Saah *et al.*, 1994), younger age at diagnosis (Ragni and Kingsley, 1990; Schinaia *et al.*, 1993; Whitmore-Overton *et al.*, 1993; Saah *et al.*, 1994), an AIDS-defining disease not associated with the central nervous system (Ragni and Kingsley, 1990; Schinaia *et al.*, 1993; Whitmore-Overton *et al.*, 1993), and PCP as the AIDS-defining disease (Jacobson *et al.*, 1993). In addition to survival after AIDS, studies have shown a significant relationship between mortality and low CD4$^+$ lymphocyte count (Phillips *et al.*, 1992; Mills and Jones, 1993; Ehmann *et al.*, 1994).

At present, the three leading causes of death in persons with hemophilia are AIDS, liver disease and hemorrhage, with or without stroke (Diamondstone *et al.*, 1995). In the MHCS, 411 deaths occurred between 1982 and 1995 (390 in HIV-1-infected patients and 21 in HIV-1-uninfected patients). Of these, 258 (63%) were due to AIDS alone, 32 (8%) were due to liver disease alone, 27 (7%) were due to both AIDS and liver disease, 40 (10%) were due to hemorrhage or stroke, 11 (3%) were due to miscellaneous HIV-1-related causes, 40 (10%) were due to common causes such as cancer, heart disease and trauma, and four (1%) were unknown.

This distribution is in stark comparison to the proportion of deaths due to specific causes which occurred in 1982 (Johnson *et al.*, 1985). In this study, 52 deaths were reported) of which five (10%) were due to AIDS, 22

(42%) were due to hemorrhage, two (4%) were due to liver disease, and 21 (40%) were due to common or other causes. This dramatic shift in cause-specific mortality is undoubtedly due to the HIV-1 epidemic, competing causes of death in an aging population and the long-term effects of infection with hepatitis viruses. The current trends in cause-specific mortality are expected to continue for many years.

Management and complications

The management of and options for treating HIV-infected patients changes frequently. State-of-the-art reviews on antiretroviral therapy (Roundtable Proceedings, 1994), as well as opportunistic infection prevention and prophylaxis (Gallant, Moore and Chaisson, 1994; CDC, 1995) and treatment (Sande and Volberding, 1992; Sepkowitz and Armstrong, 1995; Table 25.4) have been published recently. Therefore, this section will focus primarily on pharmacologic therapies for HIV infection and its complications in hemophilic patients. The three basic principles are:

1. Chronic, active HIV-1 infection is the primary disease.
2. HIV-1 causes progressive immune deficiency in most patients through slow but steady depletion of $CD4^+$ lymphocytes.
3. Most of the morbidity and mortality results from opportunistic infectious diseases and, less frequently, malignancies that occur with very advanced immune deficiency.

ZIDOVUDINE (AZT): EARLY VERSUS LATE TREATMENT

Two double-blind, placebo-controlled randomized trials of the safety and effficacy of zidovudine for asymptomatic hemophilic subjects with relatively low CD4 counts (100–400 cells/µl) have been reported. The European–Australian study of 143 subjects found that those subjects who were randomized to receive 1000 mg of zidovudine in two divided doses per day tended to have a delayed fall in CD4 counts to less than 200 cells/µl but there were no differences with respect to development of opportunistic infections or malignancies (Mannucci *et al.*, 1994). The American study randomized 193 hemophilic subjects

Table 25.4 Comparison of treatment of choice for opportunistic infection, 1981 versus 1995*

Opportunistic infections	First-line agents, 1981	First-line agents, 1995	New second-line agents
Pneumocystosis	Co-trimoxazole Pentamidine	Co-trimoxazole Pentamidine	Dapsone–trimethoprim Trimetrexate Atovaquone Clindamycin-primaquine
Toxoplasmosis	Sulfadiazine-pyrimethamine	Sulfadiazine-pyrimethamine	Clindamycin-pyrimethamine
Cryptosporidiosis	None	None	None
Tuberculosis	Isoniazid Rifampin Pyrazinamide Streptomycin Ethambutol	Isoniazid Rifampin Pyrazinamide Streptomycin Ethambutol	Ofloxacin
Cytomegalovirus disease	None	*Ganciclovir* *Foscarnet*	None
Disseminated MAC	Rifampin Clofazamine Ethambutol Amikacin	Rifampin/*rifabutin* Clofazamine Ethambutol Amikacin *Macrolides*† *Ciprofloxacin*	None
Fungal infections			
Candidosis	Amphotericin B	*Fluconazole*‡	
Other infections§	Amphotericin B	Amphotericin B *Fluconazole*** *Itraconazole***	Fluconazole Itraconazole

Adapted from Sepkowitz and Armstrong (1995), with permission.
MAC = *Mycobacterium avium* complex.
*New first-line agents are in italic.
†Macrolides include clarithromycin and azithromycin.
‡First-line agent for mucosal infections.
§Includes cryptococcosis, histoplasmosis and coccidioidomycosis.
**First-line agent for maintenance therapy and second-line agent for acute therapy

to receive either placebo or a high dose of zidovudine, 300 mg five times a day (Merigan *et al.*, 1991). Clinical end-points, including death, opportunistic infection, malignancy or symptoms of AIDS related complex, were reached by 22 placebo recipients and 13 zidovudine recipients, but the results were not statistically significant. Because older persons have more rapid progression of disease and, in this study, had lower CD4 counts, a subgroup analysis was performed. Among subjects over age 30, there were five placebo recipients who developed AIDS or died versus none of the zidovudine recipients ($P = 0.02$). Similarly, among subjects over age 30 years, zidovudine recipients had higher CD4 counts and better weight gain compared to placebo recipients at 24 weeks after randomization.

The European–Australian study found that 4% of the zidovudine recipients developed a hemoglobin concentration below 8 g/dl. Likewise, 5% of this group developed neutropenia below 750 cells/µl. Alanine aminotransferase levels were more than 10 times the upper normal limit in 3% of the zidovudine recipients and also in 4% of the placebo recipients (Mannucci *et al.*, 1994). Zidovudine-related toxicity was more frequent and more severe with the higher zidovudine dose used in the American study, in which 25 subjects withdrew before completing the study, usually because of asthenia, malaise and nausea. Granulocytopenia and anemia were also more severe in subjects of all ages.

Thus, among HIV-infected persons with hemophilia, zidovudine treatment appears to be effective in reducing the risk of AIDS and death among those who are at highest risk. Toxicity is seldom severe and appears to be reversible, even at doses of 1000 mg/day as used in the Concorde Study (Concorde Coordinating Committee, 1994), which is higher than the equally efficacious lower dose of 500–600 mg/day recommended in the USA.

DIDANOSINE (DDI) AND ZALCITABINE (DDC)

Yarchoan and colleagues (1994) have suggested that the combination of simultaneous didanosine and zidovudine is superior to zidovudine alone. Results from the AIDS Clinical Trail Group (ACTG) 116 trial suggests that didanosine is more efficacious than zidovudine in patients with at least 8 weeks of previous exposure to zidovudine (Dolin *et al.*, 1995). It should be noted, however, that improved survival has not been observed in either study. Rather, there has been more weight gain, CD4$^+$ lymphocyte increases and p24 antigenemia decreases. Perhaps because hemophilic patients have a high prevalence of chronic hepatitis, preliminary reports suggest that they are at higher risk of hepatotoxicity with combined zidovudine and didanosine, as well as smaller increases in CD4$^+$ lymphocyte counts compared to non-hemophiliacs (Ragni *et al.*, 1992, 1993).

The ACTG has recently published the results of a large study of 1001 HIV-1-infected patients who had fewer than 300 CD4$^+$ lymphocytes/µl and who had tolerated zidovudine therapy for at least 6 months (Fischl *et al.*, 1995). They were randomized to receive continued zidovudine alone, zalcitabine alone, or the two drugs combined. Overall, there were no significant differences between the treatment groups. Among patients with more than 150 CD4$^+$ lymphocytes/µl, however, the rate of progression to AIDS or death was slightly lower with combination therapy.

Practical problems in hemophilia

THROMBOCYTOPENIA AND BLEEDING

As noted above, thrombocytopenia, defined as a platelet count below 100 000 cells/µl was noted to have occurred at least once in 43% of adult and 27% of pediatric HIV-infected persons with hemophilia (Eyster *et al.*, 1993). Although most of these were not episodes of severe thrombocytopenia (i.e. fewer than 20 000 platelets/µl), the risk of spontaneous hemorrhage was increased because of the underlying coagulopathy, as vividly shown by Ragni and colleagues (1990). Consequently, platelet counts should be monitored carefully and, if low, often can be treated successfully with zidovudine and probably didanosine (Lim, Lee and Kernoff, 1990; Rarick *et al.*, 1991; Landonio *et al.*, 1993; Piketty, Gilquin and Kazatchkine, 1994).

GROWTH AND PUBERTY

HIV-1 infection appears to retard the statural growth and weight gain in children and adolescents, resulting in a diagnosis of 'small for age.' As part of the Hemophilia Growth and Development Study, 300 boys (62% HIV-1-infected) were studied to determine the impact of HIV-1 on skeletal and sexual maturity, as measured by radiologic films of the hand and Tanner stage scoring, respectively (Gertner *et al.*, 1994). The mean age-adjusted bone age was significantly reduced in the HIV-infected group compared to the uninfected group. By age 16, 61% of the HIV-uninfected hemophilic adolescents had reached Tanner stage 5, compared to only 40% of the HIV-infected adolescents. Likewise, by age 18, 73% of the HIV-uninfected hemophiliacs had reached Tanner stage 5, compared to 53% of the HIV-infected group – differences that were highly significant.

HEPATIC INSUFFICIENCY

Infection with HCV is associated with serious liver disease in persons with hemophilia. Coinfection with HIV-1 accelerates the progression to hepatic insufficiency

(Eyster *et al.*, 1993a; Telfer *et al.*, 1994a). Eyster and colleagues reported that in those coinfected, the cumulative incidence of liver failure was 17% 10 years after HIV-1 seroconversion. In this population, they also observed that lymphocytopenia, decreased CD4$^+$ cell counts, thrombocytopenia and antiretroviral therapy were associated with advanced liver disease. HCV RNA levels increase over time (Eyster *et al.*, 1994; Telfer *et al.*, 1994b) and HIV-1 infection probably enhances HCV replication. Eyster and colleagues observed an eightfold increase in the HCV RNA levels of HIV-1-infected patients compared to HIV-1-uninfected patients (Eyster *et al.*, 1994). The effects of HIV-1 on the progression of liver disease are discussed further in Chapter 24.

References

AIDS-Haemophilia French Study Group (1985) Immunologic and virologic status of multitransfused patients: role of type and origin of blood products. *Blood*, 66, 896–901.

Allain, J-P., Laurian, Y., Paul, D. *et al.* (1987) Long-term evaluation of HIV antigen and antibodies to p24 and gp41 in patients with hemophilia. *New England Journal of Medicine*, 317, 1114–1121.

Aronson, D.L. (1979a) Factor VIII (antihemophilic globulin). *Seminars in Thrombosis and Hemostasis*, 6, 12–27.

Aronson, D.L. (1979b) Factor IX complex. *Seminars in Thrombosis and Hemostasis*, 6, 28–43.

Ball, S.E., Hows, J.M., Worsley, A.M. *et al.* (1985) Seroconversion of human T cell lymphotrophic virus III (HTLV-III) in patients with hemophilia: a longitudinal study. *British Medical Journal*, 290, 1705–1706.

Barre-Sinoussi, F., Chermann, J.C., Rey, F. *et al.* (1983) Isolation of a T-lymphotropic retrovirus from a patient at risk for acquired immune deficiency syndrome (AIDS). *Science*, 220, 868–871.

Beral, V., Peterman, T.A., Berkelman, R.L. and Jaffe, H.W. (1990) Kaposi's sarcoma among persons with AIDS: a sexually transmitted infection? *Lancet*, 335, 123–128

Berntorp E., Hansson, B.G., Bottiger, B. *et al.* (1987) HIV seroconversion in Swedish haemophiliacs: relation to type and dosage of factor concentrate. *European Journal of Haematology*, 38, 256–260.

Biggar, R J. and International Registry of Seroconverters (1990) AIDS incubation in 1891 HIV seroconverters from different exposure groups. *AIDS*, 4, 1059–1066.

Blattner, W.A. (1991) HIV epidemiology: past, present, and future. *FASEB Journal*, 5, 2340–2348.

Blaxhult, A., Granath, F., Lidman, K. and Giesecke, J. (1990) The influence of age on the latency period to AIDS in people infected by HIV through blood transfusion. *AIDS*, 4, 125–129.

Blombäck, M., Kjellman, H., Schulman, S. *et al.* (1987) Immunoglobulin levels in haemophiliacs at HIV seroconversion and during follow up. *Infection*, 15, 248–252.

Bray, G.L., Kroner, B.L., Arkin, S. *et al.* (1993) Loss of high-responder inhibitors in patients with severe hemophilia A and human immunodeficiency virus type 1 infection: a report from the Multi-Center Hemophilia Cohort Study. *American Journal of Hematology*, 42, 375–379.

Centers for Disease Control (1981a) *Pneumocystis* pneumonia – Los Angeles. *Morbidity and Mortality Weekly Report*, 30, 250–252.

Centers for Disease Control (1981b) Kaposi's sarcoma and *Pneumocystis* pneumonia among homosexual men – New York City and California. *Morbidity and Mortality Weekly Report*, 30, 305–308.

Centers for Disease Control (1981c) Follow-up on Kaposi's sarcoma and *Pneumocystis* pneumonia. *Morbidity and Mortality Weekly Report*, 30, 409–410.

Centers for Disease Control (1982a) *Pneumocystis carinii* pneumonia among persons with hemophilia A. *Morbidity and Mortality Weekly Report*, 31, 365–367.

Centers for Disease Control (1982b) Update on acquired immune deficiency syndrome (AIDS) among patients with hemophilia A. *Morbidity and Mortality Weekly Report*, 31, 644–652.

Centers for Disease Control (1982c) Opportunistic infections and Kaposi's sarcoma among Haitians in the United States. *Morbidity and Mortality Weekly Report*, 31, 353–361.

Centers for Disease Control (1982d) Update on acquired immune deficiency syndrome (AIDS) – United States. *Morbidity and Mortality Weekly Report*, 31, 507–514.

Centers for Disease Control (1982e) Possible transfusion-associated acquired immune deficiency syndrome (AIDS) – California. *Morbidity and Mortality Weekly Report*, 31, 652–654.

Centers for Disease Control (1982f) Unexplained immunodeficiency and opportunistic infections in infants – New York, New Jersey, California. *Morbidity and Mortality Weekly Report*, 31, 665–667

Centers for Disease Control (1989) AIDS and human immunodeficiency virus infection in the United States: 1988 update. *Morbidity and Mortality Weekly Report*, 38, 1–38.

Centers for Disease Control (1990a) HIV-1 infection and artificial insemination with processed semen. *Morbidity and Mortality Weekly Report*, 39, 249–256.

Centers for Disease Control (1990b) Nosocomial transmission of multidrug-resistant tuberculosis to health-care workers and HIV-infected patients in an urban hospital – Florida. *Morbidity and Mortality Weekly Report*, 39, 718–722.

Centers for Disease Control (1992a) HIV infection in two brothers receiving intravenous therapy for hemophilia. *Morbidity and Mortality Weekly Report*, 41, 228–231.

Centers for Disease Control (1992b) 1993 revised classification system for HIV infection and expanded surveillance case definition for AIDS among adolescents and adults. *Morbidity and Mortality Weekly Report*, 41, 1–19.

Centers for Disease Control (1992c) Recommendations for prophylaxis against *Pneumocystis carinii* pneumonia for adults and adolescents infected with human immunodeficiency. *Morbidity and Mortality Weekly Report*, 41, 1–11.

Centers for Disease Control (1993a) *HIV/AIDS Surveillance Report*, 5, 1–23.

Centers for Disease Control (1993b) HIV transmission between two adolescent brothers with hemophilia. *Morbidity and Mortality Weekly Report*, 42, 948–951.

Centers for Disease Control (1994) *HIV/AIDS Surveillance Report*, 6, 1–39.

Centers for Disease Control and Prevention (1995) USPHS/IDSA guidelines for the prevention of opportunistic infections in persons infected with human immunodeficiency virus: a summary. *Morbidity and Mortality Weekly Report*, 44, 1–34.

Chang, S.Y., Bowman, B.H., Weiss, J.B. *et al.* (1993) The origin of HIV-1 isolate HTLV-IIIB. *Nature*, 363, 466–469.

Cheingsong-Popov, R., Weiss, R.A., Dalgleish, A. *et al.* (1984) Prevalence of antibody to human T-lymphotropic virus type III in AIDS and AIDS-risk patients in Britain. *Lancet*, 2, 477–480.

Chermann, J.C., Donker, G., Yahi, N. *et al.* (1991) Discrepancies in AIDS virus data. *Nature*, 351, 277–278.

Choi, S., Lagakos, S.W., Schooley, R.T. and Volberding, P.A. (1993) CD4$^+$ lymphocytes are an incomplete surrogate marker for clinical progression in persons with asymptomatic HIV infection taking zidovudine. *Annals of Internal Medicine*, 118, 674–680.

Concorde Coordinating Committee (1994) Concorde: MRC/ANRS randomised double blind controlled trial of immediate and deferred zidovudine in symptom-free HIV infection *Lancet*, 343, 871–881.

Croen, K D. (1991) Latency of the human herpes viruses. *Annual Review of Medicine*, 42, 61–67.

Darby, S.C., Doll, R., Thakrar, B. *et al.* (1990) Time from infection with HIV to onset of AIDS in patients with haemophilia in the UK. *Statistics in Medicine*, 9, 681–689.

de Biasi, R., Rocino, A., Miraglia, E. *et al.* (1991) The impact of a very high purity factor VIII concentrate on the immune system of human immunodeficiency virus-infected hemophiliacs: a randomized, prospective two-year comparison with an intermediate purity concentrate. *Blood*, 78, 1919–1922.

Diamondstone, L.S., Blakley, S.A., Rice, J.C. *et al.* (1995) Prognostic factors for all-cause mortality among hemophiliacs infected with human immunodeficiency virus. *American Journal of Epidemiology*, 142, 304–313.

Dodd, R.Y. (1994) Donor screening for HIV infection – United States model, in *Blood, Blood Products, and AIDS*, 2nd edn (eds R. Madhok, C.D. Forbes and B.L. Evatt), Chapman and Hall, London, pp. 183–205.

Dolin, R., Amato, D.A., Fischl, M.A. *et al.* (1995) Zidovudine compared to didanosine in patients with advanced HIV type 1 infection and little or no previous experience with zidovudine. *Archives of Internal Medicine*, 155, 961–974.

Dublin, S., Rosenberg, P.S. and Goedert, J.J. (1992) Patterns and predictors of high-risk sexual behavior in female partners of HIV-infected men with hemophilia. *AIDS*, 6, 475–482.

Dublin, S., Blattner, W.A., White, G.C. II and Goedert, J.J. (1993) Procreation and HIV. *Lancet*, 342, 1241–1242.

Dumitrescu, O., Kalish, M.L., Kliks, S.C. *et al.* (1994) Characterization of human immunodeficiency virus type 1 isolates from children in Romania: identification of a new envelope subtype. *Journal of Infectious Diseases*, 169, 281–288.

Ehmann, W.C., Eyster, M.E., Wilson, S.E. *et al.* (1994) Relationship of CD4 lymphocyte counts to survival in a cohort of hemophiliacs infected with human immunodeficiency virus. *Journal of Acquired Immune Deficiency Syndromes*, 7, 1095–1098.

Evatt, B.L., Gomperts, E.D., McDougal, J.S. and Ramsey, R.B. (1985) Coincidental appearance of LAV/HTLV-III antibodies in hemophiliacs and the onset of the AIDS epidemic. *New England Journal of Medicine*, 312, 483–486.

Eyster, M.E., Goedert, J.J., Sarngadharan, M.G. *et al.* (1985) Development and early natural history of HTLV-III antibodies in persons with hemophilia. *Journal of the American Medical Association*, 253, 2219–2223.

Eyster, M.E., Gail, M.H., Ballard, J.O. *et al.* (1987) Natural history of human immunodeficiency virus infections in hemophiliacs: effects of T-cell subsets, platelet counts, and age. *Annals of Internal Medicine*, **107**, 1–6.

Eyster, M.E., Ballard, J.O., Gail, M.H. *et al.* (1989) Predictive markers for the acquired immunodeficiency syndrome (AIDS) in hemophiliacs: persistence of p24 antigen and low T4 cell count. *Annals of Internal Medicine*, **110**, 963–969.

Eyster, M.E., Alter, H.J., Aledort, L.M. *et al.* (1991) Heterosexual co-transmission of hepatitis C virus (HCV) and human immunodeficiency virus (HIV). *Annals of Internal Medicine*, **115**, 746–768.

Eyster, M.E., Diamondstone, L.S., Lien, J.M. *et al.* (1993a) The natural history of hepatitis C virus infection in multitransfused hemophiliacs: effect of coinfection with human immunodeficiency virus. *Journal of Acquired Immune Deficiency Syndromes*, **6**, 602–610.

Eyster, M.E., Rabkin, C.S., Hilgartner, M.W. *et al.* (1993b) Human immunodeficiency virus-related conditions in children and adults with hemophilia: rates, relationship to CD4 counts, and predictive value. *Blood*, **81**, 828–834.

Eyster, M.E., Fried, M.W., Di Bisceglie, A.M. and Goedert, J.J. (1994) Increasing hepatitis C virus RNA levels in hemophiliacs: relationship to human immunodeficiency virus infection and liver disease. *Blood*, **84**, 1020–1023.

Fahey, J.L., Taylor, J.M.G., Detels, R. *et al.* (1990) The prognostic value of cellular and serological markers in infection with human immunodeficiency virus type 1. *New England Journal of Medicine*, **322**, 166–172.

Fischl, M.A., Dickinson, G.M., Scott, G.B. *et al.* (1987) Evaluation of heterosexual partners, children, and household contact of adults with AIDS. *Journal of the American Medical Association*, **257**, 640–644.

Fischl, M.A., Stanley, K., Collier, A.C. *et al.* (1995) Combination and monotherapy with zidovudine and zalcitabine in patients with advanced HIV disease. *Annals of Internal Medicine*, **122**, 24–32.

Fricke, W., Augustyniak, L., Lawrence, D. *et al.* (1992) Human immunodeficiency virus infection due to clotting factor concentrates: results of the Seroconversion Surveillance Project. *Transfusion*, **32**, 707–709.

Friedman-Kien, A.E. (1981) Disseminated Kaposi-like sarcoma syndrome in young homosexual men. *Journal of the American Academy of Dermatology*, **5**, 468–471.

Gallant, J.E., Moore, R.D. and Chaisson, R.E. (1994) Prophylaxis for opportunistic infections in patients with HIV infection. *Annals of Internal Medicine*, **120**, 932–944.

Gallo, R.C. (1990) Mechanism of disease induction by HIV. *Journal of Acquired Immune Deficiency Syndromes*, **3**, 380–389.

Gallo, R.C., Salahuddin, S.Z., Popovic, M. *et al.* (1984) Frequent detection and isolation of cytopathic retroviruses (HTLV-III) from patients with AIDS and at risk for AIDS. *Science*, **224**, 500–503.

Gange, R.W. and Jones, E.W. (1978) Kaposi's sarcoma and immunosuppressive therapy: an appraisal. *Clinical and Experimental Dermatology*, **3**, 135–146.

Gayle, H.D., Keeling, R.P., Garcia-Tunon, M. *et al.* (1990) Prevalence of the human immunodeficiency virus among university students. *New England Journal of Medicine*, **323**, 1538–1541.

Gertner, J.M., Kaufman, F.R., Donfield, S.M. *et al.* (1994) Delayed somatic growth and pubertal development in human immunodeficiency virus positive hemophiliac boys: the Hemophilia Growth and Development Study. *Journal of Pediatrics*, **124**, 896–902.

Gjerset, G.F., Clements, M.J., Counts, R.B. *et al.* (1991) Treatment type and amount influenced human immunodeficiency virus seroprevalence of patients with congenital bleeding disorders. *Blood*, **78**, 1623–1627.

Goedert, J.J., Eyster, M.E., Biggar, R.J. and Blattner, W.A. (1987) Heterosexual transmission of human immunodeficiency virus: association with severe depletion of T-helper lymphocytes in men with hemophilia. *AIDS Research and Human Retroviruses*, **3**, 355–361.

Goedert, J.J., Kessler, C.M., Aledort, L.M. *et al.* (1989) A prospective study of human immunodeficiency virus type I infection and the development of AIDS in subjects with hemophilia. *New England Journal of Medicine*, **321**, 1141–1148.

Goedert, J.J., Cohen, A.R., Kessler, C.M. *et al.* (1994) Risks of immunodeficiency, AIDS, and death related to purity of factor VIII concentrate. *Lancet*, **344**, 791–792.

Goldsmith, J.M., Deutsche, J., Tang, M. and Green, D. (1991) CD4 cells in HIV-1 infected hemophiliacs: effect of factor VIII concentrates. *Thrombosis and Haemostasis*, **66**, 415–419.

Gottlieb, M.S., Schroff, R., Schanker, H.M. *et al.* (1981) *Pneumocystis carinii* pneumonia and mucosal candidiasis in previously healthy homosexual men: evidence of a new acquired cellular immunodeficiency. *New England Journal of Medicine*, **305**, 1425–1431.

Gringeri, A., Mannucci, P.M. and the Medical–Scientific Committee of the Fondazione dell'Emofilia (1988) National survey of human immunodeficiency virus infection in Italian hemophiliacs: 1983–1987. *La Ricercain Clinica e in Laboratorio*, **18**, 275–280.

Guo, H.G., Chermann, J.C., Waters, D. *et al.* (1991) Sequence analysis of original HIV-1. *Nature*, **349**, 745–746.

Gürtler, L.G., Wernicke, D., Eberle, J. *et al.* (1984) Increase in prevalence of anti-HTLV-III in haemophiliacs. *Lancet*, **2**, 1275–1276.

Gwinn, M., Pappaioanou, M., George, J.R. *et al.* (1991) Prevalence of HIV infection in childbearing women in the United States. Surveillance using newborn blood samples. *Journal of the American Medical Association*, **265**, 1704–1708.

Haas, J.S., Bolan, G., Larsen, S.A. *et al.* (1990) Sensitivity of treponemal tests for detecting prior treated syphilis during human immunodeficiency virus infection. *Journal of Infectious Diseases*, **162**, 862–866.

Hahn, B.H. (1992) Viral genes and their products, in *Textbook of AIDS Medicine* (eds S. Broder, T.C. Jr. Merigan and D. Bolognesi), Williams & Wilkins, Baltimore, MD, pp. 21–43.

Haim, S., Shafrir, A., Better, O.S. *et al.* (1972) Kaposi's sarcoma in association with immunosuppressive therapy. Report of two cases. *Israel Journal Medical Science*, **8**, 1993–1997.

Henrard, D.R., Phillips, J., Muenz, L.R. *et al.* (1995) Natural history of HIV-1 cell-free viremia. *Journal of the American Medical Association*, **274**, 554–558.

Heredia, A., Guo, Z.P., Yu, M.W. *et al.* (1994) Detection of HIV-1 by RNA PCR in factor VIII concentrates. *Vox Sanguinis*, **67**, 402–403.

Hilgartner, M.W., Buckley, J.D., Operskalski, E.A. *et al.* (1993) Purity of factor VIII concentrates and serial CD4 counts. *Lancet*, **341**, 1373–1374.

Holmes, E.C., Zhang, L.Q., MacKenzie, P. *et al.* (1992) Molecular epidemiology of HIV-1 in Edinburgh. *International Conference on AIDS*, **8**, abstract WeC 1026.

Horsburgh, C.R. and Selik, R.M. (1989) The epidemiology of disseminated nontuberculous mycobacterial infection in the acquired immunodeficiency syndrome (AIDS). *American Review of Respiratory Diseases*, **139**, 4–7.

Hoshaw, R.A. and Schwartz, R.A. (1980) Kaposi's sarcoma after immuno-suppressive therapy with prednisone. *Archives of Dermatology*, **116**, 1280–1282.

Hymes, K.B., Cheung, T., Greene, J.B. *et al.* (1981) Kaposi's sarcoma in homosexual men – a report of eight cases. *Lancet*, **2**, 598–600.

Jackson, J.B., Sannerud, K.J., Hopsicker, J.S. *et al.* (1988) Hemophiliacs with HIV antibody are actively infected. *Journal of the American Medical Association*, **260**, 2236–2239.

Jacobson, L.P., Kirby, A.J., Polk, S. *et al.* (1993) Changes in survival after acquired immunodeficiency syndrome (AIDS): 1984–1991. *American Journal of Epidemiology*, **138**, 952–964.

Jason, J. and Evatt, B.L. (1990) Pregnancies in human immunodeficiency virus-infected sex partners of hemophilic men. *American Journal of Diseases of Children*, **144**, 485–490.

Jason, J., Holman, R.C., Dixon, G. *et al.* (1986) Effects of exposure to factor concentrates containing donations from identified AIDS patients. A matched cohort study. *Journal of the American Medical Association*, **256**, 1758–1761.

Johnson, J.E. (1992) Detection of human immunodeficiency virus type 1 antibody by using commercially available whole-cell viral lysate, synthetic peptide, and recombinant protein enzyme immunoassay systems. *Journal of Clinical Microbiology*, **30**, 216–218.

Johnson, A.M. and Laga, M. (1988) Heterosexual transmission of HIV. *AIDS*, **2**, S49–S56.

Johnson, R.E., Lawrence, D.N., Evatt, B.L. *et al.* (1985) Acquired immuno-deficiency syndrome among patients attending hemophilia treatment centers and mortality experience of hemophiliacs in the United States. *American Journal of Epidemiology*, **121**, 797–810.

Johnson, P.D.R., Graves, S.R., Stewart, L. *et al.* (1991) Specific syphilis serological tests may become negative in HIV infection. *AIDS*, **5**, 419–423.

Kasper, C.K., Lusher, J.M. and the Transfusion Practices Committee (1993) Recent evolution of clotting factor concentrates for hemophilia A and B. *Transfusion*, **33**, 422–434.

Klepp, O., Dahl, O. and Stenwig, J.T. (1978) Association of Kaposi's sarcoma and prior immunosuppressive therapy: a 5-year material of Kaposi's sarcoma in Norway. *Cancer*, **42**, 2626–2630.

Krämer, A., Biggar, R.J., Fuchs, D. *et al.* (1990) Levels of CD4$^+$ lymphocytes, neopterin and beta-2-microglobulin are early predictors of acquired immunodeficiency syndrome, in *Human Immunodeficiency Virus: Innovative Techiniques. Monographs in Virology* (eds N.C. Khan and J.L. Melnick), S. Karger, Basel, pp. 61–73.

Kroner, B.L., Rosenberg, P.S., Aledort, L.M. *et al.* (1994) HIV-1 infection incidence among persons with hemophilia in the United States and Western Europe, 1978–1990. *Journal of Acquired Immune Deficiency Syndromes*, **7**, 279–286.

Kroner, B.L., Goedert, J.J., Blattner, W.A. *et al.* (1995) Concordance of human leukocyte antigen haplotype-sharing, CD4 decline and AIDS in hemophilic siblings. *AIDS*, **9**, 275–280.

Landonio, G., Cinque, P., Nosari, A. *et al.* (1993) Comparison of two dose regimens of zidovudine in an open, randomized, multicentre study for severe HIV-related thrombocytopenia. *AIDS*, **7**, 209–212.

Lawrence, D.N., Jason, J.M., Bouhasin, J.D. *et al.* (1985) HTLV-III/LAV-antibody status of spouses and household contacts assisting in home infusion of hemophilia patients. *Blood*, **66**, 703–705.

Lim, S.G., Lee, C.A. and Kernoff, P.B.A. (1990) The treatment of HIV associated thrombocytopenia in haemophiliacs. *Clinical Laboratory Haematology*, **12**, 237–245.

Lissen, E., Wichmann, I., Jimenez, J.M. and Andreu-Kern, F. (1983) AIDS in haemophilia patients in Spain. *Lancet*, **1**, 992–993.

Louwagie, J., Delwart, E.L., Mullins, J.I. *et al.* (1994) Genetic analysis of HIV-1 isolates from Brazil reveals presence of two distinct genetic subtypes. *AIDS Research and Human Retroviruses*, **10**, 561–567.

Ludlam, C.A., Tucker, J., Steel, C.M. *et al.* (1985) Human T-lymphotropic virus type III (HTLV-III) infection in seronegative haemophiliacs after transfusion of factor VIII. *Lancet*, **2**, 233–236.

McFadden, T., Jason, J.M. and Feorino, P. (1986) HTLV-III/LAV-seronegative, virus negative sexual partners and household contacts of hemophiliacs. *Journal of the American Medical Association*, **255**, 1702.

MacKenzie, W.R., Davis, J.P., Peterson, D.E. *et al.* (1992) Multiple false-positive serologic tests for HIV, HTLV-I, and hepatitis C following influenza vaccination, 1991. *Journal of the American Medical Association*, **268**, 1015–1017.

Magallon, M.M., Ortega, F. and Pinilla, J. (1992) AIDS and hemophilia: experience in the La Paz Hemophilia Center. *Haemostasis*, **22**, 281–292.

Malebranche, R., Arnoux, E., Guerin, J.M. *et al.* (1983) Acquired immuno-deficiency syndrome with severe gastrointestinal manifestations in Haiti. *Lancet*, **2**, 873–878.

Mann, D.L., Carrington, M.N. and Kroner, B.L. (1994) The human major histo-compatibility complex and HIV-1 pathogenesis. *AIDS*, **8** (suppl. 1), S53–S60.

Mannucci, P.M., Gringeri, A., Ammassari, M. *et al.* (1984) Abnormalities of lymphocyte subsets are correlated with concentrate consumption in asympto-matic Italian hemophiliacs treated with concentrates made from American plasma. *American Journal of Hematology*, **17**, 167–176.

Mannucci, P.M., Gringeri, A., Savidge, G. *et al.* (1994) Randomized double-blind, placebo-controlled trial of twice-daily zidovudine in asymptomatic haemo-philiacs infected with the human immunodeficiency virus type 1. *British Journal of Haematology*, **86**, 174–179.

Mariotto, A., Mariotti, S., Pezzotti, P. *et al.* (1992) Estimation of the acquired immunodeficiency syndrome incubation period in intravenous drug users: a comparison with male homosexuals. *American Journal of Epidemiology*, **135**, 428–437.

Marx, J.L. (1983) Acquired immune deficiency syndrome abroad. The new immune deficiency disease is now found in several countries: links to Central Africa and Haiti may provide clues to its origin. *Science*, **222**, 998–999.

Masur, H., Michelis, M.A., Greene, J.B. *et al.* (1981) An outbreak of community-acquired *Pneumocystis carinii* pneumonia: initial manifestation of cellular immune dysfunction. *New England Journal of Medicine*, **305**, 1431–1434.

Masur, H., Michelis, M.A., Wormeser, G.P. *et al.* (1982) Opportunistic infection in previously healthy women: initial manifestations of a community-acquired cellular immunodeficiency. *Annals of Internal Medicine*, **97**, 533–539.

Medical and Scientific Advisory Council (1982) *AIDS: Implications Regarding Blood Product Use*, National Hemophilia Foundation, New York.

Melbye, M., Froebel, K.S., Madhok, R. *et al.* (1984) HTLV-III seropositivity in European haemophiliacs exposed to factor VIII concentrate imported from the USA. *Lancet*, **2**, 1444–1446.

Merigan, T.C., Amato, D.A., Balsley, J. *et al.* (1991) Placebo-controlled trial to evaluate zidovudine in treatment of human immunodeficiency virus infection in asymptomatic patients with hemophilia. *Blood*, **78**, 900–906.

Meropol, N.J., Krause, P.R., Ratnoff, O.D. *et al.* (1989) Tendency to serious sequelae of infection with the human immunodeficiency virus in sibships with hemophilia. *Archives of Internal Medicine*, **149**, 885–888.

Mills, G.D. and Jones, P.D. (1993) Relationship between CD4 lymphocyte count and AIDS mortality, 1986–1991. *AIDS*, **7**, 1383–1386.

Moss, A.R., Bacchetti, P., Osmond, D. *et al.* (1988) Seropositivity for HIV and the development of AIDS or AIDS related conditions: three year follow up of the San Francisco General Hospital cohort. *British Medical Journal*, **296**, 745–750.

Muñoz, A., Schrager, L.K., Bacellar, H. *et al.* (1993) Trends in the incidence of outcomes defining acquired immunodeficiency syndrome (AIDS) in the Multicenter AIDS Cohort Study: 1985–1991. *American Journal of Epidemiology*, **137**, 423–438.

Myers, G., Korber, B., Smith, R.F. *et al.* (1992) *Human Retroviruses and AIDS 1992*, Los Alamos National Laboratory, Los Alamos, NM.

Nightingale, S.D., Byrd, L.T., Southern, P.M. *et al.* (1992) Incidence of Myco-bacterium avium intracellulare complex bacteremia in human immunodeficien-cy virus-positive patients. *Journal of Infectious Diseases*, **165**, 108–125.

Nunn, P., Mungai, M., Nyamwaya, J. *et al.* (1994) The effect of human immuno-deficiency virus type 1 on the infectiousness of tuberculosis. *Tuberculosis and Lung Diseases*, **75**, 25–32.

O'Brien, T.R., Busch, M.P., Donegan, E.A. *et al.* (1994) Heterosexual transmission of human immunodeficiency virus type 1 from transfusion recipients to their sex partners. *Journal of Acquired Immune Deficiency Syndromes*, **7**, 705–710.

Orgad, S., Malone, G., Zaizov, R. *et al.* (1987) Antibodies to HIV in Israeli hemophiliacs: relationship between serological profile and disease development. *AIDS Research and Human Retroviruses*, **3**, 323–332.

Pape, J.W., Liautaud, B., Thomas, F. *et al.* (1983) Characteristics of the acquired immunodeficiency syndrome (AIDS) in Haiti. *New England Journal of Medicine*, **309**, 945–950.

Phillips, A.N., Elford, J., Sabin, C. *et al.* (1992) Immunodeficiency and the risk of death in HIV infection. *Journal of the American Medical Association*, **268**, 2662–2666.

Piketty, C., Gilquin, J. and Kazatchkine, M.D. (1994) Successful treatment of HIV related thrombocytopenia with didanosine (DDI). *Journal of Acquired Immune Deficiency Syndromes*, **7**, 521–522.

Pitchenik, A.E., Fischl, M.A., Dickinson, G.M. *et al.* (1983) Opportunistic infections and Kaposi's sarcoma among Haitians: evidence of a new acquired immunodeficiency state. *Annals of Internal Medicine*, **98**, 277–284.

Pitchenik, A.E., Shafron, R.D., Glasser, R.M. and Spira, T.J. (1984) The acquired immunodeficiency syndrome in the wife of a hemophiliac. *Annals of Internal Medicine*, **100**, 62–65.

Pizzo, P.A., Wilfert, C.M. and the Pediatric AIDS Sienna Workshop II (1995) Markers and determinants of disease progression in children and HIV infection. *Journal of Acquired Immune Deficiency Syndromes and Human Retrovirology*, **8**, 30–44.

Pluda, J.M., Yarchoan, R., Jaffe, E.S. *et al.* (1990) Development of non-Hodgkin lymphoma in a cohort of patients with severe HIV infection on long-term antiretroviral therapy. *Annals of Internal Medicine*, **113**, 276–282.

Popovic, M., Sarngadharan, M.G., Read, E. and Gallo, R.C. (1984) Detection, isolation, and continuous production of cytopathic retroviruses (HTLV-III) from patients with AIDS and pre-AIDS. *Science*, **224**, 497–500.

Potts, K.E., Kalish, M.L., Lott, T. *et al.* (1993) Genetic heterogeneity of the V3 region of the HIV-1 envelope glycoprotein in Brazil. *AIDS*, **7**, 1191–1197.

Rabkin, C.S., Hilgartner, M., Hedberg, K.W. *et al.* (1992) Incidence of lymphomas and other cancers in HIV-infected and HIV-uninfected patients with hemophilia. *Journal of the American Medical Association*, **267**, 1090–1094.

Ragni, M.V. (1988) AIDS and the treatment of hemophilia patients. *Plasma Therapy and Transfusion Technology*, **9**, 173–191.

Ragni, M.V. and Kingsley, L.A. (1990) Cumulative risk for AIDS and other HIV outcomes in a cohort of hemophiliacs in Western Pennsylvania. *Journal of Acquired Immune Deficiency Syndromes*, **3**, 708–713.

Ragni, M.V., Tegtmeier, G.E., Levy, J.A. *et al.* (1986) AIDS retrovirus antibodies in hemophiliacs treated with factor VIII or factor IX concentrates, cryoprecipitate, or fresh frozen plasma: prevalence, seroconversion rate, and clinical correlations. *Blood*, **67**, 592–595.

Ragni, M.V., Winkelstein, A., Kingsley, L. *et al.* (1987) 1986 update of HIV seroprevalence, seroconversion, AIDS incidence, and immunologic correlates of HIV infection in patients with hemophilia A and B. *Blood*, **70**, 786–790.

Ragni, M.V., Kingsley, L.A., Nimorwicz, P. *et al.* (1989) HIV heterosexual transmission in hemophilia couples: lack of relation to T4 number, clinical diag-nosis, or duration of HIV exposure. *Journal of Acquired Immune Deficiency Syndromes*, **2**, 557–563.

Ragni, M.V., Bontempo, F.A., Myers, D.J. *et al.* (1990) Hemorrhagic sequelae of immune thrombocytopenic purpura in human immunodeficiency virus infected hemophiliacs. *Blood*, **75**, 1267–1272.

Ragni, M., Dafni, R., Amato, D.A. *et al.* (1992) Combination zidovudine and dideoxyinosine in asymptomatic HIV(+) patients (abstract no. MoB 0055). VIII International Conference on AIDS, Amsterdam, July 1992, Final Program and Oral Abstracts, p. Mo15.

Ragni, M., Amato, D., LoFaro, M. *et al.* (1993) CD4 response to antiviral therapy in HIV+ hemophilic men. *Blood*, **82** (suppl. 1), 413a.

Rarick, M.U., Espina, B., Montgomery, T. *et al.* (1991) The long-term use of zidovudine in patients with severe immune-mediated thrombocytopenia secondary to infection with HIV. *AIDS*, **5**, 1357–1362.

Rechavi, G., Ben-Bassat, M., Berkowicz, U. *et al.* (1987) Molecular analysis of Burkitt's leukemia in two hemophilic brothers with AIDS. *Blood*, **70**, 1713–1717.

Rosenberg, P.S., Biggar, R.J., Goedert, J.J. and Gail, M.H. (1991) Backcalculation of the number with human immunodeficiency virus infection in the United States. *American Journal of Epidemiology*, **133**, 276–285.

Rosenberg, P.S., Goedert, J.J. and Biggar, R.J. (1994) Effect of age at sero-conversion on the natural AIDS incubation distribution. *AIDS*, **8**, 803–810.

Roundtable Proceedings (1994) Clinical consensus on the management of HIV infection and disease. San Francisco, California, March 18–19, 1994. *Journal of Acquired Immune Deficiency Syndromes*, **7** (suppl. 2), S1–S49.

Rouzioux, C., Chamaret, S., Montagnier, L. *et al.* (1985) Absence of antibodies to AIDS virus in haemophiliacs treated with heat-treated factor VIII concentrate. *Lancet*, **1**, 271–272.

Saah, A.J., Hoover, D.R., He, Y. *et al.* (1994) Factors influencing survival after AIDS: report from the Multicenter AIDS Cohort Study (MACS). *Journal of Acquired Immune Deficiency Syndromes*, **7**, 287–295.

Safrin, S. (1994) Herpes simplex and varicella-zoster virus infections in HIV-infected individuals, in *Textbook of AIDS Medicine* (eds S. Broder, T.C. Merigan Jr. and D. Bologne), Willliams & Wilkins, Baltimore, MD, pp. 373–383.

St Louis, M.E., Rauch, K.J., Petersen, L.R. *et al.* (1990) Seroprevalence rates of human immunodeficiency virus infection at sentinel hospitals in the United States. *New England Journal of Medicine*, **323**, 213–218.

St Louis, M.E., Conway, G.A., Hayman, C.R. *et al.* (1991) Human immunodeficiency virus infection in disadvantaged adolescents. Findings from the US Job Corps. *Journal of the American Medical Association*, **266**, 2387–2391.

Sande, M.A. and Volberding, P.A. (1992) *Pneumocystis carinii* pneumonia – current concepts, in *Medical Management of AIDS*, 3rd edn (eds M.A. Sande and P.A. Volberding), W.B. Saunders, Philadelphia, pp. 261–283.

Sarngadharan, M.G., Popovic, M., Bruch, L. *et al.* (1984) Antibodies reactive with human T-lymphotropic retroviruses (HTLV-III) in the serum of patients with AIDS. *Science*, **224**, 506–508.

Sayers, M. H. (1988) Acquired immune deficiency syndrome and blood banking. *Plasma Therapy and Transfusion Technology*, **9**, 161–172.

Schinaia, N., Ghirardini, A., Chiarotti, F. *et al.* (1991) Progression to AIDS among Italian HIV-seropositive haemophiliacs. *AIDS*, **5**, 385–391.

Schinaia, N., Bellocco, R., Arcieri, R. and Zaccarelli, M. (1993) Time from diagnosis of acquired immune deficiency syndrome (AIDS) to death among persons with blood borne AIDS in Italy. *Transfusion*, **33**, 509–514.

Schüpbach, J., Popovic, M., Gilden, R.V. *et al.* (1984) Serological analysis of a subgroup of human T-lymphotropic retroviruses (HTLV-III) associated with AIDS. *Science*, **224**, 503–505.

Semple, M.G., Loveday, C., Preston, E. and Tedder, R.S. (1991) Detection of HIV-1 RNA in factor VIII concentrate. *AIDS*, **5**, 597–598.

Sepkowitz, K.A. and Armstrong, D. (1995) Treatment of opportunistic infections in AIDS. *Lancet*, **346**, 588–589.

Seremetis, S.V., Aledort, L.M., Bergman, G.E. *et al.* (1993) Three-year randomised study of high-purity or intermediate-purity factor VIII concentrates in symptom-free HIV seropositive haemophiliacs: effects on immune status. *Lancet*, **342**, 700–703.

Simonds, R.J. and Chanock, S. (1993) Medical issues related to caring for HIV-infected children in and out of the home. *Pediatric Infectious Disease Journal*, **12**, 845–852.

Smiley, M.L., White, G.C. II, Becherer, P. *et al.* (1988) Transmission of human immunodeficiency virus to sexual partners of hemophiliacs. *American Journal of Hematology*, **28**, 27–32.

Smith, R.S. and Parks, D.E. (1990) Synthetic peptide assays to detect human immunodeficiency virus types 1 and 2 in seropositive individuals. *Archives of Pathology and Laboratory Medicine*, **114**, 254–258.

Staszewski, S., Rehmet, S., Hofmeister, W.D. *et al.* (1988) Analysis of transmission rates in heterosexual transmitted HIV infection (abstract no. 4068). *IV International Conference on AIDS*, Stockholm, June 1988, Program and Abstracts, p. 276.

Telfer, P., Sabin, C., Devereux, H. *et al.* (1994a) The progression of HCV-associated liver disease in a cohort of haemophilic patients. *British Journal of Haematology*, **87**, 555–561.

Telfer, P.T., Brown, D., Devereux, H. *et al.* (1994b) HCV RNA levels and HIV infection: evidence for a viral interaction in haemophilic patients. *British Journal of Haematology*, **88**, 397–399.

Thorn, R.M., Beltz, G.A., Hung, C.H. *et al.* (1987) Enzyme immunoassay using a novel recombinant polypeptide to detect human immunodeficiency virus env antibody. *Journal of Clinical Microbiology*, **25**, 1207–1212.

US Department of Defense (1992) *Prevalence of HIV-1 Antibody In Civilian Applicants For Military Service, October 1985–March 1992*. Tables prepared by the Division of HIV/AIDS, Centers for Disease Control, Atlanta, Georgia.

Vieira, J., Frank, E., Spira, T.J. and Landesman, S.H. (1983) Acquired immune deficiency in Haitians: opportunistic infections in previously healthy Haitian immigrants. *New England Journal of Medicine*, **308**, 125–129.

Walzer, P.D., Perl, D.P., Krogstad, D.J. *et al.* (1974) *Pneumocystis carinii* pneumonia in the United States. Epidemiologic, diagnostic, and clinical features. *Annals of Internal Medicine*, **80**, 83–93.

Weiss, S.H., Goedert, J.J., Sarngadharan, M.G. *et al.* (1984) Screening test for HTLV-III (AIDS-agent) antibodies: specificity, sensitivity, and applications. *Journal of the American Medical Association*, **253**, 221–225.

Whitmore-Overton, S.E., Tillett, H.E., Evans, B.G. and Allardice, G.M. (1993) Improved survival from diagnosis of AIDS in adult cases in the United Kingdom and bias due to reporting delays. *AIDS*, **7**, 415–420.

Wolfs, T.F.W., Breederveld, C., Krone, W.J.A. *et al.* (1988) HIV-antibody seroconversions in Dutch haemophiliacs using heat-treated and non heat-treated coagulation factor concentrates. *Thrombosis and Haemostasis*, **59**, 396–399.

Yarchoan, R., Lietzau, J.A., Nguyen, B.Y. *et al.* (1994) A randomized pilot study of alternating or simultaneous zidovudine and didanosine therapy in patients with symptomatic human immunodeficiency virus syndrome. *Journal of Infectious Diseases*, **169**, 9–17.

Zhang, L.Q., Simmonds, P., Ludlam, C.A. and Brown, A.J.L. (1991) Detection, quantification and sequencing of HIV-1 from the plasma of seropositive individuals and from factor VIII concentrates. *AIDS*, **5**, 675–681.

26 NON-INFECTIOUS COMPLICATIONS OF HEMOPHILIA

C.R.M. Hay and P.H.B. Bolton-Maggs

The principal non-infectious complications of the use of clotting factor concentrates are transfusion reactions and modulation of immune function. Thrombosis, myocardial infarction and disseminated intravascular coagulation (DIC) have been reported following the use of factor IX and prothrombin complex concentrates. Hemolysis following large doses of factor VIII concentrate has also been reported but does not complicate treatment with more recent products of higher specific activity.

These are problems associated largely, but not exclusively, with the use of low-purity blood products such as cryoprecipitate or plasma, or intermediate-purity lyophylized freeze-dried clotting factor concentrates (specific activity of <2 iu/mg protein) rather than higher-purity concentrates (>150 iu/mg protein). All of these complications might be expected to become less common as high-purity clotting factor concentrates replace intermediate-purity products.

Immune-mediated

TRANSFUSION REACTIONS

Mild transfusion reactions occur relatively frequently following the administration of low- or intermediate-purity factor VIII concentrate and are found in up to 19% of infusions (Ahrons *et al.*, 1970; Eyster, Bowman and Haverstick, 1977; Ratnoff, 1984). These reactions may include symptoms of mild fever, nausea, rigors, headache and urticaria. Muscle cramps, backache and bronchospasm occur during more severe reactions. Severe pulmonary edema has also been reported after infusion of fresh frozen plasma and cryoprecipitate (Kernoff *et al.*, 1972; Reese, McCullough and Craddick, 1975). Such reactions were very common and often severe following plasma infusions and cryoprecipitate. Anaphylaxis occurs rarely, most often in patients with factor VIII inhibitors and particularly following the use of porcine factor VIII (Erskine and Davidson, 1981; Gringeri *et al.*, 1991; Hay *et al.*, 1996a).

Reactions are now rare, since high-purity factor VIII concentrates have largely superseded intermediate-purity products (Hay *et al.*, 1996b; Brown, 1990). Fewer than 15 reactions per year have been reported within the UK during the past 2 years, almost all following the use of intermediate-purity factor VIII concentrate, although occasional batches giving rise to reactions in a number of individuals have been withdrawn by the manufacturer over the years.

Reactions to porcine factor VIII fall into one of two patterns. Mild allergic idiosyncratic reactions occur in a minority of patients. Most reactions appear to be dose-related, occurring with large doses only, not recurring following subsequent infusions of smaller dose (Hay *et al.*, 1996a). Low doses of porcine factor VIII are rarely followed by reactions. Small doses (<50 u/kg) may safely be used as home therapy but larger doses should be administered under hospital supervision (Hay *et al.*, 1990, 1996a). This dose relationship may also be a reflection that larger doses tend to be given at a more rapid dose rate (Kernoff *et al.*, 1984).

No such dose relationship has been demonstrated with human factor VIII, although it is a common observation that some patients have repeated reactions with some brands of concentrate but not with other, apparently similar, products. A number of precipitating factors have been implicated in these reactions. Reactions may be commoner if the concentrate is infused very rapidly (Kernoff *et al.*, 1984). Class-specific anti-immunoglobulin A (IgA) antibodies found in IgA-deficient subjects may cause anaphylaxis when they are infused with plasma (Vyas, Perkins and Fudenberg, 1968). Occasional

Hemophilia. Edited by C.D. Forbes, L. Aledort and R. Madhok. Published in 1997 by Chapman & Hall, London. ISBN 0 412 63820 7

antibodies to Gm determinants of the immunoglobulin molecule may cause acute reactions (Prentice *et al.*, 1971). These antibodies are usually of low titer and are probably not a common cause of reactions (Kernoff and Bowell, 1973). Leukoagglutinins in donor plasma may also cause febrile reactions and pulmonary infiltrates (Mollison, 1979). Reactions may also be caused by particulate matter in clotting factor concentrates, and filter needles have been included with home treatment packs for many years to minimize this risk (Reese, McCullough and Craddoick, 1975; Eyster and Nau, 1978). There are reports that, despite the use of these filters, carbon monoxide diffusing capacity is impaired following factor VIII infusion, suggesting that the pore size may be too large (Boese, Tantum and Eyster, 1979; Chediak *et al.*, 1984). This transfer factor impairment was eliminated in one study by the use of a finer filter (Boese, Tantum and Eyster, 1979). The clinical significance of this small and clinically undetectable change in pulmonary function remains obscure.

Reactions may also occur following the administration of prothrombin complex concentrates, where activation products of the kinin system may be responsible. These give symptoms of flushing, tachycardia, headache and blood pressure changes, particularly if the concentrate is infused too rapidly or if the reconstituted product is left standing. Many clinicians administer prophylactic antihistamine before giving activated prothrombin complex concentrates, such as Autoplex, for this reason.

Mild reactions generally respond to stopping or slowing the rate of the factor VIII or IX infusion, or to intravenous antihistamine. It is doubtful whether the addition of intravenous hydrocortisone adds to the efficacy of the antihistamine, since it is slow-acting. Patients suffering repeated reactions should be changed from intermediate- to high-purity factor VIII or IX or to a different brand of high-purity concentrate. Alternatively, antihistamines may be administered before the infusion, but this may fail to prevent anaphylaxis in patients whose reactions are becoming progressively more severe.

Patients who have suffered anaphylaxis with porcine factor VIII or repeated minor reactions with every administration of this product should probably avoid further porcine factor VIII therapy altogether (Hay *et al.*, 1996a). Mild isolated reactions to large doses of porcine factor VIII are not a contraindication to further treatment with this product.

IMMUNE COMPLEXES IN HEMOPHILIA

Circulating immune complexes have been detected in up to 94% of patients with hemophilia using non-specific methods (McVerry *et al.*, 1977; Kazatchine *et al.*, 1980; Gomperts *et al.*, 1981; Poskitt *et al.*, 1981; Verroust *et al.*, 1981; Celada *et al.*, 1984; Passaleva *et al*, 1983; Hilgartner, 1984). Methods used to detect immune complexes are not specific to the antigen and provide no clue as to the origin or clinical significance of these circulating immune complexes.

Although complex-bound factor VIII activity and antifactor VIII activity have been detected in some patients (Kazatchine *et al.*, 1980; Nilsson *et al.*, 1990), the identity of the majority of such antigens remains unknown. This may be due to the technical difficulty encountered in retaining functionally active and immunologically intact immunoglobulin following dissociation of the immune complex. It is possible that most of these immune complexes are factor VIII–immunoglobulin complexes or factor VIII in non-inhibitor patients. Nilsson *et al.* (1990) demonstrated that such complexes arise following successful immune-tolerance induction and they may also circulate in patients in whom tolerance to factor VIII has developed naturally.

Immune complexes may also arise as a side-effect of the chronic liver disease which affects a high proportion of patients with severe hemophilia. Although immune complexes and immunoglobulins are infused in factor VIII and IX concentrate, their presence in the circulation does not correlate with the severity of the hemophilia, the intensity of treatment or the patient's age (McVerry *et al.*, 1977; Kazatchine *et al.*, 1980; Gomperts *et al.*, 1981; Poskitt *et al.*, 1981; Celada *et al.*, 1984), suggesting that the complexes detected in patients' plasma are not those infused with the concentrate. This does not exclude the possibility that circulating immune complexes may arise in relation to chronic antigenic stimulation from infused alloantigens in the concentrate. Impaired monocyte function, described in greater detail below (Mannhalter *et al.*, 1986; Eible *et al.*, 1987; Pasi and Hill, 1990), may also lead to impaired clearance of immune complexes.

The clinical significance of these circulating immune complexes remains obscure. Some hemophilic patients show clinical features similar to those found in systemic lupus erythematosus and rheumatoid arthritis, both of which may be associated with circulating immune complexes. Arthropathy and renal dysfunction may also relate to circulating immune complexes in some patients, but arthropathy is usually caused by repeated hemarthroses and renal disease is uncommon. Hilgartner (1984) has shown a correlation between the presence of circulating immune complexes and synovitis, although the synovial fluid from these patients contained very few immune complexes. Hilgartner also showed that the presence of immune complexes correlated with factor VIII inhibitor status and hematuria – an observation indirectly confirmed by Nilsson *et al.* (1990). Clinical experience tends to suggest that these immune complexes generally lack the size and capacity to activate complement since overt immune complex-disease, glomerulonephritis and vasculitis are not commonly observed in patients with hemophilia.

IMPAIRED CELL-MEDIATED IMMUNITY

In-vitro observations

Abnormalities of immune function have been observed to occur independently of human immunodeficiency virus (HIV) infection in hemophilic patients (Menitove *et al.*, 1983; Carr *et al.*, 1984; Madhok *et al.*, 1986). These abnormalities are not observed in untreated patients and do not appear to arise in patients treated with the latest generation of high-purity and recombinant concentrates (Teitel *et al.*, 1989; Cuthbert, Ludlam and Tucker, 1990; Evans *et al.*, 1991; Fukutake, Fujimaki and Hanabusa, 1991). Teitel and Evans have both suggested that the absence of immune modulation may be connected with the non-infectivity of these concentrates for hepatitis C. Immune dysfunction is first discernible during childhood and adolescence, but appears to remain stable through long periods during adult life (Kessler *et al.*, 1984; Shannon *et al.*, 1986; Cuthbert, Ludlam and Tucker, 1990). Although abnormalities of almost every aspect of immune function have been described, they are milder than those observed in patients symptomatic from HIV infection, and are not associated with susceptibility to opportunist pathogens.

The defects observed include decreased T-helper cell and increased T-suppressor cell numbers (Menitove *et al.*, 1983; Carr *et al.*, 1984; Madhok *et al.*, 1986), impaired cell-mediated immunity, as reflected by cutaneous anergy (Froebel *et al.*, 1983; Brettler *et al.*, 1986), monocyte dysfunction (Eible *et al.*, 1987; Pasi and Hill, 1990) and B-cell dysfunction (Madhok *et al.*, 1991). Many of these earlier reports should be interpreted with some caution because they antedate the discovery of the HIV virus, and include an unknown proportion of HIV-seropositive patients.

The degree to which different brands of factor VIII concentrate inhibit lymphocyte transformation following stimulation with lectins or phorbol esters varies considerably. Intermediate-purity concentrates exhibit up to 80% inhibition whilst monoclonally immunopurified plasma-derived and recombinant concentrates have little effect on this system (Hay and McEvoy, 1989, 1992). Concentrates fractionated by ion-exchange chromatography (specific activity > 150 iu/mg protein) and intermediate-purity concentrates (specific activity 2–5 iu/mg protein) inhibit lymphocyte transformation to the same degree (Hay and McEvoy, 1992).

Decreased lymphocyte secretion of interleukin-2 has also been demonstrated by several groups, both *in vivo* (Madhok *et al.*, 1990) and *in vitro* following incubation of mononuclear cells with factor VIII concentrates (Lederman *et al.*, 1986; Thorpe *et al.*, 1989; Wadwa *et al.*, 1992). The degree to which different types of factor VIII concentrate inhibit interleukin-2 (IL-2) secretion *in vitro* varies considerably and appears to reflect not only product purity as reflected by specific activity but also the method of fractionation used (Thorpe *et al.*, 1989). Concentrates purified by ion-exchange chromatography are far more inhibitory than concentrates of a similar specific activity purified using monoclonal immuno-affinity chromatography (Thorpe *et al.*, 1989). This suggests that if an impurity in the concentrate impairs lymphocyte function, this co-purifies with factor VIII during fractionation using ion-exchange chromatography, but not using monoclonal immunoaffinity chromatography (Hay and McEvoy, 1992).

Factor VIII concentrates also inhibit lymphocyte expression of Tac, the low mecular-weight moiety of the IL-2 receptor (Hay *et al.*, 1990). IL-2 secretion is inextricably linked by a positive-feedback loop to IL-2-receptor expression, since increased IL-2 secretion is dependent upon up-regulation of the IL-2 receptor and vice versa (Smith, 1984).

B-cell abnormalities include an increased concentration of B-cell growth and differentiation factors (Matheson *et al.*, 1987), the presence of partially activated B-cells (Madhok *et al.*, 1991). An increased incidence of auto-antibodies has also been described (Llopis *et al.*, 1986). These abnormalities may relate to the presence of chronic hepatitis C, and in some cases to HIV infection (Madhok *et al.*, 1991).

Eible and Mannhalter have shown that factor VIII concentrate inhibits monocyte phagocytosis, Fc-receptor production, antigen presentation and free radial production (Mannhalter *et al.*, 1986; Eible *et al.*, 1987; Pasi and Hill, 1990). Decreased red-cell phagocytosis was observed within an hour of factor VIII infusion, may be cumulative and appeared to be dose related (Pasi and Hill, 1990). Decreased Fc-receptor expression and decreased oxygen radial production are also observed *in vitro* when monocytes are incubated with factor VIII concentrate for as little as an hour (Mannhalter *et al.*, 1986; Eible *et al.*, 1987; Pasi and Hill, 1990). This may be caused by immunoglobulin and immune complexes or immunoglobulin aggregates, which are thought to block and down-regulate Fc-receptors (Eible *et al.*, 1987; Pasi and Hill, 1990). Mannhalter and Eible have suggested that picogram amounts of immunoglobulin aggregates, which may form during heat treatment of concentrates, may cause significant monocyte dysfunction.

Pasi and Hill have shown that concentrates differ in the degree to which they inhibit monocyte phagocytic activity. The degree of inhibition correlated roughly with product purity and immunoglobulin content; immunopurified concentrates had little effect, whereas intermediate-purity concentrates were profoundly inhibitory.

Although there is good evidence that immunoglobulin aggregates are a cause of monocyte dysfunction amongst hemophilic patients, the cause of the lymphocyte dysfunction is not known. Lymphocyte dysfunction may reflect hepatitis C infection (Evans *et al.*, 1991; Lee *et al.*, 1992), partly because hepatitis C-free hemophiliacs have not been shown to have immune dysfunction. Hemophilic patients uninfected with hepatitis C virus (HCV) have generally been treated with relatively pure factor VIII concentrates, and so it is impossible to determine whether HCV or increased product purity is responsible for the absence of immune dysfunction amongst these patients. Others have pointed to the importance of chronic exposure to alloantigens (Brettler and Levine, 1989) or to some other contaminant in the concentrate. Although the contaminant responsible remains to be identified, inhibition of lymphocyte function *in vitro* by chromatographically separated fractions of the concentrate indicates that most intermediate-purity and ion-exchange purified high-purity concentrates contain inhibitory activity in low-molecular-weight and high-molecular-weight fractions (Eible *et al.*, 1987; Wadwa *et al.*, 1992; Hay *et al.*, 1995b). This may be associated with transforming growth factor-β_1 (Wadwa *et al.*, 1992) or with amidolytic activity associated with high-molecular-weight kalkrein – α_2-macroglobulin complexes (Jones *et al.*, 1991; Hay *et al.*, 1995). The presence of either of these activities correlates well with the degree to which different brands of concentrate inhibit either lymphocyte transformation or IL-2 secretion.

The degree to which such *in vitro* experiments can be extrapolated to the clinical situation is always in some doubt, and so interest has increasingly focused upon epidemiologic evidence of immunomodulation, and clinical trials.

Clinical studies

Effect on the natural history of HIV infection. Following the suggestion of Margolick *et al.* (1987) that activation of the immune system may increase the rate of HIV viral replication, several groups have investigated the effect of high-purity factor VIII concentrates on immune-function and outcome in hemophiliacs infected with HIV. Several controlled trials have now shown that the CD4 count declines more rapidly in HIV-seropositive hemophiliac patients treated with intermediate-purity factor VIII concentrate than amongst those treated with monoclonally immunopurified factor VIII concentrate (Goldsmith *et al.*, 1991; de Biasi *et al.*, 1991; Seremetis *et al.*, 1993).

The longest-running and largest such trial is that of Seremetis *et al.*, in which 20 patients randomized to receive monoclonal factor VIII and 15 randomized to receive intermediate-purity factor VIII have completed 3 years' follow-up. A further 25 patients failed to complete

the follow-up. The CD4 count stabilized in the monoclonal arm but fell to half of the starting value in the intermediate-purity arm ($P = 0.007$). Stabilization of the CD4 count is not normally observed either in non-hemophiliacs with HIV infection or in hemophilic patients treated with high-purity factor VIII (Hilgartner *et al.*, 1993; Sabin *et al.*, 1994), suggesting that the data may have been biased by the 25 patients who failed to complete 3 years' follow-up. De Biasi *et al.* also reported similar results in two groups of 10 non-randomized patients matched for CD4 count at the outset following 2 years' treatment with either intermediate-purity or monoclonal immunopurified factor VIII (de Biasi *et al.*, 1991). This contrasts with the study of Mannucci *et al.*, who compared patients treated with intermediate-purity concentrate with patients treated with high-purity concentrate prepared by ion-exchange, rather than monoclonal immunoaffinity, chromatography. This study showed no significant difference in CD4 count between the two treatment arms after 2-year follow-up (Mannucci *et al.*, 1992). It is possible that the impurity responsible for immune modulation may copurify with factor VIII with ion-exchange but not immunoaffinity chromatography.

Both Hilgartner (1984), in a large cohort study of 498 hemophiliacs infected with HIV, and Sabin *et al.* (1994) in a much smaller study, have shown that the rate of decline of the CD4 count is reduced following the change from intermediate- to high-purity concentrate. The difference between the two treatment periods was not great, even when corrected for the intensity of treatment, and barely achieved statistical significance in either study. The Multicenter Hemophilia Cohort study has confirmed this slowing in the rate of decline of CD4 cells following the change from intermediate- to high-purity concentrate (Goedert *et al.*, 1994). Studies of this design suffer the weakness that they have historical controls, and also that there may be a natural slowing of the rate of decline of CD4 cell count as low values are reached. This change may not be attributable to the change in factor VIII concentrate. None of these three studies has shown any survival advantage from the change to high-purity concentrate even after prolonged follow-up, despite the widespread assumption that patients with higher CD4 counts will be less likely to develop an acquired immunodeficiency syndrome (AIDS)-defining illness. Extended clinical trials of zidovudine have also shown that the CD4 count is an imperfect predictor of the risk of AIDS and death (Concorde Coordinating Committee, 1994, Choi *et al.*, 1993).

Several large controlled studies have shown that hemophiliacs do not have a more rapid progression to AIDS than other AIDS risk groups, despite repeated exposure to the impurities in factor VIII concentrate (Jason *et al.*, 1989; Lee *et al.*, 1989; Berntorp, 1994). An effect of factor VIII concentrate on HIV disease progression cannot be dismissed on this basis, however, since the prevalence of other cofactors for HIV progression, such as cytomegalovirus (CMV) differs between AIDS risk groups. Coinfection with CMV, which is much commoner amongst homosexuals than amongst hemophiliacs (Lee *et al.*, 1989), may have a similar effect to that of factor VIII concentrate so that the two risk groups progress to AIDS at the same rate, affected by different cofactors for disease progression. Whether the purity of factor VIII concentrate affects the natural history of HIV or not, other factors such as age and genetically determined host-response appear to be more important (Simmonds *et al.*, 1991).

Effects in HIV-seronegative hemophilic patients. The *in vitro* defects of cellular immunity observed in hemophiliacs are comparable, although probably less marked, than those observed following blood transfusion. One might expect, for this reason, that hemophiliacs might have an increased tendency to develop malignancy and an increased susceptibility to infections, as has been observed following blood transfusion (Burrows and Tartter, 1982; Blumberg, Heal and Murphy, 1986; Tartter *et al.*, 1986; Dawes *et al.*, 1986; Quinter and Barron, 1986).

Mortality statistics from the pre-HIV era suggest that factor VIII concentrate may influence the cause of death in hemophiliacs who died between 1968 and 1979. Pneumonia accounted for 38% of deaths amongst patients under the age of 45 years – well in excess of the 8% of deaths which might have been expected from pneumonia in this age group (Aronson, 1988). A number of other unexpected and unusual causes of death were reported including two from *Candida albicans*, one from glandular fever and one from measles. This survey was based upon death certification data and should therefore be interpreted with caution. Rizza and Spooner (1983) also noted an unexpectedly high incidence of death from pneumonia amongst hemophilic patients dying in the UK between 1976 and 1980.

Blood transfusion has been reported to be an independent risk factor for postoperative infection in non-hemophilic patients (Dawes *et al.*, 1986; Tartter, Quintero and Barron, 1986). This risk may relate to the effect on the immune system of blood transfusion or to the degree of operative manipulation which is indirectly affected by the need for blood transfusion. Hemophiliacs might also be expected to have an increased risk of postoperative infection, if the risk of postoperative infection is related to immune dysfunction, although there are few published data to support this. Buehrer *et al.* (1990) found that HIV-positive patients had a 1.4% risk of postoperative infection but that none of the HIV-negative patients in their series of 102 patients undergoing orthopedic surgery suffer postoperative infection. Buehrer *et al.* reported only infections within the immediate postoperative period, whereas Green also reported late infections in 60 HIV-positive and HIV-negative hemophilic patients undergoing orthopedic surgery compared with a non-hemophilic control group (Green, DeGnore and White, 1990). The 10% of HIV-positive and 2% of HIV-negative hemophilic patients suffered an infection in the operative area (usually infected arthroplasty), compared with 0.5% amongst HIV-negative non-hemophilic patients. This would imply a fourfold increase in postoperative infection amongst HIV-negative hemophilic patients – a risk nevertheless much smaller than that observed amongst HIV-positive patients. All but one of these infections were late infections, often occurring years after the joint arthroplasty, usually with common pathogens such as staphylococci, *haemophilus* and pneumococci. Early postoperative infections are rare, even amongst HIV-positive hemophilic patients, but late infections appear significantly increased, even amongst HIV-negative patients. Although this has been attributed in the past to hematogenous spread of bacteria following hemarthroses, these joints usually bleed far less frequently following arthroplasty, and it seems more probable that this is evidence of a mild but clinically significant degree of immunosuppression.

An outbreak of pulmonary tuberculosis on a pediatric ward in 1981 provides provides further evidence that immune dysfunction in hemophilic patients may predispose to infection (Beddal *et al.*, 1985). In all, 126 children (30 hemophilia, 21 oncology and 75 general pediatric) were exposed to the index case, the mother of an inpatient with open tuberculosis who visited the ward over a 3-week period. Primary tuberculosis developed in 38% of the hemophiliac children, 48% of the oncology children and only 4% of the general pediatric children. This suggest that the children with hemophila were immunosuppressed to the same degree as the children with hematologic malignancy. This is particularly remarkable when one considers that most of the hemophilic children were outpatients who were only fleetingly in contact with the index case.

Hemophilic patients may be more susceptible to virus infections. Ludlam *et al.* (1985), reporting an outbreak of HIV related to a single batch of contaminated concentrate in a previously HIV-negative population, were able to show that those patients with the lowest CD4 cell count prior to exposure to HIV were most likely to become infected with the virus. This may be a reflection of inherited rather than acquired host factors, as subsequently suggested by the same group (Simmonds *et al.*, 1991).

There is no conclusive evidence that the immune dysfunction observed in HIV-negative hemophilic patients causes a clinically significant degree of immunosuppression. Such patients do not generally suffer infections with opportunist pathogens, and if they are more susceptible to infections with standard pathogens, then this is not obvious or marked.

Patients with hemophilia may have an increased risk of malignancy (Madhok *et al.*, 1987). Aronson noted a high incidence of carcinoma, particularly of the lung, but lacked the data necessary to assess whether the age-adjusted mortality from malignancy was increased. Given the median age at death of only 44 years in his series, one suspects that it was (Aronson, 1988). Rizza and Spooner (1983) also observed that 1% of UK hemophilic patients died from carcinoma – a higher incidence than one would expect from a population with a median age at death of 45 years. Rosendaal *et al.* (1989) observed a 2.5-fold age-adjusted excess incidence of carcinoma, particularly carcinoma of the lung, amongst 43 Dutch hemophiliacs who died between 1973 and 1986. Although these authors initially attributed this to smoking, a subsequent analysis showed that their patients did not smoke more than the population from which they were drawn. This suggests that hemophilic patients have an increased cancer risk which may relate to immune dysfunction. The evidence is not conclusive, however, and there is no evidence that tumors more usually associated with immune disturbance such as lymphomas and leukemias are increased in hemophiliacs.

The clinical significance of the defects of immune function detected *in vitro* remains the subject of debate. The evidence that patients with hemophilia who are not infected with HIV are significantly immunosuppressed is inconclusive and fragmentary, consisting of a series of observations open to other interpretations.

HEMOLYSIS

Low- and intermediate-purity blood products contain small quantities of blood group-specific isoagglutinins which may cause immune hemolysis. Immune-mediated hemolysis due to immune anti-A and anti-B has been described following the use of factor VIII concentrate, cryoprecipitate and pooled plasma (Seeler *et al.*, 1972; Orringer *et al.*, 1976). Most cases of hemolysis occurred following the administration of massive doses of factor VIII concentrate in inhibitor patients because of the relatively small amounts of isoagglutinins found in factor VIII concentrate (Oberman, Barnes and Ginther, 1966; Rosati *et al.*, 1970; Orringer *et al.*, 1976). Hemolysis has not been shown to complicate the administration of small doses of factor VIII (Orringer *et al.*, 1976).

The falling hemoglobin, reticulocytosis and mild fever which may accompany hemolysis may be misinterpreted as bleeding. The Coombs test is positive and spherocytes are commonly seen in the blood film. Other blood group substances may also potentially lead to sensitization in patients lacking that particular antigen (Hussain *et al.*, 1983).

Most reports of blood product-related hemolysis date from the 1970s and relate to the use of low-purity factor VIII concentrate or cryoprecipitate. These products were significantly contaminated with immunoglobulin. High-purity concentrates, whether prepared by ion-exchange or monoclonal immunoaffinity chromatography, contain only trace amounts of immunoglobulin and they do not cause immune hemolysis for this reason.

Non-immune-mediated

THROMBOSIS, MYOCARDIAL INFARCTION AND DIC

Thromboembolism, DIC and myocardial infarction associated with the use of factor IX and prothrombin complex concentrates (PCCs) have been recognized for more than 20 years (Kasper, 1973, 1975; Lusher, 1991; Thompson, 1993). Such complications are believed to be caused by the presence in PCCs of activated factor IX and X and VIIa (Seligsohn *et al.*, 1979; Hultin, 1983; Gray *et al.*, 1992). Intermediate-purity factor IX concentrates contain large quantities of factor II, IX and X and traces of activated factors Xa and IXa. Infusion of these additional factors and activated coagulation factors are thought to produce a hypercoagulable state contributing to the thrombotic tendency and disseminated intravascular coagulation which are clearly associated with the use of these products. The factor IXa concentration increases markedly on standing after reconstitution, and so these products should be administered immediately, to minimize the risk of thrombosis. The prothrombotic effect of PCCs and factor IX concentrates appear to be dose related, and thrombotic complications have not been reported in relation to the small doses of factor IX commonly used to treat routine hemarthroses.

Thrombotic problems occur most commonly in patients with other risk factors, or with underlying cardiovascular disease. Thrombosis is particularly common in factor IX-deficient patients who are elderly, undergoing surgery with intensive replacement therapy (Kasper, 1973; Machin and Miller, 1978), and those who are immobile for prolonged periods. The release of thromboplastic substances following head injury, intracerebral bleeding or crush injuries also appears to predispose certain individuals to thrombosis following the use of PCCs and factor IX concentrate. Patients with pre-existing liver disease (Gazzard *et al.*, 1974; Kasper, 1975; Davey, Shashaby and Rath, 1976; Cederbaum, Blatt and Roberts, 1976) and premature infants (Kasper, 1975) seem particularly susceptible to develop DIC when treated with PCCs or factor IX concentrate.

Thrombotic problems have been reported in patients as young as 6 years of age. Several such serious and alarming cases are described by Lusher (1991). These cases include a child of 4 who developed DIC after treatment for a circumcision; a 9-year-old who developed renal failure and extensive femoral and iliofemoral thrombosis with DIC following treatment for a gangrenous appendix; and a 6-year-old who died from complications, including DIC, venous thrombosis and pulmonary embolism, following treatment for a displaced fracture of the elbow. These complications followed the use of a variety of different PCCs, and were not associated with supraphysiologic factor IX levels. More recently, eight cases of thromboembolism were reported to the UK Haemophilia Centre Directors Adverse Events Working Party over a $2^1/_2$-year period. All of these events followed surgery. No thrombotic events were reported following the use of small doses of intermediated-purity factor IX for hemarthroses (Preston, 1991).

There have been 20 reported instances of myocardial infarction in inhibitor patients treated with PCCs or activated PCCs (Agarwal, 1981; Fuerth, 1981; Gruppo *et al.*, 1983; Sullivan, 1984; Chavin, 1988; Lusher, 1991). Rather alarmingly, most occurred in young patients; the first four cases were reported between the ages of 15 and 22 years (Agarwal, Zelkowitz and Hletko, 1981; Gruppo *et al.*, 1983; Sullivan and Loyer 1993). Several died: transmural myocardial hemorrhage was the most striking pathologic feature on postmortem examination. Some, but not all, of these patients had been given very large doses of PCC and one or two had also been given antifibrinolytic treatment; however, most had been treated fairly conventionally with repeated doses of PCC or activated PCC. These infarcts were presumably thrombotic, the transmural hemorrhage being a reflection of the underlying bleeding disorder.

THE PREVENTION OF THROMBOSIS WITH FACTOR IX AND PCCS

The addition of 5–10 u/ml of heparin to the concentrate was found to reduce thrombogenicity in the Wessler stasis model (Kingdon *et al.*, 1975), leading the International Society of Thrombosis and Haemostasis (ISTH) Taskforce to recommend addition of heparin to the concentrates (Menache and Roberts, 1975). Antithrombin III (ATIII) has also been added to some concentrates, but has little effect on the Wessler stasis model (Prowse *et al.*, 1979), whereas the addition of both heparin and ATIII appears to have an increased effect on the NAPTT, an *in vitro* screen for thrombogenicity still routinely used by the manufacturers but falling into disrepute (White *et al.*, 1977; Chandra and Wickerhauser, 1978; Prowse *et al.*, 1979).

The addition of heparin, with or without ATIII, does not offer full protection from the thrombotic risks of PCCs and intermediate-purity factor IX concentrates (Campbell *et al.*, 1978). These risks may be minimized by avoiding large and repetitive dosing of PCC or activated PCC in inhibitor patients and using high-purity factor IX concentrate in patients with hemophilia B. If a hemarthrosis in an inhibitor patient fails to respond to two or three doses of PCC then the patient should be offered an alternative treatment, since it is unlikely that he will respond to further treatment with PCCs. Muscle bleeds in such patients, which would require relatively prolonged and intensive treatment with PCCs to obtain a clinical response, should be treated with human or porcine factor VIII or recombinant VIIa. PCCs should only be used with the greatest caution in neonates and patients with liver disease. The concentrate should be infused immediately after reconstitution to minimize activation of factor IX *in vitro*. PCCs should not be used in combination with antifibrinolytic therapy, which may theoretically increase the thrombotic risk.

Patients treated with factor IX concentrate who undergo orthopedic or general surgery are at least as great a risk of thromboembolism as non-hemophilic patients, and should be offered appropriate thromboprophylaxis including subcutaneous heparin (Goudemand *et al.*, 1993).

The use of intermediate-purity factor IX concentrates has been abandoned in favor of newer high-purity products in many countries. As early as 1991, the evidence that high-purity factor IX concentrates were not thrombogenic was considered sufficiently compelling that the UK Haemophilia Centre Directors Organization (UKHCDO) recommended that hemophilia B only be treated with high-purity factor IX concentrates (UKHCDO, 1992).

These high-purity factor IX concentrates are purified using metal chelate or immunoaffinity chromatography (Feldman *et al.*, 1991; Goldman *et al.*, 1992; Kim *et al.*, 1992; Thomas *et al.*, 1995). They have been used extensively for surgery in patients with hemophilia B without thrombotic complications (Bardin and Sultan, 1990; Goldsmith *et al.*, 1992; Tengborn *et al.*, 1993; Thomas *et al.*, 1995). They do not cause measurable activation of coagulation, in contrast with PCCs. Plasma concentrations of fibrinopeptide A (FPA), thrombin–antithrombin complexes (TAT) and prothrombin peptide F1+2 (F1+2) increase significantly following infusion of PCCs, indicating activation of coagulation and thrombin generation, but do not change following the infusion of high-purity factor IX concentrate (Mannucci *et al.*, 1990, 1991; Hampton *et al.*, 1993; Thomas *et al.*, 1995). There is now considerable clinical experience with these high-purity concentrates.

Although intermediate-purity factor IX concentrates are much less widely used for hemophilia B than they were, PCCs continue to be used for the treatment of patients with hemophilia A and factor VIII inhibitors. These patients remain at risk of thromboembolism, DIC and myocardial infarction, although this risk may be reduced in the future, should recombinant VIIa replace PCC. Recombinant VIIa appears to be substantially free from prothrombotic complications.

FACTOR XI DEFICIENCY AND ITS TREATMENT

Factor XI deficiency (hemophilia C) is autosomally inherited, and even in its most severe form (factor XI level below 1%) is associated with a mild and variable bleeding tendency which is only evident after surgery or injury. Spontaneous bleeding has been reported but is rare.

In the past, fresh frozen plasma was the treatment of choice to cover surgical procedures, but had the major disadvantage of volume and the risk of transfusion-associated viruses. Three different factor IX concentrates have been produced in recent years and used with varying results (Gitel *et al.*, 1991; Bolton-Maggs *et al.*, 1992; Burnouf-Radesovich and Burnouf, 1992). The alarming report of Gitel *et al.* described the treatment of 3 patients. Two of these showed elevated D-dimers. One received the product to cover coronary bypass grafting, but died postoperatively with all grafts occluded. No manufacturing details were given in this short report (Gitel *et al.*, 1991).

Since 1985 a factor XI concentrate has been available on a named-patient basis manufactured in the UK (Bioproducts Ltd. UK). Activated factor XI is known to be very thrombogenic, but cannot be detected in this concentrate. Nevertheless, small amounts of heparin and large amounts of ATIII have been added to this concentrate to reduce the thrombotic risk which might be associated with its use. Initial clinical experience in 30 patients showed that it was hemostatically effective and that there were no significant adverse events (Bolton-Maggs *et al.*, 1992). The patients, aged 5–79 years, had baseline factor XI levels of <1% to 47%.

More recent experiments have shown that doses two to four times greater than those recommended showed a thrombotic effect in the Wessler venous stasis model equivalent to that found with intermediate-purity factor IX concentrates (Winkelman *et al.*, 1993). Although there is no published evidence, there have been a number of adverse events reported in recent years, some difficult to evaluate, which suggest that this concentrate may be thrombogenic (Bolton-Maggs *et al.*, 1994). Four patients have been reported, including a 61-year-old female who developed a probable pulmonary embolism 21 days after coronary artery bypass grafting. Three other patients, aged 66, 74 and 85 years, died of cardiovascular complications, two with myocardial infarction and one from a stroke, within a few days of factor XI concentrate administration. Both patients who suffered myocardial infarction were known to have pre-existing ischemic heart disease. In the light of these cases, the manufacturer's recommended maximum dose was reduced to 30 iu/kg. Formal *in vivo* thrombogenicity trials similar to those already conducted for factor IX concentrates are urgently needed. In the meanwhile, this concentrate should be used with caution in the elderly and in those with pre-existing ischemic heart disease.

A third factor XI concentrate is manufactured in France (CRTS Lille, France; Radosevich and Burnouf 1992). This product has not been shown to contain factor XIa and contains no added ATIII, but does not apparently cause thrombosis in the Wessler rabbit ear model. When infused into two patients with severe factor XI deficiency (factor XI level <1%), there was clear evidence of activation of coagulation (Mannucci *et al.*, 1992). One patient was a 19-year-old undergoing surgery for a pilonidal sinus and the other a 69-year-old undergoing mastectomy for carcinoma of the breast. Both showed elevation of fibrinopeptide A, F1+2 levels and D-dimers. The second patient had more severe derangements, with a fall in platelet count and fibrinogen. Neither patient had clinical evidence of thrombosis or DIC.

While there are factor XI concentrates available that are hemostatically effective, it is clear that they cause activation of coagulation and thrombosis in some patients. Until safer factor XI concentrates become available it may be prudent to use the currently available concentrates with caution. Heparin deep venous thrombosis prophylaxis should be offered. The concentrates should probably only be used in homozygotes with low baseline factor XI levels and should be used with great caution in the elderly.

Conclusion

Although low- and intermediate-purity blood products are still widely used worldwide, they have been largely superseded in Europe, North America and other areas by high-purity concentrates prepared using ion-exchange or monoclonal immunoaffinity chromatography. Transfusion reactions are rare and usually very mild following the use of these products. These concentrates also have little effect on immune function. The recently introduced high-purity factor IX preparatins and recombinant VIIa also appear to be free from the thrombogenic risk observed with the use of PCCs. High-purity clotting factor concentrates are significantly more expensive to manufacture than intermediate- or low-purity products. It is likely, therefore, that the intermediate-purity products will be widely used for some time to come.

References

Agarwal, B.L., Zelkowitz, L. and Hletko, J. (1981) Acute myocardial infarction in a young hemophiliac patient during therapy with factor IX concentrate and epsilon aminocaproic acid. *Journal of Pediatrics*, 98, 931–933.
Ahrons, S., Glavind-Kristensen, S., Drachmann, O. and Kissmeyer-Nillson, F. (1970) Severe reactions after cryoprecipitated human factor VIII. *Vox Sanguinis*, 18, 181–186.
Aronson, D.L. (1988) Cause of death in hemophilia A patients in the United States from 1968–1979. *American Journal of Haematology*, 27, 7–12.
Bardin, J.M. and Sultan, Y. (1990) Faactor IX concentrate versus prothrombin complex concentrate for the treatment of haemophilia B during surgery. *Transfusion*, 30, 441–443.
Beddal, A.C., Hill, F.G.H., George, R.H. *et al.* (1985) Unusually high incidence of tuberculosis among boys with haemophilia during an outbreak of the disease in hospital. *Journal of Clinical Pathology*, 38, 1163–1165.

Berntorp, E. (1994) Impact of replacement therapy on the evolution of HIV infection in hemophiliacs. *Thrombosis and Haemostasis*, **71**, 678–683.

Blumberg, N., Heal, J.M. and Murphy, P. (1986) Association between transfusion of whole blood and recurrence of cancer. *British Medical Journal*, **293**, 530–533.

Brettler, D.B. and Levine, P.H. (1989) Factor concentrates for the treatment of hemophilia: which one to choose? *Blood*, **73**, 2067–2073.

Brettler, D.B., Forsberg, A.D., Brewster, F. *et al.* (1986) Delayed cutaneous hypersensitivity reactions in hemophilic subjects treated with factor concentrate. *American Journal of Medicine*, **81**, 607–611.

Boese, E.C., Tantum, K.R. and Eyster, M.E. (1979) Pulmonary function abnormalities after infusion of antihemophilic factor (AHF) concentrates. *American Journal of Medicine*, **67**, 474–478.

Bolton-Maggs, P.H.B., Wensley, R.T., Kernoff, P.B.A. *et al.* (1992) Production and therapeutic use of factor XI concentrate from plasma. *Thrombosis and Haemostasis*, **67**, 314–319.

Bolton-Maggs, P.H.B., Colvin, B.T., Satchi, G. *et al.* (1994) Thrombogenic potential of factor XI concentrate. *Lancet*, **344**, 748–749.

Brown, C.P. (1990) Adverse events reported in association with the use of monoclonal antibody purified factor VIIIC: Monoclate. *Seminars in Haematology*, **27** (suppl. 2), 16–17.

Buehrer, J.L., Weber, D.J., Meyer, A.A. *et al.* (1990) Wound infection rates after invasive procedures in HIV-1 seropositive versus HIV-seronegative hemophiliacs. *Annals of Surgery*, **211**, 492–498.

Burnouf-Radosevich, M. and Burnouf, T. (1992) A therapeutic highly purified factor XI concentrate from human plasma. *Transfusion*, **32**, 861–867.

Burrows, L. and Tartter, P.I. (1982) Effect of blood transfusion on colonic malignancy recurrence rate. *Lancet*, **ii**, 662–665.

Carr, R., Edmond, E., Prescott, R.J. *et al.* (1984) Abnormalities of circulating lymphocyte subsets in haemophiliacs in an AIDS-free population. *Lancet*, **i**, 1431–1434.

Cederbaum, A.I., Blatt, P.M. and Roberts, H.R. (1976) Intravascular coagulation with use of human prothrombin complex concentrates. *Annals of Internal Medicine*, **84**, 683–684.

Celada, A., Agudo, M.T., Maire, M. *et al.* (1984) Effect of circulating immune complexes on transfusional therapy in patients with hemophilia or von Willebrand's disease. *Transfusion*, **24**, 46–50.

Chandra, S. and Wickerhauser, M. (1978) Large scale preparation of nonthrombogenic prothrombin complex. *Thrombosis Research*, **12**, 571–577.

Chavin, S.I., Siegel, D.M. and Rocco, T.A. (1988) Acute myocardial infarction during treatment with an activated prothrombin complex concentrate in a patient with factor VIII deficiency and a factor VIII inhibitor. *American Journal of Medicine*, **85**, 245–249.

Chediak, J., Chaisow, A., Solarski, A. and Telfer, M.C. (1984) Pulmonary function in hemophilic patients treated with commercial factor VIII concentrates. *American Journal of Medicine*, **77**, 293–297.

Choi, S., Lagakos, S.W., Schooley, R.T. and Volberding, P.A. (1994) CD4⁺ lymphocytes are an incomplete surrogate marker for clinical progression in persons with asymptomatic HIV infection taking zidovudine. *Annals of Internal Medicine*, **118**, 675–680.

Concorde Coordinating Committee (1994) Concorde: MRC/ANRS randomised double-blind controlled trial of immediate and deferred zidovudine in symptom-free HIV infection. *Lancet*, **343**, 871–881.

Cuthbert, R.J.G., Ludlam, C.A. and Tucker, J. (1990) Five year prospective study of HIV infection in the Edinburgh haemophilic cohort. *British Medical Journal*, **301**, 956–961.

Davey, R.J., Shashaty, G.G. and Rath, C.E. (1976) Acute coagulopathy following infusion of prothrombin complex concentrates. *American Journal of Medicine*, **60**, 719–722.

David, J. (1987) Immune response mechanisms, in: *Scientific American Medicine* vol. 4 (eds E. Rubenstein and D.D. Federman), Scientific American, New York, pp. 41–50.

Dawes, L.G., Aprahamian, C., Conoin, R.E. and Malangoni, M.A. (1986) The risk of infection after colon injury. *Surgery*, **100**, 796–803.

De Biasi, R., Rocino, A., Miraglia, E. *et al.* (1991) The impact of very high purity factor VIII concentrate on the immune system of HIV infected haemophiliacs: a randomised prospective, 2 year comparison with intermediate purity concentrate. *Blood*, **78**, 1919–1923.

Eible, M.M., Ahmad, R., Wolf, H.M. *et al.* (1987) A component of factor VIII preparations which can be separated from factor VIII activity down modulates human monocyte functions. *Blood*, **69**, 1153–1160.

Erskine, J.G. and Davidson, J.F. (1981) Anaphylactic reaction to low molecular weight porcine factor VIII concentrates. *British Medical Journal*, **282**, 654–655.

Evans, J.A., Pasi, K.J., Williams, M.D. and Hill, F.G.H. (1991) Consistently normal CD4⁺, CD8⁺ levels in haemophilic boys only treated with a virally safe factor VIII concentrate. *British Journal of Haematology*, **79**, 457–461.

Eyster, M.E. and Nau, M.E. (1978) Particulate material in antihaemophilic factor (AHF) concentrates. *Transfusion*, **18**, 576–580.

Eyster, M.E., Bowman, H.S. and Haverstick, J.N. (1977) Adverse reactions to factor VIII infusions. *Annals of Internal Medicine*. **87**, 248–251.

Feldman, P.A., Harris, L., Evans, D.R. and Evans, H.E. (1991) Preparation of a high-purity factor IX concentrate using metal chelate affinity chromatography,

in *Biotechnology of Blood Proteins*, vol. 227 (eds C. Rivat and J.F. Stolz), Inserm/Libbey, Eurotext, pp. 63–68.

Froebel, K.S., Madhok, R., Forbes, C.D. *et al.* (1983) Immunological abnormalities in haemophilia: are they caused by American factor VIII concentrate? *British Medical Journal*, **287**, 1091–1093.

Fuerth, J.H. and Maher, P. (1981) Myocardial infarction after factor IX therapy. *Journal of the American Medical Association*, **245**, 1455–1456.

Fukutake, K., Fujimaki, M. and Hanabusa, S. (1991) Multicentre study on the influence of long term continuous use of ultrapurified factor VIII preparation on the immunological status of HIV infected and non-infected haemophilia A₂ patients. *Thrombosis and Haemostasis*, **65**, 996.

Gazzard, B.G., Lewis, M.L., Ash, G. *et al.* (1974) Coagulation factor concentrate in the treatment of the haemorrhagic diathesis of fulminant hepatic failure. *Gut*, **15**, 993–996.

Gitel, S.N., Varon, D., Schulman, S. and Martinowitz, U. (1991) Clinical experience with a FXI concentrate: possible side-effects. *Thrombosis and Haemostasis*, **65**, 1157.

Goedert, J.J., Cohen, A.R., Kessler, C.M., Eichinger, S., Seremetis, S.V., Rabkin, C.S., Yellin, F.J., Rosenberg, P.S. and Aledort, L.M. (1994) Risks of immunodeficiency, AIDS and death related to purity of factor VIII concentrate. *Lancet*, **344**, 791–792.

Goldsmith, J.M., Deutche, J., Tang, M. and Green, D. (1991) CD4 cells in HIV-1 infected hemophiliacs: effect of factor VIII concentrates. *Thrombosis and Haemostasis*, **66**, 415–419.

Goldsmith, J.M., Kasper, C.K., Blatt, P.M. *et al.* (1992) Coagulation factor IX: successful surgical experience with a purified factor IX concentrate. *American Journal of Haematology*, **40**, 210–215.

Gomperts, E.D., Jordan, S., Berg, D. *et al.* (1981) Circulating immune complexes pre and post clotting factor infusion in hemophilia. *Thrombosis and Haemostasis*, **46**, 694–698.

Goudemand, J., Marey, A., Caron, C. *et al.* (1993) Clinical efficacy of a highly purified SD-treated factor IX concentrate prepared by conventional chromatography. *Transfusion Medicine*, **3**, 299–305.

Gray, E., Tubbs, J., Cesmeli, S. and Barrowcliffe, T.W. (1992) Thrombogenicity of factor IX concentrates: *in vitro* and *in vivo* results. *British Journal of Haematology*, **80** (suppl. 1), 20.

Green, W.B., DeGnore, L.T. and White, G.C. (1990) Orthopaedic procedures and prognosis in hemophilic patients who are seropositive for human immunodeficiency virus. *Journal of Bone and Joint Surgery*, **72**, 2–11.

Gringeri, A., Santagostino, E., Tradati, F. and Mannucci, P.M. (1991) Adverse effects of treatment with porcine FVIII. *Thrombosis and Haemostasis*, **65**, 245–247.

Gruppo, R.A., Bove, K.E. and Donaldson, V.E. (1983) Fatal myocardial necrosis associated with prothrombin complex concentrate therapy in hemophilia A. *New England Journal of Medicine*, **309**, 242–243.

Hampton, K.K., Preston, F.E., Lowe, G.D.O. *et al.* (1993) Reduced coagulation activation following infusion of a highly purified factor IX concentrate compared to a prothrombin complex concentrate. *British Journal of Haematology*, **84**, 279–284.

Hay, C.R.M. and McEvoy, P. (1989) The variable effect of diverse clotting factor concentrates on lymphocyte function *in vitro*. *Thrombosis and Haemostasis*, **62**, 452.

Hay, C.R.M. and McEvoy, P. (1992) Purity of factor VIII concentrates. *Lancet*, **339**, 1613.

Hay, C.R.M., Preston, F.E., Triger, D.R. and Underwood, J.C.E. (1985) Progressive liver disease in haemophilia: an understated problem? *Lancet*, **i**, 1495–1498.

Hay, C.R.M., Laurian, Y., Verroust, F., Preston, F.E. and Kernoff, P.B.A. (1990) Induction of immune-tolerance in patients with hemophilia A and inhibitors treated with porcine FVIII:C by home therapy. *Blood*, **76**, 882–886.

Hay, C.R.M., McEvoy, P. and Duggan-Keen, M. (1990) Inhibition of lymphocyte IL2 receptor expression by factor VIII concentrate: a possible cause of immunosuppression in haemophiliacs. *British Journal of Haematology*, **75**, 278–281.

Hay, C.R.M., McKernan, A.M., Winter, M., Galimore., M. and Jones, W. (1995) Lymphocyte dysfunction related to amidolytic activity of factor VIII concentrates. *Thrombosis and Haemostasis*, **73**, 1017.

Hay, C.R.M. Lozier, J.N., Lee, C.A., Laffan, M., Tradati, F., Santagostino, E., Ciavarella, N., Shiavoni, M., Fukui, H., Yoshioka, A., Teitel, J., Mannucci, PM. and Kasper, C.K. (1996a) Porcine factor VIII therapy for patients with haemophilia A and inhibitors. *Thrombosis and Haemostasis*, **75**, 25–29.

Hay, C.R.M., Lee, C.A. and Savidge, G.F. (1996b) A post marketing survcillance study of a high-purity, monoclonally immunopurified factor VIII concentrate. *Haemophilia*, **2**, 32–36.

Hilgartner, M. (1984) Antigen–antibody complexes in hemophilia. *Scandinavian Journal of Haematology*, **33**, 335–340.

Hilgartner, M.W., Buckley, J.D., Operskalski, E.A. *et al.* (1993) Purity of factor VIII concentrates and serial CD4 counts. *Lancet*, **341**, 1373–1374.

Hultin, M.B. (1983) Studies of factor IX concentrate therapy in haemophilia. *Blood*, **62**, 797–801.

Jason, J., Lui, K.J., Ragni, M.V. *et al.* (1989) Risk of developing AIDS in HIV-infected cohorts of hemophilic and homosexual men. *Journal of the American Medical Association*, **261**, 725–724.

Jones, D.W., Winter, M. and Gallimore, M. (1991) Proteolytic activity in commercial factor VIII concentrates. *British Journal of Haematology*, 77, 41.

Kasper, C.K. (1973) Postoperative thromboses in hemophilia. *New England Journal of Medicine*, 289, 160.

Kasper, C.K. (1975) Thromboembolic complications. *Thrombosis et Diathesis Haemorrhagica*, 33, 640–644.

Kazatchine, M.D., Sultan, Y., Burton-Kee, E.J. and Mowbray, J.F. (1980) Circulating immune complexes containing anti-VIII antibodies in multi-transfused patients with haemophilia A. *Clinical and Experimental Immunology*, 39, 315–320.

Kernoff, P.B.A. and Bowell, P.J. (1973) Gm types and antibodies in multitransfused haemophiliacs. *British Journal of Haematology*, 24, 443–447.

Kernoff, P.B.A., Durrant, I.J., Rizza, C.R. and Wright, F.W. (1972) Severe allergic pulmonary oedema after plasma transfusion. *British Journal of Haematology*, 23, 777–781.

Kernoff, P.B.A., Thomas, N.D., Lilley, P.A. et al. (1984) Clinical experience with polyelectrolyte-fractionated porcine factor VIII concentrate in the treatment of haemophiliacs with antibodies to factor VIII. *Blood*, 63, 31–41.

Kessler, C.M., Schulof, R.S., Alibaster, O. et al. (1984) Inverse correlation between age-related abnormalities of T-cell immunity and circulating thymosin alpha-1 levels in haemophilia A. *British Journal of Haematology*, 58, 325–336.

Kim, H.C., McMillan, C.W., White, G.C. et al. (1992) Purified factor IX prepared using monoclonal immunoaffinity technique: clinical trials in haemophilia B and comparisons to prothrombin complex concentrates. *Blood*, 79, 568–575.

Kingdon, H.S., Lundblad, R.C., Veltkamp, J.J. and Aronson, D.L. (1975) Potentially thrombogenic materials in factor IX concentrates. *Thrombosis et Diathesis Haemorrhagica*, 33, 617–621.

Koretz, R.L., Stone, D. and Gitnick, G.L. (1980) The long-term course of non-A, non-B hepatitis. *Gastroenterology*, 79, 893–898.

Lederman, M.M., Saunders, C., Toosi, Z. et al. (1986) Antihaemophilic factor preparations inhibit lymphocyte proliferation and production of interleukin 2. *Journal of Laboratory and Clinical Medicine*, 107, 471–478.

Lee, C.A., Kernoff, P/B/A/, Karayiannis, P. et al. (1985) Interactions between hepatotropic viruses in patients with haemophilia. *Journal of Hepatology*, 1, 379–384.

Lee, C.A., Phillips, A.N., Elford, J. et al. (1989) The natural history of human immunodeficiency virus infection in a haemophilic cohort. *British Journal of Haematology*, 73, 228–234.

Llopis, F., Gonzalez-Molina, A., Aznar, J.A. et al. (1986) Autoantibodies in haemophilia A and B. *Thrombosis and Haemostasis*, 55, 292.

Ludlam, C.A., Tucker, J., Steel, C.M. et al. (1985) Human T-lymphocyte virus type III (HTLV-III) infection in seronegative haemophiliacs after transfusion of factor VIII. *Lancet*, ii, 233–236.

Lusher, J.M. (1991) Thrombogenicity associated with factor IX complex concentrates. *Seminars in Haematology*, 28 (suppl. 6), 3–5.

Machin, S.J. and Miller, B.R. (1978) Thrombosis and factor IX concentrate. *Lancet*, i, 1367.

McVerry, B.A., Voke, J., Mohammed, I. et al. (1977) Immune complexes and abnormal liver function in haemophilia. *Journal of Clinical Pathology*, 30, 1142–1146.

Madhok, R., Gracie A., Lowe, G.D.O. et al. (1986) Impaired cell mediated immunity in haemophilia in the absence of infection with human immuno-deficiency virus. *British Medical Journal*, 293, 978–980.

Madhok, R., Lowe, G.D.O., Forbes, C.D. and Stewart, C.J.R. (1987) Extranodal lymphoma in a haemophiliac negative for antibody to HIV-1. *British Medical Journal*, 294, 679–680.

Madhok, R., Gracie, J.A., Smith, J. et al. (1990) Capacity to produce interleukin 2 is impaired in haemophilia in the absence and presence HIV 1 infection. *British Journal of Haematology*, 76, 70–74.

Madhok, R., Gracie, J.A., Forbes, C.D. and Lowe, G.D.O. (1991) B cell dysfunction in haemophilia in the absence and presence of HIV-1 infection. *Thrombosis and Haemostasis*, 65, 7–10.

Mannhalter, J.W., Zlabinger, G.J., Ahmad, R. et al. (1986) A functional defect in the early phase of the immune-response observed in patients with haemophilia A. *Clinical Immunology and Immunopathology*, 38, 390–397.

Mannucci, P.M., Gringeri, A., De Biasi, R. et al. (1992) Immune status of asymptomatic HIV-infected haemophiliacs: randomised comparison of treatment with high-purity with intermediate-purity factor VIII concentrate. *Thrombosis and Haemostasis*, 67, 310–313.

Margolick, J.B., Volkman, D.J., Folks, T.M. and Fauci, A.S. (1987) Amplification of HTLV-III/LAV infection by antigen-induced activation of T-cells by antigen-induced activation of T-cells and direct suppression by virus of lymphocyte blastogenic responses. *Journal of Immunology*, 138, 1719–1723.

Matheson, D.S., Green, B.J., Fritzler, M.J. et al. (1987) Humoral immune response in patients with haemophilia. *Clinical Immunology and Immuno-pathology*, 4, 41–50.

Menache, D. and Roberts, H.R. (1975) Summary and recommendations of the Task Force members and consultants. *Thrombosis et Diathesis Haemorrhagica*, 33, 645–646.

Menitove, J.E., Aster, R.H., Kasper, J.T. et al. (1983) T-lymphocyte subpopulations in patients with classical hemophilia treated with cryoprecipitate and lyophylised concentrates. *New England Journal of Medicine*, 308, 83–86.

Mollison, P.L. (1979) Some unfavourable effects of transfusion, in *Blood Transfusion and Clinical Medicine*, 6th edn, Blackwell Scientific, Oxford.

Nilsson, I.M., Berntorp, E., Zettervall, O. et al. (1990) Noncoagulation inhibitory factor VIII antibodies after induction of tolerance to factor VIII in hemophilia A patients. *Blood*, 75, 378–383.

Oberman, H.A., Barnes, B.A. and Ginther, P.L. (1966) Erythrocyte sensitisation and anaemia due to isoantibodies in lyophilised pooled plasma. *Journal of the American Medical Association*, 198, 233–235.

Orringer, E.P., Koury, M.J., Blatt, P.M. and Roberts, H.R. (1976) Haemolysis caused by factor VIII concentrates. *Archives of Internal Medicine*, 136, 1018–1020.

Pasi, K.J. and Hill, F.G.H. (1990) *In vitro* and *in vivo* inhibition of monocyte phagocytic function by factor VIII concentrates: correlations with concentrate purity. *British Journal of Haematology*, 76, 88–93.

Passaleva, A., Massai, G., Morlini, M. et al. (1983) Circulating immune-complexes in haemophilia and von Willebrand's disease. *Scandinavian Journal of Haematology*, 31, 466–470.

Poskitt, T.R., Poskitt, P.K.F. Bean, C.A. and Arkel, Y.S. (1981) Immune complexes in hemophilia. *American Journal of Hematology*, 11, 147–149.

Prentice, C.R.M., Izzat, M.M., Adams, J.F. et al. (1971) Amyloidosis associated with the nephrotic syndrome and transfusion reactions in a haemophiliac. *British Journal of Haematology*, 21, 305–308.

Proud, G., Shenton, B.K. and Smith, B.M. (1979) Blood transfusion and renal transplantation. *British Journal of Surgery*, 66, 678–682.

Prowse, C.V., Boffa, M.C., Guthrie, C., and Pepper, D.S. (1979) *In vitro* thrombogenicity tests of factor IX concentrates II: effects of phospholipids and heparin. *Thrombosis and Haemostasis*, 42, 1368–1372.

Ratnoff, O.D. (1984) Some complications of therapy of classical haemophilia. *Journal of Laboratory and Clinical Medicine*, 103, 653–659.

Reese, E.P., McCullough, J.J. and Craddoick, P.R. (1975) An adverse pulmonary reaction to cryoprecipitate in a haemophiliac. *Transfusion*, 15, 583–584.

Rizza, C. and Spooner, R.J.D. (1983) Treatment of haemophilia and related disorders in Britain and Northern Ireland during 1976–80: report on behalf of the directors of haemophilia centres in the United Kingdom. *British Medical Journal*, 286, 829–833.

Rosati, L.A., Barnes, B., Oberman, H.A. et al. (1970) Haemolytic anaemia due to anti-A in concentrated antihaemophilic factor preparation. *Transfusion*, 10, 139–141.

Rosendaal, F.R., Varekamp, I., Smit, C. et al. (1989) Mortality and causes of death in Dutch haemophiliacs, 1973–86. *British Journal of Haematology*, 71, 71–76.

Sabin, C., Pasi, J., Phillips, A. et al. (1994) CD4[+] counts before and after switching to monoclonal high-purity factor VIII concentrate in HIV-infected haemophilic patients. *Thrombosis and Haemostasis*, 72, 214–217.

Seeler, R.A. (1972) Haemolysis due to an anti-A and anti-B in factor VIII preparations. *Archives of Internal Medicine*, 130, 101–103.

Seligsohn, U., Kasper, C.K., Oserud, B. and Rapaport, S.I. (1979) Activated factor VIIL presence in factor IX concentrates and persistence in the circulation after infusion. *Blood*, 53, 828–833.

Seremetis, S., Aledort, L., Bergman, G.E. et al. (1993) Three year randomised study of high-purity or intermediate-purity factor VIII concentrates in symptom-free HIV-seropositive haemophiliacs: effects on immune-status. *Lancet*, 342, 700–703.

Shannon, B.T., Roach, J., Cheek-Luten, M. et al. (1986) progressive change in lymphocyte distribution and degree of hypogammaglobulinaemia with children with haemophilia. *Journal of Clinical Immunology*, 6, 121–129.

Simmonds, P., Beatson, D., Cuthbert, R.J.G. et al. (1991) Determinants of HIV disease progression: six-year longitudinal study in the Edinburgh haemophilia/HIV cohort. *Lancet*, 338, 1156–1159.

Smith, K.A. (1984) Interleukin 2. *Annual Reviews of Immunology*, 2, 319–333.

Spero, J.A., Lewis, J.H., Van Thiel, D.H. et al. (1978) Asymptomatic structural liver disease in haemophiliacs. *New England Journal of Medicine*, 31, 779–783.

Sullivan, Y. and Loyer, F. (1993) *In vitro* evaluation of factor VIII bypassing activity of activated prothrombin complex concentrate, and factor VIIa in the plasma of patients with factor VIII inhibitors: thrombin generation test in the presence of collagen-activated platelets. *Journal of Laboratory and Clinical Medicine*, 121, 444–452.

Tartter, P.I., Quintero, S. and Barron, D.M. (1986) Perioperative blood transfusion associated with infectious complications after colorectal cancer operations. *American Journal of Surgery*, 152, 479–482.

Teitel, J.M., Freedman, J.J., Garvey, M.B. and Kardish, M. (1989) Two year evaluation of clinical and laboratory variables of immune function in 117 hemophiliacs seropositive or seronegative for HIV-1. *American Journal of Hematology*, 32, 262–272.

Tengborn, I., Stigendal, L., Gustafsson, G. et al. (1993) Treatment with factor IX concentrate in a patient with factor IX concentrate in a patient with moderate haemophilia B undergoing bilateral total hip replacement. *Transfusion*, 33, 936–939.

Thomas, D.P., Lee, C.A., Colvin, B.T. et al. (1995) Clinical experience with highly purified factor IX concentrate in patients undergoing surgical operations. *Haemophilia*, 1, 17–23.

Thompson, A.R. (1993) Factor IX concentrates for clinical use. *Seminars in Thrombosis and Haemostasis*, 19, 25–36.

Thorpe, R., Dilger, P., Dawson, N.J. and Barrowcliffe, T.W. (1989) Inhibition of interleukin-2 secreted by factor VIII concentrates: a possible cause of immunospression in haemophiliacs. *British Journal of Haematology*, **71**, 387–391.

UK Haemophilia Centre Directors Organization (1992) Recommendation on choice of therapeutic products for the treatment of patients with haemophilia A, haemophilia B and von Willebrand's disease. *Blood Coagulation and Fibrinolysis*, **3**, 205–214.

Verroust, F., Adam, C., Kourilski, O. *et al.* (1981) Circulating immune complexes and complement levels in hemophilic children. *Journal of Clinical and Laboratory Immunology*, **6**, 127–131.

Vyas, G.N., Perkins, H.A. and Fudenberg, H.H. (1968) Anaphylactoid transfusion reactions associated with anti-IgA. *Lancet*, **ii**, 312–314.

Wadwa, M., Dilger, P., Tubbs, J. *et al.* (1992) Mechanisms of inhibition of T cell IL-2 secretion by factor VIII concentrates. *British Journal of Haematology*, **82**, 578–583.

Wadwa, M., Dilger, P., Thorpe, R. *et al.* (1993) TGF-Beta 1 as an immunosuppressive contaminant of factor VIII concentrate. *Blood Coagulation and Fibrinolysis*, **4** (suppl. 8).

White, G.C., Roberts, H.R., Kingdon, H.S and Lundblad, R.L. (1977) Prothrombin complex concentrates: potentially thrombogenic materials and clues to the mechanism of thrombosis *in vivo. Blood*, **49**, 159–162.

Winkelman, L., McLaughlin, L.F., Gray, E. and Thomas, S. (1993) Heat treated factor XI concentrate: evaluation of *in vivo* thrombogenicity in two animal models. *Thrombosis and Haemostasis*, **69**, 538–545.

27 SAFER CLOTTING FACTOR CONCENTRATES

P.R. Foster, B. Cuthbertson, R.V. McIntosh and A.J. MacLeod

A range of products are available for the treatment of hemophilia (Drohan and Hoyer, 1994), including various concentrates of factor VIII and of factor IX derived from human plasma and biosynthetic factor VIII products prepared in animal cell culture using recombinant DNA technology. The latter products are currently being introduced into clinical practice and a biosynthetic factor IX concentrate is under development (Keith *et al.*, 1994) There have been major changes since the early 1980s in the processing of plasma-derived products (Kasper *et al.*, 1993) aimed primarily at removing the risk of viral infection and increasing substantially the specific activity of factor VIII or factor IX.

Although significant advances have been made in the manufacture of coagulation factor concentrates, their safety can still be improved and issues which remain to be resolved include:

- The possible residual risk of viral infection, especially from hepatitis B virus (HBV), hepatitis A virus (HAV), B19 parvovirus (B19) or any unknown or emerging infectious agents (Murphy, 1994).
- The formation of inhibitors to factor VIII and the possibility that the incidence or the severity of those inhibitors may be product-related.
- A risk of product-related thromboembolic complications in the treatment of hemophilia B.

In this chapter the greatest attention will be given to the risk of viral infection as this aspect of safety remains the most important issue in the manufacture and selection of products for clinical use (Bray and Aledort, 1994). In considering the risks of product-related infection, the manufacturing procedures that are being used to address the possibility of virus contamination will be outlined, instances of continuing product-related virus transmission will be examined, the limitations of some of the manufacturing procedures will be described and developments to enhance product safety further will be identified.

Methods and procedures for the elimination or inactivation of viruses in the manufacture of coagulation factor concentrates

SELECTION OF BLOOD OR PLASMA DONATIONS

Testing for the presence of viruses

The first viral disease known to be transmitted by plasma derivatives was hepatitis and a correlation between the Australia antigen and posttransfusion hepatitis (Gocke, Greenberg and Kavey, 1970) led to the introduction, in the early 1970s of the first-generation tests for hepatitis B surface antigen (HBsAg) for the screening of blood donations. The current enzyme immunoassay method is sensitive to antigen levels of about 0.1–0.3 iu/ml, but some carriers of HBV have antigen levels below this limit of detection and the risk of an infectious donation from the USA testing negative has been estimated to be 1 in 200 000 (Center for Disease Control, 1991; Dodd, 1992).

During the 1970s it became evident that HBV was not the only cause of posttransfusion hepatitis and in the mid-1980s two surrogate tests aimed at detecting non-A non-B hepatitis (NANBH) became available. These were the hepatitis B core antibody (HBcAb) test (Koziol *et al.*, 1986) and the alanine aminotransferase test (ALT), a measure of liver function (Aach *et al.*, 1981). These surrogate tests have been largely superseded by a test for hepatitis C virus antibody (HCV Ab) which became

Hemophilia. Edited by C.D. Forbes, L. Aledort and R. Madhok. Published in 1997 by Chapman & Hall, London. ISBN 0 412 63820 7

available in 1990 (Kuo *et al.*, 1989). With the introduction of a second-generation enzyme-linked immunosorbent assay (ELISA), the risk of an HCV Ab-negative blood donation in the USA being infectious has been estimated to be about 1 in 4000 (Alter, 1995). A third-generation assay is now available, and its use should reduce this figure further (Buffet *et al.*, 1994)

The epidemic of acquired immunodeficiency syndrome (AIDS) and the isolation of a viral agent, the human immunodeficiency virus (HIV), resulted in an HIV antibody test becoming available in 1985. A more sensitive assay, which could detect HIV-2 as well as HIV-1, was subsequently developed using recombinant DNA-derived antigen (Lelie *et al.*, 1989) and with this type of assay, the risk of an HIV Ab-negative blood donation being infectious has been estimated to be about 1 in 400 000 (Lackritz *et al.*, 1995). Donor screening is not yet undertaken routinely for the other viruses known to be transmissible by plasma derivatives, i.e. HAV, HDV and B19 (Table 27.1).

Other selection criteria

In addition to tests for the viral infections noted above, donors are also tested for syphilis and questioned to discover if they may be at risk from infection, for example, recipients of human growth hormone should be excluded because of a possible risk of infection with Creutzfeldt–Jakob disease (CJD), which may be transmissible by blood products (Nau, 1995). An increased risk of infection may also be associated with intravenous drug abuse, sexual behavior and travel in areas where an infectious disease is endemic, therefore the self-exclusion of donors who fall into a defined risk category is encouraged (Pindyck, Waldman and Zang, 1985). For similar

reasons, donations collected from prison inmates carry a higher risk of infection and should also be excluded. In general, plasma obtained from non-remunerated donors carries a lower risk of transmitting a viral infection (Leikola, 1993) and, for this reason, it has been recommended that all plasma products should be prepared from plasma of this type (EEC, 1989).

Coagulation factor concentrates are prepared from relatively large volumes of plasma obtained by pooling individual donations and in some instances over 15 000 donations may be used to prepare a single batch of concentrate. In these circumstances the risk of a plasma pool being infectious depends on the number and volume of donations used, as well as on the effectiveness of donation testing and selection procedures. When individual plasma pools have been examined for evidence of HCV infection, most pools from paid donors have been found to be contaminated, whereas pools derived from non-remunerated donors tested negative (Minor *et al.*, 1990; Simmonds *et al.*, 1990). Similarly, HCV was detectable by polymerase chain reaction (PCR) in 10 of 13 batches of FVIII prepared from the plasma of paid donors compared with 1 of 5 from unpaid donors (Garson *et al.*, 1990). A requirement for the routine testing of plasma pools for the absence of HBsAg and antibodies to HIV and HCV has since been introduced in Europe (EEC Ad Hoc Working Party on Biotechnology/Pharmacy, 1994).

TESTING AND SELECTION OF OTHER BIOLOGIC SUBSTANCES

A number of biological substances other than human plasma may be used in the manufacture of coagulation factor concentrates (Table 27.2) This is especially the case with recombinant product and with plasma-derived

Table 27.1 Features of viruses known to be transmissable by plasma derivatives

Virus	Classification	Nucleic acid	Lipid-enveloped	Size (nm)
Human immuno-deficiency virus-1–2 (HIV-1–2)	Retrovirus	ss-RNA	Yes	80–100
Hepatitis A virus (HAV)	Picornavirus	ss-RNA	No	25–30
Hepatitis B virus (HBV)	Hepadna virus	Partly ds-DNA	Yes	42
Hepatitis C virus (HCV)	Flavivirus	ss-RNA	Yes	40–50
Hepatitis D virus (HDV)	Deltavirus	ss-RNA	Yes	32
Human parvovirus (B19)	Parvovirus	ss-DNA	No	20

ss = Single-stranded; ds = double-stranded.
Data from White, D.O. and Fenner, F.J. (1994) *Medical Virology*, 4th edn, Academic Press, San Diego.

Table 27.2 Biologic substances used in the manufacture of factor VIII (FVIII) concentrates

Biologic substance	Source of substance	Purpose	*Use in the manufacture of FVIII*		
			Conventional plasma products	*Immunopurified plasma products*	*Recombinant products*
Human plasma	Blood or plasma donors	Source of natural FVIII	+	+	–
Transfected cells	Hamster ovaries or kidneys	Source of recombinant FVIII	–	–	+
Monoclonal antibodies	Murine ascites or cultured cells	Protein purification	–	+	+
Serum and/or serum proteins	Bovine plasma	Cell growth supplements	–	(+)	+
Insulin	Bovine pancreas	Cell growth supplement	–	(+)	+
Aprotinin	Bovine lung	Protease inhibitor	–	(+)	+
Heparin	Bovine or porcine mucosa	Protein purification and stabilizer	(+)	(+)	(+)
Albumin	Human plasma	Stabilizer	(+)	+	+

+ = Normally used; – = not normally used; (+) = may be used by some manufacturers.

products where monoclonal antibodies are used for immunopurification. The cell lines used in these processes are screened for a wide range of animal viruses (Feldman *et al.*, 1992; Koplove, 1994) because of the possibility of contamination with pathogenic agents (Food and Drug Administration, 1993, 1994). Bovine cell culture supplements used in the preparation of recombinant products (Adamson, 1994; Koplove, 1994) must be obtained from disease-free sources, to avoid contamination with the infectious agent responsible for bovine spongiform encephalopathy (BSE).

PROCESSES FOR THE PREPARATION OF COAGULATION FACTOR CONCENTRATES

Factor VIII concentrates

Products for the treatment of hemophilia A were first prepared from human plasma over 40 years ago by cold-ethanol precipitation of a factor VIII-rich fraction (fraction I) from pooled donations of plasma (Cohn *et al.*, 1946; Blomback and Blomback, 1956; van Creveld *et al.*, 1959; McMillan, Diamond and Surgenor, 1961). These products were normally freeze-dried and, although stable with a factor VIII activity (VIII:C) of about 1 iu/ml, carried a risk of bacterial contamination because of the absence of sterilizing filtration (Cumming *et al.*, 1965). The use of cryoprecipitate (Hershgold, Pool and Pappenhagen, 1966), together with developments in its extraction and clarification when obtained from large

pools of plasma (Newman *et al.*, 1971), enabled more concentrated solutions of VIII:C to be filtered to 0.2 μm, prior to aseptic dispensing and freeze-drying. The convenience of preparations of this type, the assurance of freedom from bacterial contamination and the applicability of these processes to large-scale manufacture led to their widespread use from the early 1970s to the mid-1980s. This type of product (product A, Table 27.3) was the starting point for a number of developments, with additional process steps being incorporated to inactivate potential viral contaminants, and to obtain more highly purified and potent preparations. The integration of additional protein separation technology into earlier manufacturing methods required the stability of VIII:C during processing to be increased (Foster *et al.*, 1983a, 1988a), suitable chromatographic media and procedures to be developed (Hrinda, Feldman and Schreiber, 1990; Burnouf *et al.*, 1991; Griffin, 1991; Brockway and Seng, 1994; Josic *et al.*, 1994) and solution formulations suitable for highly purified preparations to be devised (McIntosh and Foster, 1990).

A large number of manufacturers prepare factor VIII:C from plasma, in both commercial and not-for-profit operations (World-Wide Directory of Plasma Fractionators, 1990; Foster, 1994a), and a variety of process methods are used (Kasper *et al.*, 1993). The principal processing steps employed and their purpose are summarised in Table 27.4 where the type of product (Table 27.3) obtained by a given combination of process steps is also indicated.

Table 27.3 Different types of factor VIII concentrate prepared from human plasma

Type	Product description
A	Typical concentrates prior to 1984, specific activity 0.5–2.0 iu/mg, e.g. Factorate (Armour), Hemofil (Baxter), Koate (Cutter), 8A (BPL), NY (PFC)
B	Terminal (dry) heat-treated concentrates from 1983, specific activity 0.5–2.0 iu/mg, e.g. HT-Factorate (Armour), Hemofil T (Baxter), Koate HT (Cutter), NY-HT (PFC)
C	Severe terminally (dry) heat-treated concentrates from 1985, specific activity 0.5–5.0 iu/mg, e.g. 8Y (BPL), Z8 (PFC)
D	Pasteurized concentrates, from 1981, specific activity 15 iu/mg, e.g. Haemate-P (Behringwerke), Koate-HS (Cutter)
E	Solvent/detergent-treated, from 1985, specific activity 1 iu/mg, e.g. FVIII-SD (NYBC)
F	Solvent/detergent-treated and ion-exchange-purified, from 1988, specific activity 50–200 iu/mg, e.g. Melate (NYBC), Octa VI (Octapharma), Innovate (Lille), Liberate (PFC), Emoclot (AIMA)
G	Solvent/detergent-treated and immuno/affinity purified from 1988, specific activity 2–20 iu/mg (inclusive of added albumin), e.g. Hemofil M (Baxter), Alpha-8 HP (Alpha), 8SM (Kabi), Replenate (BPL)
H	Pasteurized and immunopurified, from 1990, specific activity 5–10 iu/mg (inclusive of added albumin), e.g. Monoclate-P (Armour)

Table 27.4 Principal steps used in the manufacture of plasma-derived factor VIII (FVIII) concentrates

Step	Purpose of step	Use by type of product*							
		A	B	C	D	E	F	G	H
Cryoprecipitation	Removal and concentration of FVIII from plasma	+	+	+	+	+	+	+	+
Precipitation of protein from FVIII solution	Separation of FVIII from least soluble proteins	+	+	+	+	+	+	+	+
Adsorption of protein from FVIII solution with aluminium hydroxide	Removal of residual coagulation factors II, VII, IX and X. Clarification and stabilization of the FVIII solution	(+)	(+)	(+)	(+)	(+)	(+)	(+)	(+)
Heating 60°C 10 h	Virus inactivation	–	–	–	+	–	–	–	+
Solvent/detergent treatment	Virus inactivation	–	–	–	–	+	+	+	–
Immuno/affinity chromatography	Removal of process reagents and further purification of FVIII	–	–	–	–	–	–	+	+
Ion-exchange chromatography	Removal of process reagents and further purification of FVIII	–	–	–	(+)	–	+	+	–
Size exclusion chromatography	Product formulation	–	–	(+)	(+)	–	–	–	–
Filtration to 0.2 μm	Removal of bacteria	+	+	+	+	+	+	+	+
Freeze-drying	Stabilization	+	+	+	+	+	+	+	+
Heating 60–68°C	Virus inactivation	–	+	–	–	–	–	–	–
Heating 80°C	Virus inactivation	–	–	+	–	–	–	–	–

*See Table 27.3 for a description of the product type.
+ = Step used; – = step not used; (+) = step used for some products of this type.

Manufacturing processes for the preparation of recombinant factor VIII have been designed to separate factor VIII from cell culture supernatant and depend predominantly on a series of chromatographic steps including immunoaffinity, anion exchange, cation exchange and size exclusion (Griffin *et al.*, 1991; Boedeker, 1992; Lawrence, 1994). This extensive processing is required to remove cell-derived proteins, media components, potential viral contaminants and cellular DNA, which may be oncogenic (World Health Organization, 1987; Avest *et al.*, 1992; Ng and Mitra, 1994).

Factor IX Concentrates

Factor IX concentrates for the treatment of hemophilia B were first developed over 30 years ago. The earliest products were prepared via calcium phosphate adsorption of plasma anticoagulated with ethylenediaminetetraacetic acid (EDTA; Didisheim *et al.*, 1959) and contained coagulation factors II, VII and X as well as factor IX (Soulier, 1984). However, EDTA-plasma was unsuitable for the recovery of factor VIII and, following the introduction of citrate-based anticoagulants, alternative procedures were developed for the preparation of factor IX concentrates involving ion-exchange adsorption of the plasma supernatant which remained following the removal of cryoprecipitate or fraction I (Fig. 27.1). The composition of this type of product was determined by the particular adsorbent used (Pejaudier *et al.*, 1987), with factors II, VII and X co-purifying with factor IX when a stronger ion-exchange matrix was used (Hoag *et al.*, 1969; Heystek, Brummelhuis and Krijnen, 1973) or only factors II and X when a weaker ion-exchange matrix was used (Casillas, Simonetti and Pavlovsky, 1969; Middleton, Bennett and Smith, 1973). The three- or four-factor concentrates prepared in this manner were used for the treatment of hemophilia B for almost 20 years, although the cold-ethanol precipitate Cohn fraction IV (Fig. 27.1) was developed as a source of factor IX by one manufacturer (Gilchrist *et al.*, 1969; Fekete, Shanbrom and Shanbrom, 1971).

Recently, further purification has been introduced involving affinity chromatography (Menaché *et al.*, 1984; Burnouf *et al.*, 1989; Herring *et al.*, 1993) or immunoaffinity chromatography (Hrinda *et al.*, 1991). This additional processing was introduced to incorporate virus inactivation procedures and to provide factor IX free from factors II, VII and X.

METHODS OF VIRUS INACTIVATION

A number of procedures have been developed with the objective of inactivating viruses which can contaminate plasma-derived coagulation factor concentrates, and these have been reviewed previously (Cuthbertson, Reid and Foster, 1991; Burnouf, 1992; Suomela, 1993;

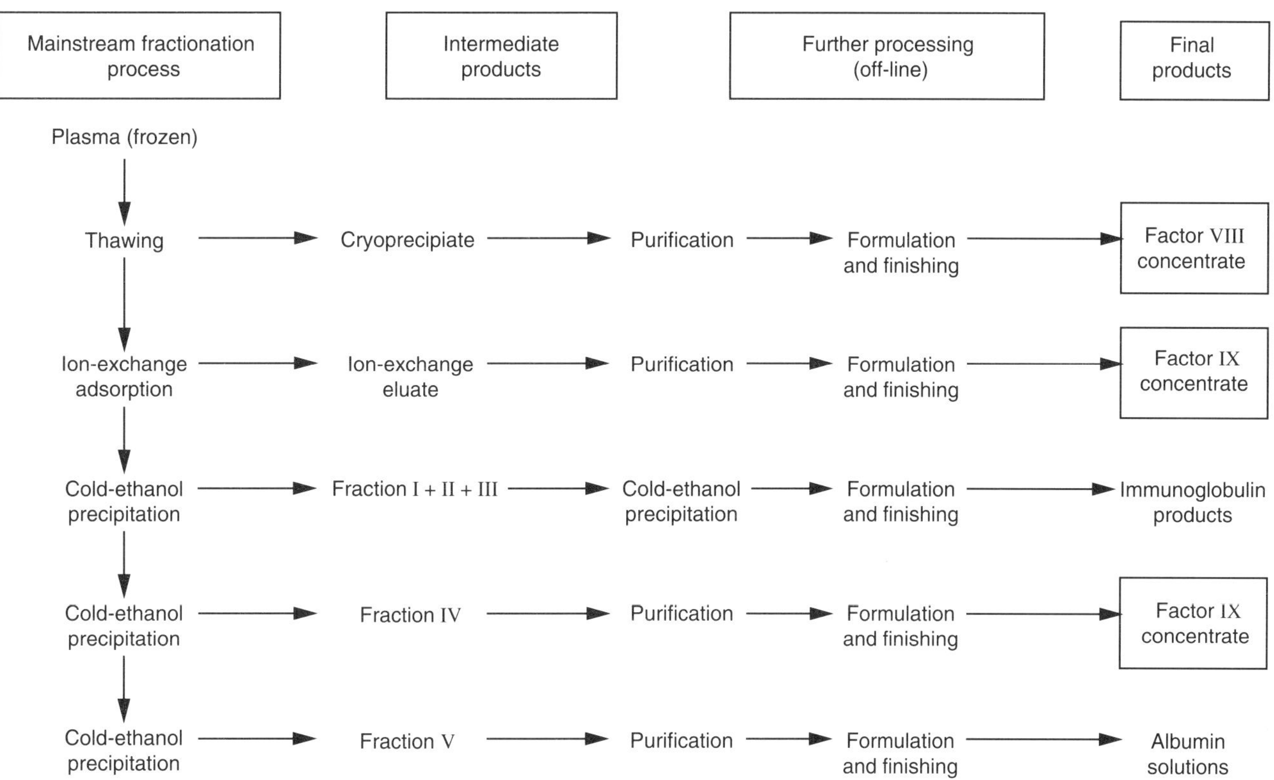

Fig. 27.1 Routes used for the preparation of factor VIII and factor IX concentrates from plasma.

Prodouz and Fratantoni, 1994) Some of these methods have now been abandoned and others are no longer applied routinely. The methods described below have been well-established and involve either heat treatment (with different methods of protein stabilization) or various chemical treatments (Table 27.5).

Heat treatment of freeze-dried products

Freeze-drying (lyophilization) is normally employed to stabilize coagulation factor concentrates so that their biological activity is retained throughout their shelf-life. Heat treatment of coagulation factors already stabilized in this manner was widely adopted when it was reported that HIV could be inactivated following dry heat treatment at 60 or 68°C (Heldebrant *et al.*, 1985; Levy *et al.*, 1985; McDougal *et al.*, 1985; Piskiewicz *et al.*, 1986, 1987). Dry-heat treatment at 60°C for 30 h was also reported to inactivate 3.5 $\log_{10}$ of NANBH virus but not HBV or HDV (Purcell *et al.*, 1985). In this procedure the heating conditions are constrained by changes to product characteristics, such as the reconstitution time and factor VIII potency, which may become unacceptable. Although these limitations resulted in initial heating procedures being generally restricted to temperatures of 60–68°C (product B, Table 27.3), this was the first virus inactivation method to be introduced into widespread use in the manufacture of coagulation factor concentrates.

The method of stabilization (freeze-drying) is influenced by a number of parameters, including the composition of the solution, the method of freezing, the freeze-drying cycle and the residual water content of the product (Williams and Polli, 1984). By carefully specifying and controlling these parameters it has been possible to heat freeze-dried products at 80°C (product type C, Table 27.3) whilst retaining acceptable product characteristics (McIntosh *et al.*, 1987; Winkelman *et al.*, 1989; Knevelman *et al.*, 1994). Treatment at 80°C has been reported to inactivate ⩾4.0 $\log_{10}$ HAV within 24 h in both factor VIII and factor IX concentrates (Hart *et al.*, 1994b). Currently all factor VIII concentrates subjected to terminal (dry) heat treatment are heated at a temperature of 80°C or higher.

Terminal (dry) heat treatment has also been applied to factor IX concentrates where the absence of proteins with a low solubility, such as fibrinogen, means that the product reconstitution time is less likely to be adversely affected. However, as unheated factor IX concentrates carried a risk of inducing thromboembolic reactions, safety studies were undertaken in animals to insure that the terminal (dry) heat treatment did not exacerbate this potential (Littlewood *et al.*, 1987). All factor IX concentrates subjected to terminal (dry) heat treatment are heated at a temperature of 80°C or higher, except for Proplex T and Autoplex T (Hyland-Baxter), which are heated at 60°C for 144 h (Kasper *et al.*, 1993).

In general, the principal advantage of heat-treating the freeze-dried product is that it can be carried out when the product is sealed in its final container, thereby avoiding the risk of subsequent contamination, which applies to all virus elimination procedures carried out prior to the dispensing of the final product (Foster *et al.*, 1988b).

Table 27.5 Methods of virus inactivation used in the preparation of coagulation factor concentrates

Method (manufacturer)	Procedure	References
Terminal (dry) heat treatment (various, see Tables 27.3 and 27.4)	Heating of the lyophilized product in its sealed final container	Winkelman, Feldman and Evans (1989) Winkelman *et al.* (1989) McIntosh *et al.* (1987)
Suspension heating (Alpha Therapeutic)	Heating of the lyophilized product suspended in an organic solvent, at an intermediate stage of manufacture	Heldebrant (1984)
Moist heating (Immuno)	Heating of the lyophilized product under pressure in the presence of steam, at an intermediate stage of manufacture	Eibl and Kasser (1988)
Pasteurization (various, see Tables 27.3 and 27.4)	Heating in solution in the presence of stabilizers, at an intermediate stage of manufacture	Schwinn *et al.* (1981) Fernandes and Lundblad (1984) Feldman *et al.* (1989)
Solvent/detergent treatment (various, see Tables 27.3 and 27.4)	Incubation of the solution in a mixture of organic solvent and detergent, at an intermediate stage of manufacture	Horowitz *et al.* (1985a) Horowitz *et al.* (1993)
β-Propiolactone–ultraviolet treatment (Biotest)	Ultraviolet irradiation of the solution in the presence of β-Propiolactone, at an intermediate stage of manufacture	Prince, Stephan and Brotman (1983) Stephan (1989)

Other heating procedures applied to dried products

Two other methods have been devised for the heat treatment of coagulation factor concentrates in a freeze-dried state. In the first method, used by Alpha Therapeutic Corp., the dried powder, in the form of an insoluble suspension in an organic solvent, is heated at 60°C for 24 h (Heldebrant, 1984). Following heat treatment the dried material must be further purified, dispensed into vials and freeze-dried again, making this procedure an in-process rather than a terminal method.

In the second procedure, used by Immuno AG, the dried powder is heated at 60°C for 10 h in the presence of steam at 1190 mbar (Eibl and Kasser, 1988), with some products (e.g. factor IX concentrates) subsequently being heated for a further period of 1 h at 80°C and 1375 mbar (Kasper *et al.*, 1993). The purpose of all of these methods is to heat-treat a full product batch as a single homogeneous mass with an even distribution of temperature and moisture throughout the material.

Heating in solution (pasteurization)

To heat-treat coagulation factors in solution it is necessary to avoid protein denaturation and to minimize the loss of clotting factor activity by stabilizing the proteins present. High concentrations of a carbohydrate, such as sucrose, together with an amino acid, such as glycine (Schwinn *et al.*, 1981; Fernandes and Lundblad, 1984) or a neutral salt such as sodium sulfate (Feldman *et al.*, 1989) have been used to stabilize coagulation factors for this purpose.

Heating conditions of 60°C for 10 h were selected for the bulk pasteurization of coagulation factors because these are the conditions used for the pasteurization of human albumin solutions (Gellis *et al.*, 1948). However, the excellent safety record of human albumin (Hoofnagle *et al.*, 1976; Tullis, 1977) cannot be extrapolated to the pasteurization of coagulation factors, as the reagents used to stabilize the respective proteins are entirely different and the treatment of human albumin is a terminal rather than an in-process step. In a direct comparison with albumin pasteurization, a substantial decrease in the rate of virus inactivation was observed in the presence of stabilizing reagents used with coagulation factors (Mac-Leod, Cuthbertson and Foster, 1984; Horowitz *et al.*, 1985b; Ng and Dobkin, 1985). Nevertheless, the bulk pasteurization of coagulation factors has been reported to inactivate >6.5 $\log_{10}$ HIV-1 and between 3.6 $\log_{10}$ and 5.2 $\log_{10}$ HAV (Hilfenhaus and Nowak, 1994).

The reagents used for stabilization must be largely removed following pasteurization so that the products can be supplied in a physiologically acceptable formulation. In the original method (Heimburger *et al.*, 1981b) this was achieved by an extensive dilution of the solution followed by precipitation of the protein, resulting in an overall factor VIII yield of only 8% (Heimburger *et al.*, 1981a). Subsequently, chromatographic procedures were developed to remove the stabilizers more efficiently and, more recently, pasteurization at 63°C for 10 h has been introduced to obtain a greater degree of inactivation of HAV (Josic *et al.*, 1994).

Solvent/detergent treatment

The viruses of most concern, which may be present in human blood plasma (HIV-1, HIV-2, HBV, HCV), have a viral nucleus surrounded by a lipid-containing envelope. Removal of lipid by extraction in appropriate solvents generally results in the inactivation of the virus particle (Neurath *et al.*, 1970, 1972). The application of this principle to the treatment of coagulation factors involves the addition of the non-volatile organic solvent tri(n-butyl) phosphate (TnBP) in conjunction with a suitable detergent such as Tween-80 or Triton X-100 (Horowitz *et al.*, 1985a). The rate of virus inactivation is influenced by the temperature of the solution, therefore the time and temperature of the treatment must be specified and controlled as well as the concentrations of the solvent and the detergent. The most commonly used conditions are incubation in 0.3% TnBP + 1% Tween-80 at 25°C for at least 6 h (Horowitz, 1989) but 0.3% TnBP + 1% Triton X-100 at room temperature for 15 min has also been used (Griffin, 1991). The former conditions have been reported to inactivate ≥11 $\log_{10}$ HIV-1, ≥6 $\log_{10}$ HIV-2, ≥6 $\log_{10}$ HBV and ≥5 $\log_{10}$ HCV as well as inactivating a wide range of lipid-enveloped marker viruses (Horowitz *et al.*, 1993).

The toxicity of the solvent and detergent reagents means that they must be removed following completion of the virus inactivation procedure (Guillaume, 1991). Typically this is achieved by column chromatography using either an ion-exchange matrix (Burnouf *et al.*, 1991; Josic *et al.*, 1994) or an immobilized monoclonal antibody (Griffin, 1991) to adsorb the product, allowing the unwanted reagents to be washed from the packed bed. As with bulk pasteurization, the in-process nature of the virus inactivation procedure requires that all subsequent processing be carried out in a contained manner to prevent any recontamination of the process stream.

Other chemical treatments

Although viruses may be inactivated by a range of different procedures involving chemical treatment (Prodouz and Fratantoni, 1994) only two methods, other than solvent detergent treatment, have been applied in the preparation of coagulation factors. As further processing is required to remove the chemical agents, both of these methods must also be carried out at an intermediate stage of processing.

The first method, used exclusively by Armour, involves exposure to 3 mol/l sodium thiocyanate, which is used to desorb factor IX bound to a monoclonal antibody ligand. This exposure to sodium thiocyanate has been found to inactivate 8 $\log_{10}$ HIV but its effectiveness against non-lipid-enveloped viruses is not clear (Hrinda *et al.*, 1991).

The second method, used exclusively by Biotest Pharma, combined the effect of the chemical agent β-propiolactone (β-PL) with ultraviolet irradiation and was introduced in the preparation of a factor IX concentrate in 1975 (Stephan, 1989). Validation studies demonstrated the inactivation of 8.2 $\log_{10}$ HAV (Frösner, Stephan and Dichtelmuller, 1983), 6.9 $\log_{10}$ HBV (Prince, Stephan and Brotman, 1983), >4.5 $\log_{10}$ NANBH (Prince *et al.*, 1985) and >3.5 $\log_{10}$ HIV (Dichtelmuller *et al.*, 1987). The transmission of HIV by a product prepared using this technology subsequently led to this method being abandoned.

SEPARATION TECHNOLOGY AND VIRUS REMOVAL

In the preparation of coagulation factor concentrates, separation technology is utilized to concentrate selectively and to formulate the active component (see Table 27.4 for factor VIII concentrates). Although most of the technologies available were not designed to remove viruses (Foster and Cuthbertson, 1994), a reduction in the concentration of viral contaminants may occur in an adventitious manner. However, the mechanisms which determine the behavior of viruses may not be well-appreciated and the processes may not be monitored and controlled for virus removal. Consequently the use of protein separation technology alone is not regarded as a secure means of insuring product safety (FDA, 1994).

Precipitation

Differences in protein solubility are used to separate factor VIII from other plasma proteins and there are two precipitation stages in widespread use in factor VIII processes: first, cryoprecipitation, in which factor VIII partitions into the solids phase and second, a reduction of the fibrinogen and fibronectin content, by precipitation from the redissolved cryoprecipitate, with factor VIII remaining in solution (Wagner *et al.*, 1964; Newman *et al.*, 1971; Fekete and Shanbrom, 1972; Hagen and Glaser, 1976; Schwinn *et al.*, 1981; Foster *et al.*, 1983b; Winkelman *et al.*, 1989). A number of investigators have studied the partitioning of viruses across these precipitation steps.

The degree of HIV reduction following cryoprecipitation has been reported to vary from about 1 $\log_{10}$ (Levy *et al.*, 1985; Wells *et al.*, 1986) to 2.8 $\log_{10}$ (Hilfenhaus and Nowak, 1994) and HAV reduction has ranged from 1.5 $\log_{10}$ (Mitra *et al.*, 1994) to 2.7 $\log_{10}$ (Lemon *et al.*, 1994). Reductions of about 2 $\log_{10}$ HBsAg. (Schroeder and Mozen, 1970) and about 1 $\log_{10}$ of HCV (Yei, Yu and Tankersley, 1992) have also been reported following cryoprecipitation.

At the second precipitation step, most investigators studying virus removal have examined virus removal across both the precipitation step and the adsorption step, which is also carried out at this stage of processing (Table 27.4). The overall degree of virus reduction reported was from 1 $\log_{10}$ to 3 $\log_{10}$ HIV (Hilfenhaus and Nowak, 1994; Levy *et al.*, 1985), 1.8 $\log_{10}$ HAV (Mitra *et al.*, 1994) and 2 $\log_{10}$ HBV (Heimburger, Schwinn and Mauler, 1980).

Ion-exchange and hydrophobic interaction chromatography

Ion-exchange chromatography is currently employed in virtually all processes used for the manufacture of coagulation factor products. A difference in net charge is the principal property used to separate the different solution constituents. Typically, the desired coagulation factor (factor VIII or factor IX) is adsorbed to an anion exchange gel in a packed-bed format (column). The column is then washed to remove unbound and lightly bound material, before the coagulation factor of interest is desorbed by increasing the ionic strength. If the product protein is to be separated from any contaminating viruses, then the viruses of concern must bind either less strongly or more strongly than the product protein. Most studies concerning the removal of viruses across ion-exchange chromatography do not describe which of these mechanisms is involved, although B19 parvovirus was reported to bind more strongly than factor VIII to the ion-exchange resin DEAE-Fractogel (Schwarz *et al.*, 1991). A similar anion exchange step has also been reported to result in the clearance of 3 $\log_{10}$ HIV-1 (Burnouf, 1992) but it is not clear if this virus was adsorbed to the resin or not. Further studies using the same ion-exchange method have demonstrated a reduction of HAV of about 1 $\log_{10}$ but with some virus being detected in all of the fractions as well as being retained after elution of the factor VIII (Lemon, Murphy, Smith *et al.*, 1994).

In the preparation of factor IX concentrates, ion-exchange adsorption using DEAE-Sephadex has been found to remove 3.5 $\log_{10}$ HBV (Prince, Stephan and Brotman, 1983) and 5.0 $\log_{10}$ HBsAg (Suomela, Myllyla and Raaska, 1977). However, in clinical use, the latter product caused HBV seroconversions in 5 of 29 recipients (Suomela, 1993). The use of hydrophobic interaction chromatography in the preparation of a factor IX concentrate was also found to be capable of removing 4 $\log_{10}$ to 5 $\log_{10}$ HBsAg (Einarsson *et al.*, 1981). However, this product was associated with the transmission of hepatitis and HIV in subsequent clinical use (Mannucci and Colombo, 1988).

Affinity chromatography

Highly selective separation technology, using immobilized bio-specific ligands (e.g. monoclonal antibodies) has been employed in the preparation of plasma-derived factor VIII (Griffin, 1991; Hrinda, Feldman and Schrieber, 1990), recombinant factor VIII (Griffin *et al.*, 1991) and plasma-derived factor IX (Hrinda *et al.*, 1991). In factor VIII processing, immunopurification has been reported to provide a 3 $\log_{10}$ to 4 $\log_{10}$ reduction of HIV (Piszkiewicz, Sun and Tondreau, 1989; Schrieber *et al.*, 1989). The use of other affinity ligands, such as aminohexyl, have been reported to give a 1 $\log_{10}$ reduction of HIV (Schrieber *et al.*, 1989).

Model viruses have also been utilized to establish the degree of virus removal by these methods, with a 4 $\log_{10}$ reduction of both an enveloped and a non-enveloped virus being described following extensive washing of an immunoaffinity column before desorption of factor VIII (Griffin, 1991). In other reports, the degree of removal has been shown to depend on the particular model virus used, ranging from 1.2 $\log_{10}$ to 6.3 $\log_{10}$ (Schreiber *et al.*, 1989; Chtourou *et al.*, 1993). Similarly, in the manufacture of recombinant products, immunoaffinity chromatography used in the purification of factor VIII has been reported to remove from 2 $\log_{10}$ to 5 $\log_{10}$ of virus according to the particular marker viruses used (Griffin *et al.*, 1991).

Membrane filtration

In contrast to the separation methods described above, which were designed according to the behavior of the proteins to be separated, membrane filtration systems are being developed specifically for the removal of viruses from protein solutions. The principal systems designed for this purpose are the Viresolve membranes of Millipore, which operate in a tangential-flow mode (DiLeo, Allegrezza and Builder, 1992) and the BMM membranes of Asahi which can be operated in either a tangential-flow or dead-end mode (Hamamoto *et al.*, 1989). With all of these filtration systems, the viruses are believed to be retained by a sieving mechanism whilst the product proteins pass through the membrane (DiLeo, Vacante and Deane, 1993; Tsurumi *et al.*, 1990). Some viruses of concern are relatively small (Table 27.1) and filtration of protein solutions using membranes with a pore diameter sufficiently small to retain them is not necessarily straightforward. For this reason the technology has been largely restricted to date to the filtration of factor IX solutions, as these are generally less difficult to filter than solutions containing factor VIII. In factor IX processing, a 35 nm BMM filter has been reported to remove 7.8 $\log_{10}$ HIV and from $\geqslant 5.9$ $\log_{10}$ $\geqslant 7.8$ $\log_{10}$ of model viruses (Burnouf-Radosevich *et al.*, 1994). Alternatively a traditional 10 kDa membrane ultrafilter has been reported to give from 4 $\log_{10}$ to 11.2 $\log_{10}$ reduction of marker viruses according to the size of the virus (Hrinda *et al.*, 1991).

Progress to date in eliminating the risk of viral infection

TRIALS IN SUSCEPTIBLE PATIENTS

To establish the degree of safety or risk associated with a particular coagulation factor product. it is necessary to undertake the surveillance of patients who are susceptible to the infection concerned. A protocol for detecting hepatitis transmission has been recommended by the International Society of Thrombosis and Haemostasis (Mannucci and Colombo, 1989) and a further protocol is available for B19 parvovirus transmission (Mannucci, 1994). A number of studies of this type have been reported, dealing predominantly with HIV, NANBH (HCV) and HBV. A summary of data from studies on products with a relatively high degree of safety with regard to these infections is given in Table 27.6. It should be noted that a smaller number of patients were susceptible to HBV infection, because many hemophiliacs have been vaccinated against this virus. All of these studies involved previously untreated patients only, and the results suggest that considerable progress has been made towards eradicating the risk of serious viral infection previously associated with these products. Of the viral inactivation methods listed in Table 27.6, only the heat treatment of the lyophilized powder with steam was associated with virus transmission (see below).

In recent reviews (Mannucci, 1993, 1995) the risk associated with each virucidal method has been calculated from the total numbers of patients treated in prospective safety studies (Hanley and Lippman-Hand, 1983; Araújo and Araújo, 1994), with risk estimates for HBV and HCV transmission being 0–2% for pasteurization, 0–3% for solvent/detergent treatment and 0–6% for both dry and vapor heating. This approach may underestimate the risk of viral infection for a number of reasons. First, the many procedures required to achieve a non-infectious product (Foster and Cuthbertson, 1994) may not be carried out or controlled in exactly the same manner by all manufacturers who are ostensibly using the same virucidal procedure. Second, in the absence of appropriate control tests on the final product, an infective batch would only be detected by continued surveillance in patients. The reproducibility of each manufacturer's procedures and controls can only be

Table 27.6 Validation of the effectiveness of different virus inactivation methods in clinical studies involving previously untreated patients

Virus inactivation method	Manufacturer		Number of batches used in study	Number of patients infected/total				References
				HIV	HBV	HCV	NANBH	
Solvent/detergent (TnBP/Tween-80)	New York Blood Center	(USA)	10	0/14			0/14	Horowitz *et al* (1988)
	Biotransfusion	(France)	12	0/10			0/10	Gazengel *et al.* (1988)
			N/A			0/16		Noel *et al.* (1989)
			N/A	0/55	0/4	0/55		Guérois *et al.* (1993)
	Santa Caterina	(Brazil)	N/A	0/20	0/14		0/20	Gongaga and Bonecker (1990)
	AIMA	(Italy)	41	0/31	0/14	0/31	0/30	Mariani *et al.* (1993)
	Alpha	(USA)	10	0/10		0/10	0/10	Becton *et al.* (1994)
Solvent/detergent (TnBP/Triton X-100)	Hyland/Baxter	(USA)	N/A	0.41		0/21	0/28	Addiego *et al.* (1992)
Heating in solution 60°C, 10 h	Behringwerke	(Germany)	32	0/26	0/10		0/26	Schimpf *et al.* (1987)
			N/A	0/155				Schimpf *et al.* (1989)
			13	0/29	0/15	0/29	0/29	Mannucci *et al.* (1990b)
			72			0/98	0/98	Kreuz *et al.* (1992)
			N/A	0/36		0/36	0/26	Pollmann and Richter (1994)
	Armour	(USA)	N/A	0/13			0/12	Mauser-Bunschoten *et al.* (1993)
Moist heating of lyophilized powder	Immuno	(Austria)	9	0/28	4/14		0/24	Mannucci *et al.* (1988b)
			20	0/31	0/17	0/20	0/28	Mannucci *et al.* (1992)
			N/A	0/13	0/2	0/9	0/14	Shapiro *et al.* (1993)
Terminal (dry) heating 80°C, 72 h	Bio-Products Laboratory	England	30	0/32	0/16	0/32	0/19	Colvin *et al.* (1988), Colvin (1990)
			9			0/18	0/18	Pasi *et al.* (1990)
			24	0/27	0/6	0/27	0/27	Rizza, Fletcher and Kernoff (1993)
	PFC	Scotland	25	0/13			0/13	Bennett *et al.* (1993)

HIV = Human immunodeficiency virus; HBV = hepatitis B virus; HCV = hepatitis C virus; NANBH = non-A non-B hepatitis; N/A = not available.

determined if patients are monitored after receiving a large number of consecutive batches. However, in some of the studies listed, the number of batches used was not given. Third, it is not always clear whether each report represents a new set of patients, or if later reports simply represent the updating of earlier studies. Despite these points, it can be concluded that products manufactured using any of the virucidal methods listed in Table 27.6 should not normally be infectious with regard to HIV nor HCV, although safety with regard to HBV is less certain because of the smaller number of susceptible patients that have been monitored.

INSTANCES OF VIRUS TRANSMISSION ASSOCIATED WITH COAGULATION FACTOR CONCENTRATES WHICH HAD BEEN TREATED TO INACTIVATE OR REMOVE VIRUSES

In addition to data from prospective safety studies (Table 27.6), a number of reports have described a variety of instances of viral infection associated with the clinical use of coagulation factor concentrates.

HIV infection

Following the widespread introduction of virucidal steps into the preparation of coagulation factor concentrates, episodes of HIV transmission have been attributed to three particular products, all of which were subsequently withdrawn from use.

HT Factorate, an intermediate-purity factor VIII concentrate manufactured by Armour, which was terminally (dry) heat-treated at 60°C for 30 h, has been the subject of a number of reports (Table 27.7). The effectiveness of terminal (dry) heat-treated at 60°C for 30 h, is dependent on a number of product and process parameters, particularly the residual water content of the product, as well as the temperature and time of heat treatment and the quantity of virus to be inactivated. Data concerning viral inactivation with HT Factorate suggested that, according to the model virus Sindbis, less virus was inactivated than in the other products studied (Menaché and Aronson, 1985; Horowitz and Prince, 1987).

Two factor IX concentrates have also transmitted HIV (Table 27.7). One product, prepared by Kabi, utilized hydrophobic chromatography which had been developed for HBV removal (Einarsson *et al.*, 1981). Unfortunately, the product transmitted both HIV and hepatitis in clinical use (Mannucci and Colombo, 1988), despite extensive validation studies (Einarsson and Morgenthaler, 1989) and a satisfactory prospective clinical trial (Mannucci *et al.*, 1988a).

A prothrombin complex concentrate prepared by Biotest using β-PL ultraviolet treatment as the virucidal step has also transmitted HIV (Table 27.7). This particular product had been manufactured since 1975 and had been regarded as secure following trials in susceptible patients (Heinrich *et al.*, 1987) and a long record of safety (Stephan, 1989). Only one product batch appears to have been implicated and it is circumstances such as these (one batch failure in 15 years) that suggest that a breakdown in the control of the manufacturing operation may have occurred. Alternatively, it has been suggested that the capacity of the method to inactivate HIV was not as high as reported previously (Norley, Löwer and Kurth, 1993). However the validity of this investigation is uncertain as the β-PL treatment appears to have been studied in the absence of ultraviolet irradiation.

Table 27.7   Human immunodeficiency virus infection associated with coagulation factor concentrates which had been treated to inactivate or remove viruses

Product (manufacturer)	Method of virus inactivation or removal	Number of patients infected	Reference
FVIII concentrate (not reported)	Terminal (dry) heat	1	Van den Berg *et al.* (1986)
		1	White *et al.* (1986)
		1	Weisser (1988)
HT Factorate (Armour)	Terminal (dry) heat 60°C, 30 h	1	Wolfs *et al.* (1988)
		6	Dietrich *et al.* (1990)
		8	Remis *et al.* (1990)
		≥1 (4)	Williams, Skidmore and Hall (1990a)
FVIII concentrate (not reported)	Pasteurization	2	Kleim *et al.* (1990)
FIX concentrate (Kabi)	Hydrophobic Chromatography	4	Mannucci *et al.* (1988a)
FIX concentrate, PPSB (Biotest)	β-Propiolactone/ultraviolet treatment	6	Kleim *et al.* (1990)
		10	Karcher (1991)

FVIII = factor VIII; FIX = factor IX.

HBV infection

The transmission of HBV has been attributed to factor VIII concentrates manufactured by Behringwerke and Immuno AG and to a factor IX concentrate manufactured by Behringwerke (Table 27.8) It is possible that the pasteurization method of Beringwerke may not be capable of inactivating HBV to the extent required, despite many validation studies concerning this procedure (Heimburger and Karges, 1989). Similar considerations apply to the steam-heating method of Immuno AG. Alternatively, HBV contamination of these batches could have taken place after the virucidal treatment had been completed, due to the in-process nature of the virucidal methods concerned.

HCV and NANBH infection

The transmission of NANBH or HCV has been associated with products treated using a number of different virucidal methods, including terminal (dry) heat treatment at 60–68°C, steam heating of the freeze-dried powder, heating the freeze-dried powder in the presence of an organic solvent and heating in solution at 60°C in the presence of stabilizers (Table 27.9). HCV transmission has also been attributed to a factor VIII concentrate which was immunopurified and terminally (dry) heat-treated at 60°C for 30 h (Berntorp *et al.*, 1990). Since HCV can be transmitted by other routes (Allander *et al.*, 1995), the exact cause of virus transmission in one instance has been the subject of some debate (Anderle, Eder and Eible, 1991; Mannucci *et al.*, 1991).

Although the early terminal (dry) heat treatment procedures did not eliminate NANB (HCV) transmission, a reduction in the incidence of infection was noted (Parquet *et al.*, 1988; Kolho, Ebeling and Rasi, 1992; Morfini *et al.*, 1994), suggesting that the method may have been partially effective against this virus. However, for the products described in Table 27.6 terminal (dry) heat treatment at 80°C appears to have been effective in inactivating HCV.

HAV infection

Transmission of HAV has been associated with factor VIII concentrates prepared by three different manufacturers (Table 27.10). These episodes of infection were unexpected because HAV transmission had not been associated previously with factor VIII concentrates, despite the widespread use for almost 20 years of products not subjected to a virucidal treatment. Why should these earlier products have been non-infectious with regard to HAV? The products implicated all have two features in common. First, they used the same virucidal method, solvent/detergent treatment, a procedure which was not designed to inactivate non-lipid-enveloped viruses such as HAV, and second, they all utilized chromatographic purification to remove the virucidal chemicals and further purify the factor VIII.

A number of theories have been postulated to explain HAV transmission by these products, including a high degree of contamination of the plasma pool in conjunction with an insufficient content of neutralizing immunoglobulin, or by the dissociation of virus-antibody complexes during manufacturing (Mannucci *et al.*, 1994). In examining this latter theory a reversal of antibody-mediated neutralization was not observed, but it was noted that 0.1–1% of cell culture-derived HAV was not neutralized by the antibody present in the plasma pool, possible because the added virus was aggregated by the method of preparation (Lemon, 1994).

It should be noted that earlier products, not associated with transmission of HAV, were prepared without chromatographic purification (Tables 27.3 and 27.4) and, as a consequence, contained a significant quantity of immunoglobulin (e.g. IgG) which co-purified with factor VIII (Allain, 1984; Nilsson *et al.*, 1984; Wadsworth *et al.*, 1989). Normal immunoglobulin is effective in neutralizing HAV and is used prophylactically for this purpose (Gerety *et al.*, 1983; Lerman *et al.*, 1993). The IgG present in factor VIII concentrates could have provided passive protection to recipients (Peerlinck *et al.*, 1994) or its presence throughout the manufacturing process could have provided protection to the products through-

Table 27.8   Hepatitis B virus infection associated with coagulation factor concentrates which had been treated to inactivate or remove viruses

Product (manufacturer)	Method of virus inactivation or removal	Number of patients infected	Reference
Haemate HS (Behringwerke)	Heated in solution 60°C, 10 h	2	Brackman and Egli (1988)
Kryobulin TIM-3 (Immuno)	Steam-heated 60°C, 10 h	4	Mannucci *et al.* (1988b)
Beriplex HS (FIX) (Behringwerke)	Heated in solution 60°C, 10 h	22	Arzneimittelkommission (1994)

Table 27.9   Hepatitis C virus and non-A non-B hepatitis infection associated with coagulation factor concentrates which had been treated to inactivate or remove viruses

Product (manufacturer)	Method of virus inactivation or removal	Number of patients infected	Reference
Hemofil-T (Hyland/Baxter)	Terminal (dry) heat 60°C, 72 h	11	Colombo *et al.* (1985)
Kryobulin TIM-1 (Immuno)	Heated suspension in chloroform	3	Mannucci, Colombo and Rhodeghiero (1985)
Profilate HT (Apha)	Heated 60°C, 24 h in heptane suspension	≥ 1 (3)	Carnelli *et al.* (1987)
Profilate HT (Alpha)	Heated 60°C, 24 h in heptane suspension	5	Kernoff *et al.* (1987)
Monoclate (Armour)	Monoclonal immunoaffinity chromatography and terminal (dry) heat 60°C, 30 h	1	Berntorp *et al.* (1990)
Kryobulin TIM-3 (Immuno)	Steam heat, 60°C, 10 h	1	Mannucci *et al.* (1990c) Mannucci *et al.* (1991)
FVIII and FIX concentrates (not given)	Terminal (dry) heat	2	Blanchette *et al.* (1991)
Haemate HS (Behringwerke)	Heated in solution 60°C, 10 h	1	Gerritzen *et al.* (1992a)
Haemate P (Behringwerke)	Heated in solution 60°C, 10 h	1	Schulman *et al.* (1992)

FVIII = factor VIII; FIX = factor IX.

Table 27.10   Hepatitis A virus infection associated with coagulation factor concentrates which had been treated to inactivate or remove viruses

Product (manufacturer)	Method of virus inactivation or removal	Number of patients infected	Reference
Emoclot, Octa V1 (AIMA)	Solvent/detergent treatment	1	Mariani *et al.* (1991)
Emoclot, Octa V1 (AIMA)	Solvent/detergent treatment	52	Mannucci (1992) Mannucci *et al.* (1994)
Octa Vl (Octapharma)	Solvent/detergent treatment	13	Gerritzen *et al.* (1992b)
Octa V1 (Octapharma)	Solvent/detergent treatment	17	Temperley *et al.* (1992)
Octa V1 (Octapharma)	Solvent/detergent treatment	6	Peerlinck and Vermylen (1993)
FVIII concentrate (Natal BTS)	Solvent/detergent treatment	7	Cohn *et al.* (1994)

FVIII = factor VIII.

out their manufacture. In a process similar to those associated with HAV transmission, 0.25 mg IgG/iu VIII C was measured up to the chromatographic step – a quantity which should be sufficient to neutralize HAV present in the starting plasma (Hart *et al.*, 1994a). However, the removal of immunoglobulin over chromato-graphic purification means that the process would be vulnerable to any subsequent HAV contamination.

Despite these various theories, the precise cause of these HAV infections is not yet known. However, it should be noted that solvent/detergent treatment has been adopted by over 50 organizations worldwide

(Horowitz *et al.*, 1993) and that HAV transmission was not associated with similar factor VIII concentrates from other manufacturers (Gonzaga, Bonecker and Dantas, 1994; Goudemand, Parquet, d'Oiron *et al.*, 1994; Watson, Ludlam, McOmish *et al.*, 1995). Therefore, the risk of HAV transmission by coagulation factor concentrates appears to be very low and is most likely to be eliminated only by a return to products containing neutralizing antibodies to HAV or by the use of an effective terminal virucidal step.

B19 Parvovirus infection

The human B19 parvovirus is a highly infectious non-lipid-enveloped virus to which a significant proportion of the adult population has been exposed (Anderson, 1987; Adler *et al.*, 1993; Seng *et al.*, 1994). Occasional transmission of B19 via blood components has also been noted (Luban, 1994). Studies of the incidence of B19 infection amongst hemophiliacs indicate that patients infused with earlier concentrates, which had not been treated to eliminate viral contaminants, have a relatively high rate of seroconversion to B19 compared to control groups (Table 27.11). However, in one study, a much higher incidence of seroprevalence to B19 was found in the age-matched control group, with an increase in hemophilia A patients being significant only with those under 25 years of age (Peerlinck *et al.*, 1995).

The incidence of B19 in patients susceptible to infection who were treated only with concentrates subjected to viral inactivation has been reported for a number of products (Table 27.12). Of the virucidal methods studied, terminal heat treatment of a factor VIII:C at 80°C for 72 h was associated with the lowest incidence of infection, suggesting the possibility that B19 infectivity may have been eliminated – or at least reduced – by this treatment. The transmission of parvovirus by both monoclonal antibody-immunopurified products and by recombinant products has also been reported, possibly via the human albumin used as an excipient (Kasper, 1995). The interpretation of all of these data on the transmission of B19 by coagulation factor products is complicated by the fact that as a community-acquired infection it tends to be seasonal, with an incidence that may vary in different countries, making it difficult to determine whether or not a B19 infection in a hemophiliac is product-related and therefore to demonstrate that a particular virucidal method is effective in eliminating B19 infectivity (Prowse, 1994).

Immunoglobulin has been used to treat B19 infection (Finkel *et al.*, 1994) and it has been reported that anti-B19 antibody activity can be found in the immunoglobulin fraction remaining present in a factor VIII process up to the chromatographic purification stage (Hart *et al.*, 1994a). This observation raises the possibility that, as with HAV, B19 present in a pool of plasma may be at least partially neutralized, thereby protecting the product in those parts of the process where immunoglobulin is present.

Developments required to reduce further the risk of viral infection from coagulation factor concentrates

Despite a dramatic reduction in the transmission of viral infections by coagulation factor concentrates, the clinical reports listed in Tables 27.7–27.12 indicate that

Table 27.11 Incidence of B19 paravovirus infection in hemophiliacs infused with products not treated to eliminate viruses and in non-hemophilic controls

			Anti B19+ve		
Product (manufacturer)	*Group tested*	*Number of subjects*	*No.*	*%*	*Reference*
Various	Hemophiliacs	33	29	88	Mortimer *et al.* (1983)
	Age-matched surgical patients	53	9	17	
Various	Hemophiliacs	30	28	93	Bartolomei Corsi *et al.* (1988)
	Blood donors	58	17	29	
IP FVIII (Armour and BPL)	Hemophiliacs	45	40	89	Williams *et al.* (1990)
	Age-matched hospital patients	135	53	39	
Various	Hemophiliacs	136	94	69	Grosse-Bley *et al.* (1994)
	Age and sex-matched, healthy with no recent B19 infection	50	16	32	

IP = Intermediate-purity;
FVIII = factor VIII.

Table 27.12   Seroconversion against B19 parvovirus in patients treated with virally inactivated concentrates only

Product (manufacturer)	Virucidal method	Number of subjects	Anti-B19+ve No.	%	Reference
Koate HT (Cutter)	Terminal (dry) heating 68°C, 72 h	N/A	1*		Bartolomei Corsi *et al.* (1988)
Kryobulin TIM3 (Immuno)	Moist heating	15	3	20	Bartolomei Corsi *et al.* (1988)
FIX concentrate (BPL)	Terminal (dry) heating 80°C, 72 h	N/A	2*		Lyon *et al.* (1989)
BPL 8Y (BPL)	Terminal (dry) heating 80°C, 72 h	11	1	9.0	Williams *et al.* (1990)
Beriate-P (Behringwerke)	Pasteurization 60°C, 10 h	13	4	31	Azzi *et al.* (1992)
Emoclot, Octa VI (AIMA)	Solvent/detergent	7	5	71	Azzi *et al.* (1992)
Various	Heat-treated, mainly pasteurized 60°C, 10 h	32	20	63	Grosse-Bley *et al.* (1994)
Various	Solvent/detergent	16	12	75	Grosse-Bley *et al.* (1994)
VIII THPSD (Biotransfusion)	Solvent/detergent	53	43	81	Laurian *et al.* (1994)
Emoclot DI (AIMA)	Solvent/detergent + dry heat	6	3	50	Santagostino *et al.* (1994)

*Denotes report of individual patients seroconverting to B19.
FIX = factor IX; N/A = not applicable.

residual risks remain. Infections associated with current products appear to have been due either to a failure associated with a virucidal method which had previously been effective or to an absence of suitable methods for the elimination of non-lipid-enveloped viruses such as HAV and B19 parvovirus. The development, implementation and operation of procedures that eliminate or prevent viral contamination of coagulation factor concentrates is a complex undertaking with many different elements requiring to be validated and controlled (Foster and Cuthbertson, 1994) and it is unlikely that all of these elements will have been dealt with in the same manner by all manufacturers. Even where a degree of harmonization has been achieved, such as in the testing of blood donations, improvements may still be possible that would increase the margin of product safety further.

This section will describe the procedures which are required to insure that all products meet the level of safety which is currently achievable. The principal elements involved in the introduction of a virus elimination procedure into a manufacturing process are summarized in Figure 27.2, whilst those required for the routine operation of the technology are summarized in Figure 27.3.

SELECTION OF BLOOD AND PLASMA DONATIONS

Ideally, a comprehensive set of tests should be available which will detect all donations of blood or plasma which may be infectious. Currently there are no suitable tests available for the mass screening of donations for HDV, HAV and B19 parvovirus, all of which are known to be transmissible via coagulation factor concentrates, or the infectious agent of CJD which may be transmissible by blood products. Where mass screening is in place, the possibility that errors may occur in the testing or administrative procedures associated with the selection or rejection of donations must also be appreciated (Linden, 1994; Sazama, 1995).

Current tests used for screening donations for HIV-1–2 and HCV are indirect in that they detect antibody produced in response to the infection. Even where a test measures virus directly, the identification of an infectious donation is dependent on viral particles being expressed into the plasma of the donor at a detectable concentration (Löwer, 1990). Both of these factors result in a delay between the onset of infection and the development of viral markers which are detectable by current screening tests. Estimates of the resultant 'window' period and the consequent risk of a blood donation being infectious for HIV, HBV or HCV in the USA, despite testing

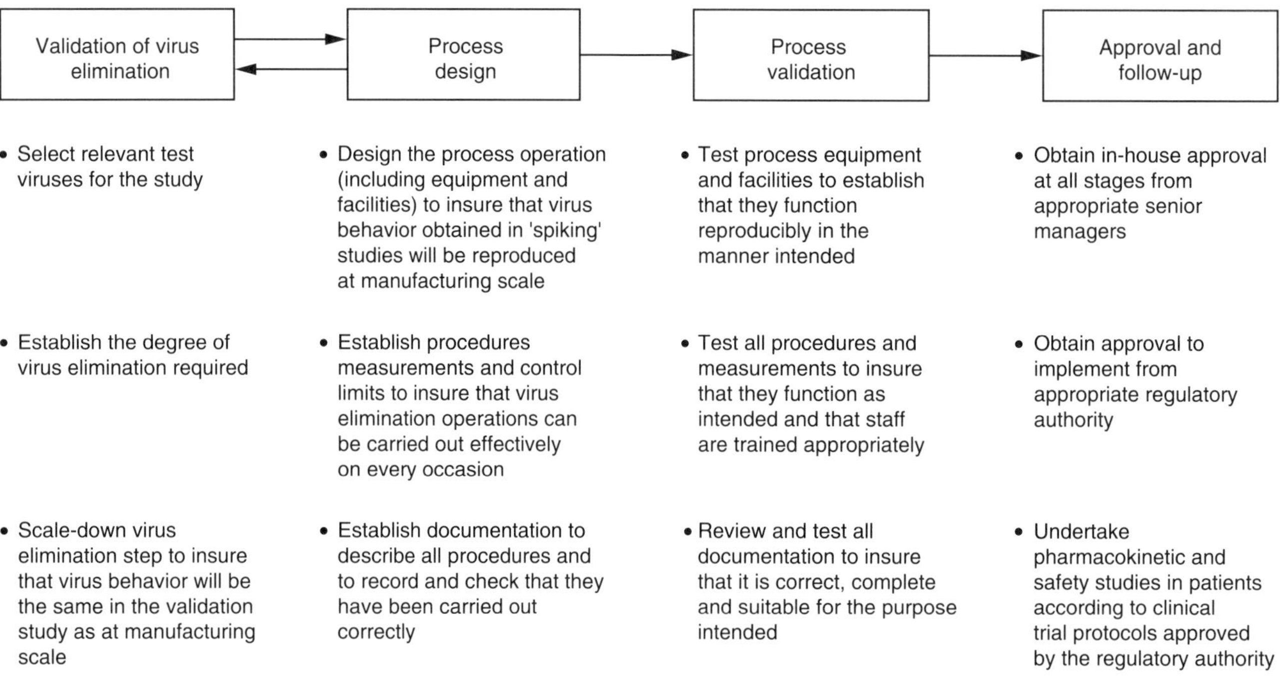

Fig. 27.2 Summary of key stages in the introduction of a step for virus elimination into a manufacturing process.

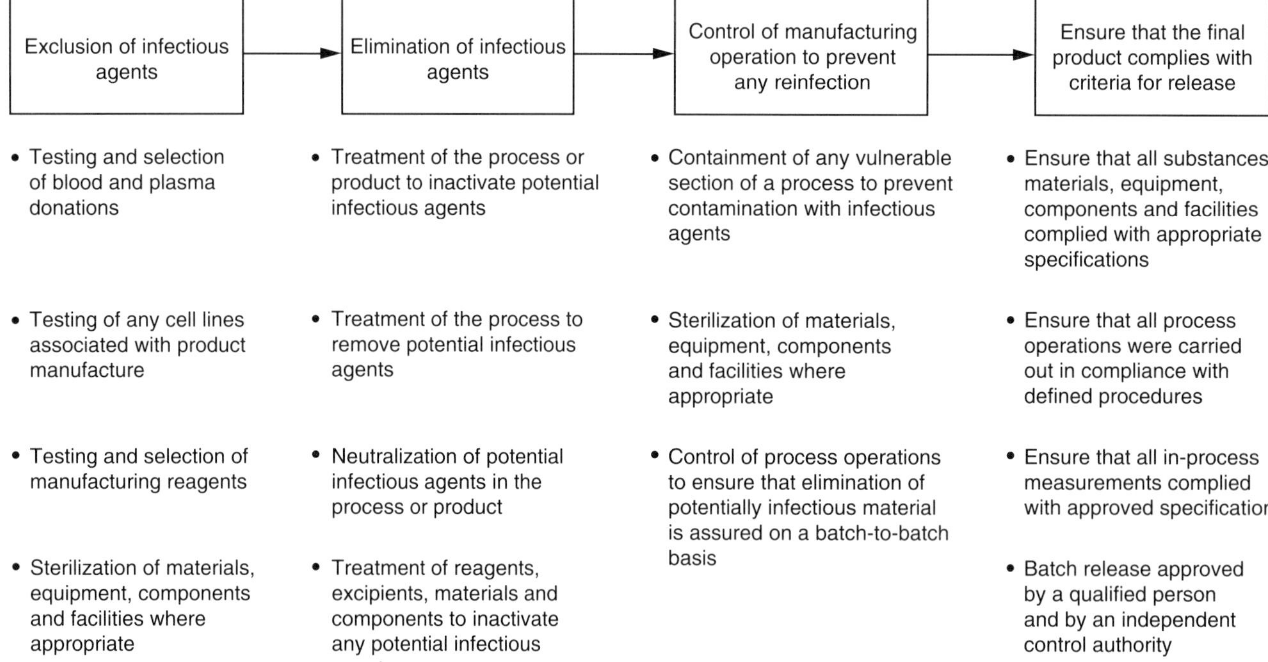

Fig. 27.3 Summary of manufacturing and control procedures on which the safety of coagulation factor products depends.

negative, are summarized in Table 27.13 (Busch, 1995; Busch *et al.*, 1995). It should be noted that these figures refer to non-remunerated repeat blood donors and that equivalent data are not available for paid donors. The number of infectious particles per milliliter plasma which remain undetected during the window period have been estimated to be 2 $\log_{10}$ to 4 $\log_{10}$ for HIV-1, 2 $\log_{10}$ for HCV and <5 $\log_{10}$ for HBV (Friedman, Stromberg and Wagner, 1995)

The amplification of viral nucleic acid by the PCR has been applied to the detection of HAV, HDV and B19 parvovirus as well as to HIV-1–2, HBV and HCV

Table 27.13 Estimates of the risk of infective donations from repeat USA blood donors being undetected as a consequence of the seroconversion window period

Virus	Test marker	Annual risk of a donor giving an infective donation	Window period (days)		Annual risk of a donor giving an infective donation which is not detected
			Mean	Range	
HIV-1–2	Anti-HIV-1–2	1 in 25 000	22	6–38	1 in 416 667
HBV	HBsAg	1 in 23 500	56	24–128	1 in 153 194
HCV	Anti-HCV	1 in 16 550	98	56–189	1 in 61 639

HIV = Human immunodeficiency virus; HBV = hepatitis B virus; HBsAg = hepatitis B surface antigen; HCV = hepatitis C virus. Calculated from Busch, M.P. (1995) Incidence of infectious disease markers in blood donors implications for residual risk of viral transmission by transfusion, in *Proceedings of NIH Consensus Development Conference on Infectious Disease Testing for Blood Transfusions* (eds P.R. McCurdy and J.M. Elliot), National Institute of Health, Bethesda, Maryland, pp. 29–30.

(Birkenmeyer and Mushahwar, 1994; Vyas, Yang and Murphy, 1994). Although the technology is not yet suitable for the routine screening of individual blood donations (McOmish, Yap, Jordan *et al.*, 1993), developments in control, standardization and automation may address current limitations. As with all methods for the detection of viruses, the testing of donations would be the most suitable point to apply PCR technology as it is here, prior to dilution in a plasma pool, that greater sensitivity will be obtained.

SELECTION OF OTHER BIOLOGICAL SUBSTANCES

Considerations similar to those which apply to blood plasma also apply to the testing of the cell lines and other biological materials used in the manufacture of products by recombinant technology. Concerns with recombinant products include the potential for contamination with viruses (FDA, 1993), retrovirus-like particles (Chan, 1994; Lie *et al.*, 1994) and infectious agents responsible for transmissible spongiform encephalopathies, such as BSE in substances of bovine origin (Danner, 1993; Jungbauer and Boschetti, 1994) and scrapie in cell lines derived from rodents (Priola *et al.*, 1994). Ideally, the development of specific and sensitive tests for the infectious agents of BSE and scrapie would enable biological substances for use in the manufacture of recombinant products (Table 27.2) to be selected on the basis of controlled tests.

VALIDATION OF VIRUS INACTIVATION AND ELIMINATION

Virological methods

To establish that a given process operation will provide an appropriate degree of virus elimination, it is necessary to measure the capability and the capacity of the operation using relevant viruses. HIV and HAV replicate in mammalian cell culture and high-titer preparations can be obtained for test purposes, whereas other viruses of concern (HBV, HCV, HDV and B19) cannot be cultured as easily, so various model or marker viruses have been employed to obtain data that might be representative of these types of virus. A total of over 20 different viruses have been used for this purpose by different investigators but, even where the same virus is used, differences may exist in the strain or in the methods used to culture and detect the virus. Therefore, in the absence of any standardization and control in this area, and in the absence of common methodology for data presentation and analysis, all virus validation data must be interpreted with caution. The possibility also exists that the viruses cultured *in vitro* may behave differently to the equivalent wild *in vivo* strain; for example, viruses prepared via cell culture may be more highly aggregated, a feature which would influence their behavior in chromatographic and filtration studies.

Scale-down of virus inactivation and elimination procedures

Virus validation studies are carried out in containment laboratories at a scale of operation substantially smaller than the full-scale routine manufacturing method under consideration. Typically, virus validation studies will be carried out using product or process fluid volumes ranging from 1 to 100 ml, compared to full-scale volumes ranging from 1 to 5000 l depending on the particular process technology involved. To scale down a procedure as accurately as possible it is necessary to establish that the product and the appropriate viruses will behave in the same way in the small-scale procedure as in the full-scale process. To achieve this, the parameters which determine virus and product behavior must be defined. For example, in the scale-down of terminal (dry) heat treatment the production freeze-drying cycle should be simulated as closely as possible to obtain a product with an equivalent residual water content and the heating conditions must also be defined and reproduced accurately.

Accurate scale-down may be particularly difficult to achieve when the mechanisms which determine the outcome are not well-defined, or where laboratory equipment is very different to that used at industrial scale. In chromatographic procedures,changes to a gel on re-use (Bessos *et al.*, 1991; Seeley *et al.*, 1994) should be taken into consideration, as should any influence of non-specific binding (Nishikawa and Bailon, 1975). In studying the removal of viruses by membrane filtration it is necessary to be aware of the influence that concentration polarization can have on the sieving coefficient (Iritani *et al.*, 1991; Opong and Zydney, 1991; Balakrishnan, Agarwal and Cooney, 1993) and also of changes that can occur with progressive fouling or when membranes are re-used (Jonsson and Johansen, 1991; Meireles, Aimar and Sanchez, 1991). The observation that a virus smaller than the nominal pore size of the membrane can be retained by that membrane (Burnouf-Radesovich *et al.*, 1994) may be explained at least in part, by the effect of concentration polarization (DiLeo, Vacante and Deane, 1993) a feature which, for cross-flow operation, is normally more pronounced at small scale (Bell and Cousins, 1994).

These examples have been cited to illustrate the difficulty of accurately scaling down operations which at first sight may seem straightforward. Unfortunately, essential details of scale-down are rarely given in publications concerning the effectiveness of virus elimination procedures, placing the validity of the data in question. Ideally, a standard set of validated protocols should be established for the scale-down of each unit operation.

PROCESS DESIGN AND VALIDATION

When introducing a virus removal or inactivation technology into a routine manufacturing process it is necessary to design the equipment, the facilities and the procedures to insure that the virus behavior or the process conditions that were validated in small-scale studies are reproduced on every occasion in the full-scale operation.

Precipitation

Protein precipitation can be affected by mixing conditions and other relevant parameters, such as pH and temperature (Foster, 1994b). Mixing conditions and the geometric relationships of the equipment cannot be scaled-up in the same manner (Leng, 1991). Therefore, operating parameters cannot always be predicted from small-scale experiments and may have to be finalized by monitoring the behavior of the different proteins at

full-scale, with the assumption that viruses of concern will behave in the same manner. Industrial centrifuges used to recover protein precipitates are normally very different in their design and operation to small-scale laboratory machines (Bell, Hoare and Dunnill, 1983); therefore, their selection and operational specifications cannot be easily predicted and must normally be determined following pilot or large-scale trials (Records, 1986; Belter, Cussler and Hu, 1988).

Heating in solution (pasteurization)

Pasteurization equipment must be designed to insure that every element of the solution reaches the desired temperature and remains there for the correct length of time. Mixing, heat transfer and precise details of the geometry of a vessel and its fittings are all-important. Temperature mapping of pasteurization vessels is also required to establish that the equipment is suitable for use. A failure to achieve suitable conditions throughout a vessel used for bulk pasteurization is believed to have been responsible for a plasma derivative (Plasma Protein Fraction) remaining infectious for HBV following heat treatment (Pattison *et al.*, 1976).

Solvent/detergent treatment

Mixing is equally important in solvent/detergent treatment as in bulk pasteurization. As well as avoiding cold spots, the design must also insure that the virucidal chemicals are distributed homogeneously and that every element of the solution is treated appropriately. Temperature mapping in vessels used for solvent/detergent treatment and tracer studies to measure mixing performance (Edwards, 1985) are required to establish that the equipment is functioning correctly. Procedures must also be established to insure that the correct concentration of solvent and detergent is added on every occasion.

Chromatography

In chromatography it is not possible to scale-up all of the parameters in the same manner. Normally, the solution velocity through the bed, sometimes called the linear flow rate, is maintained constant and in this situation the geometric relationships (e.g. height/diameter ratio) and the mean residence time will change as a consequence. Validation studies are necessary therefore to demonstrate that the degree of separation obtained at small scale is also achieved at large-scale (Null, 1987). Studies of this type necessarily focus on the behavior of the proteins and chemicals which the technology was designed to separate. The behavior of added viruses cannot be validated at this scale, although endogenous viruses, such as B19, which may be present in the normal process solution, could be used to make a direct comparison of virus partitioning between the full-scale process and the small-scale model procedure. Other considerations in the scale-up of chromatography include the possibility of channeling as a result of distortions or cracks in the bed, or from an uneven distribution of solutions across the much larger cross-sectional area. Procedures for cleaning chromatography columns must also be established to inactivate and remove viruses which may adsorb to the gel.

Terminal (dry) heat treatment

In terminal (dry) heat treatment, virus inactivation takes place in the final container, with the size of the vial and the quantity of material in each vial being independent of the scale of operation. However, the number of vials being treated will be much greater than the number used in virus inactivation studies, as will the size of the freeze-drier and the oven or bath used for heat treatment. The range in product residual water content must be determined at full scale, as should the temperature distribution across the load in the heat treatment apparatus.

PROCESS OPERATION AND CONTROL

In-process controls

Once a virus elimination procedure has been established at full-scale, it is necessary to insure that the technology functions correctly on every occasion. All relevant conditions and procedures must be monitored and checked with every batch of product to insure compliance with predetermined specifications and limits. For methods involving heat inactivation, representative temperatures and the time of measurement must be recorded throughout the period of treatment. Where a chemical treatment is used, the appropriate quantity of reagents must be calculated, measured and recorded. Monitoring should also be carried out to check that correct concentrations were achieved.

For the removal of viruses by separation technology, such as precipitation or chromatography, some of the parameters responsible for partitioning behavior (e.g. pH) can be monitored and recorded but other conditions (e.g. fluid mechanic) or properties (e.g. charge or size differentials) which determine or influence the outcome may not be easily monitored or controlled. In these circumstances, in-process controls tend to focus on the protein separation for which the technology was designed, with virus partitioning being assumed to be satisfactory so long as the protein separation remains within limits. The performance of cross-flow filtration is also difficult to monitor and control for virus removal on a batch-to-batch basis, as the degree of virus retention will be determined by the mechanical operation of the

equipment as well as by the sieving properties of the membrane (Murkes and Carlsson, 1988; Bell and Cousins, 1994)

Process segregation and containment

To avoid the introduction of viral contaminants after the virus elimination step has been completed, it is necessary to insure that all relevant equipment, tools, instruments, services and facilities are free from viral contamination. The control of personnel is also vital in this regard, as is the control of reagents and excipients being used at this point in the process and thereafter. The containment of a section of a manufacturing process in this manner is not straightforward when operating in a plant which will be handling a variety of processes and products, all of which at some stage may be potentially infectious (Fig. 27.1).

If this route of contamination has been responsible for any of the reported instances of virus transmission (Tables 27.7–27.12) then the safety of these products will be increased either by improved product containment following virus inactivation, or by the use of a further virus inactivation procedure which is carried out on the product sealed in its final container. The introduction of additional in-process virus elimination steps would not necessarily address the problem and, by increasing the length and complexity of a process, may even increase the opportunity for contamination to occur.

PRODUCT CONTROL

Before a batch of coagulation factor concentrate is released for clinical use, documentation must have been completed and checked to insure:

1. That all substances, materials, equipment, components and facilities complied with their defined specifications.
2. That all process operations were carried out by trained personnel in compliance with defined procedures and that all in-process control measurements were within defined limits.
3. That the characteristics of the final product comply fully with the approved product specification.

For this last point, a range of analytical measurements and other tests must be performed on representative samples from the batch of product. This will include measurements of the active substance, the protein composition, sterility, biologic safety and the concentration of excipients. Acceptable residual levels of chemicals or other potentially toxic substances used in virus inactivation and elimination procedures must also be demonstrated. Substances controlled in this way can include TnBP, Tween-80 or Triton X-100 used in solvent/detergent treatment and murine monoclonal antibodies, cyanogen bromide, ethylene glycol, sodium thiocyanate and sodium azide associated with the use of immuno-purification methods (Griffin, 1991; Hrinda *et al.*, 1991; Feldman *et al.*, 1992)

The testing of final products for viral safety on the basis of antibody detection (e.g. HIV, HCV) is limited by the presence of little or no immunoglobulin in current coagulation factor products and is therefore of little relevance. The detection of a greater range of viruses at an increased sensitivity should be obtainable using PCR methods to test final products. However, there are problems of assay standardization which must be overcome before such methods could be introduced on a routine basis. In addition, there are problems in data interpretation, because non-infective viruses can still be PCR-reactive (Hart *et al.*, 1993; Hart *et al.*, 1994b).

Most of the testing considerations above also apply to recombinant products derived from transfected cell lines. However, additional testing is required with these products to measure possible contamination with cellu-lar protein, nucleic acids and media components, as well as to confirm the integrity of the molecular structure of the active component, e.g. factor VIII (Griffin *et al.*, 1991).

Product pharmacology

There are two pharmacologic aspects of coagulation factor concentrates which are of particular concern with respect to product safety. These are the potential of products to induce either inhibitors or thrombogenic reactions.

INHIBITORS

Plasma-derived concentrates

The development of antibodies (inhibitors) to factor VIII or to factor IX is a serious complication of hemophilia treatment. For many years it was believed that 5–15% of hemophiliacs would develop inhibitors according to their genetic susceptibility (Gill, 1984). However, a relatively high incidence of inhibitors to factor VIII following the use of an immunopurified product (Lusher and Salzman, 1990) led to this earlier view being questioned (Aledort, 1994). An outbreak of inhibitors associated with one particular product (Peerlinck *et al.*, 1993; Mauser-Bunschoten *et al.*, 1994) has also led to concerns that the incidence of inhibitors may be product-related.

Recent data from trials in previously untreated patients tend to support this possibility, as the incidence of inhibitors reported in trials of different products has ranged from 0/25 (0%; Williams, O'Brien and Hill, 1994), 5/56 (9%; Guérois *et al.*, 1995), 2/23 (9%;

Addiego *et al.*, 1992) through 1/7 (14%; de Biasi *et al.*, 1994) to 6/38 (16%; Lusher and Salzman, 1990). If inhibitor formation is product-related (Littlewood *et al.*, 1991), it will be necessary to identify the product characteristics responsible (Lubahn *et al.*, 1989; Healey *et al.*, 1994; Lubin *et al.*, 1994) and to establish analytical tests that would be suitable for the development and control of products that would be less prone to causing inhibitors.

Recombinant factor VIII

In studies of two recombinant factor VIII products in previously untreated patients, inhibitors were identified in 19/99 (19%; Lusher *et al.*, 1993) and in 17/71 (24%; Bray *et al.*, 1994) of patients respectively, with about half of these being high-titer responses, i.e. exceeding 10 Bethesda units/ml (Lusher, 1994).

New antigenic sites can be formed by the genetic instability inherent in recombinant systems (Berthold, 1994). Recombinant factor VIII also undergoes extensive posttranslation modifications (Kaufman, 1991; Pittman, Wang and Kaufman, 1992) which are sensitive to small variations in cell culture conditions (Goochee *et al.*, 1992) and which could also influence the immuno-genicity of a product. Whether or not variations of this type will be of any clinical significance remains to be determined. Safety studies with recombinant factor VIII have begun to address the subject of genetic instability, with no adverse events being observed (Gomperts *et al.*, 1994). However, the recent report of an anaphylactic reaction to recombinant factor VIII (Shopnick *et al.*, 1994), in conjunction with the apparently high incidence of inhibitor formation, suggests that recombinant prod-ucts should be used with caution until long-term safety studies have been completed.

THROMBOGENICITY

The treatment of hemophilia B with factor IX concen-trates is associated with a risk of thromboembolic compli-cations and disseminated intravascular coagulation (Ratnoff, 1974; Abilgaard, 1981). For example, in one study, 72 cases of thromboembolic disease, including five cases of myocardial infarction, were associated with the use of factor IX concentrates over a 3-year period (Lusher, 1991). A number of theories have been postulated to explain this behavior, including the presence of phospholipid with activated coagulation factors (Giles *et al.*, 1982), degraded or activated factor IX (Gray *et al.*, 1993) or the infusion of factors II, VII and X in patients deficient only in factor IX (Menaché *et al.*, 1984). Despite these theories, the precise characteristics of factor IX concentrates responsible for these reactions have not yet been determined.

Studies with more highly purified factor IX preparations have indicated that these products may carry a much reduced thrombogenic risk (Mannucci *et al.*, 1990a; Kim *et al.*, 1991; Hampton *et al.*, 1993). However, to insure that this reduced risk of thrombogenicity is achieved consistently it will be necessary to define fully those product characteristics responsible, so that suitable tests for thrombogenic potential can be established to control products on a batch-to-batch basis.

Conclusions

The safety of plasma-derived coagulation factor concentrates has increased substantially over the last decade with respect to the risk of virus transmission. The use of highly purified factor IX concentrates has also substantially reduced the thrombogenic risks associated with the treatment of hemophilia B. However, a similar reduction in the risk of inhibitor formation requires further knowledge of product characteristics which may be involved in eliciting inhibitor antibodies.

Instances of virus infection associated with coagulation factor concentrates continue to be reported. Where an infectious agent (e.g. HAV, B19) was not screened out, or specifically removed or inactivated by the manufacturing process, then this should not be surprising. However, where screening and inactivation procedures have been in place, the sporadic nature of the failures reported suggests that the technology may not always have been applied correctly. In these circumstances, greater consideration must be given to the design, containment and control of relevant process operations.

To reduce the risk of contamination with infectious agents further, there are a number of developments which could be applied to plasma-derived and recombinant products alike. These include:

1. Improved screening of source materials and other biologic substances for the presence of infectious agents, e.g. the screening of blood donations for HAV, B19 and possible HDV, and increasing the sensitivity of current testing for HIV, HBV and HCV.
2. The development of effective virus inactivation methods that can be applied to the final product.
3. A better understanding of the potential role of immunoglobulin, where present, in neutralizing viral contaminants.
4. The development of viral inactivation methods which will inactivate non-lipid-enveloped viruses.
5. The harmonization, standardization and control of methods for measuring the inactivation or partitioning behaviour of viruses.
6. The preparation of validated protocols for the scale-down and scale-up of methods for virus inactivation and removal.
7. The development of sensitive tests for detecting infectivity which could be used for the control of products and process operations.
8. The development of guidelines for the design, containment and control of process operations used for the inactivation or removal of viruses.

Acknowledgements

We would like to thank Dr H. Hart, Dr J. Gillon, Dr J. Löwer, Dr Y. Laurian, Dr C. Prowse and Ms D. Rodger for providing helpful information. The typing skills of Mrs K. Glass were also greatly appreciated.

References

Aach, R.D., Szmuness, W., Mosley, J.W. *et al.* (1981) Serum alanine aminotransferase of donors in relation to the risk of non-A, non-B hepatitis in recipients. *New England Journal of Medicine*, **304**, 989–994.

Abildgaard, C.F. (1981) Hazards of prothrombin-complex concentrates in treatment of haemophilia. *New England Journal of Medicine*, **304**, 670–671.

Adamson, R. (1994) Design and operation of a recombinant mammalian cell manufacturing process for rFVIII. *Annals of Hematology*, **68** (suppl. III), S9–S14; S25–S28.

Addiego, J.E., Gomperts, E., Liu, S.L *et al.*, (1992) Treatment of hemophilia A with a highly purified factor VIII concentrate prepared by anti-FVIIIC immunoaffinity chromatography. *Thrombosis and Haemostasis*, **67**, 19–27.

Adler, S.P., Manganello, A.M.A., Koch, W.C. *et al.* (1993) Risk of human parvovirus B19 infections among school and hospital employees during endemic periods. *Journal of Infectious Diseases*, **168**, 361–368.

Aledort, L. (1994) Inhibitors in hemophilia patients: current status and management. *American Journal of Hematology*, **47**, 208–217.

Allain, J.P. (1984) Non factor VIII related constituents in concentrates. *Scandanavian Journal of Haemotology*, **33** (suppl. 41), 173–180.

Allain, J.P., Verroust, F. and Soulier, J.P. (1980) *In vitro* and *in vivo* characterization of factor VIII preparations. *Vox Sanguinis*, **38**, 68–80.

Allander, T., Gruber, A., Naghavi, M. *et al.* (1995) Frequent patient-to-patient transmission of hepatitis C virus in a haematology ward. *Lancet*, **345**, 603–607.

Alter, M.J. (1995) Residual risk of transfusion-associated hepatitis, in *Proceedings of NIH Consensus Development Conference on Infectious Disease Testing for Blood Transfusions* (eds P.R. McCurdy and J.M. Elliot), National Institute of Health, Bethesda, Maryland, pp. 23–27.

Anderle, K., Eder, G. and Eibl, J. (1991) Antibody to hepatitis C virus after a vapour heated factor VIII concentrate – lack of evidence. *Thrombosis Haemastosis*, **66**, 620.

Anderson, L.J. (1987) Role of parvovirus B19 in human disease. *Pediatric Infectious Diseases Journal*, **6**, 711–718.

Araújo, F. and Araújo, A.R. (1994) How to calculate the maximum risk. *Blood Coagulation and Fibrinolysis*, **5**, 849–850.

Arzneimittelkommission (1994) Information Beriplex HS250 and 500. *Pharmazeutische Zeitung*, **139**, 2192–2193.

Avest, A.R., van Zoelen, E.J.J., Spijkers, I.E.M., *et al.* (1992) Purification process monitoring on monoclonal antibody preparation: contamination with viruses, DNA and peptide growth factors. *Biologicals*, **20**, 177–186.

Azzi, A., Ciappi, S., Zakvrzewska, K. *et al.* (1992) Human parvovirus B19 infection in hemophiliacs first infused with two high-purity, virally attenuated factor VIII concentrates. *American Journal of Hematology*, **39**, 228–230.

Balakrishnan, M., Agarwal, G.P. and Cooney, C.L. (1993) Study of protein transmission through ultrafiltration membranes. *Journal of Membrane Science*, **85**, 111–128.

Bartolomei Corsi, O., Azzi, A., Morfini, M. *et al.* (1988) Human parvovirus infection in haemophiliacs first infused with treated clotting factor concentrates. *Journal of Medical Virology*, **25**, 165–170.

Becton, D., Manno, C., Green, D. *et al.* (1994) Viral safety of an affinity-purified coagulation factor IX concentrate (Alphanine S D). *Blood*, **84** (suppl. 4), 198a.

Bell, G. and Cousins, R.B. (1994) Membrane separation processes, in *Engineering Processes for Bioseparations* (ed. L.R. Weatherley), Butterworth-Heinemann, Oxford, pp. 135–165.

Bell, D.J., Hoare, M. and Dunnill, P. (1983) The formation of protein precipitates and their centrifugal recovery, in *Advances in Biochemical Engineering*, vol. 26 (ed. A. Fiechter), Springer-Verlag, New York, pp. 1–72.

Belter, P.A., Cussler, E.L. and Hu, W.S. (1988) *Bioseparations Downstream Processing for Biotechnology*, John Wiley, New York

Bennet, B., Dawson, A.A., Gibson, B.S. *et al.* (1993) Study of viral safety of Scottish National Blood Transfusion Service factor VIII/IX concentrate. *Transfusion Medicine*, 3, 295–298.

Berntorp, E., Nilsson, I.M., Ljung, R. *et al.* (1990) Hepatitis C virus transmission by monoclonal purified factor VIII concentrate. *Lancet*, 335, 1531–1532.

Berthold, W. (1994) Gene stability in mammalian cells and protein consistency. in *Developments in Biological Standardization*, Karger, Basel, World Federation of Hemophilia, Montreal, Canada, 83, 67–80.

Bessos, H., Appleyard, C., Micklem, C.R. and Pepper, D.S. (1991) Monolonal antibody leakage from gels: effect of support, activation and eluant composition. *Preparative Chromatography*, 1, 207–220.

Birkenmeyer, L.G. and Mushahwar, I.K. (1994) Detection of hepatitis A, B and D virus by the polymerase chain reaction. *Journal of Virological Methods*, 49, 101–112.

Blanchette, V., Vortstmon, E., Shore, A. *et al.* (1991) Hepatitis C infection in children with haemophilia A and B. *Blood*, 78, 285–289.

Blomback, B. and Blomback, M. (1956) Purification of human and bovine fibrinogen. *Arkiv For Kemi*, 10, 415–443.

Boedeker, B.G.D. (1992) Production of Kogenate, in *Process Testing and characterization of Recombinant Factor VIII*. Proceedings of XXth International Congress of the World Federation of Hemophilia. Abstracts, Athens, p. 81.

Brackman, H.H. and Egli, H. (1988) Acute hepatitis B infection after treatment with heat inactivated factor VIII concentrate. *Lancet*, ii, 967.

Bray, G.L. and Aledort, L.M. (1994) Considerations governing factor IX product choice in hemophilia B. *Transfusion*, 34, 554.

Bray, G., Gomperts, E.D., Courter, S. *et al.* (1994) A multicentre study of recombinant factor VIII (Recombinate): safety, efficacy and inhibitor risk in previously untreated patients with hemophilia A. *Blood*, 83, 2428–2435.

Brockway, W.J. and Seng, R.I. (1994) *Gel Filtration of Factor VIII*. US patent, no. 5356878.

Buffet, C., Charnaux, N., Laurentpuig, P. *et al.* (1994) Enhanced detection of antibodies to hepatitis C virus by use of a third-generation recombinant immunoblot assay. *Journal of Medical Virology*, 43, 259–261.

Burnouf, T. (1992) Safety aspects in the manufacture of plasma-derived coagulation factor concentrates. *Biologicals*, 20, 91–100.

Burnouf, T., Michalski, C., Goudemand, M. *et al.* (1989) Properties of a highly purified human plasma factor IX: therapeutic concentrate prepared by conventional chromatography. *Vox Sanguinis*, 57, 225–232.

Burnouf, T., Burnouf-Radesovich, M., Huart, J.J. and Goudemand, M. (1991) A highly purified factor VIII:C concentrate prepared from cryoprecipitate by ion-exchange chromatography. *Vox Sanguinis*, 60, 8–15.

Burnouf-Radesovich, M., Appourchaux, P., Huart, J.J. and Burnouf, T., (1994) Nanofiltration, a new specific virus elimination method applied to high purity factor IX and factor XI concentrates. *Vox Sanguinis*, 67, 132–138.

Busch, M.P. (1995) Incidence of infectious disease markers in blood donors: implications for residual risk of viral transmission by transfusion, in *Proceedings of NIH Consensus Development Conference on Infectious Disease Testing for Blood Transfusions* (eds P.R. McCurdy and J.M. Elliot), National Institute of Health, Bethesda, Maryland, pp. 29–30.

Busch, M.P., Lee, L.L.L., Satton, G.A. *et al.* (1995) Time course of detection of viral and serologic markers preceding human immunodeficiency virus type 1 seroconversion: implications for screening of blood and tissue donors. *Transfusion*, 35, 91–97.

Carnelli, V., Gomports, E.D., Friedman, A. *et al.* (1987) Assessment for evidence of non-A, non-B hepatitis in patients given n-heptane suspended heat treated clotting factor concentrates. *Thrombosis Research*, 46, 827–834.

Casillas, G., Simonetti, C. and Pavlovsky, A. (1969) Chromatographic behaviour of clotting factors. *British Journal of Haematology*, 16, 363–372.

Centers for Disease Control (1991) Public Health Service inter-agency guidelines for screening donors of blood, plasma organs, tissues and semen for evidence of hepatitis B and hepatitis C. *Morbidity and Mortality Weekly Report*, 40, (RR-4) 1–17.

Chan, S.Y. (1994) Characterisation of recombinant BHK-21 endogenous particles: R-type particles *Biologicals*, 22, 121–125.

Chtourou, S., Nogré, M., Olivier, B. and Perissé, C. (1993) Virological safety of a new plasma-derived immunopurifed FVIII. *Thrombosis Haemostasis*, 69, 1101.

Cohn, E.J., Strong, C.E., Hughes, W.L. *et al.* (1946) Preparation and properties of serum and plasma proteins IV: a system for the separation into fractions of the protein and lipoprotein components of biological tissues and fluids. *Journal of the American Chemical Society*, 68, 459–475.

Cohn, R.J., Schwyzer, R., Field, S.P. *et al.* (1994) Acute hepatitis A in haemophiliacs. *Thrombosis and Haemostasis*, 72, 782–786.

Colombo, M., Carnelli, V., Gazengel, C. *et al.* (1985) Transmission of non-A, non-B hepatitis by heat treated factor VIII concentrate. *Lancet*, ii, 1–4.

Colvin, B.T. (1990) Prevention of hepatitis C infection in haemophiliacs. *Lancet*, 335, 1474.

Colvin, B.T., Rizza, C.R., Hill, F.G.H. *et al.* (1988) Effect of dry-heating of coagulation factor concentrates at 80°C for 72 hours on transmission of non-A, non-B hepatitis. *Lancet*, ii, 814–816.

Cumming, R.A., Davies, S.H., Ellis, D. and Grant, W. (1965) Red cell banking and the production of a factor VIII concentrate *Vox Sanguinis*, 10, 687–699.

Cuthbertson, B., Reid, K.G. and Foster, P.R. (1991) Viral contamination of human plasma and procedures for preventing virus transmission by plasma products. in *Blood Separation and Plasma Fractionation* (ed. J.R. Harris), Wiley-Liss, New York, pp. 385–435.

Danner, K. (1993) BSE – a risk for man through pharmaceutical products? Position and politics of the German pharmaceutical industry. *Developments in Biological Standardization*, S. Karger, Basel, World Federation of Hemophilia, Montreal, Canada, 80, 199–205.

de Biasi, R., Rocino, A., Papa, M.L. *et al.* (1994) Incidence of factor VIII inhibitor development in hemophilia A patients treated with less pure plasma derived concentrates. *Thrombosis and Haemostasis*, 71, 544–547.

Dichtelmuller, H., Stephan, W., Prince, A.M. *et al.* (1987) Inactivation of HIV in plasma derivatives by β-propiolactone and UV irradiation. *Infection*, 15, 367–369.

Didisheim, P., Loeb, J., Blatrix, C. and Soulier, J.P. (1959) Preparation of a human plasma fraction rich in prothrombin, proconvertion, stuart factor, and PTC and a study of its activity and toxicity in rabbits and man. *Journal of Laboratory and Clinical Medicine*, 53, 322–330.

Dietrich, S.L., Mosley, J.W., Lusher, J.M. *et al* (1990) Transmission of human immunodeficiency virus type I by dry-heated clotting factor concentrates. *Vox Sanguinis*, 59, 129–135.

DiLeo, A.J., Allegrezza, A.E. and Builder, S.E. (1992) High resolution removal of virus from protein solutions using a membrane of unique structure. *Biotechnology*, 10, 182–188.

DiLeo, A.J., Vacante, D.A. and Deane, E.F. (1993) Size exclusion removal of model mammalian viruses using a unique membrane system, part I: Membrane qualification. part II: Module qualification and process simulation. *Biologicals*, 21, 275–286: 287–296.

Dodd, R.Y. (1992) The risk of transfusion transmitted infection. *New England Journal of Medicine*, 327, 419–421.

Drohan, W.N. and Hoyer, L.W. (1994) Plasma protein products, in *Scientific Basis of Transfusion Medicine* (eds K.C. Anderson and P.M. Ness), W.B. Saunders, Philadelphia, pp. 381–402.

Edwards, M.F. (1985) Mixing of low-viscosity liquids in stirred tanks, in *Mixing in the Process Industries* (eds N. Harnby, M.F. Edwards and A.W. Nienow), Butterworths, London, pp. 131–144.

EEC (1989) Council directive 89/381/EEC. *Official Journal of the European Communities* L181, 44–46.

EEC Ad Hoc Working Party on Biotechnology/Pharmacy (1994) Note for guidance: Plasma pool testing EEC III/5, 193/94.

Eibl, J. and Kasser, A. (1988) Ways to reduce the risk of transmission of viral infections by plasma and plasma products. *Vox Sanguinis*, 54, 228–230.

Einarsson, M. and Morgenthaler, J.J. (1989) Removal of viruses from plasma fractions by chromatography, in *Virus Inactivation in Plasma Products. Current Studies in Hematology and Blood Transfusion* (ed. J.J. Morgenthaler), Karger, Basel, pp. 138–145.

Einarsson, M., Kaplan, L., Nordenfelt, E. *et al.* (1981) Removal of hepatitis B virus from a concentrate of coagulation factor II, VII, IX and X by hydrophobic interaction chromatography. *Journal of Virological Methods*, 3, 213–228.

Fekete, L.F. and Shanbrom, E. (1972) *Fractionation of Plasma using Glycine and Polyethylene Glycol*. US patent, no. 3682881.

Fekete, L.F., Shanbrom, V. and Shanbrom, E. (1971) *Prothrombin Complex Prepared by Precipitation with Polyethylen Glycol*. US patent, no. 3560475.

Feldman, F., Klekamp, M.S., Hrinda, M.E. *et al.* (1989) *Stabilization of Biologicals and Pharmaceutical Products during Thermal Inactivation of Viral and Bacterial Contaminants*. US patent, no. 4876241.

Feldman, F., Chandra, S., Hrinda, M.E. and Schrieber, A.B. (1992) Quality assurance in production of plasma proteins, in *Quality Assurance in Transfusion Medicine*, vol. II, *Methodological Advances and clinical Aspects* (eds G. Rock and M.J. Seghatchian), CRC Press, Boca Raton, pp. 259–284.

Fernandes, P.M. and Lundblad, J.L. (1984) *Pasteurised Therapeutically Active Protein Compositions*. US patent, no. 4440679.

Finkel, T.H., Török, T.J., Ferguson, P.J. *et al.* (1994) Chronic parvovirus B19 infection and systemic necrotising vasculitis: opportunistic infection or aetiological agent. *Lancet*, 343, 1255–1258

Food and Drug Administration (1993) *Draft Points to Consider in the Characterization of cell Lines used to Produce Biologicals*. Center for Biologic Evaluation and Research, FDA, Rockville, Maryland.

Food and Drug Administration (1994) *Draft Points to Consider in the Manufacture and Testing of Monoclonal Antibody Products for Human Use*. Center for Biologics Evaluation and Research, FDA, Rockville, Maryland.

Foster, P.R. (1994a) Fractionation, blood plasma fractionation, in *The Kirk–Othmer Encyclopaedia of Chemical Technology*, 4th edn, vol. 11. John Wiley, New York, pp. 990–1021.

Foster, P.R. (1994b) Protein precipitation, in *Engineering Processes for Bioseparations* (ed. L.R. Weatherley), Butterworth-Heinemann, Oxford, pp. 73–109.

Foster, P.R. and Cuthbertson, B. (1994) Procedures for the prevention of virus transmission by blood products, in *Blood, Blood Products and HIV* (eds R. Madhok, C.D. Forbes and B.L. Evatt), Chapman & Hall Medical, London, pp. 207–248.

Foster, P.R., Dickson, I.H., McQuillan, T.A. and Dawes, J. (1983a) Factor VIII stability during the manufacture of a clinical concentrate. *Thrombosis Haemostasis*, **50**, 117.

Foster, P.R., Dickson, I.H., MacLeod, A.J. *et al.* (1983b) Zinc fractionation of cryoprecipitate. *Thrombosis and Haemostasis*, **50**, 117.

Foster, P.R., Dickson, I.H., McQuillan, T.A. *et al.* (1988b) Studies on the stability of VIII:C during the manufacture of a factor VIII concentrate for clinical use. *Vox Sanguinis*, **55**, 81–89.

Foster, P.R., Cuthbertson, B., Perry, R.J. and McIntosh, R.V. (1988a) Coagulation factor VIII concentrates and the market place. *Lancet*, **ii**, 43.

Friedman, L.I., Stromberg, R.R. and Wagner, S.J. (1995) Reducing the infectivity of blood components – what have we learned? *Immunological Investigations*. **24**, 49–71.

Frösner, G., Stephan, W. and Dichtelmuller, H. (1983) Inactivation of heptitis A virus seeded in pooled human plasma by β-propiolactone- and UV-irradiation. *European Journal of Clinical Microbiology*, **2**, 355–357.

Garson, J.A., Preston, F.E., Makris, M. *et al.* (1990) Detection by PCR of hepatitis C virus in factor VIII concentrates. *Lancet*, **335**, 1473.

Gazengel, C., Torcher, M.F., Boneu, B. *et al.* (1988) Viral safety of solvent/detergent treated FVIII concentrate. Results of a French multicenter study, in *Proceedings of 18th International Congress of the World Federation of Hemophilia* (Abstracts), Madrid (eds G. Papaevangelon and W. Hennessen), p. 59.

Gellis, S.S., Neefe, J.R., Stokes, J. *et al.* (1948) Chemical, clinical and immunological studies on products of human plasma fractionation; inactivation of virus of homologous serum albumin by means of heat. *Journal of Clinical Investigation*, **27**, 239–244.

Gerety, R.J., Smallwood, L.A., Finlayson, J.S. and Tabor, E. (1983) Standardization of the antibody to hepatitis A virus (anti-HAV) content of immunoglobulin. *Developments in Biological Standardization*, World Federation of Hemophilia, Montreal, Canada, S. Karger, Basel, **54**, 411–416.

Gerritzen, A., Scholt, B., Kaiser, R. *et al.* (1992a). Acute hepatitis C in haemophiliacs due to "virus inactivated" clotting factor concentrates. *Thrombosis and Haemostasis*, **68**, 781.

Gerritzen, A., Schneweis, K.E., Brackmann, H.H. *et al.* (1992b) Acute hepatitis A in hemophiliacs. *Lancet*, **340**, 1231–1232.

Gilchrist, G.S., Eckert, H., Shanbrom, E. *et al.*, (1969) Evaluation of a new concentrate for the treatment of a factor IX deficiency. *New England Journal of Medicine*, **280**, 291–295.

Giles, A.R., Nesheim, M.E., Hoogendorn, H. *et al.* (1982) The coagulant active phospholipid content is a major determinant of *in vitro* thrombogenicity of prothrombin complex (factor IX concentrates) in rabbits. *Blood*, **59**, 401–407.

Gill, F.M. (1984) The natural history of factor VIII in patients with hemophilia A, in *Factor VIII Inhibitors* (ed. L.W. Hoyer), Alan R. Liss, New York, pp. 19–29.

Gocke, D.J., Greenberg, H.B. and Kavey, N.B. (1970) Correlation of Australia antigen with post-transfusion hepatitis. *Journal of the American Medical Association*, **212**, 877–879.

Gomperts, E.D., Courter, S.G., Lynes, M.D. and Baker, D.A. (1994) A clinical evaluation of genetic stability. *Developments in Biological Standardization*, World Federation of Hemophilia, Montreal, Canada, Karger, Basel, **83**, 111–120.

Gonzaga, A.L. and Bonecker, C. (1990) Follow-up of hemophiliacs using solvent/detergent treated FVIII and FIX concentrates, in *Proceedings of 19th International Congress of the World Federation of Hemophilia* (abstracts), Washington (eds F. Brown and A.S. Lubiniecki), p. 25.

Gonzaga, A.L., Bonecker, C. and Dantas, W.V. (1994) Hepatitis A transmission in Brazilian hemophiliacs. *Vox Sanguinis*, **67** (suppl. I), 29–30.

Goochee, C.F., Gramer, M.J., Andersen, D.C. and Bahr, J.B. (1992) The oligosaccharides of glycoproteins: factors affecting their synthesis and their influence on glycoprotein properties, in *Frontiers in Bioprocessing II* (eds P. Todd, S.K. Sikdar and M. Bier), American Chemical Society, Washington, pp. 199–240.

Goudemand, J., Parquet, A., d'Oiron, R. *et al.* (1994) Hepatitis A in French hemophiliacs. *Vox Sanguinis*, **67** (suppl. I), 9–13.

Gray, E., Tubbs, J., Cesmeli, S. and Barrowcliffe, T.W. (1993) Thrombogenicity of FIX concentrates: *in vitro* and *in vivo* results. *Thrombosis and Haemostasis*, **69**, 1285.

Griffin, M. (1991) Ultrapure plasma factor VIII produced by anti-FVIIIC immunoaffinity chromatography and solvent/detergent viral inactivation. Characterization of the Method M process and Hemofil M antihemophilic factor (human). *Annals of Hematology*, **63**, 131–137.

Griffin, M., Kingdon, H., Liu, S.L. and Burkart, W. (1991) In-process controls and characterization of recombinate antihemophilic factor (recombinant). *Annals of Hematology*, **63**, 166–171.

Grosse-Bley, A., Eis-Hubinger, A.M., Kaiser, R. *et al.* (1994) Serological and virological markers of human parvovirus B19 infection in sera of hemophiliacs. *Thrombosis and Haemostasis*, **72**, 503–507.

Guérois, C., Laurian, Y., Rothschild, C. *et al.* (1995) Incidence of inhibitors specific for factor VIII (FVIII) or IX (FIX) in severe hemophiliacs A and B only treated with very high purity FVIII or FIX SD concentrates. *Thrombosis and Haemostasis*, **69**, 852.

Guérois, C., Rothschild, C., Laurian, Y. *et al.* (1993) Incidence of inhibitors specific for factor VIII Inhibitor development in severe haemophilia A patients treated with only one brand of highly purified plasma-derived concentrate *Thrombosis and Haemostasis*, **73**, 215–218.

Guillaume, T.A. (1991) Potential accumulation of tri(n-butyl) phosphate in solvent–detergent virus inactivated plasma products. *Transfusion*, **31**, 871.

Hagen, J.J. and Glaser, C. (1976) *Antihemophilic Factor*. US patent, no. 3973002.

Hamamoto, Y., Horada, S., Kobayashi, K. *et al.* (1989) A novel method for removal of human immunodeficiency virus: filtration with porous polymeric membranes. *Vox Sanguinis*, **56**, 230–236.

Hampton, K.K., Preston, F.E., Lowe, G.D.O. *et al.* (1993) Reduced coagulation activation following infusion of a highly purified factor IX concentrate compared to a prothrombin complex concentrate. *British Journal of Haematology*, **84**, 279–284.

Hanley, J.A. and Lippman-Hand, A. (1983) If nothing goes wrong, is everything all right? Interpreting zero numerators. *Journal of the American Medical Association*, **249**, 1743–1745.

Hart, H., McOmish, F., Hart, W.G. *et al.* (1993) A comparison of polymerase chain reaction and an infectivity assay for human immunodeficiency virus type I titration during virus inactivation of blood components. *Transfusion*, **33**, 838–841.

Hart, H., Jones, A., Cubie, H. *et al* (1994a). Distribution of hepatitis A antibody over a process for the preparation of a high-purity factor VIII concentrate. *Vox Sanguinis,* **67** (suppl. I), 51–55.

Hart, H.F., Hart, W.G., Crossley, J. *et al.* (1994b) Effect of terminal (dry) heat treatment on non-enveloped viruses in coagulation factor concentrates. *Vox Sanguinis*, **67**, 345–350.

Healy, J.F., Lubin, I.M., Scandella, D. and Lollar, P. (1994) Residues 484–509 contain a major determinant of the inhibiting epitope in the A2 domain of human factor VIII. *Blood*, **84** (suppl. I), 240a.

Heimburger, N. and Karges, H.E. (1989) Strategies to produce virus-safe blood derivatives, in *Virus Inactivation in Plasma Products. Current Studies in Hematology and Blood Transfusion* (ed. J.J. Morgenthaler), Karger, Basel, pp. 23–33.

Heimburger, N., Schwinn, H. and Mauler, R. (1980) Factor VIII concentrate – now free from hepatitis risk: progress in the treatment of haemophilia. *Die gelben Hefte*, **4**, 165–174.

Heimburger, N., Schwinn, H., Gratz, P. *et al.* (1981a) A factor VIII concentrate, highly purified and heated in solution. *Haemostasis*, **10** (suppl. I), 204.

Heimburger, N., Schwinn, H., Gratz, P. *et al.* (1981b) Factor VIII concentrate highly purified and heated in solution. *Arzneimittel – Forschung/Drug Research*, **31**, 619–622.

Heinrich, D., Sugg, U., Brackmann, H.H. *et al.* (1987) Virus safety of β-propiolactone treated plasma preparations. *Developments in Biological Standardization*, World Federation of Hemophilia, Montreal, Canada, S. Karger, Basel, **67**, 313–317.

Heldebrant, C.M. (1984) *Virus inactivating Heat Treatment of Plasma Fractions*. US patent, no. 4490361.

Heldebrant, C.M., Gomperts, E.D., Kasper, C.K. *et al.* (1985) Evaluation of two viral inactivation methods for the preparation of safer factor VIII and factor IX concentrates. *Transfusion*, **25**, 510–515.

Herring, W.S., Abilgaard, C., Shitanishi, K.T. *et al.* (1993) Human coagulation factor IX: assessment of thrombogenicity in animal models and viral safety. *Journal of Laboratory and Clinical Medicine*, **121**, 394–405.

Hershgold, E.J., Pool, J.G. and Pappenhagen, A.R. (1966) The potent antihemophilia globulin concentrate derived from a cold insoluble fraction of human plasma: charactcrization and further data on preparation and clinical trial. *Journal of Laboratory and Clinical Medicine*, **67**, 23–32.

Heystek, J., Brummelhuis, H.G.J. and Krijnen, H.W. (1973) Contributions to the optimal use of human blood. II. The large-scale preparation of prothrombin complex. A comparison between two methods using the anion exchanges. DEAE-cellulose DE52 and DEAE-sephadex A-50. *Vox Sanguinis*, **25**, 113–123.

Hilfenhaus, J. and Nowak, T. (1994) Inactivation of hepatitis A virus by pasteurisation and elimination of picornaviruses during manufacture of factor VIII concentrate. *Vox Sanguinis*, **67** (suppl. I), 62–66.

Hoag, M.S., Johnson, F.F., Robinson, J.A. and Aggeler, P.M. (1969) Treatment of hemophilia B with a new clotting factor concentrate. *New England Journal of Medicine*, **280**, 581–586.

Hoofnagle, J.H., Barker, L.F., Thiel, J. and Gerety, R.J. (1976) Hepatitis B virus and hepatitis B surface antigen in human albumin products. *Transfusion*, **16**, 141–147.

Horowitz, B. (1989) Investigations into the application of tri(n-butyl) phosphate/detergent mixtures to blood derivatives, in *Virus Inactivation in Plasma Products* (ed. J.J. Morgenthaler), Karger, Basel, pp. 83–96.

Horowitz, B. and Prince, A.M. (1987) Laboratory and preclinical evaluation of the virus safety of coagulation factor concentrates. in *Developments in Biological Standardization*, World Federation of Hemophilia, Montreal, Canada, Karger, Basel, **67**, 291–302.

Horowitz, B., Wiebe, M.E., Lippin, A. and Stryker, M.H. (1985a) Inactivation of viruses in labile blood derivatives. I. Diruption of lipid-enveloped viruses by tri(n-butyl) phosphate detergent combinations *Transfusion*, **25**, 516–522.

Horowitz, B., Wiebe, M.E., Lippin, A. *et al.* (1985b) Inactivation of viruses in labile blood derivatives. II. Physical methods *Transfusion*, **25**, 523–527.

Horowitz, M.S., Rooks, C., Horowitz, B. and Hilgartner, M. (1988) Virus safety of solvent-detergent treated antihemophilic factor concentrate. *Lancet*, **ii**, 186–189.

Horowitz, B., Prince, A.M., Horowitz, M.S. and Watklevicz, C. (1993) Viral safety of solven/detergent treated blood products, in *Biotechnology of Blood Proteins*, vol. 227 (eds C. Rivat and J.F. Stoltz), Colloque INSERM, Montronge, France, pp. 237–247.

Hrinda, M.E., Feldman, F. and Schreiber, A.B. (1990) Preclinical characterization of a new pasteurised monoclonal antibody purified factor VIIIC. *Seminars in Hematology*, 27 (suppl. 2), 19–24.

Hrinda, H.E., Huang, C., Tarr, G.C. *et al.* (1991) Preclinical studies of a monoclonal antibody-purified factor IX, Mononine. *Seminars in Hematology*, 28 (suppl. 6), 6–14.

Iritani, E., Nakatsaka, S., Aoki, H. *et al.* (1991) Effect of solution environment on unstirred dead-end ultrafiltration characteristics of proteinaceous solutions. *Journal of Chemical Engineering Japan*, 24, 117–183.

Jonsson, G. and Johansen, P.L. (1991) Selectivity of ultrafiltration membranes. Influence of fouling and cleaning conditions. *Filtration and Separation*, **28**, 21–23.

Josic, D., Schwinn, H., Stadler, M. and Strancor, A. (1994) Purification of factor VIII and von Willebrand factor from human plasma by anion-exchange chromatography. *Journal of Chromatography B*, **662**, 181–190.

Jungbauer, A. and Boschetti, E. (1994) Manufacture of recombinant proteins with safe and validated chromatographic sorbents. *Journal of Chromatography B*, **662**, 143–179.

Karcher, H. (1991) German haemophilic patients infected with HIV. *British Medical Journal*, 303, 1352–1353.

Kasper, C.K. (1995) Report of the National Hemophilia Foundation Symposium 'Liver disease in hemophilia', Atlanta, in *The Hemophilia Bulletin* (ed. C.K. Kasper), Orthopaedic Hospital, Los Angeles, pp. 1–7.

Kasper, C.K., Lusher, J.M., Silberstein, C.E. *et al.* (1993) Recent evolution of clotting factor concentrates for haemophilia A and B. *Transfusion*, 33, 422–434.

Kaufman, R.J. (1991) Insight into the structure, function and biosynthesis, of factor VIII through recombinant DNA technology. *Annals of Hematology*, 63, 155–165.

Keith, J.C., Ferranti, J.T, Misra, B. *et al.* (1994) Evaluation of recombinant human factor IX: pharmacokinetic studies in the rat and the dog. *Thrombosis and Haemostasis*, 73, 101–105.

Kernoff, P.B.A., Miller, E.J., Savidge, G.F. *et al.* (1987) Reduced risk of non-A, non-B hepatitis after a first exposure to 'wet heated' factor VIII concentrate. *British Journal of Haematology*, 67, 207–211.

Kim, H.C., Matts, L., Eisele, J. *et al.* (1991) Monoclonal antibody-purified factor IX – comparative thrombogenicity to prothrombin complex concentrate. *Seminars in Hematology*, 28 (suppl. 6), 15–19.

Kleim, J.P., Bailly, E., Schneweis, K.E. *et al.* (1990) Acute HIV-1 infection in patients with haemophilia B treated with β-propiolactoe-UV-inactivated clotting factor. *Thrombosis Haemostasis*, 64, 336–337.

Knevelman, A., de Wit, H.J.C., Griffin, B. *et al.* (1994) Effect of monosaccharides during severe dry heat treatment of coagulation factor VIII concentrates. *Vox Sanguinis*, 66, 96–103.

Kolho, E., Ebeling, F. and Rasi, V. (1992) Risk of HCV infection in haemophiliacs treated with a dry-heated factor VIII concentrate. *Thrombosis Haemostasis*, 67, 728.

Koplove, H.M. (1994) Cell culture and purification process – purity and safety testing. *Annals of Hematology*, 68 (suppl. III), S15–S20.

Koziol, D.E., Holland, P.V., Alling, D.W. *et al.* (1986) Antibody to hepatitis B core antigen as a paradoxical marker for non-A, non-B hepatitis agents in donated blood. *Annals of Internal Medicine*, 104, 488–495.

Kreuz, W., Auerswald, G., Bruckmann, C. *et al.* (1992) Prevention of hepatitis C virus infection in children, with hemophilia A and B and von Willebrand's disease. *Thrombosis and Haemostasis*, 67, 728.

Kuo, G., Choo, Q.L., Alter, H.J. *et al.* An asssay for circulating antibodies to a major etiologic virus of human non-A, non-B hepatitis. *Science*, 244, 362–364.

Lackritz, E.M., Satten, G.A., Kennedy, M.B. *et al.* (1995) Residual risk of transfusion-associated HIV transmission, in *Proceedings of NIH Consensus Development Conference on Infectious Disease Testing for Blood Transfusions* (eds P.R. McCurdy and J.M. Elliot), National Institute of Health, Bethesda, Maryland, p. 21.

Laurian, Y., Dussaix, E., Parquet, A. *et al.* (1994) Transmission of human parvovirus B19 by plasma derived factor VIII concentrates. *Nouvelle Revue Française Hématologie*, 36, 449–453.

Lawrence, J. (1994) Recombinate: viral safety and final product manufacturing testing and specifications. *Annals of Hematology*, 68 (suppl. III), S21–S24.

Leikola, J. (1993) Non-remunerated donations. in *Developments in Biological Standardization* (ed. F. Brown), World Federation of Hemophilia, Montreal, Canada, Karger, Basel, 81, 51–56.

Lelie, P.N., van der Poel, C.L., Reesink, H.W. *et al.* (1989) Efficacy of the latest generation of antibody assays for (early) detection of HIV1 and HIV2 infection. *Vox Sanguinis*, 56, 59–61.

Lemon, S.M. (1994) The natural history of hepatitis A: the potential for transmission by transfusion of blood or blood products. *Vox Sanguinis*, 67 (suppl. 4), 19–23.

Lemon, S.M., Murphy, P.C., Smith, A. *et al* (1994) Removal/neutralisation of HAV during manufacture of high purity, solvent/detergent factor VIII concentrate. *Journal of Medical Virology*, 43, 44–49.

Leng, D.E. (1991) Mixing. Succeed at scale-up. *Chemical Engineering Progress*, 87(6), 23–31.

Lerman, Y., Shohat, T., Ashkenazi, S. *et al.* (1993) Efficacy of different doses of immune serum globulin in the prevention of hepatitis A – a 3 year prospective study. *Clinical Infectious Diseases*, 17, 411–414.

Levy, J.A., Mitra, G.A., Wong, M.F. and Mozen, M.M. (1985) Inactivation by wet and dry heat of AIDS-associated retroviruses during FVIII purification from plasma. *Lancet*, i, 1456–1457.

Lie, Y.S., Penuel, E.M., Low, M.A.L. *et al.* (1994) Chinese hamster ovary cells contain transcriptionally active full-length type C proviruses. *Journal of Virology*, 68, 7840–7858.

Linden, J.V. (1994) Error contributes to the risk of transmissable disease. *Transfusion*, 34, 1016.

Littlewood, J.D., Dawes, J., Smith, J.K. *et al.* (1987) Studies on the effect of heat treatment on the thrombogenicity of factor IX concentrates in dogs. *British Journal of Haematology*, 65, 463–468.

Littlewood, J.D., Bevan, S.A., Kemball-Cook, G. *et al.* (1991) Variable inactivation of human factor VIII from different sources by human factor VIII inhibitors. *British Journal of Haematology*, 77, 535–538.

Löwer, J. (1990) Virological aspects of the quality control of biologicals: quantitative considerations, in *Developments in Biological Standardization* (eds F. Horand and F. Brown), World Federation of Hemophilia, Montreal, Canada, Karger, Basel, 75, 221–226.

Lubahn, B.C., Ware, J., Stafford, D.W. and Reisner, H.M. (1989) Identification of a F.VIII epitope recognized by a human hemophilic inhibitor. *Blood*, 73, 497–499.

Luban, N.C.L. (1994) Human parvoviruses: implications for transfusion medicine. *Transfusion*, 34, 821–827.

Lubin, I.M., Healey, J.F., Scandella, D. *et al.* (1994) Elimination of a major inhibitor epitope in factor VIII. *Journal of Biological Chemistry*, 269, 8639–8641.

Lusher, J.M. (1991) Thrombogenicity associated with factor IX complex concentrates. *Seminars in Hematology*, 28 (suppl. 6), 3–5.

Lusher, J.M. (1994) Human antibodies to recombinant factor VIII in hemophiliacs. *Journal of Interferon Research*, 14, 173–174.

Lusher, J.M. and Salzman, P.M. (1990) Monoclate study group: viral safety and inhibitor development associated with factor VIIIC ultra-purified from plasma in hemophiliacs previously unexposed to factor VIIIC concentrates. *Seminars in Hematology*, 27 (suppl. 2), 1–7.

Lusher, J.M., Arkin, S., Abilgaard, C.F. *et al.* (1993) Inhibitor development in previously untreated patients (PUPS) with hemophilia receiving Kogenate: 4.5 year fullow-up data, including response to immune tolerance (IT) with Kogenate. *Blood*, 82 (suppl. 1), 153.

Lyon, D.J., Chapman, C.S., Martin, C. *et al.* (1989) Symptomatic parvovirus B19 infection and heat treated factor IX concentrate. *Lancet*, i, 1085.

McDougal, J.S., Martin, L.S., Court, S.P. *et al.* (1985) Thermal inactivation of the acquired immunodeficiency syndrome virus, human T-cell lymphotrophic virus-III/lymphadenopathy-associated virus, with special reference to antihemophilic factor. *Journal of Clinical Investigation*, 76, 875–877.

McIntosh, R.V. and Foster, P.R. (1990) The effect of solution formulation on the stability and surface interactions of factor VIII during plasma fractionation. *Transfusion Science*, 11, 55–66.

McIntosh, R.V., Docherty, N., Fleming, D. and Foster, P.R. (1987) A high yield factor VIII concentrate suitable for advanced heat treatment. *Thrombosis Haemostasis*, 58, 306.

McMillan, C.W., Diamond, C.L. and Surgenor, D.M. (1961) Treatment of classic hemophilia: the use of fibrinogen rich in factor VIII for hemorrhage and for surgery. *New England Journal of Medicine*, 265, 224–230.

McOmish, F., Yap, P.L., Jordan, A. *et al.* (1993) Detection of parvovirus B19 in donated blood: a model system for screening by polymerase chain reaction. *Journal of Clinical Microbiology*, 31, 323–328.

MacLeod, A.J., Cuthbertson, B. and Foster, P.R. (1984) Pasteurisation of factor VIII and factor IX concentrates, in *Abstracts of 18th Congress of the International Society of Blood Transfusion*, Karger, Basel, p. 34.

Mannucci, P.M. (1992) Outbreak of hepatitis A among Italian patients with haemophilia. *Lancet*, 339, 819.

Mannucci, P.M. (1993) Clinical evaluation of viral safety of coagulation factor VIII and IX concentrates. *Vox Sanguinis*, 64, 197–203.

Mannuci, P.M. (1994) Viral safety of factor VIII concentrates. Reply. *Vox Sanguinis*, 66, 248.

Mannucci, P.M. (1995) Viral safety of plasma-derived and recombinant products used in the management of haemophilia A and B. *Haemophilia*, 1 (suppl. 1), 14–20.

Mannucci, P.M. and Colombo, M. (1988) Virucidal treatment of clotting factor concentrates. *Lancet*, ii, 782–785.

Mannucci, P.M. and Colombo, M. (1989) Revision of the protocol recommended for studies of safety from hepatitis of clotting factor concentrates. *Thrombosis Haemostasis*, 62, 532–534.

Mannucci, P.M., Colombo, M. and Rhodeghiero, F. (1985) Non-A, non-B hepatitis after factor VIII concentrate treated by heating and chloroform. *Lancet*, ii, 1013.

Mannucci, P.M., Morfini, M., Gatti, L. *et al.* (1988a) No hepatitis after treatment with a modified factor IX concentrate in previously untreated haemophiliacs. *Annals of Internal Medicine*, 103, 226–227.

Mannucci, P.M., Zanetti, A.R., Colombo, M. *et al.* (1988b) Prospective study of hepatitis after factor VIII exposed to hot vapour. *British Journal of Haematology*, 68, 427–430.

Mannucci, P.M., Bauer, K.A., Gringeri, A. *et al.* (1990a) Thrombin generation is not increased in the blood of hemophilia B patients after the infusion of a purified factor IX concentrate. *Blood*, 76, 2540–2545.

Mannucci, P.M., Schimpf, K., Brettler, D.B. *et al.* (1990b) Low-risk for hepatitis in hemophiliacs given a high-purity, pasteurized factor VIII concentrate. *Annals of Internal Medicine*, 113, 24–32.

Mannucci, P.M., Zanetti, A.R., Colombo, M. *et al.* (1990c) Antibody to hepatitis C virus after a vapour-heated factor VIII concentrate. *Thrombosis and Haemostasis*, 64, 232–234.

Mannucci, P.M. Colombo, M., Zanetti, A.R. *et al.* (1991) Antibody to hepatitis C virus after a vapour heated factor VIII concentrate – lack of evidence – rebuttal. *Thrombosis Haemostasis*, 66, 621–622.

Mannucci, P.M., Schimpf, K., Abe, T. *et al.* (1992) Low risk of viral infection after administration of vapour-heated factor VIII concentrate. *Transfusion*, 32, 134–138.

Mannucci, P.M., Gdovin, S., Gringeri, A. *et al.* (1994) Transmission of hepatitis A to patients with hemophilia by factor VIII concentrates treated with organic solvent and detergent to inactivate viruses. *Annals of Internal Medicine*, 120, 1–7.

Mariani, G., Di Paolantonio, T., Baklaya, R. and Mannucci, P.M. (1991) Prospective hepatitis C safety evaluation of a high purity solvent detergent treated FVIII concentrate. *Blood*, 78 (suppl. 1), 55a.

Mariani, G., Di Paolantonio, T., Baklaya, R. *et al.* (1993) Prospective study of the evaluation of hepatitis C virus infectivity in a high-purity; solvent/detergent-treated factor VIII concentrate: parallel evaluation of other markers for lipid-enveloped and non-lipid-enveloped virus. *Transfusion*, 33, 814–818.

Mauser-Bunschoten, E.P., Varon, D., Savidge, G.F. and Bergman, G.E. (1993) Effects of chronic use of Monoclate, pasteurized in patients with hemophilia A previously unexposed to factor VIII concentrate or other blood products. *Blood*, 82 (suppl. 1), 153.

Mauser-Buschoten, E.P., Rosendaal, F.R., Nieuwenhuis, H.K. *et al.* (1994) Clinical course of factor VIII inhibitors developed after exposure to a pasteurised Dutch concentrate compared to classic inhibitors in hemophilia A. *Thrombosis and Haemostasis*, 71, 703–706.

Meireles, M., Aimar, P. and Sanchez, V. (1991) Effects of protein fouling on the apparent pore size distribution of sieving membranes. *Journal of Membrane Science*, 56, 13–28.

Menaché, D. and Aronson, D.L. (1985) Measures to inactivate viral contaminants of pooled plasma products, in *Infection, Immunity and Blood Transfusion* (eds R.Y. Dodd and L.F. Barker), Alan R. Liss, New York, pp. 407–423.

Menaché, D., Behre, H.E., Orthner, C.L. *et al.* (1984) Coagulation factor IX concentrate: method for preparation and assessment of potential *in vivo* thrombogenicity in animal models. *Blood*, 64, 1220–1227.

Middleton, S.H., Bennett, I.H. and Smith, J.K. (1973) A therapeutic concentrate of coagulation factors II, IX and X from citrated, factor VIII-depleted plasma. *Vox Sanguinis*, 24, 441–456.

Minor, P., Pipkin, P., Thorpe, R. *et al.* (1990) Antibody to hepatitis C in plasma pools. *Lancet*, 326, 188.

Mitra, G., Dobkin, M., Dumas, M. *et al.* (1994) Hepatitis A viral safety of plasma-derived factor VIII concentrate. *Vox Sanguinis*, 67 (suppl. 1), 80–82.

Morfini, M., Mannucci, P.M., Ciaverella, N. *et al.* (1994) Prevalence of infection with the hepatitis C virus among Italian hemophiliacs before and after the introduction of virally inactivated clotting factor concentrates: a retrospective evaluation. *Vox Sanguinis*, 67, 178–182.

Mortimer, P.P., Luban, N.L.C., Kelleher, J.F. and Cohen, B.J. (1983) Transmission of parvovirus-like virus by clotting factor concentrates. *Lancet*, ii, 482–484.

Murkes, J. and Carlsson, C.G. (1988) *Crossflow Filtration, Theory and Practice*, John Wiley, London.

Murphy, F.A. (1994) New, emerging and reemerging infectious disease, in *Advance in Virus Research*, vol. 43 (eds K. Maramorosch, F.A. Murphy and A.J. Shatkin), Academic Press, San Diego, pp. 1–52.

Nau, J.Y. (1995) CJD and albumin? *Lancet*, 345, 442.

Neurath, A.R., Stasny, J.T., Rubin, B.A. *et al.* (1970) The effects of nonaqueous solvents on the quaternary structure of viruses: properties of haemagglutinins obtained by diruption of influenza viruses with tri(n-butyl) phosphate. *Microbios*, 2, 209.

Neurath, A.R., Vernon, K.S., Dobkin, M.B. and Rubin, B.A. (1972) Characterization of subviral components resulting from treatment of rabies virus with tri(n-butyl) phosphate. *Journal of General Virology*, 14, 33–48.

Newman, J., Johnson, A.J., Karpatkin, M.H. *et al.* (1971) Methods for the production of clinically effective intermediate – and high purity factor VIII concentrates. *British Journal of Haematology*, 21, 1–20.

Ng, P.K. and Dobkin, M.B. (1985) Pasteurisation of antihemophilic factor and model virus inactivation studies. *Thrombosis Research*, 39, 439–447.

Ng, P. and Mitra, G. (1994) Removal of DNA contaminants from therapeutic protein preparations. *Journal of Chromatography A*, 658, 459–463.

Nilsson, I.M., Borge, L., Gunnarsson, M. and Kristoffersson, A.C. (1984) Factor VIII related activities in concentrates. *Scandinavian Journal of Haematology*, 33 (suppl. 41), 157–172.

Nishikawa, A.H. and Bailon, P. (1975) Affinity purification methods. Non specific adsorption of proteins due to ionic groups in cyanogen bromide treated agarose. *Archives of Biochemistry and Biophysics*, 168, 576–584.

Noel, L., Guerois, C., Maisonneuve, P. *et al.* (1989) Antibodies to hepatitis C virus in hemophilia. *Lancet*, ii, 560.

Norley, S.G., Löwer, J. and Kurth, R. (1993) Insufficient inactivation of HIV-1 in human cryo poor plasma by beta-propiolactone: results from a highly accurate virus detection method. *Biologicals*, 21, 251–258.

Null, H.R. (1987) Selection of a separation process, in *Handbook of Separation Process Technology* (ed. R.W. Rousseau), John Wiley, New York, pp. 982–995.

Opong, W.S. and Zydney, A.L. (1991) Diffusive and convective protein transport through asymetric membranes. *American Institute of Chemical Engineers Journal*, 37, 1497–1510.

Parquet, A., Boneu, B., Bosser, C. *et al.* (1988) Clinical and biological survey of haemophilia A and B patients infused with French heat treated concentrates. *Nouvelle Revue Française d'Hématologie*, 30, 205–207.

Pasi, K.J., Evans, J.A., Skidmore, S.J. and Hill, F.G.H. (1990) Prevention of hepatitis C infection in haemophiliacs. *Lancet*, 335, 1473–1474.

Pattison, C.P., Klein, C.A., Leger, R.T. *et al.* (1976) An outbreak of type B hepatitis associated with transfusion of Plasma Protein Fraction. *American Journal of Epidemiology*, 103, 399–407.

Peerlinck, K. and Vermylen, J. (1993) Acute hepatitis A in patients with hemophilia A. *Lancet*, 341, 189.

Peerlinck, K., Arnout, J., Gilles, J.G. *et al.* (1993) A higher than expected incidence of factor VIII inhibitors in multitransfused haemophilia A patients treated with an intermiediate purity pasteurised factor VIII concentrate. *Thrombosis and Haemostasis*, 69, 115–118.

Peerlinck, K., Goubau, P., Coppens, G. *et al.* (1994) Is the apparent outbreak of hepatitis A in Belgian haemophiliacs due to a loss of previous passive immunity? *Vox Sanguinis*, 67 (suppl. 1), 14–17.

Peerlinck, K., Goubau, P., Reybrouck, R. *et al.* (1995) Parvovirus B19 antibodies in patients with haemophilia A. *Thrombosis and Haemostasis*, 73, 555–556.

Pejaudier, L., Kichenin-Martin, V., Boffa, M.C. and Steinbuch, M. (1987) Appraisal of the protein composition of prothrombin complex concentrates of different origin. *Vox Sanguinis*, 52, 1–9.

Pindyck, J., Waldman, A. and Zang, E. (1985) Measures to decrease the risk of acquired immunodeficiency syndrome by blood transmission: evidence of volunteer blood donor cooperation. *Transfusion*, 25, 3–9.

Piskiewicz, D., Thomas, W., Lieu, M. *et al.* (1986) Heat inactivation of human immunodeficiency virus in lyophilised anti-inhibitr coagulant complex (Autoplex). *Thrombosis Research*, 44, 701–707.

Piskiewicz, D., Bourret, L., Lieu, C. *et al.* (1987) Heat inactivation of human immunodeficiency virus in lyophilised factor VIII and factorIX concentrates. *Thrombosis Research*, 47, 235–241.

Piskiewicz, D., Sun, C.S. and Tondreau, S.C. (1989) Inactivation and removal of human immunodeficiency virus in monoclonal purified antihemophilic factor (human) (Hemofil M). *Thrombosis Research*, 55, 627–634.

Pittman, D.D., Wang, J.H. and Kaufman, R.J. (1992) Identification and functional importance of tyrosine sulphate residues within recombinant factor VIII. *Biochemistry*, 31, 3315–3325.

Pollmann, H. and Richter, H. (1994) Prevalence of hepatitis and HIV in a group of haemophiliacs, in *Proceedings of the 21st International Congress of the World Federation of Hemophilia*, Mexico City, p. 309.

Prince, A.M., Stephan, W. and Brotman, B. (1983) β-Propiolactone/ultraviolet irradiation: a review of its effectiveness for inactivation of viruses in blood derivatives. *Review of Infectious Diseases*, 5, 92–107.

Prince, A.M., Stephan, W., Dichtelmüller, H. *et al.* (1985) Inactivation if the Hutchinson strain of non-A, non-B hepatitis by combined use of β-propiolactone and ultraviolet irradiation. *Journal of Medical Virology*, 16, 119–125.

Priola, S.A., Caughey, B., Raymond, G.J. and Chesebro, B. (1994) Prion protein and the scrapie agent: *in vitro* studies in infected neuroblastoma cells. *Infectious Agents and Disease*, 3, 54–58.

Prodouz, K. and Fratantoni, J.C. (1994) Viral inactivation of blood products, in *Scientific Basis of Transfusion Medicine* (eds K.C. Anderson and P.M. Ness), W.B. Saunders, Philadelphia, pp. 852–871.

Prowse, C.V. (1994) Parvovirus B19 and blood products. *Lancet*, 343, 1101.

Purcell, R.H., Gerin, J.L., Popper, H. *et al.* (1985) Hepatitis B virus hepatitis non-A, non-B virus and hepatitis delta virus in lyophilized antihemophilic factor: relative sensitivity to heat. *Hepatology*, 5, 1091–1099.

Ratnoff, O. (1974) Prothrombin complex preparations: a cautionary note. *Annals of Internal Medicine*, 81, 852–853.

Record, F.A. (1986) Sedimenting centrifuges, in *Solid/Liquid Separation Scale-up*, 2nd edn (eds D.B. Purchas and R.J. Wakeman), Uplands Press, London, pp. 253–292.

Remis, R.S., O'Shaughnessy, M., Tsoukas, C. *et al.* (1990) HIV transmission to patients with hemophilia by heat-treated donor screened factor concentrate. *Canadian Medical Association Journal*, 142, 1247–1254.

Rizza, C.R., Fletcher, M.L. and Kernoff, P.B.A. (1993) Confirmation of viral safety of dry heat treated factor VIII concentrate (8Y) prepared by Bio Products Laboratory (BPL): a report on behalf of UK haemophilia centre directors. *British Journal of Haematology*, **84**, 269–272.

Santagostino, E., Gringeri, A., Muleo, G. *et al.* (1994) Human parvovirus B19 transmission by double inactivated (solvent/detergent plus terminal super-dry heating) clotting factor concentrates, in *Proceedings of 21st International Congress of the World Federation of Hemophilia*, Mexico City, p. 75.

Sazama, K. (1995) Existing problems in the testing for infectious diseases. *Immunological Investigations*, **24**, 131–146.

Schimpf, K., Mannucci, P.M., Kreuz, W. *et al.* (1987) Absence of hepatitis after treatment with a pasteurized factor VIII. *New England Journal of Medicine*, **316**, 918–922.

Schimpf, K., Brackmann, H.H., Kreuz, W. *et al.* (1989) Absence of anti-human immunodeficiency virus types 1 and 2 seroconversion after the treatment of hemophilia A and B or von Willebrand's disease with pasteurized factor VIII concentrate. *New England Journal of Medicine*, **321**, 1148–1152.

Schrieber, A.B., Hrinda, M.E., Newman, J. *et al.* (1989) Removal of viral contaminants by monoclonal antibody purification of plasma proteins, in *Virus Inactivation in Plasma Products. Current Studies in Hematology and Blood Transfusion* (ed. J.J. Morgenthaler), Karger, Basel, pp. 146–153.

Schroeder, B.D. and Mozen, M.M. (1970) Australia antigen, distribution during Cohn ethanol fractionation of human plasma. *Science*, **168**, 1462–1464.

Schulman, S., Lindgren, A.C., Petrini, P. and Allander, T. (1992) Transmission of hepatitis C with pasteurised factor VIII. *Lancet*, **340**, 305–306.

Schwarz, T.F. Roggendorf, M., Hottenräger, B. *et al.* (1991) Removal of parvovirus B19 from contaminated factor VIII during fractionation. *Journal of Medical Virology*, **35**, 28–31.

Schwinn, H., Heimberger, N., Kumpe, G. and Herchenhan, B. (1981) *Blood coagulation Factors and Process for their Manufacture.* US patent, no. 4297344.

Seeley, R.J., Wight, H.D., Fry, H.H. *et al.* (1994) Biotechnology product validation part 7: validation of chromatography resin useful life. *Biopharm*, **7**(7), 41–48.

Seng, C., Watkins, P., Morse, D. *et al.* (1994) Parvovirus B19 outbreak on an adult ward. *Epidemiology and Infection*, **113**, 345–353.

Shapiro, A. and the International Factor Safety Group (1993) Vapour heated intermediate-purity factor IX concentrated tested in a safety study monitoring transfusion-related viral infection in previously untreated hemophiliacs. *Thrombosis and Haemostasis*, **69**, 943.

Shopnick, R.I., Brettler, D.B., Kazemi, M. and Gomperts, E.D. (1994) Anaphylaxis following the use of recombinant factor VIII (Recombinate, Baxter/Hyland). *Blood*, **84** (suppl. 1), 467a.

Simmonds, P., Zhang, L.R., Watson, H.G. *et al.* (1990) Hepatitis C quantification and sequencing in blood products, haemophiliacs, and drug users. *Lancet*, **336**, 1469–1472.

Soulier, J.P. (1984) The history of PPSB. *Vox Sanguinis*, **46**, 58–61.

Stephan, W. (1989) Inactivation of hepatitis viruses and HIV in plasma and plasma derivatives by treatment with β-propiolactone/UV irradiation, in *Virus Inactivation in Plasma Products. Current Studies in Hematology and Blood Transfusion* (ed. J.J. Morgenthaler), Karger, Basel, pp. 275–336.

Suomela, H. (1993) Inactivation of viruses in blood and plasma products. *Transfusion Medicine Reviews.*

Suomela, H., Myllyla, G. and Raaska, E. (1977) Preparation and properties of a therapeutic factor IX concentrate. *Vox Sanguinis*, **33**, 37–50.

Temperley, I.J., Cotter, K.P., Walsh, T.J. *et al.* (1992) Clotting factors and hepatitis A. *Lancet*, **340**, 1466.

Tsurumi, T., Osawa, N., Hitaka, H. *et al.* (1990) Structure of cuprammonium regenerated cellulose hollow fibre (BMM hollow fibre) for virus removal. *Polymer Journal*, **22**, 751–758.

Tullis, J.L. (1977) Albumin1. Background and use. *Journal of American Medical Association*, **237**, 355–360.

Van Creveld, S., Veder, H.A., Pascha, C.N. and Kroeze, W.F. (1959) The separation of AHF from fibrinogen. *Thrombosis et Diathesis Haemorrhagica*, **3**, 572–577.

Van den Berg, W., Ten Cate, J.W., Breederveld, C. and Goudsmit, J. (1986) Seroconversion to HTLV-III in haemophiliac given heat treated factor VIII concentrate. *Lancet*, **I**, 803–804.

Vyas, G.N., Yang, G. and Murphy, E.L. (1994) Transfusion-related transmissable diseases: detection by polymerase chain reaction–amplified genes of the microbial agents. *Transfusion Medicine Reviews*, **8**, 253–266.

Wadsworth, C., Hanson, L.A., Kjellman, H. *et al.* (1989) Some characteristics of aggregates and proteins in heat treated factor VIII concentrates. *Blut*, **58**, 133–141.

Wagner, R.H., McLester, W.D., Smith, M. *et al.* (1964) Purification of anti-hemophilic factor (factor VIII) by amino acid precipitation. *Thrombosis et Diathesis Haemorraghica*, **11**, 64–74.

Watson, W.G., Ludlam, C.A., McOmish, F. *et al.* (1995) Absence of hepatitis A virus transmission by high-purity solvent detergent treated coagulation factor concentrates in Scottish haemophiliacs. *British Journal of Haematology*, **89**, 214–216.

Weisser, J. (1988) Transmission of the human immunodeficiency virus by a dry heat treated factor VIII concentrate. *Klinische Pediatrie*, **200**, 307–309.

Wells, M.A., Wittek, A.E., Epstein, J.S. *et al.* (1986) Inactivation and partitioning of human T-cell lymphotropic virus, type III, during ethanol fractionation of plasma. *Transfusion*, **26**, 210–213.

White, D.O. and Fenner, F.J. (1994) *Medical Virology*, 4th edn, Academic Press, San Diego.

White, G.C., Matthews, T.J., Weinhold, K.J. *et al.* (1986) HTLV-III seroconversion associated with heat-treated factor VIII concentrate. *Lancet*, **i**, 611–612.

Williams, N.A. and Polli, G.P. (1984) The lyophilization of pharmaceuticals: a literature review. *Journal of Parenteral Science and Technology*, **38**, 48–59.

Williams, M.D., O'Brien, S.O. and Hill, F.G.H (1994) Prospective study of the frequency of factor VIII inhibitor formation following the use of a single heat treated intermediate purity concentrate (BPL 8Y) in haemophilic boys. *British Journal of Haematology*, **86** (suppl. 1), 59.

Williams, M.D., Skidmore, S.J. and Hill, F.G.H. (1990) HIV seroconversion in haemophilia boys receiving heat treated factor VIII concentrate. *Vox Sanguinis*, **58**, 135–136.

Williams, M.D., Cohen, B.J., Beddal, A.C. *et al.* (1990) Transmission of human parvovirus B19 by coagulation factor concentrates. *Vox Sanguinis*, **58**, 177–181.

Winkelman, L., Feldman, P.A. and Evans, D.R. (1989) Severe heat treatment of lyophilised coagulation factors, in *Virus Inactivation in Plasma Products. Current Studies in Hematology and Blood Transfusion* (ed. J.J. Morgenthaler), Karger, Basel, pp. 55–69.

Winkelman, L., Owen, N.E., Evans, D.R. *et al.* (1989) Severely heated therapeutic factor VIII concentrate of high specific activity. *Vox Sanguinis*, **57**, 97–103.

Wolfs, T.F., Breederveld, C., Krone, W.J. *et al.* (1988) HIV-antibody seroconversions in Dutch haemophiliacs using heat-treated and non-heat-treated coagulation factor concentrates. *Thrombosis and Haemostasis*, **59**, 396–399.

World Health Organization (1987) Acceptability of cell substrates for production of biologicals. *WHO Technical Report Series*, no. 747, World Health Organization, Geneva.

World-Wide Directory of Plasma Fractionators (1990) Marketing Research Bureau, Laguna Beach, California.

Yei, S., Yu, M.W. and Tankersley, D.L. (1992) Partitioning of hepatitis C virus during Cohn-Oncley fractionation of plasma. *Transfusion*, **32**, 824–828.

PART FOUR

Psychosocial Aspects

It seems to me that so much of my life has been wasted. There is so much that I may have done or attempted if I had money, proper training and education. The mind is young but the body feels older.

Hemophiliac, aged 25 years
Quoted by Professor A.H. Katz, 1970

28 THE FAMILY AND HEMOPHILIA

I. Marková

Viewing the family as a system

In their analysis of the historical period from the Renaissance until now, Mitterauer and Sieder (1977) argued that considerable changes have taken place in the structure and function of the European family. In the context of industrialization and sociocultural changes, the family's significance as an emotional retreat and a secure place for its members has much increased. In comparison to the pre-modern age, most families in Europe are now usually small and closely knit. They have become systems of mutual relationships between individual members, of their role interdependencies and of their emotional bonds. What one member does, or what happens to him or her, affects all of them in one way or other. The young are dependent on the family for much longer than in the past, not only for their education and for financial support, but above all emotionally. While the emotional bond can be very gratifying for family members, their mutual relationships, interdependences of their roles and conflicting activities can also lead to stressful experience. Indeed, some authors claim that family relationships, today, appear to be the most common sources of stress for a large part of the population (Ilfeld, 1982).

The family system can become under particular stress if a chronic disorder or disease affects any of its members. As Massie (1985), reflecting on his life as a child growing up with hemophilia, said: 'Chronic illness does not strike individuals; it strikes the whole living unit of the family.' The concept of viewing the family as a living unit rather than as a collection of individuals has been generally accepted, in theory, by the professionals dealing with chronic illness. However, it is a difficult concept to apply in practical terms (Authier and Land, 1978; Schwenk and Hughes, 1983). It means that the actual patient is the family rather than the individual. Each problem encoun-

tered within the individual must be treated as a higher-order, i.e. a family problem. For example, if chronic illness affects the child, the family has to cope with diagnosing, treatment procedures and hospitalization, and with the resulting emotional trauma and restrictions of their joint activities (Burr, 1985; Pless and Perrin, 1985; Doherty and Campbell, 1988; Eiser, 1990, 1993). In contrast to the past, most parents in Europe and in North America expect their children to grow up healthy and to outlive them. Yet, despite such expectations, statistics show that approximately 10–15% of children under 16 years of age have some kind of a chronic, long-term condition, and approximately 1.5% of such conditions are so severe that they require continuous specialized attention (Perrin, 1985; Eiser, 1993). Chronic disease in the adult is likely to lead to changes of family roles; the division of labor must be redistributed, which the affected individual may experience as a personal loss (Bruhn, 1977).

Hemophilia, like other chronic disorders, is a family matter. Moreover, being genetically transmitted, men and women experience a different kind of trauma which, in turn, has a particular effect on family dynamics. In families with hemophilia, individual members are under various kinds of obligation with respect to decisions they must take; whether and how they should restrict the size of their families; whether to undergo prenatal diagnosing; how to restrict the child's activities; how to cope with physical pain and emotions; and so on. Moreover, there are societal factors that interact with the family's coping. These include other people's perceptions of hemophilia; the ways mass media report on and affect the public awareness of hemophilia; the understanding of new medical discoveries such as viruses interfering with treatment, e.g. hepatitis C; changes in technologic advances and in treatment.

Like other chapters in this part of the book, this chapter differs in one significant respect from the other parts

Hemophilia. Edited by C.D. Forbes, L. Aledort and R. Madhok. Published in 1997 by Chapman & Hall, London. ISBN 0 412 63820 7

of this textbook. While medical professionals can hope that with progress in science, most or all biochemical, pathologic and physiologic aspects of hemophilia will, in the end, be explained in terms of causes and effects, this is not so when one is concerned with psychosocial issues. These issues are human issues and as such they can hardly ever be explained in terms of causes and effects or be measured, quantified, predicted and controlled. One may, only in a very general sense, make predictions about human behavior, e.g. too much stress can lead to family break-up. However, each human individual is an agent and each human family is a unique system. People interact with their environment in unique ways. One cannot hope to identify general characteristics of a 'hemophilic personality' or common features of a 'hemophilic family.' Rather, the response to hemophilia by the individual or by the family is co-determined by that individual's or family's particular circumstances, by their agency and by the sociocultural conditions in which they live. Individuals respond not only to hemophilia as it affects them directly, but they also respond to others' beliefs of hemophilia. For example in his autobiography, *Touch Me Who Dares*, Shelley (1985) described how he had to cope with others' ignorance of hemophilia and with their fear that he would bleed to death from any superficial injury. Massie (1985), too, in his childhood reflections describes an unforgettable event when his schoolmaster announced that no one was to touch Bobby Massie under threat of punishment:

> My sudden transformation into an untouchable – for whatever well-intentioned reasons – filled me with a sense of powerlessness and stinging humiliation (Massie, 1985).

However, in contrast to this clearly verbalized event, many beliefs about illnesses and disabilities are not stated explicitly. Rather, they are implicit and operate under the level of awareness. People often shy away from those with chronic disease for unconscious fears of contamination, whether physical or moral (Douglas, 1966; Brandt, 1985; Jodelet, 1991). Such fears are often transmitted from generation to generation. Unconsciously held beliefs can have a very powerful negative effect on human conduct. As people are not aware of their existence and do not state them explicitly, such beliefs are resistant to change.

In this chapter I shall discuss not only how hemophilia affects individual family members and how the family copes as a unique system but also how hemophilia is represented in the culture in which that family lives. Some of the issues to be raised are common to coping with any chronic disease, others are specific to hemophilia. Moreover, individuals both respond to hemophilia in their unique ways, and are agents who try to control its direct (e.g. pain, taking precautions) and indirect (e.g. stigma) effects. It is because of the interplay between individual, family and sociocultural factors that many research findings relating to hemophilia and the family appear to provide contradictory results. Therefore, the focus of our attention will be on those factors that might explain and help us understand the differences in research findings, many of which pertain to both individual human agency and to culture.

The family life cycle

THE GENETIC NATURE OF HEMOPHILIA

Technologic advancements in prenatal diagnosing of genetic disorders now make it possible to prevent the birth of fetuses that are considered physically and/or mentally unfit. The very existence of these advancements thus confronts carriers of hemophilia and prospective parents with unprecedented kinds of decision-making and responsibilities. The abortion of affected fetuses is often justified to parents in terms of the child's and of their own poor quality of life; and on the grounds that high technology enables us to identify the most serious genetic abnormalities very early in pregnancy and that its benefits, therefore, should be used by the concerned prospective parents.

The fact that hemophilia can now be diagnosed in very early stages of pregnancy forces prospective parents to decide two things. First, they must decide whether to undergo diagnostic procedures for hemophilia. Second, if they do, and, the fetus is found to be affected by hemophilia, they must decide whether to opt for abortion. In the study by Marková, Forbes and Inwood (1984), it was found that undergoing prenatal testing is sometimes interpreted by prospective parents not as enabling them to decide freely whether or not to have a child with hemophilia, but as a commitment to abortion. A number of women felt that availing themselves of an amniocentesis committed them to abortion should the fetus prove to be affected. The study showed that about 60% of Scottish and Canadian female carriers of hemophilia, many of whom were already mothers of sons with hemophilia, claimed that hemophilia was not a sufficiently severe disorder to justify the termination of a pregnancy. Moreover, none of the men with hemophilia thought that pregnancy should be terminated in the case of hemophilia. Understandably, these patients may have realized that had amniocentesis existed years ago, they themselves might not have been born (Marková, Forbes and Inwood 1984) and, of course, this was a very offensive point of view to many of them. In a recent survey of 500 carrier women in the Netherlands, 98% women thought that carrier testing and genetic counseling was either 'very useful' or 'useful'. However, the study has found that 50% of the respondents were against termination of pregnancy in the case of hemophilia (Varekamp *et al.*, 1993).

Studies of prospective mothers' perceptions of pre-natal diagnosing in other genetic disorders support the above findings in hemophilia. For example, research by Sanden and Bjurulf (1988) indicates that many pregnant women wish to take the diagnostic test but will not consider abortion even if malformation of the fetus is found. Their reason for having an amniocentesis is to find out if the fetus is healthy. Such reasons, however, are not considered to be cost-effective from the scientific and economic points of view. As Green (1990) points out, the purpose of pre-natal diagnosis is usually presented to prospective mothers as a matter of securing the well-being of their unborn baby. In reality, however, it is a screening procedure for genetic defects and if the fetus is diagnosed as being affected, abortion is the only way of avoiding it. Pre-natal diagnosing is justified to the public in terms of reducing genetic defects and not in terms of the mother having early knowledge about the presence of a defect in the baby. Green further expresses fear that women who reject the idea of abortion and who decline pre-natal diagnosis may be viewed as being responsible for the birth of a child with disability and for the situation resulting from it. That women are conscious of such pressures has been shown not only in Markova *et al*.'s (1984) study but also in a Swedish study carried out by Sjörgen and Uddenberg (1987) about 30% of participants thought that the very existence of prenatal diagnosis can lead to more negative attitudes towards disabled people. Green (1990) argues that the availability of fetal diagnosis has changed the whole nature of pregnancy. It can never be the same, even for those mothers who decline to have tests because there will always be the knowledge that they had the opportunity and could have acted.

Clearly, the issue of prenatal diagnosing goes far beyond the parents' knowing or not knowing about their child's hemophilia. The right to choose a course of action in the case of prenatal diagnosing may be perceived by the individual as having too much choice, i.e. too many responsibilities and moral obligations resulting from his or her decisions. Marková, MacDonald and Forbes (1980a) data on diagnosis and genetic knowledge showed that a number of parents who knew about the history of hemophilia in their family did not restrict themselves to not having children. Some mothers commented that they were glad they had not known about their carrier status because if they had they would have had to make a decision regarding having a family. This may show their attempt to suppress thoughts on the possibility of having an affected child. Clearly, no matter how sophisticated methods, on their own they do not affect the course of parents' actions. The parents' decisions are determined by their personal preferences, by their ethical and cultural beliefs, as well as by pressures from the society in which they live.

BRINGING UP THE CHILD WITH HEMOPHILIA

Reading about childhood experiences of hemophilia by writers such as Shelley (1985) and Massie (1985), and examining research findings concerning family interactions that were published in the 1960s and early 1970s (e.g. Dowling, 1960; Katz and Goldy, 1963; Mattsson and Gross, 1966; Katz, 1970) highlights some of the most difficult problems of coping with hemophilia. They include excruciating pain, constant threat of internal bleeds, chronic arthritis, parental anxiety and overprotection of the child, maternal depression and guilt feelings, sometimes paternal aloofness and in some cases accusations of their wives for being 'responsible' for hemophilia.

If one excludes the effect of acquired immunodeficiency syndrome (AIDS) on families with hemophilia (see later), the findings of more recent research into psychosocial problems are less drastic. This can be attributed to two main issues: first, to factor treatment that was introduced in the mid-1960s and to home therapy and second, to improved support services that have been introduced during the last two or three decades. These include multidisciplinary comprehensive care, choices available to patients and families with respect to the management of hemophilia, the impact of parent self-help groups and the increased involvement of national hemophilia societies as support organizations.

The availability of factor treatment, prophylaxis and home therapy (see later) means that parents are encouraged by the physician to let their son explore the world as fully as possible and to participate in activities like other children. This is essential for the child's social and psychologic well-being. They are also advised that, rather than restricting the child's activities in order to prevent his injuries, they should alter the child's home environment, e.g. cover floor with soft carpets, avoid sharp edges on furniture, use nonslip floors and so on. Some severely affected children wear special outfits to protect their heads and joints, although such measures make the child different from his peers and encourage stigmatization by peers and by teachers (Marková, MacDonald and Forbes, 1980b).

However, despite the improvements in treatment, in their attempt to minimize the number of bleedings, parents experience continual uncertainty as to how to define a balance between necessary protection and unnecessary restrictions of the child (Katz, 1970; Jones, 1974; Agle, 1977; Marková, MacDonald and Forbes, 1980a). There are several stages in bringing up a child with hemophilia that parents still find particularly difficult. These are the following: coping with the diagnosis, teaching a young child to be careful in his activities; coping with stress and anxiety when the child starts school; the choice of career; the young man's anxieties concerning intimate relationships (Katz, 1970; Marková and Forbes, 1984). Children with hemophilia have often been claimed to be overprotected by their parents (Agle and Mattsson, 1970, 1972; Katz, 1970; Agle, 1975; Mattsson, 1975). However, more recent research finds parents of boys with hemophilia less indulgent than the parents of controls (Marková,

MacDonald and Forbes, 1980a; Lineberger, Hernandez and Brantley, 1984). Moreover, parents of children with milder forms of hemophilia were found to show greater awareness of child-rearing practices, e.g. reward, punishment, planning for the child, than parents of children with severe hemophilia and those of non-hemophilic children (Marková, MacDonald and Forbes, 1980a). Perhaps milder forms of hemophilia mobilize parents' effort and emotional strength to cope with the disease when it is not excessively overburdening. In contrast, it appears that if the child is severely affected, the parents find it difficult to cope with the burden of the constant threat of the child bleeding and with the uncertainty concerning his future health and well-being.

Many families are now involved in home care (see later) and they must learn to monitor the child's medical situation, assess potential and real dangers, overcome anxieties with respect to infusion, make decisions as to whether to administer treatment and to normalize the child's social life. The child's schooling and other situations when he is out of his parents' sight may encourage parents to divulge information about his hemophilia in order to evoke protection by peers or teachers (Oremland, 1988). The child, in contrast, prefers withholding information about his hemophilia for fear of rejection for being different. For this reason a child may underreport being in pain or even having a bleed.

Similar fears of being rejected by others apply to adult men. Many men with hemophilia will attempt to conceal hemophilia if at all possible (Mattsson, 1972; Marková, Lockyer and Forbes, 1977) and some data show that approximately 50% of men do not tell their employers about their hemophilia. Analyzing views of people with hemophilia on their employment prospects, Forbes *et al.* (1982) found that whether 'to tell or not to tell' remains a dilemma for many:

> First of all say nothing to employers that you suffer from hemophilia. They think you can bleed to death from a pin prick.
> Lie like hell when interviewed and pray you have enough time between bleeds to prove you can do the job as well as the next person when you are fit.

Molleman and van Knippenberg (1987) found that the individual's awareness of the visibility of his hemophilia is associated with social problems and anxiety about negative reactions from others and with difficulty in making intimate friends. The authors found that if their hemophilia is not visible, men with hemophilia would not wish to discuss their problems with others because of possible stigmatization. Such fears may interfere with men's attempts to establish intimate relationships.

Amongst the most difficult stages for a family with a hemophilic child is adolescence. Adolescence is a cultural concept. It became identified, in most western cultures,

as an age category in the life cycle, at the end of the 19th and at the beginning of the 20th century (Modell and Goodman, 1993). It spans approximately from 11 to 21 years and is associated with physiologic growth and pubertal changes. For a young person it is a time of seeking independence from the family and it is often associated with the formation of intimate relationships and friendships, with making decisions about education and/or jobs. Adolescents with hemophilia, in addition to facing the same kinds of issues as their peers, must come to terms with other problems. Hemophilia imposes limits on what they can do in terms of their physical activities, sports and jobs that are suitable for them. It may interfere with their social life, with holidays and with forming intimate relationships. For parents, it is important to understand that their son needs both the security of home and independence from it. Literature often draws attention to risk-taking of adolescents with hemophilia, i.e. involvement in activities that may lead to bleedings, such as fights or dangerous sports such as boxing or motorcycling (Agle and Mattsson, 1968; Jones, 1985). The other side of the coin is a dependent young man with excessive passivity.

So far, I have been concerned with problems associated with hemophilias A and B, affecting boys. However, families with von Willebrand disease may experience specific problems if it is a girl who is affected. Since von Willebrand disease is rare, the families in which it is a woman who is affected may feel particularly isolated because the services and the literature concerning psychosocial problems in hemophilia are all geared towards families with an affected male. It is important to acknowledge that families with von Willebrand disease may need even more individualized services and counseling than those with hemophilias A and B.

INTERACTIONS WITHIN THE FAMILY

Research findings concerning the effect of chronic disease on the family and on marital relationships provide conflicting results (Howard, 1978; Burr, 1985; Bussing and Johnson, 1992; Eiser, 1993). They range from those that show a great deal of family disruption and marital disharmony, to those that find no differences in comparison with control families, to those claiming that having a child with chronic disease or disability has brought parents closer together. In hemophilia, research reflects a variety of findings, similar to that in chronic disability in general. The differences in results depend not only on individual and cultural factors but also on methodologic issues. For example, data collected by questionnaires and by in-depth interviews provide different opportunities for parents to express their feelings and be open about the issues in question. Research in hemophilia that was published in the 1960s and the 1970s tended to find depressed, guilt-ridden and overprotective mothers (Browne, Mally and Kane,

1960; Agle and Mattsson, 1970; Katz, 1970; Mattsson, 1972; Agle, 1975), aloof fathers (e.g. Mattsson and Gross, 1966) and high marital disharmony (Salk, Hilgartner and Giranich, 1972). More recent research, however, suggests that marital disharmony in families with a chronic disease is no greater than in control families. Some claim that having a child with hemophilia actually facilitates family relationships (Marková, MacDonald and Forbes, 1980a; Handford *et al.*, 1986; Varekamp *et al.*, 1990). The study by Varekamp *et al.* (1990), using a much larger sample than previous studies, has found that in 52% of marriages hemophilia had no influence on parents' relationships; in 45% the respondents stated that having a child with hemophilia has brought them closer together. It could be argued, though, that such claims are rationalizations on parents' part and parents' attempts to find some meaning in their difficult situation. Nevertheless, whether or not such claims reflect parents' true beliefs, they form part of their social reality and, as such, they should be treated seriously.

Traditionally, it is women who usually take care and responsibility for attending to the sick in the family (King, 1981; Eiser, 1990; Wilkie, 1992). A comparative study involving men with hemophilia and carriers in the USA, Canada, Scotland and Greece (Marková *et al.*, 1986) has shown that for carrier women, coping with hemophilia means coping with severe emotional problems. Women consistently perceived pain, parental anxieties of various kinds, stress in the family and other issues to be of much greater importance then did men affected by hemophilia. Varekamp *et al.* (1990) explored family burden in families with a hemophilic child. The authors made a distinction between psychologic distress and the burden caused by daily practical problems. They found that parental psychologic distress was more significant than burden caused by practical problems. Psychologic distress was mostly caused by fears of bleedings, by concern about the child's future and by the child's general medical situation.

Literature on the effects of a chronic disease on healthy siblings is inconclusive. Some researchers have found healthy siblings to be at higher risk of psychiatric disturbance (Martino and Newman, 1974), attention-seeking, maladjusted and distressed (Drotar and Crawford, 1985; Eiser, 1993), restless and disobedient (Gath, 1973). As Eiser (1993) documents, however, siblings can show other kinds of response, such as empathy and consideration, and so on. A study by Breslau, Weitzman and Messenger (1981) explored the effects of cystic fibrosis, cerebral palsy, myelodysplasia and multiple handicaps on siblings' adjustment. The authors found that the severity of the illness was not related to the siblings' adjustment, but they were more aggressive at school than their peers.

Massie (1985) discussed the difficulties for his two sisters, arising from his hemophilia. They had to contend with the unusual amount of attention that the parents devoted to his care as well as with the curiosity of their peers. Oremland (1988) points out that siblings with hemophilia often help quite significantly to care for the brother with hemophilia. Sometimes they perform surrogate mother work by going for medical supplies, bringing homework if the brother is off school, calling for help if he has a bleed, being a sitter and so on. They also become self-conscious about having a brother with hemophilia and, more recently, with human immunodeficiency virus (HIV) infection. With respect to HIV infection, some evidence shows that they may feel left out, develop problems such as bed-wetting, refusing to go to school, having fears about their own contamination or feeling guilty for not having AIDS themselves (Miller *et al.*, 1991). As Wilkie (1992) points out, parents themselves must cope with HIV in the family and therefore, there is a tendency to neglect problems encountered by their other children.

LIVING WITH HEMOPHILIA-RELATED PHYSICAL PROBLEMS

Although plasma factor treatment has brought tremendous benefits to people with hemophilia, it was apparent by the mid-1970s that it can lead to some complications, e.g. cardiovascular and renal diseases, hepatitis, chronic liver disease and inhibitors. In addition to such life-threatening problems, families and patients have to learn to cope with a variety of problems of daily living caused by hemophilia, such as acute and chronic pain, chronic degenerative arthritis and restriction of their social life (Marková and Forbes, 1984; Marková *et al.*, 1986). Wilkie *et al.* (1990) found that, amongst the most claimed problems of daily living were pain, tiredness, impaired mobility and loss of job. Spontaneous hemorrhages prevent planning; holidays and family activities become restricted and spoilt (Varekamp *et al.*, 1990; Goldman, Miller and Lee, 1993).

Anecdotal evidence suggests the existence of a relationship between emotional state, stress and bleeding frequency, and/or between stress and severity of bleedings. For example, Katz (1970) refers to cases observed by himself and by other researchers of hemorrhages occurring in anticipation of threatening events, aggressive excitements and so on. However, there are very few well-designed studies to explore these issues. As Bussing and Johnson (1992) point out, it is very difficult to make an objective assessment of the relevant parameters. These authors have reviewed the relevant studies on the subject which, however, report conflicting evidence. They suggest that intervention, e.g. relaxation, self-hypnosis, training and education, may be most useful for patients with high frequency of bleedings.

Severe hemophilia is a painful condition. As yet there is no satisfactory analgesic available which does not lead to addiction (Dormandy, 1973; Frommer and Ingram, 1973; Harvey, 1973). Patients sometimes turn to alcohol and the misuse of prescribed drugs to relieve their pain (Wilkie *et al.*, 1990). This often leads to drug dependence. Since there are no satisfactory medical means to alleviate pain, some attempts have been made to develop psychologic interventions. Recently, a series of studies have evaluated cognitive-behavioral interventions in reducing arthritic pain of persons with hemophilia (Varni, 1981, b; Varni, Gilbert and Dietrich, 1981; Dunne *et al.*, 1991). These interventions consist of progressive muscular relaxation exercises, meditative breathing and imagery associated with past experiences of warmth and pain relief. Some overall pain alleviation has been reported, along with improved mobility and with reduction in the use of analgesics.

Hemophilia and HIV

When HIV was identified in commercially produced factor concentrates in the early 1980s, a great number of men with hemophilia worldwide had already been infected. In order to prevent further spread of HIV, health education in hemophilia has made a major effort to promote HIV/AIDS-related knowledge, hoping that this will lead to more cautious behavior on the part of people with HIV. These efforts were similar in their spirit to national campaigns, e.g. 'Don't die of ignorance', run in the UK in the mid-1980s.

HIV AND BEHAVIORAL CHANGE

Evidence has shown that in the late 1980s – although at that time blood donors were screened for the presence of HIV and blood products were heat-treated – many men with hemophilia still reduced factor treatment and waited longer before administering it for fear of HIV infection (Agle, Gluck and Pierce 1987; Rosendaal *et al.*, 1988; Overby, Lo and Litt, 1989; Wilson and Wasserman, 1989; Marková *et al.*, 1990b). Most research findings indicate that men with hemophilia and their families are well-informed about HIV infection, its natural history, transmission and precautions to be taken to prevent infection (Smiley *et al.*, 1988; Overby, Lo and Litt, 1989; Marková *et al.*, 1990b; Catalan and Klimes, 1991). Despite these results, behavioral change with respect to safer sex, in particular in the use of condoms in the young, has been disappointing (Parish *et al.*, 1988; Lawrence *et al.*, 1989; Overby, Lo and Litt, 1989; Ragni and Nimorwicz, 1989; Marková *et al.*, 1990a, b; Catalan *et al.*, 1992).

Psychosocial factors involved in the lack of use of safer sex techniques are numerous and only some of these factors will be raised here. It has been pointed out in the previous section that hemophilia has been experienced, both by patients and by their families, as a stigmatizing disease. The association of hemophilia with HIV/AIDS has led to a double stigma. Men with hemophilia revealed that they could not cope with the stigma attached to HIV

being a sexually transmitted disease (Marková *et al.*, 1990a). As far as men with hemophilia are concerned, HIV was transmitted by factor treatment on which their lives were dependent.

Men in different stages of life experience different kinds of dilemmas. Adolescents and young men who are not in stable relationships find it difficult to explain to their girlfriends why they should use a condom. The logic of their thoughts is generally as follows. Most young women are on the pill and therefore they would question the use of a condom. Therefore, the men would have to reveal to them both their hemophilia and HIV status. What girl would be interested in a man with both hemophilia and HIV? Thus it appears that for a number of patients the main reason for not using a condom has been their anxiety of being rejected by others (Mason, Olson and Parish, 1988; Mason *et al.*, 1989; Marková *et al.*, 1990a; Catalan and Klimes, 1991). The use of condoms also caused difficulties for married men who were HIV-antibody-positive, reminding them that AIDS is a 'dirty disease.'

Ordinary household contacts do not present a risk of the spread of HIV/AIDS. A case of a woman infected by HIV through eight needlestick injuries was reported by Smiley *et al.* (1988). Most men with hemophilia and other members of the household know that if care is taken with respect to needlestick injuries, there is no danger of the spread of HIV through household routines. Despite this, research findings suggest what may appear to be irrational behavior on the part of parents. For example, one mother claimed to have spent a lot of money on bleach after she had known about AIDS because she did not want anybody to think that she kept a dirty house. Another mother poured disinfectant down the toilet after her son had used it. Forty per cent of medical and of paramedical staff thought that persons with HIV should not work in food industry and handle food (Marková, Wilkie and Forbes, 1988). Like other sexually transmitted diseases, there is a tendency in the general public to associate HIV with 'dirt' and 'uncleanliness' (Brandt, 1985, 1988).

Such associations of dirt and HIV/AIDS by patients, their families and medical and paramedical staff are reminiscent of more general research findings in sociology and anthropologic research associating illness, dirt and contagion (Douglas, 1966). Jodelet's (1991) study is particularly instructive. This author studied attitudes of villagers in France who offered their homes to ex-patients from mental hospitals. Although these villagers originally responded to the governmental invitation to accept mental ex-patients as paying guests, they devised ingenious strategies to isolate themselves from them. For example, they washed their laundry separately, used different kinds of crockery and rescheduled their meal times to avoid eating together with their paying guests. As Jodelet makes it clear, the villagers had implicit fears of contagion of mental illness and adopted their irrational activities to avoid contagion.

THE FAMILY RESPONSE TO HIV

The psychosocial impact of HIV infection on the family has been unprecedented, in particular in the case of children with hemophilia infected by HIV (Agle, Gluck and Pierce, 1987; Nelson and Album, 1987). In addition to general distress, families must cope with the question as to whether children should be told of their HIV antibody status. This problem has been widely discussed and the generally accepted view today is that the child should be told. This view is based on the experience with other serious childhood diseases such as cystic fibrosis and cancer (Wilkie, 1992; Schulman and Kupst, 1980). It is now believed that education with respect to this matter should start as soon as the child can grasp the concepts of health and illness. The view that parents should be truthful with their children comes from the knowledge that children assimilate a great deal of information from parents' anxieties, non-verbal interaction, friends, mass media, and so on. Parents striving to keep HIV a secret may unwittingly magnify unnecessary uncertainty and anxiety in the child.

Another difficulty is when and what the child should be told (Miller *et al.*, 1989a, b; Wilkie, 1992; Goldman, Lee and Miller, 1993a). This depends on the child's emotional state, general medical situation, whether he or she is asymptomatic and how mature the child is. Obviously, the issue of what and how to tell is different for children of different ages, e.g. for a pre-school child and for an adolescent (Miller *et al.*, 1989a).

Another difficult issue is that of informing other children in the family. As Wilkie (1992) points out, since parents must cope with their own distress, they may neglect dealing with the distress of other children in the family who might then develop various kinds of psychosomatic problems or become disturbed (Miller *et al.*, 1991).

Parents of children with HIV must often cope with the stigma and with discrimination by others (Nelson and Album, 1987; Mason, Olson and Parish, 1988; Parish, 1991). Instances of discrimination toward school-aged children with hemophilia and HIV/AIDS infection have been publicized by the media. This may reinforce parents in their wish to keep HIV a secret not only with respect to outsiders but even with respect to members of their own family.

Anxiety about HIV has been found to be higher amongst carers of men with hemophilia than amongst the patients themselves (Agle, Gluck and Pierce, 1987). Klimes *et al.* (1992) found generally worse levels of psychologic adjustment in the partners than in the men with hemophilia. It appears, however, that there are no differences between partners of HIV-seropositive and seronegative men. This may suggest that stress, attached to hemophilia as such, is no greater when the man is HIV-antibody-positive. This could mean either that hemophilia as such already causes a high level of emotional

trauma or that the partners of HIV-seronegative men may worry about the possibility of future infection. This confirms the earlier study by Marková *et al.* (1986), showing that emotional trauma is higher in carriers of hemophilia than in the patients themselves.

Research findings show that family and spouse support for men with hemophilia who are HIV-antibody-positive moderates psychologic trauma and reduced vulnerability to psychiatric symptoms (Dew *et al.*, 1990; Catalan *et al.*, 1992). Many men with hemophilia worry about transmission of HIV to their partners. They may reduce their sexual activity and even develop a psychosexual dysfunction (Catalan *et al.*, 1989; Wilson and Wasserman, 1989).

Perhaps the most important issue is to prevent infection in the spouses and children of men with HIV. The prevalance of infection in spouses is estimated to be somewhere between 10 and 60% (Olson *et al.*, 1989; Catalan and Klimes, 1991; Aledort, 1994). Counseling couples about family planning appears to be one of the most difficult areas with respect to the spread of HIV. The wish to have a child may be so strong that some couples risk HIV transmission to the spouse. Such couples present a challenge for the counselor, and they highlight the importance of a clear definition of the aim of counseling: whether to help the couple to make an informed decision or to prevent the spread of HIV, whatever the cost (Mason, Olson and Parish, 1988).

As indicated above, some men did not inform their partners of their HIV status for fear of losing them. There remains a dilemma as to whether partners of HIV-antibody-positive men should be informed by medical staff. Such information would breach the traditional doctor–patient relationship of confidentiality (Ragni and Nimorwicz, 1989; Marková, 1990). As Ragni and Nimorwicz point out, it is now considered more and more a duty and 'the ethical responsibility of the medical profession' to inform women at risk rather than to sacrifice their lives. However, one has to deal sensitively with the inclusion of spouses and sexual partners in counseling clinics. As pointed out by Mason, Olson and Parish (1988), such involvement is perceived by some patients as an invasion of their privacy.

HEMOPHILIA, HIV AND ETHNICITY

Like everybody else, people with hemophilia and with HIV live in societies and cultures that have different images of hemophilia and of HIV. Even within a single country, among different strata of the population, one can find responses to HIV ranging from support and sympathy from a church congregation to stigmatization and discrimination, and to burning down of a family house (Parish, 1991). Moreover, professionals face problems of communication with respect to hemophilia and HIV when dealing with particular ethnic groups. Some ethnic groups have specific cultural conventions and may misunderstand the issue of hemophilia and HIV, both because of miscommunication and because of language barriers (Parish, 1991; Goldman, Miller and Lee, 1993). For example, Goldman, Miller and Lee (1993) describe a case of a Sikh family where problems have arisen due to a lack of information, secrecy, poor understanding of English and difficulty comprehending that HIV is different from hemophilia. Sikh culture expects couples to have larger families; marriages are arranged and sons will bring their wives to live in the parental home; daughters-in-law will be obedient to their husbands; and both husband and wife will respect and obey the wishes of his parents. Such cultural expectations may present particular stress to a couple with hemophilia and HIV. The authors caution, however, that although it is important for professionals to take cultural differences into account when planning counseling sessions, they should not assume differences without carefully exploring whether they affect the family's coping with hemophilia and HIV.

COMPREHENSIVE CARE

The introduction of home care programmes since the early 1970s has had several significant features. First, it has changed the traditional doctor–patient relationship by redistributing responsibilities for day-to-day hemophilia care. Second, it has led to a new concept in the management of hemophilia and of patient care – that of comprehensive therapy.

Redistribution of responsibilities

Home therapy has enabled people with hemophilia and their families to become actively involved in the day-to-day management of hemophilia. Its main feature is that treatment can be administered immediately when needed, i.e. when the bleeding occurs, or even prophylactically. Patients, relatives or friends infuse intravenous clotting factor themselves, thus avoiding delays in treatment caused by traveling to hospital, waiting, and so on. Prompt treatment reduces long-lasting crippling of joints and painful bleeding and improves the patient's and family's quality of life. It is therefore very important that the patient and/or the family make informed decisions as to when to administer the treatment, what dosage and whether they should seek further help from the specialist.

The clinic team at hemophilia units, in their turn have responsibilities, first, to carefully evaluate the suitability of patients and their families for entry into the program and second, for the subsequent monitoring of each family. The entry criteria vary between individual hemophilia centers depending on cultural, economic and political criteria. In addition to medical criteria, psychologic stability of the patient and of the family are important factors. It is essential to establish a good working relationships between the family that trusts and complies with the specialists' guidelines, and the clinic team, that is aware of possible psychosocial aspects of home care. One needs to be aware of possible stresses and anxieties of parents learning to infuse their child (Oremland, 1988). Patients on home treatment or parents are expected to maintain accurate logs of bleeding episodes and product usage.

There have been only a few studies that have evaluated the effect of home therapy on the patient's well-being and on the family relationships. The difficulty in evaluating any self-administration program depends on the researcher's and on the patient's ability to assess the wholeness of the family experience and of their quality of life. Patients on the whole have been from the start very positive about home treatment because they feel it has given them freedom they had never experienced before. One study, carried out in Scotland, registered number of bleedings by severely affected patients before and after the introduction of home treatment. However, the patients perceived home treatment so positively that they exaggerated its effect by claiming they had fewer bleeds after the home treatment, although evidence showed that this was not the case (Marková *et al.*, 1983). Those studies that have evaluated the effect of home treatment have found increased self-esteem (Lineberger, Hernandez and Brantley, 1984), less time away from school and work, shorter recovery from bleeds (Lazerson, 1972; Kaufert, 1980; Marková, Forbes and Inwood, 1984; Smith and Levine, 1984) and positive developments in social relationships (Marková *et al.*, 1983).

Home therapy, though, has its own risks. Like other regimes that are based on self-administration of treatment, home therapy in hemophilia can be mismanaged due to patient or family non-compliance (Sackett and Snow, 1979). Weiss *et al.* (1991) found that, although patients are carefully screened for home care, 71% show significant non-compliance with the requirements of medical management. It appears that at present there are no reliable criteria that would predict patient and family compliance in their home environment. As the authors point out, home treatment changes the relationship between patients and parents, requiring a new kind of cooperation within the family unit. Home therapy also changes the relationship between family and the treatment team in the hemophilia center. Successful home treatment necessarily distances the patient and the family from the medical team. While screening procedures may identify existing family conflicts and problem patients, the new kinds of responsibilities connected with infusion, and with a new kind of cooperation between parents and their children, may throw the family out of balance and present them as non-compliant.

Depending on the type and level of non-compliance, the clinician may establish different kinds of relationship with the family in the way health care is delivered. In some cases compliance can be viewed as a target for the family's behavioral change. On other occasions non-compliance can be viewed as a problem of fit between the health care and patient/family systems, and as an indicator of areas in which improvement in the fit could be made, perhaps by means of negotiation or by increasing the mutual understanding between the two parties. Weiss *et al.* (1991) conclude that, in order to insure that home therapy is fully beneficial to patients and their families, the screening procedure for home treatment must be accompanied by an assisted developmental process. This process includes education, help with social issues and individual and family therapy. A fit between the perspectives of the hemophilia team and the family with respect to the goal to be achieved should be constantly reviewed.

MODELS OF COMPREHENSIVE THERAPY

Before the introduction of home treatment, the main specialists with whom the patient dealt were the physician to control his bleedings and the psychiatrist to attend to his stress and mental problems. One immediate consequence of home treatment has been the establishment of comprehensive care clinics that now provide, through periodic multidisciplinary services and evaluations, the care of patients and their families.

Patients and their family members are invited to attend the clinic at regular intervals, at least once a year but usually every 6 months. During their visit they attend various specialized services ranging from medical (e.g. hematology, orthopedics, pediatrics, dental, rehabilitation) to psychosocial and counseling ones (e.g. educational, vocational, genetic, psychiatric, social work, about community services, financial). Psychosocial considerations are essential both in the planning and the delivery of comprehensive hemophilia care (Parish, 1991). These include, above all, viewing the individual and the family globally, in terms of an integrated unit. This in itself is a relatively new concept because the focus of comprehensive care has traditionally been on the patient rather than on the family (Mason, Olson and Parish, 1988). It has been particularly because of HIV/AIDS that the shift has taken place from patient-centered to family-centered care. With the emergence of HIV/AIDS, the already well-established comprehensive care programs have had to cope with yet another challenge – how to coordinate the needs of patients and their families with respect to both hemophilia and HIV. Different models of comprehensive care, dealing with the two issues, have recently been presented. They differ in terms of the disciplines involved, stages at which different members of the team intervene and in their emphasis on the family participation.

Following Inwood and Clegg (1992), one can identify at least three basic models of comprehensive care. First, perhaps the most familiar model is the one in which the members of a comprehensive team in a hemophilia center are also primary care-givers for HIV/AIDS (Jones, 1989). The advantage of this model is that the same professionals deal with the patient's and the family's needs relating both to the management of hemophilia and of HIV. Patients, partners, parents or siblings are brought to a regular review system and are seen by a multidisciplinary team, such as doctors, nurses and medical social workers and family therapists. If necessary, referrals are also made to other specialists, such as orthopedic surgeons and physiotherapists. General counseling and genetic counseling also form part of the review (Miller *et al.*, 1989a; Goldman *et al.*, 1993b). The disadvantage of this model could be that it might exert considerable load on already overworked staff in the hemophilia center, requesting them to deal with difficult issues, such as disclosure of HIV diagnosis, of the commencement of administration of zidovudine (AZT), coping with symptoms and so on (Tsiantis *et al.*, 1990; Tsiantis, 1991; Inwood and Clegg, 1992).

The second model is based on the operation of two systems, one providing a comprehensive HIV care and one providing comprehensive hemophilia care, with varying degrees of cooperation between these two systems. The advantage of this model is that the load of HIV/AIDS is taken away from members of the hemophilia team. However, the disadvantage could be too little communication between these two kinds of system. A variation of this model, favored by Tsiatsis (1991), involve the hemophilia care team and an interdisciplinary mental health team of child psychiatrists, psychologists and social workers. Members of both teams are involved during all stages of care intervention. For example, they deal with anxiety: they help family to adapt to the environment in the light of the HIV infection and they help cope with grief.

In choosing the second model for their own work, Inwood and Clegg (1992) put a considerable emphasis on the concept of a family-centered care program. Each family is treated as a unique system and the family-centered care program insures a personalized approach. It is recognized that each family may have different strengths and weaknesses in dealing with HIV and hemophilia. Special consideration is given to ethnic and cultural issues. An essential feature of the family-centered care system is monthly meetings of parents who experience similar kinds of problems. Figure 28.1 shows the various services available to support family-centered care. The whole system is led by a hemophilia nurse manager who coordinates services without unnecessary duplication, insures the collaborative partnership between the family and professionals and supervises ongoing assessments.

In model three, an independent practitioner provides HIV care but he or she has hardly any communication

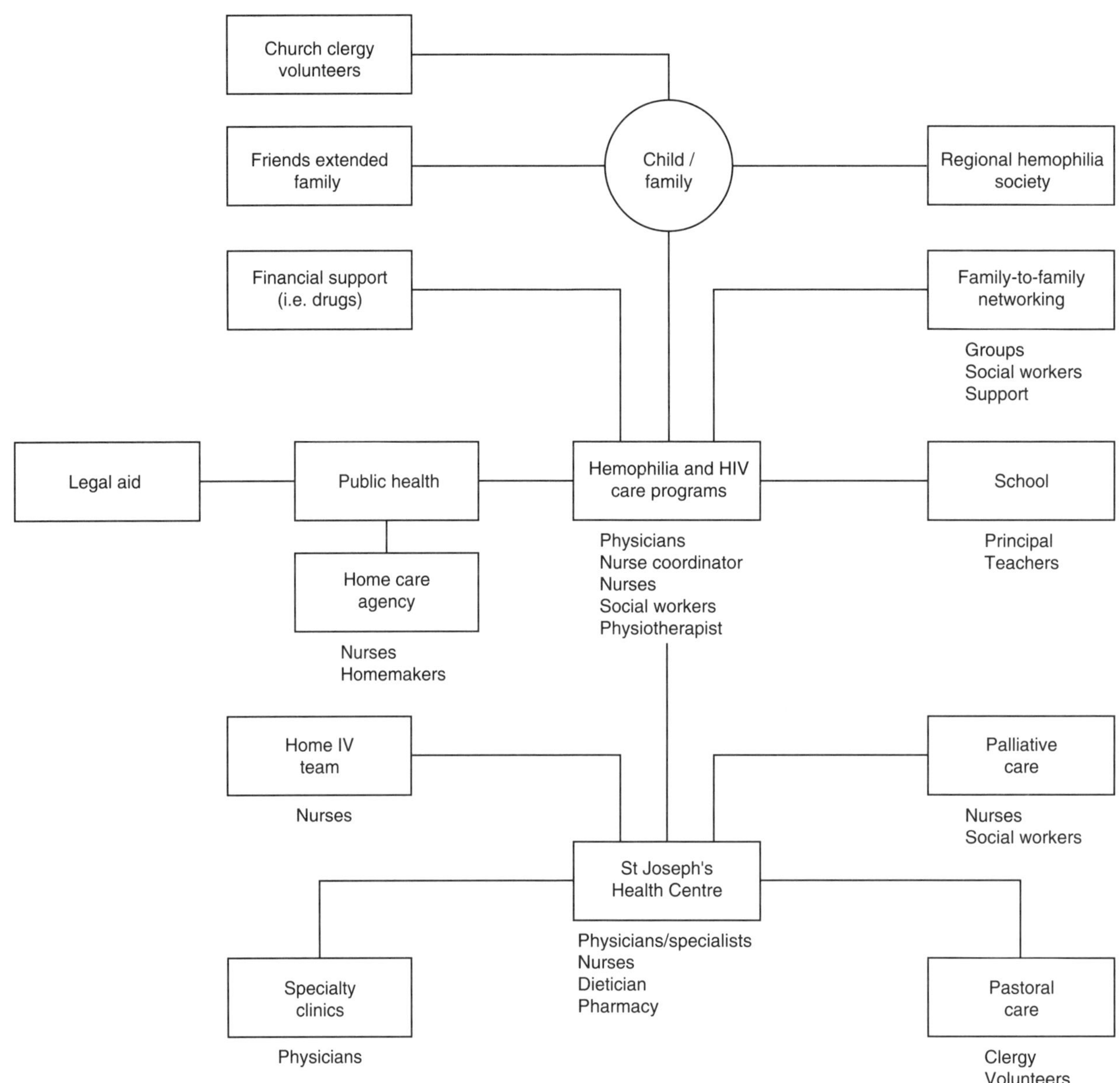

Fig. 28.1 Services available to support family-centered care. From Inwood, M.J. and Clegg, E.A. (1992) Models of care for the HIV infected adolescents hemophiliac. Paper read at the XX International Congress of the World Federation of Hemophilia, Athens, October 12–17, 1992, with permission.

with the comprehensive hemophilia center. As Inwood and Clegg (1992) point out, this model does not allow for the integration of HIV and hemophilia care.

COMPREHENSIVE THERAPY AS COMMUNICATION

The lives of families with hemophilia have been greatly altered by their involvement in the two complementary systems of care, the one of home-based emergency care and the one based on a long-term monitoring of hemophilia in treatment centers. One particular challenge for the clinic teams has been to introduce efficient methods of patient training and of health education. It appears that the mass media and the treatment centers are the most important sources of information for families with hemophilia (Olson *et al.*, 1989). Yet most educational programs and mass media campaigns rely on passive learning – providing information about HIV but not trying to change attitudes or behavior (Greenblatt *et al.*, 1989). Greenblatt *et al.* argue that, to change sexual practices, decrease drug use and improve personal health care requires more than providing information. Rather, attitude and behavioral changes require the individual's involvement in relevant activities. Their encounter programs utilize simulation games in which individuals play different roles to become aware of the dynamics of the interactive process and of different perspectives on the issue in question. Hemophilia encounters are designed to help participants improve their ability to communicate about sensitive topics related to HIV infection and AIDS.

Whatever model of comprehensive therapy is used, its success, in the end, depends on good working partnerships between families and professional teams. Comprehensive therapy takes place largely through communication and therefore, particular attention must be given to the communicative process and its goal. While participants in a communicative process may think that they are neutral with respect to what they say, communication is never neutral (Marková, 1990; Parish, 1991). Both the professional team and families enter the process of communication with their own perspectives, beliefs, roles and expectations. Their differences in perspectives and otherwise are expressed through what they say, what they do not say and what they express non-verbally. They sometimes communicate directly and explicitly, for example, when discussing AIDS, using the word 'AIDS.' However, they may talk about AIDS without using the word 'AIDS.' Individuals are rarely aware of the impression they make on each other and what the other party understands. They may think they have expressed something, yet the impression of the other is different. Yet, all messages, all understanding and all misunderstandings are always constructed by them mutually. They are both responsible for what they communicate to each other. In order to achieve a good therapeutic relationship, they both need to know a great deal about communication.

References

Agle, D. (1975) Psychological factors in hemophilia: the concept of self-care, *Annals of the New York Academy of Sciences*, **240**, 221–225.

Agle, D.P. (1977) Home care – selection and problems, in *Mental Health Services in the Comprehensive Care of Haemophiliac* (ed. D.P. Agle), The National Hemophilia Foundation, New York.

Agle, D. and Mattsson, A. (1968) Psychiatric and social care of patients with hereditary hemorrhagic disease. *Modern Treatment*, **5**, 111–124.

Agle, D. and Mattsson, A. (1970) Psychiatric factors in hemophilia: methods of parental adaption. *Haematologia*, **34**, 89–94.

Agle, D., Gluck, H. and Pierce, G.F. (1987) The risk of AIDS: psychologic impact on the hemophilic population. *General Hospital Psychiatry*, **9**, 11–17.

Aledort, L.M. (1994) Challenges in future hemophilia care, in *Blood, Blood Products and HIV* (eds R. Madhok, C.D. Forbes and B.L. Evatt), Chapman & Hall, London, p. 26.

Authier, J. and Land, T. (1978) Family: the unique component of family medicine. *Journal of Family Practice*, **7**, 1066.

Brandt, A.M. (1985) *No Magic Bullet*. Oxford University Press, Oxford.

Brandt, A.M. (1988) AIDS in historical perspective: four lessons from the history of sexually transmitted disease. *American Journal of Public Health*, **78**, 367–371.

Breslau, N., Weitzman, M. and Messenger, K. (1981) Psychological functioning of siblings of disabled children. *Pediatrics*, **67**, 344–353.

Browne, W.J., Mally, M.A. and Kane, R.P. (1960) Psychosocial aspects of hemophilia: a study of 28 hemophilic children and their families. *American Journal of Orthopsychiatry*, **30**, 730–740.

Bruhn, J.G. (1977) Effects of chronic illness on the family. *Journal of Family Practice*, **4**, 1057–1060.

Burr, C.K. (1985) Impact on the family of a chronically ill child, in *Issues in the Care of Children with Chronic Illness* (eds N. Hobbs and J.M. Perrin), Jossey-Bass, San Francisco, pp. 24–40.

Bussing, R. and Johnson, S.B. (1992) Psychosocial issues in hemophilia before and after the HIV crisis: a review of current research. *General Hospital Psychiatry*, **14**, 387–403.

Catalan, J. and Klimes, I. (1991) Psychiatric problems in HIV-infected men with haemophilia. *International Review of Psychiatry*, **3**, 373–381.

Catalan, J., Klimes, I., Bond, A. *et al.* (1989) Psychosocial and neuropsychiatric status of haemophiliacs and gay men: controlled investigation, Vth International AIDS Conference, Abstract THBP 31, p.421.

Catalan, J., Klimes, I., Bond, A. *et al.* (1992) The psychological impact of HIV infection in men with haemophilia: controlled investigation and factors associated with psychiatric morbidity. *Journal of Psychosomatic Research*, **36**, 409–416.

Dew, M.A., Ragni, M.V. and Nimorwicz, P. (1990) Infection with human immunodeficiency virus and vulnerability to psychiatric distress. *Archives of General Psychiatry*, **47**, 737–744.

Doherty, W.J. and Campbell, T.L. (1988) *Families and Health*, Sage, Beverly Hills.

Dormandy, K.M. (1973) Pain in haemophilia. *Lancet*, **1**, 931.

Douglas, M. (1966) *Purity and Danger*, Routledge and Kegan Paul, London.

Dowling, J.P. (1960) Preventing dependency patterns in chronically ill children. *Social Casework*, **41**, 395–402.

Drotar, D. and Crawford, P. (1985) Psychological adaptation of siblings of chronically ill children: research and practice implications. *Developmental and Behavioural Pediatrics*, **6**, 355–362.

Dunne, P.W., Sanders, M.R., Rowell, J.A. and McWhirter, W.R. (1991) An evaluation of cognitive–behavioural techniques in the management of chronic arthritic pain in men with haemophilia. *Behaviour Change*, **8**, 70–78.

Eiser, C. (1990) *Chronic Childhood Disease*, Cambridge University Press, Cambridge.

Eiser, C. (1993) *Growing Up with a Chronic Disease: The Impact on Children and their Families*, Jessica Kingsley, London.

Forbes, C.D., Marková, I., Stuart, J. and Jones, P. (1982) 'To tell or not to tell': haemophiliacs' views on their employment prospects. *International Journal of Rehabilitation Research*, **5**, 13–18.

Frommer, E.A. and Ingram, G.I.C. (1973) Pain in haemophilia. *Lancet*, **1**, 931–932.

Gath, A. (1973) The school age siblings of Mongol children. *British Journal of Psychiatry*, **123**, 161–167.

Goldman, E., Lee, C.A. and Miller, R. (1993) The children of HIV positive haemophilic men. *Archives of Diseases in Childhood*, **68**, 133–134.

Goldman, E., Miller, R. and Lee, C.A. (1993) A family with HIV and haemophilia. *AIDS Care*, **5**, 79–85.

Green, J. (1990) *Calming or Harming?*, Galton Institute, London.

Greenblatt, C.S., Katz, S., Gagnon, J.H. and Shannon, D. (1989) An innovative program of counselling family members and friends of seropositive haemophiliacs. *AIDS Care*, **1**, 67–75.

Handford, H.A., Mayes, S.D., Nagnato, S.J. and Bixler, E.O. (1986) Relationships between variations in parent's attitudes and personality traits of hemophilic boys. *American Journal of Orthopsychiatry*, **56l**, 424–434.

Harvey, G.P. (1973) Little relief from pain of haemophilia. *Lancet*, **1**, 776.

Howard, J. (1978) The influence of children's developmental dysfunctions on marital quality and family interaction, in *Child Influences on Marital and Family Interaction: A Life-span Perspective* (eds R.M. Lerner and G.B. Spanier), Academic Press, New York, pp. 275–298.

Ilfeld, F.W. (1982) Marital stressors, coping styles, and symptoms of depression, in *Handbook of Stress: Theoretical and Clinical Aspects* (eds L. Goldberger and S. Bereznits), Free-Press, New York, pp. 482–494.

Inwood, M.J. and Clegg, E.A. (1992) Models of care for the HIV infected adolescent hemophiliac. Paper read at the XX International Congress of the World Federation of Hemophilia, Athens, October 12–17, 1992.

Jodelet, D. (1991) *Madness and Social Representations*, Harvester Wheatsheaf, Hemel Hempstead.

Jones, P. (1974) *Living with Haemophilia*, Medical and Technical, Lancaster.

Jones, P. (1985) *AIDS and the Blood*, Haemophilia Society, London.

Jones, P. (1989) The counselling of HIV antibody positive haemophiliacs, in *Counselling in HIV Infection and AIDS* (eds J. Green and A. McCreaner), Blackwell, Oxford.

Katz, A.H. (1970) *Hemophilia – A Study in Hope and Reality*, C. C. Thomas, Springfield, Illinois.

Katz, A.H. and Goldy, F.B. (1963) Social adaptation in hemophilia. *Children*, **10**, 189–193.

Kaufert, J.M. (1980) Social and psychological responses to home treatment of hemophilia. *Journal of Epidemiology Community and Health*, **34**, 194–200.

King, E.H. (1981) Child-rearing practices: child with chronic illness and well sibling. *Issues in Comprehensive Pediatric Nursing*, **5**, 105–94.

Klimes, I., Catalan, J., Garrod, A. *et al.* (1992) Partners of men with HIV infection and haemophilia: controlled investigation of factors associated with psychological mobility. *AIDS Care*, **4**, 149–156.

Lawrence, D., Jason, J., Holman, R. *et al.* (1989) Sex practice correlates of HIV transmission and AIDS incidence in heterosexual partners and offspring of US haemophiliac men. *American Journal of Hematology*, **30**, 68–76.

Lazerson, J. (1972) Hemophilia home transfusion program: effect on school attendance. *Journal of Pediatrics*, **81**, 330–332.

Lineberger, H.P., Hernandez, J.T. and Brantley, H.T. (1984) Self concept and locus of control in hemophiliacs. *International Journal of Psychiatry and Medicine*, **14**, 243–251.

Marková, I. (1990) Medical ethics: a branch of societal psychology, in *Societal Psychology* (eds H.T. Himmelweit and G. Gaskell), Sage, Newbury Park.

Marková, I. and Forbes, C.D. (1984) Coping with haemophilia. *International Review of Applied Psychology*, **33**, 457–477.

Marková, I., Forbes, C. and Inwood, M. (1984) Consumers' views of genetic counselling in haemophilia. *American Journal of Medical Genetics*, **17**, 741–752.

Marková, I., Lockyer, R. and Forbes, C.D. (1977) Haemophilia: survey on social issues. *Health Bulletin*, **35**, 177–182.

Marková, I., MacDonald, K. and Forbes, C. (1980a) Impact of haemophilia on child-rearing practices and parental co-operation. *Journal of Child Psychology and Psychiatry*, **21**, 153–162.

Marková, I., MacDonald, K. and Forbes, C. (1980b) Integration of haemophilic boys into normal schools. Child Care. *Health and Development*, **6**, 101–109.

Marková, I., Wilkie, P.A. and Forbes, C.D. (1988) *Coping strategies of haemophilic patients who are at risk from acquired immunity deficiency syndrome (AIDS) and implications for counselling.* Unpublished final report to the Scottish Home and Health Department.

Marková, I., Forbes, C.D. Rowlands, A. *et al.* (1983) The haemophilic patient's self-perception of changes in health and lifestyle arising from self treatment. *International Journal of Rehabilitation Research*, **6**, 11–18.

Marková, I., Forbes, C.D., Aledort, L.M. *et al.* (1986): A comparison of the availability and content of genetic counselling as perceived by haemophilic men and carriers in the USA, Canada, Scotland and Greece. *American Journal of Medical Genetics*, **24**, 7–21.

Marková, I., Wilkie, P.A., Naji, S.A. and Forbes, C.D. (1990a) Self- and other awareness of the risk of HIV/AIDS in people with haemophilia and implications for behavioural change. *Social Science and Medicine*, **31**, 73–79.

Marková, I., Wilkie, P.A., Naji, S.A. and Forbes, C.D. (1990b) Knowledge of HIV/AIDS and behavioural change of people with haemophilia. *Psychology and Health*, **4**, 125–133.

Martino, M.S. and Newman, M.B. (1974) Siblings of retarded children: a population at risk. *Child Psychology and Human Development*, **4**, 168–177.

Mason, P.J., Olson, R.A. and Parish, K.L. (1988) AIDS, hemophilia, and prevention efforts within a comprehensive care program. *American Psychologist*, **43**, 971–976.

Mason, P.J., Olson, R.A., Myers, J.G. *et al.* (1989) AIDS and hemophilla: implications for interventions with families. *Journal of Pediatric Psychology*, **14**, 341–355.

Massie R.K. (1985) The constant shadow: reflections on the life of a chronically ill child. in *Issues in the Care of Children with Chronic Illness* (eds N. Hobbs and J.M. Perrin), Jossey-Bass, San Francisco, pp. 13–23.

Mattsson, A. (1972) Long-term physical illness in childhood: a challenge to psychological adaptation. *Pediatrics*, **50**, 801–810.

Mattsson, A. (1975) Psychophysiological study of bleeding and adaptation in young hemophiliacs, in *Explorations in Child Psychiatry* (ed. J. Anthony), Plenum, New York.

Mattsson, A. and Gross, S. (1966) Adaptational and defensive behavior in young hemophiliacs and their parents. *American Journal of Psychiatry*, **122**, 1349–1356.

Miller, R., Goldman, E., Bor, P. and Kernoff, P. (1989a) Counselling children and adults about AIDS/HIV: the ripple effect on haemophilia care settings. *Counselling Psychology Quarterly*, **2**, 65–72.

Miller, R., Goldman, E., Bor, P. and Kernoff, P. (1989b) AIDS and children: some of the issues in haemophilia care and how to address them. *Aids Care*, **1**, 59–65.

Miller, R., Bor, R., Salt, H. and Murray, D. (1991) Counselling patients with HIV infection about laboratory tests with predictive values. *Aids Care*, **3**, 159–164.

Mitterauer, M. and Sieder, R. (1977) *Vom Patriarchat zur Partnerschaft: Zum Strukturwandel der Familie*, C.H. Beck'sche Verlagbuchhandlung (Oscar Beck), Munchen. Translated by K. Oosterveen and M. Hörzinger (1982) as *The European Family, Patriarchy to Partnership from the Middle Ages to the Present*, Basil Blackwell, Oxford.

Modell, J. and Goodman, M. (1993) Historical perspectives, in *After the Threshold. The Developing Adolescent* (eds S.S. Feldman and G.E. Elliott), Harvard University Press, Cambridge, pp. 93–122

Molleman, E. and van Knippenberg, A.D. (1987) Social and psychological aspects of haemophilia. *Patient Education and Counselling*, **10**, 175–189.

Nelson, L. and Album, M. (1987) AIDS: children with HIV infection and their families, *Journal of Dentistry for Children*, **30**, 353–358.

Oremland, E.K. (1988) Work dynamics in family care of hemophilic children. *Social Science and Medicine*, **26**, 467–475.

Overby, K., Lo, B. and Litt, I. (1989) Knowledge and concerns about AIDS and their relationship to behaviour among adolescents with haemophilia, *Paediatrics*, **83**, 204–210.

Parish, K. (l991) Global perspectives on HIV and hemophilia: psychosocial aspects in *Hemophilia and von Willebrand's Disease in the 1990s* (eds J.M. Lusher and C.M. Kessler), Elsevier Science, Amsterdam.

Parish, K. L., Madel, J.; Thomas, J. *et al.* (1988) Psychosocial and sexual adjustment to AIDS among person with haemophilia. Paper read at the World Congress of Haemophilia, Madrid 1988.

Perrin, J.M. (1985) Introduction, in *Issues in the Care of Children with Chronic Illness* (eds N. Hobbs and J.M. Perrin), Jossey-Bass, San Francisco, pp. 1–10.

Pless, I.B. and Perrin, J.M. (1985) Issues common to a variety of illness, in *Issues in the Care of Children with Chronic Illness* (eds N. Hobbs and J.M. Perrin), Jossey-Bass, San Francisco, pp. 41–60.

Ragni M. and Nimorwicz, P. (1989) Human immunodeficiency virus transmission and haemophilia. *Archives of Internal Medicine*, **149**, 1379–1380.

Rosendaal, F.R., Smit, C., Varekamp, I. *et al.* (1988) AIDS and hemophilia: a study among Dutch hemophiliacs on the psycho-logical impact of the AIDS threat, the prevalence of HIV antibodies and the adoption of measures to prevent HIV transmission. *Haemostasis*, **18**, 73–82.

Sackett, D.L. and Snow, J.C. (1979) The magnitude of compliance and noncompliance, in *Compliance in Health Care* (eds B. Haynes, D.W. Taylor and D. Sackett), Johns Hopkins University Press, Baltimore, MD.

Salk, L., Hilgartner, M. and Granich, B. (1972) The psychosocial impact of hemophilia on the patient and his family. *Social Science and Medicine*, **6**, 491–505.

Sanden, M.L. and Bjurulf, P. (1988) Pregnant women's attitudes for accepting or declining a serum-alpha-fetoprotein test. *Scandinavian Journal of Social Medicine*, **16**, 265–271.

Schwenk, T.L. and Hughes, C.C. (1983) The family as patient in family medicine. *Social Science and Medicine*, **17**, 1–16.

Shelley, L.F. (1985) *Touch Me Who Dares*. Gomer Press, Llandsyul.

Sjörgen, B. and Uddenberg, N. (1987) Attitudes towards disabled persons and the possible effects of prenatal diagnosis. An interview study among 53 women participating in prenatal diagnosis and 20 of their husbands. *Journal of Psychosomatic Obstetrics and Gynaecology*, **6**, 187–196.

Smiley, M., White, G., Becherer, P. *et al.* (1988) Transmission of HIV to sexual partners of hemophiliacs. *American Journal of Hematology*, **28**, 27–32.

Smith, P.S. and Levine, P.H. (1984) The benefits of comprehensive care of hemophilia: 5-year study of outcomes. *American Journal of Public Health*, **74**, 616–617.

Shulmon, J.L. and Kupst (1980) *The Child with Cancer*, Thomas, Springfield, Ill.

Tsiantis, J. (1991) An interdisciplinary approach for management of the impact of seropositivity on haemophiliac children, their families and the care team: an integrating approach, in *Hemophilia and von Willebrand's Disease in the 1990s Amsterdam* (eds J.M. Lusher and C.M. Kessler), Elsevier Science, Amsterdam.

Tsiantis, J., Anastasopoulos, D., Meyer, M. *et al.* (1990) A multi-level intervention approach for care of HIV-positive haemophilic and thalassaemic patients and their families. *Aids Care*, **2**, 253–266.

Varekamp, I., Suurmeijer, Th. P.B.M., Rosendaal, F.R. *et al.* (1990) Family burden in families with a hemophilic child. *Family Systems Medicine*, **8**, 291–301.

Varekamp, I., Suurmeijer, Th. P.B.M., Rosendaal, F.R. and Bröcker-Vriends, A.H.J.T. (1993) The use of preventive health care services: carrier testing for the genetic disorder haemophilia. *Social Science and Medicine*, **5**, 639–648.

Varni, J.W. (1981a) Behavioural medicine in haemophilia arthritic pain management: two case studies. *Archives of Physical Medicine and Rehabilitation*, **62**, 183–187.

Varni, J.W. (1981b) Self regulation techniques in the management of chronic arthritic pain in haemophilia. *Behavior Therapy*, **12**, 185–194.

Varni, J.W., Gilbert, A. and Dietrich, S.L. (1981) Behavioral medicine in pain and analgesia management for the hemophilic child with factor VIII inhibitor. *Pain*, **11**, 121–126.

Weiss, H.M., Simon, R., Levi, J. *et al.* (1991) Compliance in a comprehensive hemophilia centre and its implications for home care. *Family Systems Medicine*, **9**, 111–120.

Wilkie, P. (1992) People with haemophilia and HIV, in *Reflective Helping in HIV and AIDS* (eds C. Anderson and P. Wilkie), Open University Press, Milton Keynes, pp. 237–252.

Wilkie, P.A., Marková, I., Naji, S.A. and Forbes, C.D. (1990) Daily living problems of people with haemophilia and HIV infection: implications for counselling. *International Journal of Rehabilitation Research*, **13**, 15–25.

Wilson, P.A. and Wasserman, K. (1989) Psychological responses to the threat of HIV exposure among people with bleeding disorders. *Health and Social Work*, **14**, 176–183.

29 THE COST OF HEMOPHILIA CARE

R.A. Lipton

This chapter describes the elements within health care systems that contribute to the costs of hemophilia care. It is important to differentiate within a system who assumes these costs. In short, who pays the bills? Is it the patient and his family, his health insurance company, employer, a charity or the government? How efficiently money flows through a health care system hinges on whether it is centrally configured, such as in a national health insurance program, or a diverse mixture of private and public payors and mainly for-profit providers, as is the case for the USA. The less structured or coordinated a health care system, the more the opportunities to shift costs from one component to another. But, with any system, ultimately, all costs are borne individually or collectively by households.

The single most costly aspect of hemophilia care is the price of clotting factor concentrates. Since 1984, prices have risen dramatically due to the increased costs of producing safer and purer products. Prices also rose due to production shortages that occurred with these changes. In the USA, the cost of clotting factor concentrates varies because of significant differences between the acquisition prices paid to the manufacturers of clotting factor concentrates and the final prices charged to patients, insurance companies and other third-party payors. Acquisition prices have leveled off due to a relatively stable demand for products by a diminishing patient population. However, total demand for clotting factor concentrates will soon increase as the young, non-human immunodeficiency virus (HIV)-infected patient population matures and is generally treated more intensively. Many may receive long-term or lifelong prophylaxis. Economic theory predicts that the increase in demand for clotting factor by this population will cause prices to rise once more. The anti-competitive behavior of the few firms producing plasma derivatives further assures this prediction.

Additional costs of care include lifelong expenses for other medical services related to or modified by hemophilia. Particularly in the USA, continued availability and access to comprehensive services by hemophilia patients will depend on the degree to which these direct costs will be borne by private insurance, public subsidies or the patients. Reduced access to these services could increase morbidity, leading to an increase in clotting factor use as well. There are important indirect costs to patients and families, such as lost opportunities at school and work. Generally, families experiencing serious illness incur significant care-giving and financial burdens. Ideally, costs could diminish, resulting from improvements in care that lead to a better quality of life. There are intangible benefits to patients resulting from reductions in pain and suffering (Corinsky *et al.*, 1994; Rice, 1994; Ross-Degnan *et al.*, 1996).

The adequate financing of regional hemophilia centers in the USA is sustained by monies generated through clotting factor concentrate distribution systems. In 1973 the Federal government began subsidizing regional hemophilia centers and encouraged their growth, thereby making the special medical services needed by the nation's hemophiliacs more available. Federal grants for 1994–1995 in support of hemophilia services, including HIV services, are approximately $10.4 million for 145 hemophilia centers and their affiliates. The grants pay the salaries of staff and operations, although payments for individual medical services and clotting factor concentrate are not covered (McGuckin P., personal communication). Presently, government grants cover less than half of many hemophilia centers' operating budgets. Therefore, most hemophilia treatment centers sustain their operations by varied financial linkages to clotting factor distribution and reimbursement systems.

Hemophilia. Edited by C.D. Forbes, L. Aledort and R. Madhok. Published in 1997 by Chapman & Hall, London. ISBN 0 412 63820 7

The prices for clotting factor concentrates are not just determined by the plasma industry's costs of production and marketing. The acquisition and distribution of concentrates by intermediaries result in wholesale and retail prices that are highly variable. Most clotting factor concentrate is administered at home, with its final price dependent upon the nature of the distribution system and what health insurers are willing to pay. Fully developed distribution systems provide medical coordination, shipment of concentrates and collection of used injection materials for medical waste disposal.

An informal estimate based on industry sales suggests that nearly 70% of clotting factor distribution is handled by for-profit home care companies. Considered a growth industry by investors, commercial home care companies actively seek arrangements with hemophilia treatment programs to purchase and distribute clotting factor concentrates. The difference between acquisition and final prices can be more than 150%. Profits are sufficient to offer hemophilia centers billing and collection services. Financial support by home care companies can underwrite salaries of hemophilia center staff and grants for patient and staff education.

Inflated costs to private health insurance plans allow hospitals, free-standing hemophilia centers and home care companies to underwrite otherwise uncompensated care of indigent patients. Moreover, the plasma industry supplies treatment centers with clotting factor concentrates that are used in clinical research.

There can be a significant mark-up from acquisition costs when hospital pharmacies or blood banks distribute concentrates. This money may go into a hospital's generating operating budget or directly supplement the institution's costs of hemophilia care. In the New York metropolitan area and the state of Georgia, clotting factor concentrates are purchased and distributed by not-for-profit entities. Distributions from these arrangements are used to finance operations at participating hemophilia centers.

Although the average unit cost for factor VIII actually decreased in 1993, high prices to patients continued, due to the increased disparity between acquisition prices and final charges to insurance companies. These arrangements occur because of inadequate federal support of regional hemophilia centers and because health insurers, with few objections, are willing to pay final prices.

The cost of clotting factor concentrates

In the 12-month period between July 1993 and June 1994, the New York metropolitan area's three hemophilia centers (the Long Island Jewish Medical Center, the New York Hospital–Cornell Medical Center and the Mount Sinai Medical Center) ordered for their 587 patients through the region's blood-product-purchasing consortium 46 million units of clotting factor concentrates. At an average price of $0.48 per unit (including factor VIII, factor IX and activated prothrombin complex concentrates), the total cost to third-party payors was just over $22 million. Annual consumption averaged 78 000 units, approximating $73 000 per patient. For the 288 patients on home infusion, annual consumption averaged 136 000 units or $67 000 per patient per year. In most other regions where clotting factor concentrate is commercially distributed, the final price is significantly higher than in New York. For example, in 1993 the average prices to patients at the three New York centers and their affiliates was for factor VIII products $0.31 per unit, $0.16 for factor IX and $0.75 for activated prothrombin complex concentrates (aPCCs). This is compared to the following average commercial prices: factor VIII $0.89 per unit, factor IX $0.46 per unit and aPPCs $1.26 per unit (Agnew G, personal communication).

Comprehensive hemophilia services are cost-effective

The medical and psychological benefits of comprehensive hemophilia services are significant. Specifically, the results of home infusion therapy are undisputed. Still, patients on home infusion programs generally use more clotting factor concentrates than patients receiving less coordinated and episodic care in hospital emergency rooms. The increased use of clotting factor concentrates is mainly offset by lower indirect costs to patients and families missing less work and school and documented improvements in musculoskeletal functioning (Lazarson, 1972; Smith, Keyes and Forman, 1982; Carman et al., 1984; Smit et al., 1989; Aledort et al., 1994). For patients not on home therapy there may be increased emergency room and inpatient charges. Yet, these costs may not be borne by patients if they are indigent or have limited third-party insurance that excludes coverage for home therapy.

The impact of HIV infection on people with hemophilia has been emotionally draining to patients, their families and the professionals caring for them. In addition to necessary, but costly, modifications in the manufacturing of clotting factor concentrates, the complexity and costs of clinical care have dramatically increased. Most hemophilia centers have taken on the responsibility for providing or coordinating HIV service for their patients rather than referring to acquired immunodeficiency syndrome (AIDS) clinics, although payment for these additional services generally has not covered its costs (Rickard, 1990; Hoots et al. 1991). Annual average costs for patients with AIDS alone in Massachusetts in 1986 for both inpatient and outpatient services was $40 000 (Seage et al., 1986). These costs have decreased with improvements in HIV care. Also,

Centers for Disease Control (CDC) projections on the cost of AIDS treatment appear to have been over-estimated (Green, Oppenheimer and Wintfeld, 1994).

Some problems financing comprehensive hemophilia care

In the USA, the financing of hemophilia health care services is problematic. Few hemophilia patients in the USA self-pay for clotting factor concentrates or for medical services. Those with adequate health insurance are directly shielded from paying high prices for clotting factor concentrates and specialized medical services. Still, many are impoverished by significant co-payments and deductible charges. Universal and equitable access to basic health services is not yet a reality for many Americans. Usually, health care costs are borne by private insurance plans provided as a group benefit to workers by many firms and businesses. People with hemophilia, particularly those self-employed, working part-time or full-time in low-wage industries, are not offered or cannot obtain group health insurance. Individual health insurance policies are increasingly unaffordable due to their inherent higher administrative costs and adverse risk selection because the purchasers of individual plans, collectively, include many with costly medical conditions (Harrington T, personal communication). As a result, more patients find that publicly financed health care, reserved for the indigent or disabled, is their only recourse. The hidden cost, however, is high. By foregoing wages and 'spending down' their assets or 'becoming' disabled, people with hemophilia and many others with lifelong or chronic illnesses are forced to make a needless sacrifice to support their medical care. Moreover, there is a societal cost, both from higher taxes that subsidize this care and from lost income tax revenues from potential wage earners.

Managed care

To control the rising prices for medical services, many employers in the USA that provide their workers with health benefits contract with health maintenance organizations (HMOs) or private managed-care health plans offering discounted medical services. The plans reach various arrangements with hospitals, clinics and physicians to provide discounted medical services. They further reduce their expenses by restricting referrals for specialized medical services. Under a managed-care arrangement, a patient chooses a primary care physician from a list provided by the plan. Care by specialists is controlled by the primary physician acting as a gate-keeper to higher-cost medical services. In addition, cost-sharing arrangements between a primary care physician and a managed-care plan may create financial disincen-tives to the primary physician who refers. Patients may not self-refer or, if it is allowed, there may be a higher co-payment. The referral link to the regional hemophilia center can be tenuous, as primary care physician gate-keepers consider cost control as part of their decision to refer. Moreover, the general physician may not recognize the subtle early signs and symptoms of life-threatening bleeding in hemophilia patients.

Managed-care patients frequently deny claims for payment to hemophilia centers that provide unique medical, laboratory, dental and psychosocial expertise. In a managed-care plan, a failure to recommend high-cost but uncovered medical services can be the basis of a malpractice claim against physicians of the plan, but not the plan. Although in a few instances managed-care health plans have been sued for mismanagement, generally these plans are immune from malpractice litigation due to the Employee Retirement Income Security Act (ERISA) of 1974. This federal law pre-empts any state from regulating an employee's pension benefits and has been broadly interpreted by the courts as including the provision of certain employee benefits such as a health plan. Therefore, physicians are in the unenviable position of recommending therapies to hemophilia patients that a health plan may not pay for leaving patients personally responsible for the costs of needed but uninsured services.

While gate-keeping and claims denial may result in lowered costs to a managed-care health plan, over the long term the potential for diminished quality of care to people with hemophilia and other rare diseases might eventually exact increased costs to all parties (Dona-bedian, 1985). Research to date fails to confirm the contention that managed health care arrangements will result in significant savings to the nation's health care expenditures (United States General Accounting Office, 1993).

The problem when large firms self-insure their workers' medical benefits

As more people lose their health insurance, political pres-sure in each state increases for regulated insurance reform. States may pass community rating laws that mandate that health insurance companies sell policies at a single premium rate to all people purchasing insur-ance. Because working people may have lower than average health care costs, the community rates are higher than a firm might otherwise pay to self-insure its own workers. Therefore, large employers self-insure their workers. In 1994, more than 60% of such firms in the USA self-insured. A firm that self-insures is shielded from a state's insurance regulations because its health plan is considered part of an employee's pension and benefits and not insurance (ERISA). Additionally, states may 'tax' health insurance companies in order to provide funds to hospitals that provide uncompensated care to indigent people.

The ERISA pre-emption permits self-insured firms to exercise great discretionary authority in the medical benefits they choose to offer or deny to workers and their families. People with hemophilia, employed by a company that self-insures, can be denied important medical benefits. For example, payment can be denied for health problems existing prior to employment. When people with hemophilia are unable to take advantage of group purchasing and attempt to purchase individual private insurance at community rates, they find private health insurance increasingly unaffordable.

The cost of hospital medical services

In most countries, hospitals receive operating funds from sources that are subject to a central budgetary authority. In the USA, hospitals are financed by a mix of regulated and unregulated public and private payors. Public sources include federal funds from Medicare, a health care entitlement program for all citizens over age 65 or those with permanent disabilities, and Medicaid. The Medicaid program provides health insurance to designated categories of the poor. Financial and categoric eligibility is determined by each state and the cost is shared in equal measure by the state and the federal government. Public insurers reimburse a hospital's costs prospectively according to predetermined rates, which are calculated by the average costs of caring for a person falling within a particular diagnosis-related group (DRG). There are usually several different diseases within a DRG, further compounded by different DRG lists depending on the state or the type of insurance. For example, hemophilia may be included within a more general diagnosis group, such as 'coagulation disorders.' The few hospitals with hemophilia centers generally lose money caring for this group of patients because the average reimbursement paid to all hospitals for treating 'coagulation disorders' is significantly less than the cost of treating hemophilia. This situation is further complicated when hemophilia and HIV infection coexist.

The inpatient fees paid by Medicare and Medicaid are highly discounted and cause hospitals to charge private insurance companies higher rates for the same services. But opportunities to 'cost-shift' have lessened as hospitals in the USA compete with each other to keep their beds fully occupied. Over-bedded hospitals have found it necessary to negotiate arrangements with private insurers and managed-care plans that exchange discounted hospital fees for guaranteed referrals for inpatient care. Prior to these arrangements, cost-shifting had subsidized postgraduate medical education and permitted hospitals to cover the costs of services to the uninsured.

The cost of specialized ambulatory medical services

In countries with national health insurance and global budgeting it is possible to learn the aggregate costs of hemophilia care. In the USA aggregate costs are not as easy to calculate, as payment mechanisms depend on whether medical services are provided in a hospital or on an ambulatory basis. HMOs provide payment in full for all inpatient and ambulatory services. Other managed-care plans may pay a discounted fee for each ambulatory medical service provided or pay an annual capitation fee for all services. If capitation payments are not risk-adjusted for hemophilia, or hemophilia with accompanying HIV infection, essential ambulatory services may be denied to patients. When there are high co-payment and deductible charges that accompany each medical service provided, people with chronic or lifelong conditions may forgo needed treatment (Batavia, 1993; Kinney and Steinmetz, 1994). In New York, some representative list prices include: annual comprehensive examination (including evaluations by hematologist, hemophilia nurse, social worker, dental hygienist, physical therapist and genetic counselor) $250–500; annual laboratory examination (including blood count, chemistry profile, factor assay and inhibitor assay) $400–600. The ambulatory management of HIV infection (including testing, immune system monitoring, counseling and medications) increases annual ambulatory charges by $10 000 per patient (Arno, Shenson and Siegel, 1989; Rietmeijer *et al.*, 1993). In the future, hospitals providing ambulatory services may be reimbursed by rates that are set according to the patient's diagnosis, similar to the DRG prospective payment system for inpatients previously described. It is essential that this rate-setting system be carefully crafted to cover the costs of comprehensive hemophilia care adequately.

Compensation and legal costs of hemophilia care

In addition to the already noted cost burdens to individuals with hemophilia and HIV infection, there are aggregate costs due to lawsuits against physicians, hospitals, blood banks and the plasma industry. In contrast to Canada and several European countries, the US government is unlikely to compensate or provide direct assistance to HIV-infected hemophiliacs (Schimpf, 1992). Moreover, there have been significant intangible costs to the hemophilia community whose representative organizations, now fragmented in a morass of legal and compensation issues, have diminished political influence in the health policy arena. Physicians and hospitals are exposed to significant liability costs due to the American legal system. A patient can receive large monetary awards because of successfully suing medical providers for alleged malpractice. Risk exposure and its transfer by purchasing liability insurance will continue to be a costly component of hemophilia care, as it is for American medical care in general.

Innovations in treatment will increase total clotting factor consumption

Aggressive therapeutic regimens will increase the demand for clotting factor concentrates. Prophylactic administration of clotting factor concentrates is medically effective and has been endorsed by the Medical and Scientific Advisory Council of the National Hemophilia Foundation (Nilsson, 1993; Bohn, Avom and Aledort, 1994; Manco-Johnson *et al.*, 1994). As lifelong prophylaxis is promulgated as a 'standard of care', total demand for concentrate will increase. An increased demand for concentrate will also occur as immune tolerance protocols become validated methods of managing patients with inhibitors. Depending on the choice of therapeutic material and dosing schedules, immune tolerance programs can cost between \$22 and \$114 per kg per day (Aledort *et al.*, 1984; Brettler *et al.*, 1984; Lipton, 1994). There is an increased demand for higher-purity, higher-cost concentrates, particularly recombinant products by patients and physicians concerned with viral safety (Mariani *et al.*, 1989; Cash, 1991; Mannucci and Gringeri, 1991). High-purity concentrates may be of value in the preservation of immune function in the early stages of HIV infection, although mortality may not change (Hilgartner *et al.* 1993; Seremetis *et al.*, 1993; Goedert *et al.*, 1994). Higher-purity concentrates may predispose to inhibitor occurrence and, although inhibitor titers might remain low, higher doses will be needed (Aledort, 1994).

The increased demand for clotting factor concentrates is masked, for the moment, by a steady level of total clotting factor consumption in many regions due to the deaths of older HIV-infected patients. In the New York metropolitan area, clotting factor consumption has remained steady, although there has been a trend toward the use of more costly higher-specific-activity products each year (Agnew G, personal communication). Still, as the cohort of non-infected patients matures and prophylaxis becomes widespread, total consumption of clotting factor concentrates will dramatically increase. Shifts in economic demand (to the right) will cause increased prices.

The anticompetitive nature of the plasma derivatives industry

Plasma-derived clotting factor concentrates are produced for relatively few hemophilic persons worldwide, in part because plasma is obtained mainly to manufacture more widely used plasma derivatives such as albumin and immune globulins. Its price and availability, as a by-product, are subject to economic forces operating in the much larger albumin and globulin market. Without this linkage, clotting factor concentrates would not have been available at the comparatively low costs for these products between early 1970 and early 1980. Since 1984 the costs of collection and production to increase viral safety by purification and specific virucidal technologies have caused prices for clotting factor concentrates to skyrocket (Pierce *et al.*, 1989).

Prices set by the industry for clotting factor concentrates probably exceed the estimated costs of production and marketing due to market concentration and lessened competition found in this typical oligopoly. There are very few companies currently producing clotting factor concentrates; and significant barriers to the entry of future firms. These impediments result from high fixed costs of production, large capital outlays for equipment of little salvage value and cumbersome federal regulation. Generally, similar highly concentrated industries generate large profits. There are significant economies of scale barring additional firms from entering this market. A recent example was the closing of Melville Biologics, an innovative but undercapitalized processor of plasma products.

Total production of clotting factor concentrates for distribution to American patients for 1993 was 604 million units of factor VIII and 167 million units of factor IX (including aPPCs). While national data on recombinant factor VIII are unavailable, in metropolitan New York recombinant factor VIII accounted for 7.7% of the 55 million units distributed in 1993, with an estimated 10% for 1994. However, in other regions recombinant factor VIII is more widely prescribed and in a few centers exclusively prescribed (Agnew G, personal communication).

Firms selling plasma derivatives compete by product differentiation, emphasized through aggressive advertising. Although the firms are non-cooperative, they are mutually interdependent, with each engaged in strategic decision making to maintain its market share and thereby assuring the entire industry of continued high profits. Over the long term, buyers can only discourage rising prices by ignoring product differentiation through generic buying, and encouraging competition between as many sellers as possible.

Buyers' groups, however, representing providers and patients, can achieve lower prices by bulk purchasing. By agreeing to supply a negotiated amount of clotting factor concentrate at an annually agreed price, manufacturers lower production and marketing costs. Moreover, an annual price list lowers the cost to insurance companies processing claims. Multiple bid awards by bulk purchasers to competing firms in order to accommodate patient and provider choice, in addition to the lowest prices, can be as effective in maintaining low prices over several years as a single annual award to the lowest bidder (Aledort, Lipton and Hilgartner, 1988).

A new federal law mandates discounts in the acquisition costs of clotting factor concentrates to certain government entities and hemophilia centers. But the law does not address final prices which permit an additional profit margin to the distributors of clotting factor concentrates.

National self-sufficiency in plasma resources may increase the costs of care

In Europe, the goal of national self-sufficiency in plasma collection and production may encounter barriers resulting from economies of scale. The costs of production in countries seeking self-sufficiency are likely to be high, causing local prices to rise above a more competitive international market and requiring a need for government subsidies. In a country where sufficient plasma is donated it can be processed into plasma products for that country's exclusive use by a commercial plasma derivatives firm. Alternatively, governments may spend less through continued participation in a strongly regulated international plasma derivatives market. Government support of research in safer and less costly methods of plasma fractionation may be economically more efficient than attempting national self-sufficiency (World Federation of Hemophilia, 1993).

International health reform and the cost of hemophilia care

In most developed nations, people receive their health care through established national health care systems modeled as either social insurance financed by a mix of private and government funds or national health insurance that is publicly financed. Comprehensive regional hemophilia care evolved within these systems so that the mechanisms financing hemophilia treatment are less problematic than in the USA. Still, advances in medical technology and its demand by providers and consumers of health care services worldwide have resulted in cost-cutting measures by many countries. The health reforms that impact on the sufficiency of hemophilia care involve central constraints on hemophilia center operating budgets, restrictions on the use of new technology and economic regulation of the pharmaceutical industry. In Italy, for example, recombinant factor VIII is not approved for routine clinical use. Recently, cost control and containment measures common in the USA are finding applications by European health policy makers (Spanjer, 1995).

Reduced allocations lessen the likelihood that hemophilia centers can continue clotting factor-intensive treatment protocols such as high-dose immune tolerance for inhibitor management or offer routine lifelong prophylaxis. Budget watchers will demand cost–benefit analysis in addition to scientific validation before approving high-cost treatments.

In many countries pharmaceuticals are subject to government price-setting regulations, using criteria such as the costs of research, development, production and marketing. Elsewhere, prices may be subject to an assessment of therapeutic value or a cost-effective analysis, as in Australia (Drummond, 1992). In the UK and Spain firms are given target profit ceilings that cannot be exceeded. Pharmaceutical regulations by governments limit patient and physician preferences in therapeutic products. Reference pricing or profit ceilings have led firms to practice multitiered pricing across international boundaries. This practice allows firms to compensate for lower profit margins in regulated countries through sales in countries that are less regulated. In the future, the European Agency for the Evaluation of Medicinal Produces (EMEA) may bring continuity to drug regulation in Europe (Editorial, 1995). Over the long term, pharmaceutical regulation could remove the economic incentives for companies to pursue technologic advances or continue clotting factor production altogether (Feldstein, 1994; Hutton *et al.* 1994). Therefore, it is important for governments to cultivate research in hemophilia treatment, including new therapeutic avenues such as genetic engineering.

United States health reform and the cost of hemophilia care

By the fall of 1994, President Bill Clinton's proposal for large-scale national health reform was soundly defeated, leaving uncertainties for many about the future cost and accessibility of medical care. This was particularly so for people with hemophilia. Still, the conservative political leadership now in power could propose less sweeping changes. Limited private insurance reform might attempt to regulate an amalgam of competing insurance companies, hospital and physician providers and large health care corporations. Many responsibilities and operating details would devolve to the states, subject to their local priorities, cultural values, administrative and financial capacities (Sparer, 1993). In spite of regulation, many parties are likely to be successful in avoiding patients with excessive medical costs. Hemophilia and other rare conditions in need of lifelong high cost and highly specialized medical services could escape the notice of federal and state law-makers. It would be unfortunate if the rising cost of hemophilia treatment results in increased indirect and intangible costs that burden patients and families.

Conclusion

The cost of health care depends upon the choices society makes in terms of how much and by what method household incomes are transferred and spent on medical services. People with lifelong conditions are particularly dependent on these decisions. In most countries, health care is established as a basic entitlement financed through taxation and channeled through a national health or social insurance system, whereas in the USA the right to health care is not universally guaranteed. This is because private health insurance conforms to a casualty model where premium costs are based on risk, and public insurance is categorical and means-tested. The flow of dollars from American households to these insurance funds is less direct, mainly channeled through employers and less through explicit taxes (Reinhardt, 1993).

There are significant differences between how the USA and other countries will respond to the challenge of rising costs. In other nations, cost controls can be aimed at central budgets, resource allocation, the regulation of technology transfer and the pharmaceutical industry. Centralized regulation has a greater chance of preserving equity and is more economically efficient. As health care in the USA will remain fragmented, however, the debate over future financing will be contentious. We can anticipate continued debates over income transfer and risk transfer. Unfortunately it will pit the 'haves' against the 'have nots' and the healthy against the sick, resulting in significant loss in professional and patient autonomy and yet another setback for people with hemophilia.

References

Aledort, L. (1994) Inhibitors in hemophilia patients: current status and management. *Am J Hematol*, **47**, 208–317.

Aledort, L.M., Lipton, R.A. and Hilgartner, M. (1988) A consortium for the purchase of blood products directed by physicians. *Ann Intern Med*, **108**, 754–755.

Aledort, L.M., Cohen, M., Hilgartner, M. and Lipton, R. (1984) Treatment of hemophiliacs with inhibitors: cost and effect on blood resources, in *Factor VIII Inhibitors* (ed. L. Hoyer), Alan R. Liss, New York, pp. 353–365.

Aledort, L.M., Haschmeyer, R.H., Pettersson, H. and the Orthopedic Outcome Study Group (1994) A longitudinal study of orthopaedic outcomes for severe factor VIII deficient hemophiliacs. *J Int Med*, **236**, 391–399.

Arno, P.S., Shenson, D. and Siegel, N.F. (1989) Economic and policy implications of early intervention in HIV disease. *JAMA*, **262**, 493–498.

Batavia, A. (1993) Health care reform and people with disabilities. *Health Aff*, **12**, 1, 40–57.

Bohn, R.L., Avorn, J., Aledort, L.M. (1994) Cost-effectiveness analysis of prophylactic vs. on-demand treatment for hemophilia. Paper at Proceedings of the World Federation of Hemophilia, Mexico City.

Brettler, D., Shopnick, R., Bolivar, E. and Dumas, B. (1994) The price of immune tolerance programs for factor VIII inhibitors in the New England area. Are they worth it? *Am Soc Hematol*, Nashville, Tennessee.

Carman, C.J., Britten, A.F., Ala, F. *et al.* (1984) Financial aspects of hemophilia care. *Scand J Haematol*, (suppl. 40), 529–533.

Cash, J.D. (1991) High potency factor VIII concentrates: value not proved? *Br Med J*, **303**, 633–634.

Covinsky, K.E., Goldman, L., Cook, F. *et al.* (1994) The impact of serious illness on patients' families. *JAMA*, **272**, 1839–1844.

Donabedian, A. (1985) Some thoughts on cost containment and the quality of health care. *Admin Mental Health*, **13**, 5–14.

Drummond, M.F. (1992) Basing prescription drug payment on economic analysis: the case of Australia. *Health Affairs*, **11**, 191–206.

Editorial (1995) European medicines in the 21st century. *Lancet*, **345**, 1–2.

Feldstein, P.J. (1994) The high price of prescription drugs, in *Health Policy Issues, An Economic Perspective on Health Reform*. AUPHA Press/Health Administration Press, Ann Arbor, MI, pp. 204–216.

Goedert, J.J., Cohen, A.R., Kessler, C.M. *et al.* (1994) Risks of immunodeficiency, AIDS and death related to purity of factor VIII concentrate. *Lancet*, **344**, 791–2.

Green, J., Oppenheimer, G.M. and Wintfeld, N. (1994) The $147 000 misunderstanding: repercussions of overestimating the cost of AIDS. *J Health Politics, Policy and Law*, **19**, 69–90.

Hilgartner, M.W., Buckley, J.D., Operskalski, E.A. *et al.* (1993) Purity of factor VIII concentrates and serial CD4 counts. *Lancet*, **341**, 1373–1374.

Hoots, W.K., Buchanan, G.R., Parmley, R.T. *et al.* (1991) Comprehensive care for patients with hemophilia: an expanded role in reducing risk for human immunodeficiency virus. *Tex Med*, **87**, 72–75.

Hutton J., Borowitz, M., Oleksy, I. and Luce, B.R. (1994) The pharmaceutical industry and reform: lessons from Europe. *Health Affairs*, **13**, 98–111.

Kinney, E. and Steinmetz, S.K. (1994) Notes from the insurance underground: how the chronically ill cope. *J Health, Policy, Politics and Law*, **19**, 633–642.

Lazarson, J. (1972) Hemophilia home transfusion program: effect on school attendance. *J Pediat*, **81**, 330–332.

Lipton, R.A. (1994) The economics of factor VIII inhibitor treatment. *Semin Hematol*, **31** (suppl. 4), 37–38.

McDermott, Will and Emery, attorneys, (1994) Risks involved in dealing with managed care entities. Memorandum prepared for Continental Insurance HealthCare.

Manco-Johnson, M.J., Nuss, R., Geraghty, S. *et al.* (1994) Results of secondary prophylaxis in children with severe hemophilia. *Am J Hematol*, **47**, 113–117.

Mannucci, P.M. and Gringeri, A. (1991) The use of recombinant factor VIII in the management of hemophilia. *Ric Clin Lab*, **21**, 1–7.

Mariani, G., Solinas, S., Pasqualetti, D. *et al.* (1989) Induction of immunotolerance in hemophilia for high titre inhibitor. *Thromb Haemost*, **62**, 835–839.

The Marketing Research Bureau, 352 Third Street, Suite 308, Laguna Beach, California.

Nilsson, I.M. (1993) Experience with prophylaxis in Sweden. *Semin Hematol*, **30**, 16–19.

Peirce, G.F., Lusher, J.M., Brownstein, A.P. *et al.* (1989) The use of purified clotting factor concentrates in hemophilia. Influence of viral safety, cost and supply on therapy. *JAMA*, **261**, 3434–3438.

Reinhardt, U.E. (1993) Reorganizing the financial flows in American health care. *Health Affairs*, **12** (suppl.), 172–193.

Rice, D.P. (1994) Cost-of-illness studies: fact or fiction? *Lancet*, **334**, 1519.

Rickard, K.A. (1990) The impact of HIV on health care delivery in hemophilia. *Prog Clin Cio Res*, **324**, 101–111.

Rietmeijer, C.A., Davidson, A.J., Foster, C.T. and Cohn, D.L. (1993) Cost of care for patients with human immunodeficiency virus infection. Patterns of utilization and charges in a public health care system. *Arch Intern Med*, **153**, 219–225.

Ross-Degnan, D., Soumerai, S.B., Bohn, R.L. *et al.* (1995) Hemophilia home treatment as a case study: economic analysis and implications for health policy. *Int J Technol Assess Health Care*, **11**(2), 327–344.

Schimpf, K. (1992) Financial assistance for HIV-infected persons with hemophilia worldwide. *Haemostasis*, **22**, 293–298.

Seage, G.R., Landers, S., Barry, A. *et al.* (1986) Medical care costs of AIDS in Massachusetts. *JAMA*, **256**, 3107–3109.

Seremetis, S.V., Aledort, L.M., Bergman, G.E. *et al.* (1993) Three-year randomised study of high-purity factor VIII concentrate in symptom-free HIV-seropositive hemophiliacs: effects on immune status. *Lancet*, **342**, 700–703.

Smit, C., Rosendaal, F.R., Varekamp, I. *et al.* (1989) Physical condition, longevity and social performance of Dutch hemophiliacs, 1972–85. *Br Med J*, **298**, 235–238.

Smith, P.S., Keyes, N.C. and Forman E.N. (1982) Socioeconomic evaluation of a state funded comprehensive hemophilia care program. *N Engl J Med*, **306**, 575–579.

Spanjer, M. (1995) Changes in Dutch health-care. *Lancet*, **345**, 50–51.

Sparer, M. (1993) States and the health care crisis. *J Health, Policy, Politics and Law*, **18**, 503–513.

United States General Accounting Office (1993) *Report to the Chairman, Subcommittee on Health, Committee on Ways and Means, House of Representatives. Managed Health Care: Effect on Employers' Costs Difficult to Measure*, GA0/HR0-94-3 US Govt Printing Office, Washington, DC.

World Federation of Hemophilia (1993) The EC Single Market in Plasma Products: A Question of Circulation. Executive Summary, Meeting, Brussels, April 23, 1993.

30 PSYCHOSOCIAL SERVICES IN HEMOPHILIA

L.J. Haas, J.R. Schultz and M.A. Rigdon

Introduction

This chapter focuses on the psychosocial problems and treatments likely to be of concern in the care of the hemophilia patient and family. We have oriented the chapter to medical professionals who may or may not have a background in mental health. Therefore, the chapter briefly reviews some of the existing evidence for the general effectiveness of a variety of psychosocial interventions, as there is limited evidence available regarding psychosocial interventions specifically with hemophilia patients. The chapter also includes a section on psychosocial interventions with human immunodeficiency virus (HIV)-positive patients and their partners or families. The issue of liver disease or hepatitis is somewhat more complicated. Hepatitis C in particular is endemic in the hemophilia community; and yet there appears to be no literature focused on psychosocial interventions with these patients.

This chapter takes the biopsychosocial model as its foundation, along with a family systems focus. Thus our basic tenets include the concept that biological, social and psychologic factors are interactive in their influence on medical symptoms and experiences. The theory and practice of biobehavioral interventions flow from that model's prediction that non-pharmacologic, psychosocial interventions can have a direct bearing on physical symptoms. In addition, we emphasize the need to consider different levels of intervention: in the present chapter we emphasize the **level of first choice**, although certain situations may call for less direct approaches, or multidisciplinary teamwork. We should also note that a close medical–psychosocial interrelationship demands the presence of a well-integrated multidisciplinary team which has the well being of the patients and families foremost in mind.

PSYCHOLOGIC DISTURBANCE AMONG HEMOPHILIA PATIENTS AND FAMILIES

Hemophilia is a chronic disease that requires lifelong care. Although as many as one-third of hemophilia cases arise spontaneously, it is also a genetic disease. Hemophilia may increase the risk of developmental delays. The World Health Organization has called the personal and social implications of hemophilia for patients and family members 'profound.' Nimorwicz and Klein (1982) note: 'it is virtually impossible for families to anticipate how the complex issues associated with this disease will affect their lives.' Families with newly diagnosed hemophiliac children are often confused and ill-prepared for the stresses that are about to descend upon them; family dynamics of guilt and anger can also emerge. Frequently isolated from other families with similar problems, hemophilia families may be isolated from the ongoing help available at hemophilia clinics as well. In the era of HIV acquired immunodeficiency syndrome (AIDS), fears about the safety, availability and cost of blood products can interfere with patients and family adjustment and complicate the delivery of psychosocial services.

With regard to typical personality dynamics associated with hemophilia, evidence is ambiguous. Clinical experience suggests extremes of timidity and recklessness (Wright, 1977); preoccupations with health, difficulties with intimacy, and social isolation have been noted in studies of hemophiliac patients and their families (Agle, Gluck and Pierce, 1987). However, when formal psychologic testing is employed, little evidence of abnormal personality development has emerged (Clingman, McAlister and Lushene, 1979; Bussing and Johnson, 1992; Logan *et al.*, 1993).

Many of the adjustment issues faced by hemophilia patients are the same as those which must be dealt with

Hemophilia. Edited by C.D. Forbes, L. Aledort and R. Madhok. Published in 1997 by Chapman & Hall, London. ISBN 0 412 63820 7

by non-hemophiliacs as they move through the life cycle (National Hemophilia Foundation (NHF), 1993). Hemophilia may accentuate certain developmental milestones; these crisis times may also provide 'entry points' for effective psychosocial intervention.

PSYCHOSOCIAL FEATURES OF HIV AND LIVER DISEASE

In the USA, approximately 70% of patients who have factor VIII deficiency and who received blood products before 1985 are infected with HIV (Centers for Disease Control, 1987). Parents of a hemophiliac HIV-positive child may tend to be 'ever watchful for the slightest signs of ill health' (Bor and Miller, 1988). The HIV-positive adolescent faces the issues of wondering if he will ever be able to marry and have children. Children of HIV-positive fathers may face some social stigma or rejection if the father's condition (or even the cause of death, when it occurs) becomes known. Patients in school present difficulties with regard to the need for teachers and other school staff to know of their HIV status, versus the family's wish to prevent discrimination or ostracism. Dementia (with attendant judgment problems) may be a consequence of HIV/AIDS. The grief and anger of family members (and often the patient himself) must be dealt with. In all, HIV has led to a 'crisis of faith in the medical system' among the hemophilia patients (Brown and Demaio, 1992). Anger at providers for infecting them, anger at the injustice of it all, and the frustrations from dashed hopes all contribute to this problem.

The HIV problem has also affected staff of hemophilia clinics. Because they have known hemophilia patients for many years, often close bonds are formed between providers and patients. Some staff may feel guilty about having provided factor treatment that was probably contaminated. The HIV problem has also required a change in the role of hemophilia care-providers; expertise in sexuality and sex education is now needed, in order to prevent infection of partners and children (Mason, Olson and Parish, 1988; Brown and Demaio, 1992). Although a discussion of psychosocial consultation to staff is beyond the scope of the present chapter, none the less such consultation may be essential in helping clinic staff to cope with patient deaths, to interact effectively with angry, demanding or otherwise difficult patients, and productively to fill the additional roles noted above.

Hepatitis C may also create or exacerbate psychologic difficulties, although these have not as yet been documented. Although the consequences are not as dire as those of HIV, hepatitis C is still a chronic illness, and potentially could result in fatal liver damage. The route of transmission has not been clearly identified, which makes discussion of prevention somewhat more difficult, and the symptoms are somewhat more diffuse, although

depression has been reported clinically to be a significant component of the picture. Perhaps more difficult for this already burdened population of patients is to be yet again vulnerable to an illness that results from the treatment of hemophilia. This could easily lead to a sense of frustration and further 'rebellion' against orthodox medical treatment and self-care.

THE NEED FOR PSYCHOSOCIAL SERVICES

Access to psychosocial care is an important aspect of the comprehensive treatment of hemophilia patients and their families (NHF, 1993). While the evidence for specific psychologic or psychiatric consequences of hemophilia is far from clear-cut (Bussing and Johnson, 1992; Bussing and Burhet, 1993), chronic illnesses of any sort place additional psychologic stresses and strains on the patient and family. There is undeniably some percentage of the hemophilia population which experiences lowered self-esteem as a result of developing an identity as 'crippled' or 'fragile.' These reactions, as well as other psychologic consequences of having a chronic disease, such as lowered self-confidence and difficulty initiating independent action, may place considerable burden on the partners, parents of children or hemophilia patients as well as on the patients themselves. It is also true that the incidence and prevalence of mental or emotional distress are likely to be similar in the hemophilia community to that of the population at large.

There is an additional benefit to providing psychosocial services specifically in hemophilia populations. Psychiatric disturbance (stress, depression and anxiety, etc.) can interfere with regular clinic visits, make home care more difficult, and make prophylaxis problematic. In addition, there is evidence that psychological distress may increase the frequency or severity of bleeding (Bussing and Johnson, 1992). There is also the question of whether anxiety may lead to undertreatment or overtreatment with factor. Thus, the psychologic status of the hemophilia patient's response to treatment and ability to take responsibility for adequate self-treatment interact. Among severe hemophiliacs, there may be a sense of futility that leads to excess risk-taking and poorer self-care. Problems such as these may be effectively addressed with psychosocial interventions.

With regard to family dynamics, psychosocial intervention may help in reducing the tendency of parents – mothers in particular – to 'overfunction' for their hemophiliac sons and reduce the sons' initiative. In addition, psychosocial intervention may help to reduce marital conflict which appears to have some impact on both quality of home life of the hemophiliac patient and the family's ability to care adequately for the illness.

Increasingly, psychosocial services can also play a preventive function, in decreasing the risk of acquiring or transmitting sexually transmitted diseases (STDs).

EVIDENCE FOR THE EFFECTIVENESS OF PSYCHOSOCIAL SERVICES

There is little evidence in the existing literature regarding the specific benefits of psychosocial interventions for hemophilia patients and families (Nimorwicz and Klein, 1982; Bussing and Johnson, 1992). The interventions best supported by empiric findings are hypnosis and relaxation training for the reduction of bleeds and/or reduction in the need for factor infusions (Bussing and Johnson, 1992). Other interventions have not been studied specifically within the hemophilia population or have been studied in a quasi-experimental way, which does not permit clear conclusions about effectiveness. However, we can extrapolate to some extent from the general literature which addresses the effectiveness of psychosocial interventions. This literature is extensive and, although based primarily on mental health populations, does at least allow a basis for inference (for reviews of this literature see Smith, Glass and Miller, 1980; Garfield and Bergin, 1986). In general the literature suggests that individual psychotherapy is effective in approximately three-quarters of the cases in which it is administered by competent professionals. The modal number of sessions required to obtain symptom relief significant improvement in quality of life is eight (Howard *et al.*, 1986). The difference between providers trained in different disciplines and at different levels (e.g. doctoral versus masters level) has not been extensively investigated; almost all studies have been conducted using psychotherapists with masters in social work (MSW) or doctorate in psychology (PhD) training. Increasingly, briefer or shorter-term approaches that use cognitive-behavioral techniques have been shown to be more effective than more exploratory techniques such as psychodynamic or Rogerian approaches. While symptom relief is often not the ultimate measure of psychotherapy's effectiveness, since the relevance of presenting symptoms frequently changes after therapy has begun, symptom relief certainly occurs in the majority of successful psychotherapy cases (Howard *et al.*, 1986).

The evidence of psychotherapy's effectiveness in medical conditions is fairly extensive (Pomerleau and Rodin, 1986; McDaniel, Hepworth and Doherty, 1992). To cite some notable examples, group psychotherapy has been shown to reduce the likelihood of a second myocardial infarction in controlled trials (Friedman *et al.*, 1986); family therapy has been shown to reduce the severity of brittle juvenile diabetes (Minuchin *et al.*, 1978); and group psychotherapy has been shown to increase the survival time of women who have breast cancer (Spiegel *et al.*, 1989). There is one case reported in the literature of individual psychotherapy being effective in reducing the need for factor in a hemophilia patient (Handford *et al.*, 1980).

Psychosocial services in hemophilia

In this section we discuss several foundational aspects of psychosocial services, as well as briefly review considerations with regard to several specific varieties of service.

APPROACHES TO HELPING

The basis of providing effective support to a patient who has psychosocial concerns is the patient's perception of the provider as a caring person who is interested in him or her as a person and willing to listen to his or her concerns. A hemophiliac and his parents, however, may have previous experiences with health care providers who do not understand the medical problems with which they live. The development of the patient's trust in the face of such a history depends on providers' ability to address not only the physical complaints presented, but also the psychosocial issues that typically arise, whether fear of pain, worries about what friends or neighbors will think, or concerns about the cost of treatment.

Providers who take this approach to patients will be alert for indications of serious psychosocial complications of hemophilia without assuming that all hemophiliacs will be withdrawn and underdeveloped or that all parents will be overprotective and guilt-ridden. These problems, which do occur in some cases, are best identified and treated in the context of a caring relationship that focuses on solving the ordinary day-to-day problems of living encountered similarly by patients with and without chronic illness.

In addition to psychosocial problems related to hemophilia, providers will also want to watch for signs of mental health problems that are common in the general population, particularly mood disorders and substance abuse.

For all these problems, providers will benefit from knowing when and how to make an appropriate referral. The time is ripe for a referral to a mental health professional when the situation continues to deteriorate in spite of efforts by the provider (and perhaps other members of the treatment team) to resolve the problem. Consultation with other members of the team can be sought in these instances to determine whether a referral is needed. Referral is appropriate if the team members are uncomfortable with the problem or uncertain about how to proceed. Finally, it is important to refer when the provider judges that the patient is a risk to the health or safety of himself or others, particularly if the patient refuses to address this issue.

Frequently, the most effective mental health referral involves an immediate phone call to the psychosocial professional which enables the patient to make an appointment on the spot. This is particularly important when the problem is one of alcohol or substance abuse.

PREDICTABLE DEVELOPMENTAL STRESS POINTS APPROPRIATE FOR PSYCHOSOCIAL INTERVENTION

There are relatively predictable stress points in the life cycle of the hemophilia patient and family, and psychosocial services should be available for and relevant to each of the following.

Initial diagnosis

When the disease is first diagnosed, parents and extended family should be helped to readjust the expectations they may have had for the child; feelings of grief or loss may emerge as well. Parental guilt, blaming, overprotection, denial (in families without a previous history, or in the father's family if there is no familiarity with the disease) may be issues to be resolved, and fear, uncertainty and ignorance may interfere with effective coping.

Childhood

During the childhood years, there is likely to be limited need for individual treatment and greater need for family therapy services and support groups, especially for mothers. Helping the family to care for the hemophilia effectively, so that unnecessary school absences are avoided, and encouraging appropriate sports and social involvement are key ingredients of psychosocial services during this time. As parent/child separation begins to take place and more extensive peer relationships develop, some parents may find it difficult to let go of the child at this stage, fearing potential injury. With children who are HIV-positive, there may be concern about the effects of a hostile social environment on the child.

If there are both hemophiliac and non-hemophiliac siblings in the family, fair discipline methods for both are needed. Also, developing a safe yet not smothering environment for the child is important. In the childhood phase, developing a sense of trust in the medical team is also important, as is developing an understanding of hemophilia and potential treatment complications (e.g. hepatitis, HIV, inhibitors). The parents of a young child also need to learn ways to help the child understand hemophilia and the need for treatment. The parents need to help educate siblings and extended family members plus others such as baby-sitters, preschool teachers, etc. The parents of a young hemophiliac child also need support in developing sufficient assertiveness and ego strength to cope with sometimes insensitive medical systems. Parents may also need help in thinking through what to do about having additional children.

The school-age child needs help in learning to identify bleeds early and to seek treatment effectively. The child needs to learn more about the illness and the proper limits on his physical activity. If home care is a treatment option, educating parents to take a primary role in home treatment is important too.

The effect of hemophilia on siblings should also be considered. For example, when the hemophiliac child needs attention because of a bleed, the non-hemophiliac sibling may be neglected in some respects. Miller *et al.* (1992) suggest that it is quite common for siblings of a hemophilia patient to develop problems such as bedwetting and school avoidance.

Adolescence

During these years, the need for individual psychosocial services increases, and the need for family therapy decreases. Social skills training (individual or group) becomes increasingly important. The need for home treatment may increase adolescent self-consciousness and the sense of being 'damaged.' This in turn may lead to depression or anger. In the HIV-positive hemophiliac adolescent, there is an accelerated need for sophisticated understanding of sexual behavior and methods of implementing safer sex practices as well as methods of effectively communicating about sexuality and serostatus. During the adolescent phase the task of increasing the youngster's sense of independence, knowledge of the illness and ability to take age-appropriate responsibility for self-care is important. Beginning genetic education and counseling for potential female hemophilia carriers is important in the adolescent stage also.

Adulthood

In the adult years, careful assessment of coping styles, particularly denial mechanisms, is important, to determine whether they are helping or hindering appropriate medical care of behavioral changes. If helpful self-management techniques are being used, this should be supported; if alcohol and drugs or acting out are used to deal with the illness, these must be confronted. In the HIV-positive adult, psychosocial issues may focus on such matters as encouraging healthy involvement with family and children, while at the same time recognizing that arrangements must be made for an early death.

During the adult phase, employment counseling (to help patients find jobs that provide comprehensive health benefits) is needed. Continuing to provide genetics information is important, as is patient education regarding ongoing developments in the care of hemophilia. Childbearing interventions (genetic counseling, values clarification) and partner support groups (particularly for spouses of HIV-positive patients) are also important to have available.

Family issues

Truly comprehensive services for hemophilia involve the family of the patient as well as the patient himself. Family themes that may emerge (Miller, 1987; Miller *et al.*, 1989) include the mother's isolation, fears of contaminating others and concerns about death. In the case of HIV-positive hemophiliacs, sibling bereavement (Hogan and Desantis, 1992) and spousal bereavement (Zimpfer, 1991) are issues that may well respond to support group or group counseling.

Psychotherapeutic interventions

THE RANGE OF PSYCHOSOCIAL INTERVENTIONS

Varieties of psychotherapy may focus on goals ranging from rehabilitation to prevention to expansion of personal effectiveness. Similarly, the range of therapies can be quite variable. There are more specifically focused therapies such as those for pain control and more broad-ranging personality change efforts; there are individual, couple, family and network interventions and there are interventions which focus on emotional, behavioral or cognitive aspects of individual functioning.

STAFFING

Because of the wide variety of issues and possible service options, it is important for the development of a comprehensive psychosocial service to have mental health professionals trained to deliver a wide range of interventions. It is possible to train a paraprofessional or bachelor's level person to facilitate support groups for patients and/or families, for example. It may also be useful to include a health education specialist to coordinate resources, so that hemophilia patients and families learn about available self-help materials. At the more intensive psychosocial level, staff of any number of disciplines may provide education and consultation to schools and educators. Nurses with psychiatric training, social workers and psychologists may provide parent training, especially in conjunction with health educators or child development specialist. Social work and psychology staff can provide group, marital and individual psychotherapeutic services, with appropriate training and experience or supervision. Medical and mental health staff both may provide sex education to patients and partners.

ASSESSMENT

Since psychologic or mental health services are not needed by all patients and families who come to the clinic for help, some form of assessment of their psychologic needs would be helpful. Probably the most frequent method of screening for psychological needs is self-referral. A more sophisticated program would involve informal assessment of the emotional, interpersonal and social functioning of patients in the clinic to identify those who seem distressed. At yet a further level of refinement, a number of useful screening instruments have appeared in recent years, among them the PRIME-MD (Spitzer *et al.*, 1992), or the SCL-90-R (Derogatis, 1992). An in-depth history taken by a skilled interviewer would of course be extremely useful in this regard, although it is frequently more time-consuming and expensive for the clinic to provide.

INDIVIDUAL THERAPY/COUNSELING

When is individual psychotherapy indicated? As noted, the patient who requests a referral to the psychologist, psychiatrist or social worker about some conflict or emotional distress is clearly a case when some form of psychotherapy is indicated, but often patients are quite clear that they do not want a group experience. Individual psychotherapy, although perhaps expensive for the clinic to provide, is often the treatment of choice when such preferences exist. Individual psychotherapy would be contraindicated in cases that risk fostering extreme dependence or possible decompensation. In cases of highly manipulative or substance-abusing patients, it may be helpful to put them in a group that is composed of similar individuals.

Agle (1964) notes that hemophiliac patients of his who continue in long-term psychotherapy 'did so to obtain relief from a variety of psychological symptoms including anxiety states, phobias, and depressions.' Nimorwicz and Klein (1982) cite Buchanan (1978) in warning that traditional insight-oriented psychotherapy may be highly threatening to chronically ill patients, who tend to deny their problems. As of the 1982 review that these authors conducted, no evidence was available regarding the effects of individual psychotherapy for hemophilia patients. They did find a 1980 report of a patient who received individual group and family psychotherapy for a 15-month period and who decreased his use of replacement therapy (Handford *et al.*, 1980). They note that most authors recommend short-term focused intervention for most hemophilia patients.

BIOBEHAVIORAL INTERVENTIONS IN HEMOPHILIA

Intervention by biobehavioral methods, including hypnosis, relaxation, contingency management and biofeedback, has been found to be useful in the non-pharmacologic or adjunctive management of bleeding and pain. The only contraindications identified have been severe developmental delay and psychosis, especially involving somatic delusions. For more than 40 years, there have been anecdotal reports of hypnosis affecting blood flow (Allington, 1952; Grabowska, 1971; Clawson and Swade, 1975). LaBaw (1975) found group hypnosis to be a useful adjunct to factor in the control of bleeding in patients with hemophilia. Much of his work was carried out with hemophilia summer camp participants; boys trained in hypnosis remained less anxious in the face of bleeds, required fewer transfusions than they had before the training and complained of less pain (LaBaw, 1975).

Hypnosis has been applied to a broad range of pain complaints (Chaves, 1989). Typically the literature investigating the effectiveness of hypnosis in managing pain shows great promise but relatively little experimental rigor. Other biobehavioral interventions, however, have been evaluated with greater care. Pain, whether chronic or acute, is a complex, multidimensional phenomenon involving sensory, affective, cognitive and interpersonal components (Ross and Ross, 1988). While review of this large literature is outside the scope of this chapter, applications have included treatment of pain from hemophilia-related bleeds. Varni and coworkers (Varni, 1981a; Varni and Gilbert, 1982) have developed a treatment protocol for chronic arthritic pain in hemophilia patients involving deep muscle relaxation, meditative breathing exercises and guided imagery. Findings of improved pain control with a decrease in arthritic pain and analgesic need without losing awareness of acute bleeds requiring factor replacement were obtained. Contingency management by parents, distracting pleasant imagery and relaxation were effective in reducing the pain, improving mobility and decreasing need for medication in a severely affected child with factor VIII inhibitor (Varni, Gilbert and Dietrich, 1981). Varni (1980) reports a similar case.

In hemophilia, adherence to long-term complex treatment regimens such as the home care program represents a serious challenge (Varni, 1983). Teaching of biobehavioral assessment and behavioral self-management training has been shown to be effective in maintaining adherence to proper factor replacement procedures (Sergis-Davenport and Varni, 1982, 1983), and to maintaining therapeutic exercise by children with hemophilia (Greenan, Powell and Varni, 1983).

GROUP THERAPY/COUNSELING

Clinical experience has shown that group activities can offer a tremendous benefit over individual sessions. That is, they allow patients to exchange information and discover that they are not alone in their difficulties. Group therapy can be particularly useful when the patient needs to learn social skills, may be in a state of denial about his interpersonal impact on others, or, as noted above, is likely to try and manipulate the sympathies of the therapist (Yalom, 1987). Group therapy can be more economical to provide, although it is more difficult for clinic staff to schedule and arrange times. Typically, in a working or school-involved population, group therapy must be offered in the evening, which often interferes with staff preferences. It can be difficult to engage patients in group therapy, and drop-out rates can be high, similar to patients with other chronic diseases. Patients who are extremely demanding and histrionic may not be good candidates for group therapy, as they may come to dominate a group and interfere with its effectiveness. Extremely depressed patients may either focus the entire group on themselves, or find that it is not possible to stay in the group unless it is a group specifically focused on depression. Patients with a history of being victimized or bullied, unless they are put in a group of similar individuals, can become group scapegoats without careful intervention by the therapist.

Reports of group therapy with hemophiliac patients and families suggest that decreased maladjustment, lessened feelings of isolation and increased self-esteem result (Mattson and Agle, 1972). Psychoeducational groups, which combine informational elements with therapeutic elements in a more structured and time-limited fashion, have been reported to be effective in case studies (Nimorwicz and Klein, 1982; Agle, 1984).

One issue not pursued in this chapter is the role of hemophilia camps. In a sense the camp is an intervention that is partially a support group and partially a group therapy experience. Primarily it provides access to a group of patients and allows direct intervention in their communication and interactions.

FAMILY THERAPY

As noted above, hemophilia affects the entire family – and often the extended family as well. Especially when children are younger and still living at home, difficulties that they manifest are frequently best dealt with in a family context. This allows the parents to receive support for and suggestions for improving their parenting skills, and can help to reduce the ways in which family members may be scapegoated or led to be 'symptom-bearers' for underlying conflicts in the family. Clinical evidence suggests that there are cases in which the patient's distress is encouraged by the mother (or, more rarely, the father). Cases such as this require family therapy in order to bring the underlying problems to the surface. Negative results from family therapy have not been shown. However, with late-adolescent patients, concerns have been expressed that family therapy may delay separation from the family of origin. Useful reviews of the medical family therapy literature may be found in McDaniel, Campbell and Seaburn (1990) and McDaniel, Hepworth and Doherty (1992).

MULTIPLE FAMILY GROUP THERAPY

A hybrid of family therapy and group therapy, multi-family therapy groups have been utilized in at least two formats relevant to hemophilia. All of these groups work on the assumption that living with a family member with a chronic medical condition places unusual strain on a family. One empirically evaluated intervention is the multifamily discussion group (MFDG) model described by Gonzalez, Steinglass and Reiss (1989). This format is a psychoeducationally oriented, family-focused intervention in which four or five families which have a member with chronic medical condition meet to discuss illness-related families in a structured manner. Families are generally heterogeneous with regard to medical diagnosis involved and family role so affected, so that although perhaps one family in such a group may deal with hemophilia in the father, the other families would be dealing with other medical conditions, perhaps in a child, or mother. Steinglass, Gonzalez and Reiss (1989) recommend a special training weekend for the group leaders, who have usually been psychiatrists, psychologists or social workers, but provide a detailed manual for the method. They report good success in helping families 'put the illness in its place' and yet having 'a place for the illness.'

The second, also relatively well-researched format involved groups composed of pairs of parents learning behavioral management techniques. Such interventions have resulted in reduced undesirable behavior in children, especially failure to comply with parental requests and commands (Patterson, 1974; Dangel and Polster, 1984, Forehand and Long, 1988). No studies involved parents whose child had hemophilia; however, Clark and Baker (1983) found that families of handicapped children showed improvements similar to those of other parents as a result of parent training groups.

COUPLES THERAPY

Couples therapy is most often recommended when there is marital conflict, growing psychologic distance between partners or dissatisfaction with the relationship. In general, couples therapy (sometimes called conjoint or marital counseling) is appropriate when the problem involves a relationship between committed partners (marital status or sexual orientation of the couple is not particularly relevant). Couples therapy has been embraced enthusiastically by many mental health providers; positive effects have been claimed to occur in 60–65% of treated couples. Unfortunately, different relationship problems, varying degrees of seriousness and inconsistent outcome measures utilized have made outcome studies difficult to interpret (Gurman and Kniskern, 1989). Generally, marital therapy has had better outcomes for troubled relationships than individual treatment for one member of the dyad or even both members. On the other hand, marital treatment is not entirely risk-free, as deterioration in the functioning of some couples has been noted as issues come to light. There is no consensus that a particular professional discipline has a better outcome, but there are indications that therapists who are more experienced and have training in group and family work tend to have higher rates of success. To date there have been no studies investigating the variables related to efficacy of treatment of couples in which one of the members has a bleeding disorder.

In keeping with Rolland's typology of chronic and/or life-threatening diseases (1987), the presence of HIV/AIDS or hepatitis provides very different issues than hemophilia without those complications. The HIV/AIDS related issues of almost certainly shortened lifespan and the need for precautions during sexual activity are absent, but the presence of hemophilia alone brings added stress to a couple. For couples where there has been an open discussion of hemophilia prior to marriage, preferably with consultation from a physician or other trusted health care provider, dealing with the issues normally associated with onset of a disease, prior to making the commitment to the relationship is somewhat stressful. Couples dealing with an illness that has both chronic (e.g. arthritis) and recurrent, episodic aspects (e.g. bleeds) are often able to establish a sense of normal routines and plans for future life events, such as child-bearing or professional progression. At the same time, these couples are faced with the specter of unpredictable major medical problems which could lead to death. The healthy partner may fear survivorship alone; both members of the couple may experience ambivalence about emotional intimacy and closeness (Rolland, 1989). The denial that the chronic phases allow (often an important element of coping) is punctured by the more acute phases. Anecdotal accounts often mention the altered role of the parents of the medically affected partner as overinvolved or holding the status of medical experts, which can be expressed in either supportive or critical fashion and affect marital satisfaction.

Psychoeducational interventions

Although early writers (e.g. Findlay *et al.*, 1969) emphasized the family's needs for knowledge and early understanding of hemophilia, no empirical studies have been reported of educational programs with hemophiliacs and their families. It is important to note that hemophilia patients and their families may find it difficult to absorb factual information before they have begun to feel comfortable with the staff and strategy of intervention. Hemophilia staff may be surprised that, after the enormous educational efforts undertaken in clinics, parents may still have a significant lack of information about the disease and its treatment. Miller (1987) suggests that no knowledge should be taken for granted. It is not unlikely that parents will either be too anxious to have absorbed information the first time it is presented or that denial defense mechanisms may operate to suppress existing knowledge.

PARENT SKILLS TRAINING

Because generalized parent education was not the panacea for child-related problems that it was hoped to be (Abidin and Carter, 1980), there developed programs to provide individualized, goal-oriented treatment for parents to learn skills and techniques for better managing their children's problem behaviors. The resulting literature is well beyond the scope of this chapter. Polster and Dangel (1984) and Schaefer and Briemeister (1989) both review aspects of parent training. To oversimplify and summarize this large body of work, the basic principle is that skilled parenting can influence the behavior of children in a positive way. Most interventions define skilled parenting as using principles of learning theory to reward desirable behavior in a consistent manner adapted to the age of the child. Overall, efficacy has been reported as quite positive, with improvement in about two-thirds of the families, even with such populations as delinquent preteens and teens (Patterson, 1974, children with attention deficit hyperactivity disorder (Kazdin and Lahey, 1982) and oppositional children (Forehand and Long, 1988). However, long-term efficacy has not been well-documented. Additionally, skill-based learning with observed practice has been shown to be superior to didactic training alone (Rickert *et al.*, 1988).

Providers of parent training should be thoroughly familiar with behavioral management skills, observation and shaping of parent behaviors, regardless of professional discipline. Philosophy-based programs that do not focus on skills have generally not been found to be helpful (Abidin and Carter, 1980). Although some comprehensive clinics have offered some behavioral guidance for parents (e.g. Kelly, 1991), there are no reports of efficacy of intervention for families with children with hemophilia. On the other hand, anecdotal evidence has suggested that some parents have difficulty effectively setting behavioral limits for their chronically ill children. It has been hypothesized that guilt for having an ill child, fears of further hurting a child perceived as fragile, and overcompensation to make up for the child's suffering can all be involved. Permission for and instruction in managing a child's problem behaviors may need to be combined with consciousness raising regarding the long-term social outlook for an undisciplined child.

SCHOOL CONSULTATION

For some hemophiliacs, elementary school marks the first time that their care has been entrusted to someone other than a family member. School teachers must have adequate training so that they can provide appropriate care without feeling overwhelmed by the sudden introduction of a student whose problems may seem threatening and overwhelming. Furthermore, the response of other students to the hemophiliac and his medical problems will depend on their having adequate information and an opportunity to understand his condition and to resolve their potential fears and prejudices.

School visits by members of the hemophilia treatment centre staff, with participation by hemophiliacs and parents, provide an opportunity for the hemophiliac's teachers and classmates to learn about hemophilia, thereby preventing some inappropriate reactions to the hemophilia patient and facilitating his adaptation to the school environment. Steinhart (1994) outlined the various situations in which a school visit is useful, as well as the contents of these visits. Furthermore, the NHF Nursing Network (1990) has developed a guide for presentations in schools.

Self-help resources

SUPPORT GROUPS

Self-help or support groups conducted by a veteran survivor or skilled layperson are an important aspect of psychosocial services that should be available to hemophilia patients. Frequently, the primary role which the clinic will play in such services is providing training for the leaders, providing space for the group meetings and encouraging patients to attend. Although in the HIV era some support groups run the risk of developing political agendas, if they are focused on providing emotional and informational support to patients, they are likely to be non-controversial and helpful. Participation in a support group involves less self-consciousness about being a patient, as the group consists simply of individuals who wish to make contact with others in similar situations. On the other hand, there are few data available regarding the effectiveness of self-help groups, in contrast to professionally led psychotherapy groups. However, the Alcoholics Anonymous self-help model is, of course, a clear anecdotal case of a highly successful self-help network.

Hemophilia patients and family members who are experiencing psychosocial issues that are not specific to hemophilia may well benefit from existing support groups in the community, such as grief support groups, divorce support groups, Alanon support groups (for family members of alcoholics or substance abusers) and other similar groups. Most communities have compiled lists of available self-help support group resources.

BIBLIOTHERAPY

Reading a book or listening to a tape can be done in privacy, and at the convenience of the individual. It also does not require health care insurance or entail great expense. Self-help materials are widely available on a variety of issues, and may be useful for patients and family members unwilling to come in for formal psychosocial sessions. These materials may also be useful in extending and generalizing improvements gained in the clinic. However, it should be kept in mind that almost no self-help materials have actually been tested for their effectiveness.

Although underlying theory and recommended activities can be evaluated, it is the carrying out of the activities that is likely to be the 'active ingredient' in the self-help materials, and this has proved to be the most difficult part of bibliotherapy to insure. Ineffective programs can increase emotional and behavioral problems, partially because they delay seeking effective treatment (Rosen, 1990). Clearly, if the clinic staff member is going to prescribe self-help materials (videos or books) to the patient or family members, they must match the educational level of the audience with that of the material. Clinic staff should be sure regularly to monitor the use of such materials by the patients and their families.

Psychosocial services in HIV

The introduction of factor VIII in the 1960s led to a mood of tremendous optimism in the hemophilia community; it appeared that the prospect for hemophilia patients was that they could lead normal lives. The situation changed in the mid-1980s when the links between transfusions and HIV/AIDS developed (Miller *et al.*, 1989; Hall, 1994).

APPROACHES TO HELPING

Preparing to offer psychosocial services in the HIV-positive hemophilia population means being ready to deal with issues of death and dying; being prepared for rage and despair; dealing with grief in family and partners; and having the ability none the less to help patients and family members focus on their quality of life, and on issues of protecting others from infection.

When working with HIV-positive hemophilia patients and their families, health care providers can generally assume that effective coping is occurring, because that seems to be accurate in most cases (Agle, Gluck and Pierce, 1987; Wilson and Wasserman, 1989). However,

providers should be alert to indications that HIV infection may be causing distress. Indications include reduced sexual desire, with reduced frequency of intercourse; worries about sexual transmission of HIV; and the perception that HIV status has threatened one's marriage (Agle, Gluck and Pierce, 1987; Wilson and Wasserman, 1989).

The prospect of a life shortened by AIDS can produce in some patients a process of recycling through a series of reactions, including denial, anger, hopelessness and acceptance. After the death of a patient, providers might encounter a similar cycle of reactions in partners, parents and other family members. One can also expect to encounter in both patients and family members reactions of intense rage directed at those responsible for producing and distributing the factor that caused the HIV infection as well as the nameless individuals who donated their infected blood.

Because of the stigma associated with AIDS as a 'homosexual disease,' some hemophilia patients and family members decide not to tell anyone except immediate family members about their HIV status. This decision makes responding to personal questions about HIV difficult, can produce guilt about lying to friends and family members, and can produce chronic anxiety about others somehow learning the secret.

A final important issue for providers is how to deal with the issue of preventing HIV transmsision, especially by sexual transmission. With patients, the issue is one of protecting others; with spouses and other sexual partners the issue is one of self-protection.

PSYCHOTHERAPEUTIC INTERVENTIONS: SPECIAL CONSIDERATIONS

Individual psychotherapy

Individual counseling with hemophiliacs will be similar whether the issues are HIV-related or not, although one might expect HIV-related work to be particularly intense because the issues are more starkly those of life and death. Providers can effectively respond to issues of grief and loss by listening emphatically and reflecting to patients and family members that repeated experiences of denial, anger and hopelessness are normal as one adapts to a life-threatening condition. It is particularly important to accept and validate the reactions or rage that individuals will frequently describe. If the therapeutic situation does not permit extended work on this issue, individuals may benefit from receiving information about ways to manage grief.

A common topic in individual work with HIV-positive patients is secrecy about HIV status. Providers should respect patients' need for privacy, and assist individuals who remain uncertain about divulging their status to weight the advantages and disadvantages of each alternative. Specific instruction or role-playing of methods of disclosure may be beneficial.

With respect to sexual counseling to prevent the transmission of HIV, it is clear that, in discussions with spouses or sexual partners, providers must support the right to self-protection, especially in those instances in which HIV-infected patients refuse to practice safer sex techniques. With patients it may be useful to adopt an approach based on Prochaska's stages of change model (Prochaska, DiClemente and Norcross, 1992), in which the provider can readily assess the individual's readiness to change and select an intervention that is more likely to be effective with a person at that particular stage.

HIV couples therapy

When a person with a bleeding disorder is also found to be HIV-infected, the diagnosis has profound ramifications (Agle, Gluck and Pierce, 1987). Relationships with sexual partners are among those areas deeply changed by HIV. Much has been written about the wide range of reactions of couples, ranging from strong tension between partners with a marked diminution in sexual activity to an intensification of closeness with a refusal of an informed partner to engage in safer sex activities because they 'are in this together.' Many of the hemophilia treatment centers in the USA have instituted contacts with social workers or other psychosocial professionals directly to address issues which arise between partners. While efficacy has not been established overall, there appears to be consensus that couples therapy is often necessary, if not sufficient to address issues related to safer sex, changes in sex activity, child-bearing, life-planning and grieving the loss of shared dreams.

The decision to disclose serostatus to family and/or friends often has profound meaning to both members of the couple, because of the need for support which may not be available to the spouse if the person with HIV does not choose to disclose. Whether one or both of the pair are HIV-positive, planning for the long-term emotional and practical care of any children in the family is also necessary. As the HIV progresses to AIDS and a decline in physical condition occurs, there is also a change in the dependence of the person with AIDS on the partner for physical as well as emotional needs. Therapeutic approaches for couples have included facilitating communication between partners about their emotions and concerns are well as clarifying issues in disclosure. Negotiation and communication skills have been taught as well as couples-based safe sex instruction emphasizing the pleasuring aspects of the process. These endeavors have been carried out by a variety of professionals and in peer groups.

HIV parent skills training

The presence of HIV infection does not alter the basic demands on parenting skills so much as it may change the ability of parents to carry out limit-setting. It has been noted in situations involving other life-threatening diseases (e.g. leukaemia) in children, that many parents no longer feel the need to discipline children as they had before and may become much more indulgent (Koocher and O'Malley, 1981). Given the years of survival of children with hemophilia and HIV, this crisis period could conceivably cover most of the developmental years of childhood and adolescence, shaping the whole life of the family. On the other hand, skills training is not likely to be sufficient to change the behavior of parents (if that is even deemed advisable) without much attention to the meaning of the parents' behavior and their beliefs about the child and his entitlements.

SELF-HELP RESOURCES: SPECIAL CONSIDERATIONS

HIV support groups

Group support has been an effective adjunct to individual counseling for reducing emotional distress related to HIV, particularly in the case of HIV-positive individuals and their survivors (McKusick, 1988). In the USA, support groups have been developed for members of the hemophilia community who have been affected by HIV. The Women's Outreach Network of the National Hemophilia Foundation (WONN) and the Men's Advocacy Network of the National Hemophilia Foundation (MANN), as their names indicate, are open to women and men who have been affected by HIV. A recent report (Wong-Rieger, 1993) indicated the success of national MANN training in producing leaders in the hemophilia community who will develop activities designed to provide mutual support and to lead ongoing advocacy activities for HIV-affected hemophiliacs and their families.

Bibliotherapy

For HIV-infected patients, the most useful reading material involves practical works designed to foster quality of life, health promotion and longevity (Ornstein and Sobel, 1989; Bartlett and Finkbeiner, 1991), or those that provide direction for preparing a will and making other final arrangements (Petterle, 1993).

Future directions

Clearly, a number of questions remain to be answered in the search for effective psychosocial services tailored to the hemophilia community, yet considerable gains are possible using existing psychosocial interventions and approaches. In the development of comprehensive psychosocial services, hemophilia clinics should be alert for opportunities to make outreach to the 'just hemophilia' cohort who may be reluctant to become involved with a comprehensive clinic because of the AIDS stigma. The range of possibilities and the opportunities to make a significant difference in the lives of hemophilia patients and families make careful design of a full range of psychosocial services vital to truly effective comprehensive care of this disease.

References

Abidin, R.R. and Carter, B.D. (1980) Workshops and parent groups, in *Parent Education and Intervention Handbook* (ed. R.R. Abidin), Thomas, Springfield, IL.

Agle, D.P. (1964) Psychiatric studies of patients with hemophilia and related states. *Archives of Internal Medicine*, **114**, 76–82.

Agle, D.P., Gluck, H. and Pierce, G.F. (1987) The risk of AIDS: psychologic impact on the hemophilia population. *General Hospital Psychiatry*, **9**, 11–17.

Allington, H.V. (1952) Review of the psychotherapy of warts. *Archives of Dermatology and Syphiology*, **66**, 316–326.

Bartlett, J.G. and Finkbeiner, A.K. (1991) *The Guide to Living with HIV Infection*. Johns Hopkins University Press, Baltimore, MD.

Bor, R. and Miller, R. (1988) Addressing 'dreaded issues': a description of a unique counseling intervention with patients with AIDS/HIV. *Counseling Psychology Quarterly*, **1**, 397–406.

Brown, L.K. and Demaio, D.M. (1992) The impact of secrets in hemophilia and HIV disorders. *Journal of Psychosocial Oncology*, **10**, 91–101.

Bussing, R and Burket, R.C. (1993) Anxiety and intrafamilial stress in children with hemophilia after the HIV crisis. *Journal of the American Academy of Child and Adolescent Psychiatry*, **32**, 562–567.

Bussing, R. and Johnson, S.B. (1992) Psychosocial issues in hemophilia before and after the HIV crisis: a review of current research. *General Hospital Psychiatry*, **14**, 387–403.

Chaves, J.F. (1989) Hypnotic control of clinical pain, in *Hypnosis: The Cognitive Behavioral Perspective* (eds N.P. Spanos and J.F. Chaves), Prometheus Books, Buffalo, NY.

Clark, D.B. and Baker, B.L. (1983) Predicting outcome in parent training. *Journal of Consulting and Clinical Psychology*, **51**, 309–311.

Clawson, T.A. and Swade, R.H. (1975) The hypnotic control of blood flow and pain: the cure of warts and the potential for the use of hypnosis in the treatment of cancer. *American Journal of Clinical Hypnosis*, **17**, 160–169.

Clingman, J.M., McAllister, S. and Lushene, R.L. (1979) Some psychological correlates of hemophilia. *Journal of Personality Assessment*, **43**, 629–632.

Derogatis, L. (1992) *Manual for the Symptom Checklist 90 Revised (SCL-90-R)*. Psychometric Research, Baltimore, MD.

Forehand, R. and Long, N. (1988) Outpatient treatment of the acting out child: procedures, long term follow-up data, and clinical problems. *Advances in Behavior Research and Therapy*, **10**, 129–177.

Gandil, P., Andersen, T. and Bjorner, J. (1990) A model for psycho-social support and counselling. *International Conference on AIDS*. 1990 Jun 20–23; 6(2), 479 (abstract no. 4100).

Garfield, S.L. and Bergin, A.E. (1986) *Handbook of Psychotherapy and Behavior Change*, 3rd edn, John Wiley, New York.

Gonzalez, S., Steinglass, P. and Reiss, D. (1989) Putting the illness in its place: discussion groups for families with chronic medical illnesses. *Family Process*, **28**, 69–87.

Grabowska, M.J. (1971) The effect of hypnosis and hypnotic suggestion on the blood flow in the extremities. *Polish Medical Journal*, **10**, 1044–1051.

Greenan, E., Powell, C. and Varni, J.W. (1983) Adherence to therapeutic exercise by children with hemophilia.

Gregory, M. and Foy, E. (1988) Parent attitudes and child personality traits in hemophilia: a six-year longitudinal study. *Nursing Times*, **84**, 71–72.

Gurman, A. and Kniskern, D. (1978) Research on marital and family therapy: progress, perspective and prospect, in *Handbook of Psychotherapy and Behavior Change*, 2nd edn (eds S. Garfield and A. Bergin), John Wiley, New York.

Gurman, A. and Kniskern, D. (1981), Family therapy outcome research: knowns and unknowns, in *Handbook of Family Therapy*, 2nd edn (eds A.S. Gurman and D. Kniskern), Brunner/Mazel, New York.

Hall, C.S. (1994) The experience of children with hemophilia and HIV infection. *Journal of School Health*, **64**, 16–17.

Handford, H.A., Charney, D., Ackeran, L. *et al.* (1980) Effect of psychiatric intervention on use of antihemophilic factor concentrate. *American Journal of Psychiatry*, **137**, 1254–1256.

Hogan, N. and Desantis, L. (1992) Adolescent sibling bereavement: an ongoing attachment. *Qualitative Health Research*, **2**, 159–177.

Howard, K.I., Kopta, M., Krause, M. and Orlinsky, D. (1986) The dose–response relationship in psychotherapy. *American Psychologist*, **41**, 159–164.

Kelly, L.A. (1991) *Raising a Child with Hemophilia: A Practical Guide for Parents*, Armour Pharmaceutics Co. Educational Publications, Blue Bell, PA.

Koocher, G. and O'Malley, J.E. (1981) *The Damocles Syndrome: Psychosocial Consequences of Surviving Childhood Cancer*, McGraw-Hill, New York.

LaBaw, W.L. (1975) Autohypnosis in hemophilia. *Haematologia*, **9**, 103–110.

Logan, F.A., Gibson, B., Hann, I.M. and Parry Jones, W.L. (1993) Children with hemophilia: same or different? *Child: Care, Health and Development*, **19**, 261–273.

McDaniel, S., Campbell, T.L. and Seaburn, D.B. (1990) *Family-oriented Primary Care: A Manual for Medical Providers*, Springer, New York.

McDaniel, S., Hepworth, J. and Doherty, W.J. (1992) *Medical Family Therapy: A Biopsychosocial Approach to Families with Health Problems*, Basic Books, New York.

McKusick, L. (1988) The impact of AIDS on practitioner and client. *American Psychologist*, **43**, 935–940.

Mason, P.J., Olson, R.A. and Parish, K.L. (1988) AIDS, hemophilia, and prevention efforts within a comprehensive care program. *American Psychologist*, **43**, 971–976.

Miller, R. (1987) *A Framework for Psychosocial Services in Hemophilia Care*. World Federation of Hemophilia and Alpha Therapeutics, Blue Bell, PA.

Miller, R. and Bor, R. (1988) *AIDS: A Guide to Clinical Counseling*, Science Press, London.

Miller, R., Goldman, E., Bor, R. and Kernoff, P. (1989) Aids and children: some of the issues in hemophilia care and how to address them. *AIDS Care*, **1**, 59–65.

Minuchin, S., Rosman, B. and Baker, L. (1978) *Psychosomatic Families: Anorexia Nervosa in Context*, Harvard University Press, Cambridge, MA.

National Hemophilia Foundation (1993) *Social Work Orientation Manual*, National Hemophilia Foundation, Washington, DC.

Nimorwicz, P. and Klein, R.H. (1982) Psychosocial aspects of hemophilia in families: 2: Intervention strategies and procedures. *Clinical Psychology Review*, **2**, 171–181.

Ornstein, R. and Sobel, D. (1989) *Healthy Pleasures*, Addison-Wesley, New York.

Patterson, G.R. (1974) Interventions for boys with conduct problems: multiple settings, treatments and criteria. *Journal of Consulting and Clinical Psychology*, **42**, 472–481.

Petterle, E.A. (1993) *Getting your Affairs in Order*. Shelter Publications, Bolinas, CA.

Polster, R. and Dangel, R. (1984) Behavioral parent training: where it came from and where it's at, in *Parent Training* (eds R. Dangel and R. Polster), Guilford Press, New York.

Pomerleau, O.R. and Rodin, J. (1986) Behavioral medicine and health psychology, in *Handbook of Psychotherapy and Behavior Change*, 3rd edn (eds S.L. Garfield, L. and A.E. Bergin), John Wiley, New York, pp. 483–524.

Prochaska. J., DiClemente, C.C. and Norcross, J.C. (1992) In search of how people change: applications to addictive behaviors. *American Psychologist*, **47**, 1102–1114.

Rickert, V.I., Sototalono, D.C., Parrish, J.M. *et al.* (1988) Training parents to become better behavior managers: the need for a competency-based approach. *Behavior Modification*, **12**, 325–330.

Rolland, J.S. (1987) Chronic illness and the life cycle: a conceptual framework. *Family Process*, **26**, 203–221.

Rolland, J.S. (1989) Chronic illness and the family life cycle, in *The Changing Family Life Cycle* (eds E.A. Carter and M. McGoldrick), The Changing Family Life Cycle, Allyn and Bacon, Boston, MA.

Rosen, G.M. (1990) *Psychology's Ability to Advance Self Care*. American Psychological Association Annual Convention.

Ross, D. and Ross, S. (1988) *Childhood Pain: Current Issues, Research and Management*, Urban and Schwarzenburg, Baltimore.

Schaefer, C. and Briemeister, J. (1989) *Handbook of Parent Training*, John Wiley, New York.

Sergis-Deavenport, E. and Varni, J.W. (1982) Behavioral techniques in teaching hemophilia factor replacement procedures to families. *Pediatric Nursing*, **8**, 416–419.

Sergis-Deavenport, E. and Varni, J.W. (1983) Behavioral assessment and management of adherence to factor replacement therapy in hemophilia. *Journal of Pediatric Psychology*, **8**, 367–378.

Spiegel, D., Bloom, J.R., Kraemer, H.C. and Gottheil, D. (1989) Effect of psychosocial treatment on survival of patients with metastatic breast cancer. *Lancet*, **2**, 888–891.

Spitzer, R.L., Williams, J.B.W., Kroenke, K. *et al.* (1992) *PRIME-MD: Primary Care Evaluation of Mental Disorders: Instruction Manual*, New York State Psychiatric Institute, New York.

Steinhart, B. (1994) The social worker's role in school visits, in *The National Hemophilia Foundation's Manual for Social Workers in Hemophilia*, National Hemophilia Foundation, New York.

Varni, J.W. (1980) Behavioral treatment of disease-related chronic insomnia in a hemophiliac. *Journal of Child Behavior Therapy*, 1, 171–192.

Varni, J.W. (1981a) Behavioral medicine in hemophilia arthritic pain management: two case studies. *Archives of Physical Medicine and Rehabilitation*, 62, 183–187.

Varni, J.W. (1981b) Self-regulation techniques in the management of chronic arthritic pain in hemophilia. *Behavior Therapy*, 12, 185–194.

Varni, J.W. (1983) *Clinical Behavioral Pediatrics,* Pergamon Press, New York.

Varni, J.W. and Gilbert, A. (1982) Self-regulation of chronic arthritic pain and long-term analgesic dependence in a hemophiliac. *Rheumatology and Rehabilitation*, 21, 171–174.

Varni, J.W., Gilbert, A. and Dietrich, S.L. (1981) Behavioral medicine in pain and analgesia management for the hemophilic child with factor VIII inhibitor. *Pain*, 11, 121–126.

Wong-Rieger, D. (1993) *Men's Advocacy Network of the NHF: Evaluation of One-year Impact of MANN Training Workshop*, National Hemophilia Foundation, New York.

Wright, L. (1977) Conceptualizing and defining psychosomatic disorders. *American Psychologist*, 32, 625–628.

Yalom, I.D. (1987) *The Theory and Practice of Group Psychotherapy*, 3rd edn, Basic Books, New York.

Zimpfer, D.G. (1991) Groups for grief and survivorship after bereavement: a review. *Journal for Specialists in Group Work*, 16, 46–55.

31 LIFE ASSURANCE IN HEMOPHILIA

P. Wilkie

Insurance and hemophilia

In the last 20 years there have been considerable advances in the treatment available for patients for hemophilia. These advances, discussed elsewhere in this book, have enabled young and more severely affected hemophiliacs to lead a relatively normal life. Improvement in treatment has also resulted in an increase in the expectation of life as well as an expectation of what life can bring, including a job and a home of their own. These increased expectations on the part of people with hemophilia also mean that they consider applying for life assurance. Prior to the advent of human immunodeficiency virus (HIV) in the hemophilia population, those with hemophilia had been able to get life assurance at a moderate extra premium, since the improved treatment regimes meant that their expected lifespan was approaching that of normal (Wilkie, 1987).

With the appearance of acquired immunodeficiency syndrome (AIDS) came public discussion about many of the social and psychologic problems affecting those with HIV and AIDS. In particular, the difficulties of getting life insurance and hence a mortgage were highlighted, as well as criticisms of discrimination by insurance companies of those at risk of contracting HIV. Headlines such as 'Life companies react to AIDS fears' (*Financial Times*, 7 June 1986) and 'Insurance companies refuse mortgage cover for those who may contract AIDS' (*Times*, 3 November 1986) were typical and this increased anxiety for those at risk as well as creating ethical dilemmas for doctors and counselors. There is considerable anecdotal evidence that people with hemophilia were finding it even more difficult to purchase life insurance than they would have done before the advent of HIV.

In March 1995 the Haemophilia Society (UK) announced that over 3000 people with hemophilia have now been infected with hepatitis C virus, contracted through treatment with clotting factor concentrates before 1986, and of these over 40 have died. The implications of hepatitis C virus for insurance are likely to be serious.

In 1935 R.A. Fisher, the distinguished geneticist and statistician, predicted in a paper to insurance companies that genetic markers would one day be used in assessing risks for insurance purposes. These predictions have become a reality and genetic testing for an increasing number of disorders is now possible (Harper, 1991). The increased understanding of genetic inheritance and the available of presymptomatic testing has a significant effect on life assurance. Before there was any understanding of genetic inheritance a presymptomatic individual who had no other impairment could obtain life assurance at the ordinary premium rates. The same still applied after genetic inheritance became understood, if the applicant had no knowledge of the family history that might cause him or her to be at risk, if the life assurance proposal form did not elicit this information in its questions, or if the life underwriter was insufficiently knowledgable or alert to the significance of the information that had been elicited.

Recently there have been debates about the practical and ethical issues relating to genetic testing and insurance. In their report *Heredity, Science and Society* (1989), the Health Council of the Netherlands stated that:

> we find it unacceptable that people affected from birth with a genetic predisposition should be faced with additional social obstacles and that their relatives should also be at a disadvantage in this way. At the same time, however, we recognise that insurers are entitled to protect themselves against exploitation by persons with prior knowledge of their own risks, for example, of developing a serious hereditary disease in the near future.

Hemophilia. Edited by C.D. Forbes, L. Aledort and R. Madhok. Published in 1997 by Chapman & Hall, London. ISBN 0 412 63820 7

In 1993 the Nuffield Council on Bioethics, in their report on ethical issues in genetic screening, recommended that British insurance companies should adhere to their current policy of not requiring any genetic tests as a prerequisite of obtaining insurance. They also recommended that insurance companies should accept a temporary moratorium on requiring the disclosure of genetic data with two exceptions: first, in the case of those individuals where there is a known family history of genetic disease that can be established by the conventional questions about the proposers' families, then individuals may be asked to disclose the results of any genetic tests (paragraph 7.28) and second, the moratorium should apply only to policies of moderate size. The limit would be a matter to be settled between the government and the industry in the context of arranging the moratorium.

The fact that hemophilia is genetically inherited is less important for those applying for insurance than the severity of the hemophilia. The topics emphasize the need for medical and nursing staff involved in the care of patients with hemophilia to have a clear understanding of some of the principles of insurance so that they can give appropriate advice to patients.

Types of life assurance policies

Life insurance (or assurance; both words are used) companies sell products that look, and often are, rather complicated. In principle there are three elements in these products and these provide three different types of benefit. These elements are:

1. 'Death' insurance – insuring against dying too soon.
2. Life annuities and pensions insuring against living too long.
3. Savings; however, life insurance companies are not allowed to sell savings plans on their own. These must be combined with one or other of the above insurance elements.

It is only life insurance companies that are allowed to sell death insurance or annuities. Insuring against dying too soon – death cover – is useful for someone who may die leaving dependants – a widow (or widower) or children. An important situation is where a mother still has young children to look after and is not able to go out to work. Death cover can also be used to pay off a loan, such as a house purchase loan.

There are other uses of death cover, such as to pay inheritance tax, especially on a family business; these may be for large amounts, but they are relevant to relatively few people.

Death cover can be obtained by a term assurance policy, a mortgage protection policy, as part of an endowment assurance policy, or attached to a pension policy. The last is the most tax-efficient, but the policy cannot be assigned to a lender, so it is less flexible than term assurance.

There are particular advantages and disadvantages with all of the above policies. With-profits endowment assurance life policies used to be a very tax-effective savings medium. However, this advantage ceased when tax benefits on life assurance policies (life assurance premium relief) stopped in 1984. They are now a rather expensive method of saving. These savings policies include some death cover, but this can easily be bought separately. The modern sort of endowment assurance policy is usually either a unit-linked policy or a utilized with-profits policy.

Savings (as opposed to insurance) can be done in many other ways, either directly (bank or building society deposits, or buying stocks or shares), or through other financial institutions (unit trusts, investment trusts, personal equity plans (PEPs), TESSAs, or additional voluntary contributions (AVCs) to an employer's pension scheme). Employers' pension schemes are another way in which savings for retirement can be provided.

Which method of saving is adopted depends very much on taxation, expenses and the convenience or benefit of paying for someone else to manage the investments. Many of the ways of saving, other than through life insurance, are now more tax-efficient or have lower expenses.

Pensions are still a tax-efficient savings medium, but the benefits cannot be taken until a later age, possibly at retirement, and they need to be taken mostly in the form of a pension annuity. This may not be good value for someone who might not live too long after retirement age.

A person with hemophilia may want death cover to provide for dependants and to pay off a loan. But if he has no dependants, and his house would be sold on his death, the need for death cover is less obvious.

A person with hemophilia may wish to start a savings system to provide for his retirement, or for the time when he may no longer be able to work, or to provide 'for a rainy day.' How much such a person saves privately depends on the benefits obtainable through his employer's pension scheme, if there is one. And in turn this will depend on how long he has worked there, on his salary and on the details of the rules of the scheme, especially the benefits on ill-health retirement.

If the employer has no pension scheme it may be worth considering a personal pension arranged with a life insurance company, but three-quarters of the benefit must be taken in the form of an annuity for life, and this may not be financially worth it.

Hemophilia and underwriting

Insurance companies need to assess risk, in order that income generated from premiums charged to applicants is sufficient to meet claims. Life assurance offices are organized in a variety of ways:

1. Mutual societies, which are owned by the policy-holders. All profits are distributed to the holders of with-profits policies as bonuses.
2. Traditional proprietary companies, which are owned by shareholders. These distribute the bulk of their profits to with-profits policy-holders, so are very similar to mutual companies.
3. The newer proprietary companies often sell savings policies with an annual mortality charge to pay for the death claims expected in the following year.

In each case, if there are more death claims than had been expected, other policy-holders will pay, either through lower bonuses or higher premiums (Wilkie, 1987).

Life offices have, therefore, to consider their obligation to policy-holders by avoiding unreasonable death claims. Insurers examine those whose expectation of life is reduced – what they call 'substandard' or 'impaired lives' – so that an appropriate premium can be charged. The appropriate premium for a substandard life is usually calculated by examining the mortality rates of existing policy-holders or other appropriate medical statistics (Brackenridge and Elder, 1993). Guidelines for extra premiums for all sorts of impairments are often recommended by specialist reassurance companies.

Life assurance companies require any applicant for insurance to complete an application form (a proposal form), in which a number of questions about the applicant's medical history are asked. If the answers show that the applicant is suffering from or has suffered from any more serious disorder, the life office asks for further information. The applicant with hemophilia is in a particularly exposed position. Unless he is very mildly affected, he is bound to know that he has hemophilia, and this fact would have been elicited from questions in the proposal form. Such applicants must expect further investigations.

These investigations may take the form of the life office obtaining a report from the applicant's family doctor (a medical attendant's report) and/or asking the applicant to attend for a medical examination.

If all proves to be satisfactory, then the applicant may be accepted at the normal premium rates for the type of insurance for which he or she has applied, but if there is any evidence to indicate that the applicant may have a higher than normal risk of dying prematurely then the life office may offer insurance only at higher than normal rates, or may decline the application altogether.

For hemophiliacs who have no evidence of HIV or of hepatitis C virus, the decision of a typical life office would depend on the applicant's age, on whether the hemophilia is mild, moderate or severe, and on the type of life assurance policy applied for.

Those who are only mildly affected and are rather older (say over 40) might be able to get insurance at the normal premium rates. Younger, mildly affected applicants might be asked to pay a small extra premium, as might the older, moderately affected. Younger, moderately affected and older, severely affected applicants may be offered insurance only with a substantially higher premium. The life office may decline to insure younger, severely affected hemophiliacs altogether.

A hemophiliac who is HIV-positive or infected with hepatitis is most unlikely to be acceptable for life insurance.

Since term assurance or mortgage protection insurance is quite cheap, the extra premium for such a policy may be a high proportion of the normal premium. Endowment assurances have much higher premiums (typically, the annual premium for a with-profits type of endowment assurance is roughly equal to the sum assured divided by the number of years for which the policy will run), so the extra premium may be quite a small proportion of the normal premium.

It is clear that it is necessary for insurance companies to collect sufficient information about the morbidity and mortality of a particular condition before they can assess premiums. This can be problematic for people affected by conditions such as HIV in its early days and now hepatitis C virus, for which adequate information is not yet available. In these circumstances insurers will tend to err on the side of caution and either charge higher premiums or not accept certain applicants.

Conclusion

As each life office makes its own decisions, without reference to what other offices might do, it is worth advising applicants to shop around for life insurance cover (there are 450 UK insurance companies) or to ask an independent financial adviser (an insurance broker) to advise which the most favorable companies might be. In addition, the Haemophilia Society may be able to advise.

It is also important to remember that many building societies and all direct insurance salesmen work for only one life company and can only offer that company's policies. Only independent financial advisers can give advice about the choice of life companies, and they are supposed to give best advice. But the number of such independent advisors has reduced considerably as a consequence of the Financial Services Act 1986.

Life insurance contracts have traditionally been based on the principle of *uberrima fides* or utmost good faith

– on both sides. Thus, failure to disclose information which may be relevant to the contract may justify the insurance company in repudiating the claim. However, if an individual who has already taken a life insurance contract later discovers, for example, that he is hepatitis C-positive, provided the person completed the proposal form correctly to the best of his knowledge and belief, that policy should be valid regardless of what diseases the individual has since contracted.

The diversity and potential seriousness of some of the recent medical problems of hemophilia have created considerable challenges for the patients as well as those looking after them. While some of the difficulties for those with hemophilia in acquiring life insurance are peculiar to hemophilia, the principles of insurance discussed in this chapter are applicable to many other genetic or chronic conditions.

References

Brackenridge, R.D.C. and Elder, W.J. (1993) *Medical Selection of Life Risks*, 3rd edn, Macmillan.

The Bulletin (1995) Leading article. The Haemophilia Society, Number 1, March.

Fisher, R.A. (1935) Linkage studies and the prognosis of hereditary ailments. International congress of life assurance medicine 1–3, London.

Harper, P. (1991) Genetic Testing and Insurance. Paper presented to seminar at The Mercantile and General Reinsurance Co. plc, 6–8 November, 1991.

Heredity, Science and Society (1989) Health Council of Netherlands, The Hague.

Nuffield Council on Bioethics (1993) *Genetic Screening and Ethical Issues*, Nuffield Council.

Wilkie, P.A. (1987) Life assurance, HIV seropositivity and hemophilia. *Scottish Medical Journal*, 32, 119–121.

INDEX

Page numbers appearing in **bold** refer to figures and page numbers appearing in *italic* refer to tables.